Breast Cancer

Adnan Aydiner • Abdullah Igci • Atilla Soran
Editors

Breast Cancer

A Guide to Clinical Practice

Springer

Editors
Adnan Aydiner
Internal Medicine, Medical Oncology
Istanbul Medical Faculty
Department of Medical Oncology
Institute of Oncology, Istanbul University
Istanbul, Turkey

Abdullah Igci
General Surgery
Istanbul Medical Faculty
Department of Surgery
Istanbul University
Istanbul, Turkey

Atilla Soran
Surgical Oncology
Magee-Women's Hospital
University of Pittsburgh Medical Centre
Pittsburgh, PA
USA

ISBN 978-3-030-07277-3 ISBN 978-3-319-96947-3 (eBook)
https://doi.org/10.1007/978-3-319-96947-3

Softcover re-print of the Hardcover 1st edition 2019

This Springer imprint is published by the registered company Springer Nature Switzerland AG
The registered company address is: Gewerbestrasse 11, 6330 Cham, Switzerland

Preface

This guidebook is focused on providing a practical approach to the allocation of available diagnostic procedures and therapies to individual patients in light of the most recent and reliable information from clinical trials and international guidelines. It reviews substantial new evidence on locoregional and systemic therapies for early and advanced breast cancer and in situ carcinoma. In breast cancer, the treatment strategy is chosen based on the features and biology of the tumor and on the patient's age, general health status, and personal preferences. The decision options in this edition of the book are based on the best evidence-based recommendations available. The majority of breast cancer deaths now occur in less developed regions of the world. The gold standard for breast cancer care includes an integrated multidisciplinary team approach comprising pathologists, radiologists, surgical oncologists, medical oncologists, radiation oncologists, oncology nurses, and plastic surgeons. The first chapter comprises decision pathways outlining the step-by-step clinical decision-making process for patient management. In the subsequent chapters, the recommendations are discussed in light of randomized trials.

Istanbul, Turkey — Adnan Aydiner
Istanbul, Turkey — Abdullah Igci
Pittsburgh, PA, USA — Atilla Soran

Contents

Contributors

Naziye Ak Internal Medicine, Medical Oncology, Istanbul Medical Faculty, Department of Medical Oncology, Institute of Oncology, Istanbul University, Istanbul, Turkey

Adnan Aydiner Internal Medicine, Medical Oncology, Istanbul Medical Faculty, Department of Medical Oncology, Institute of Oncology, Istanbul University, Istanbul, Turkey

Soley Bayraktar Department of Medical Oncology, Memorial Hospital, Istanbul, Turkey

Neslihan Cabioglu Department of General Surgery, Istanbul Medical Faculty, Istanbul University, Istanbul, Turkey

Irfan Cicin Department of Medical Oncology, Faculty of Medicine, Balkan Oncology Hospital, Trakya University of Medicine, Edirne, Turkey

Maktav Dincer Gayrettepe Florence Nightingale Hospital, Department of Radiation Oncology, Istanbul, Turkey

Rian Disci Istinye University, Medical Faculty, Department of Biostatistics and Medical Informatics, Istanbul, Turkey

Istanbul University, Istanbul Medical Faculty, Department of Biostatistics and Medical Informatics, Istanbul, Turkey

Yesim Eralp Internal Medicine, Medical Oncology, Istanbul University, Institute of Oncology, Istanbul Medical Faculty, Department of Medical Oncology, Istanbul, Turkey

Ece Esin Department of Medical Oncology, Dr. A. Y. Ankara Oncology Education and Research Hospital, Ankara, Turkey

Merdan Fayda Istinye University, Faculty of Medicine, Department of Radiation Oncology, Istanbul, Turkey

Nilufer Guler Hacettepe University Cancer Institute, Department of Medical Oncology, Ankara, Turkey

Kamuran Arslan Ibis Istanbul Medical Faculty, Department of Radiation Oncology, Istanbul University, Institute of Oncology, Istanbul, Turkey

Abdullah Igci General Surgery, Istanbul Medical Faculty, Department of Surgery, Istanbul University, Istanbul, Turkey

Hasan Karanlik Department of Surgical Oncology, Institute of Oncology, Istanbul University, Istanbul, Turkey

Serkan Keskin Internal Medicine, Department of Medical Oncology, Memorial Hospital, Istanbul, Turkey

Seden Kucucuk Istanbul Medical Faculty, Department of Radiation Oncology, Istanbul University, Institute of Oncology, Istanbul, Turkey

Mahmut Muslumanoglu Istanbul University, Istanbul Medical Faculty, Department of General Surgery, Istanbul, Turkey

Leyla Ozer Internal Medicine, Department of Medical Oncology, Mehmet Ali Aydinlar University Hospital, Istanbul, Turkey

Fatma Sen Department of Medical Oncology, Avrasya Hospital, Istanbul, Turkey

Atilla Soran Surgical Oncology, Magee-Women's Hospital, University of Pittsburgh Medical Centre, Pittsburgh, PA, USA

Cuneyt Turkmen Istanbul Medical Faculty, Department of Nuclear Medicine, Istanbul University, Istanbul, Turkey

Makbule Tambas Department of Radiation Oncology, University of Health Sciences, Okmeydanı Training and Research Hospital, Istanbul, Turkey

Sitki Tuzlali Istanbul University, Istanbul Medical Faculty, Department of Pathology, Istanbul, Turkey

Tuzlali Private Pathology Laboratory, Istanbul, Turkey

Ekrem Yavuz Department of Pathology, Istanbul Medical Faculty, Istanbul University, Istanbul, Turkey

Ibrahim Yildiz Internal Medicine, Department of Medical Oncology, Acibadem Hospital, Istanbul, Turkey

Part I
Review of the Breast Cancer Management

Chapter 1
Decision Pathways in Breast Cancer Management

Adnan Aydiner, Abdullah Igci, Neslihan Cabioglu, Leyla Ozer, Fatma Sen, Serkan Keskin, Mahmut Muslumanoglu, Hasan Karanlik, Kamuran Arslan Ibis, Seden Kucucuk, Maktav Dincer, Ekrem Yavuz, Sitki Tuzlali, and Atilla Soran

A. Aydiner (✉)
Internal Medicine, Medical Oncology, Istanbul Medical Faculty, Department of Medical Oncology, Institute of Oncology, Istanbul University, Istanbul, Turkey

A. Igci
General Surgery, Istanbul Medical Faculty, Department of Surgery, Istanbul University, Istanbul, Turkey
e-mail: aigci@istanbul.edu.tr

N. Cabioglu · M. Muslumanoglu
Istanbul Medical Faculty, Department of General Surgery, Istanbul University, Istanbul, Turkey
e-mail: mahmutm@istanbul.edu.tr

L. Ozer
Internal Medicine, Department of Medical Oncology, Mehmet Ali Aydinlar University Hospital, Istanbul, Turkey

F. Sen
Department of Medical Oncology, Avrasya Hospital, Istanbul, Turkey

S. Keskin
Internal Medicine, Department of Medical Oncology, Memorial Hospital, Istanbul, Turkey
e-mail: serkan.keskin@memorial.com.tr

H. Karanlik
Department of Surgical Oncology, Istanbul University, Institute of Oncology, Istanbul, Turkey

K. Arslan Ibis · S. Kucucuk
Istanbul Medical Faculty, Department of Radiation Oncology, Istanbul University, Institute of Oncology, Istanbul, Turkey

M. Dincer
Department of Radiation Oncology, Gayrettepe Florence Nightingale Hospital, Istanbul, Turkey
e-mail: dincer@superonline.com

E. Yavuz
Istanbul Medical Faculty, Department of Pathology, Istanbul University, Istanbul, Turkey
e-mail: yavuze@istanbul.edu.tr

A. Aydiner et al. (eds.), *Breast Cancer*, https://doi.org/10.1007/978-3-319-96947-3_1

S. Tuzlali
Tuzlali Private Pathology Laboratory, Istanbul, Turkey

Istanbul University, Istanbul Medical Faculty, Department of Pathology, Istanbul, Turkey

A. Soran
Surgical Oncology, Magee-Women's Hospital, University of Pittsburgh Medical Centre, Pittsburgh, PA, USA
e-mail: asoran@upmc.edu

Introduction

The decision options in this edition of the book are based on the best evidence-based recommendations available. This chapter is focused on providing a practical approach to the allocation of available diagnostic procedures and therapies to individual patients in light of the most recent and reliable information from clinical trials and international guidelines. As new information is obtained from randomized clinical trials, the decision options will change over time. In this chapter, the proposal 1 and proposal 3 recommendations are noted. Unless otherwise stated, the level of evidence for the other recommendations is generally 2.

Recommendation level	Definition
Proposal 1	There is a common consensus based on level 1 evidence
Proposal 3	There is no consensus based on level III evidence

Level of Evidence

Level I Evidence from at least one *well-designed controlled clinical randomized trial* and/or *meta analyses* and/or *systematic reviews.*

Level II (1) Evidence from a single randomized trial and/or well-designed non-randomized clinical trials. (2) Evidence from well-designed cohort or case-control studies (studies conducted by more than one research group or center are preferred). (3) Evidence obtained from case series with or without intervention.

Level III Descriptive studies, expert committee reports, or *respected authority opinions* based on clinical experience.

Breast Disease: Management *(Fig. 1.1)*

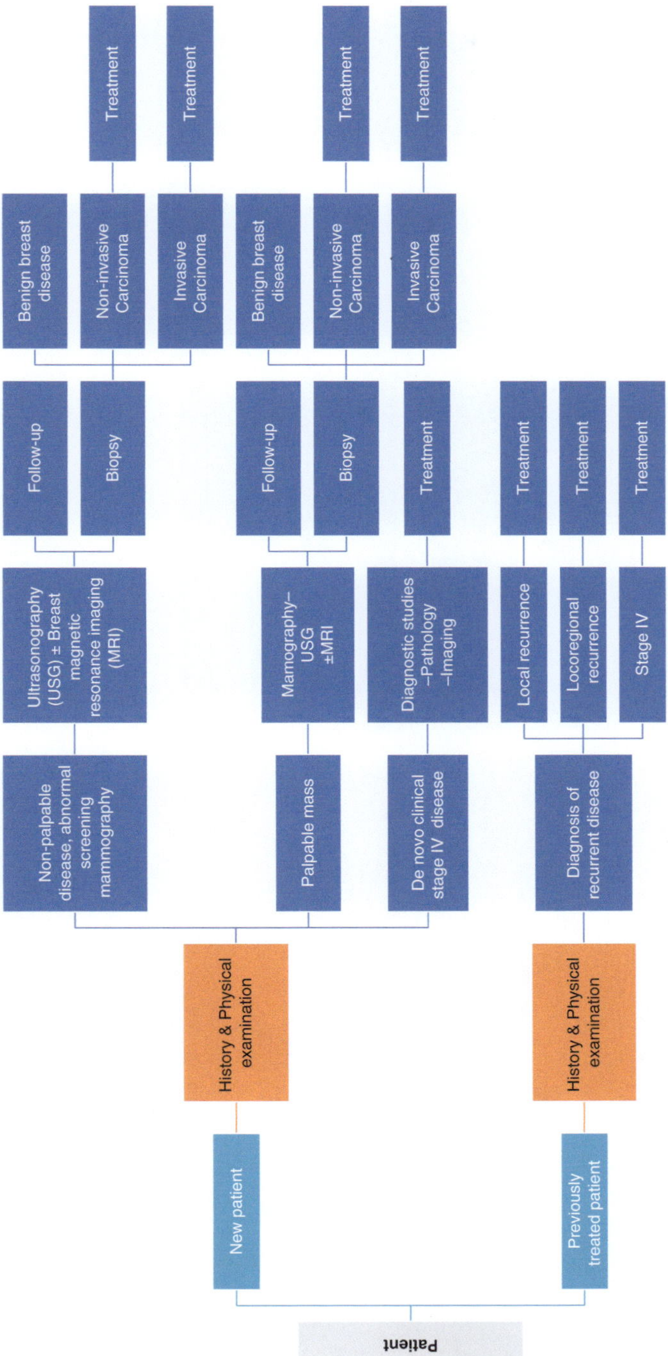

Fig. 1.1 Summary of the step-by-step clinical decision-making process in patient management (see Table 1.1)

Breast Disease: Approach to Benign Disease of the Breast (Fig. 1.2)

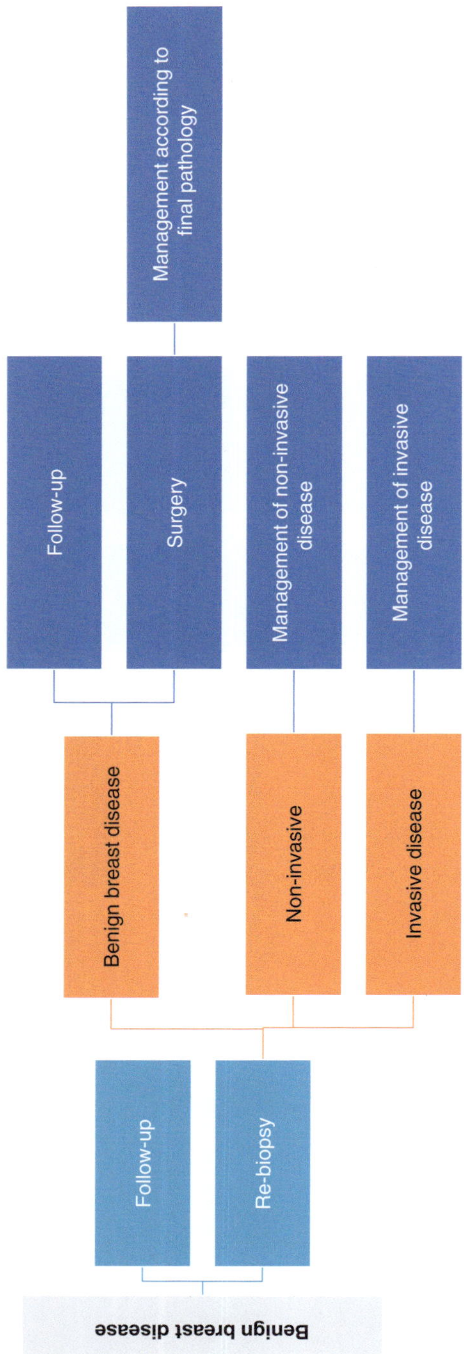

Fig. 1.2 Approach to benign breast disease after biopsy

Breast Disease: Diagnosis and Staging

Table 1.1 Diagnostic procedures for non-invasive (in situ) and invasive breast carcinoma

	In situ carcinoma	Invasive breast cancer		Inflammatory breast cancer
	Stage 0	Stage I, IIA, IIB, IIIA	Stage IIIA (N2), IIIB, IIIC	Stage T4d, N0–N3, M0
Medical history and physical examination	☑	☑	☑	☑
Mammography (MMG)	☑	☑	☑	☑
Ultrasonography (USG)		☑	If necessary ☑	If necessary ☑
Breast magnetic resonance imaging (MRI)	If necessary ☑	☑ Optional[a]	☑ Optional[a]	☑ Optional[b]
Pathological evaluation	☑	☑	☑	☑
Hormone receptors (HR) [Estrogen receptor (ER) and progesterone receptor (PgR)] determination	☑	☑	☑	☑
Assessment of tumor HER2 status		☑	☑	☑
Genetic counseling for patients at high risk for hereditary breast cancer	☑	☑	☑	☑
If required, fertility counseling	☑	☑	☑	☑
Blood tests (complete blood count, liver function tests, renal function tests, alkaline phosphatase (ALP), calcium, glucose)		☑	☑	☑
Serum tumor markers: CEA, CA153			☑	☑
Serum tumor marker: Ca125 (for young patients)		☑	☑	☑
In the case of localized bone pain or high ALP: bone scintigraphy (if PET/CT scan is not necessary)		☑	☑	☑
In the presence of high ALP, abnormal liver function tests, abdominal symptoms, or abnormalities upon abdominopelvic physical examination: abdomen ± pelvic computed tomography (CT) or MRI (or PET/CT scan)		☑	☑	☑
In the presence of pulmonary symptoms: CHEST CT		☑	☑	☑
FDG positron emission tomography (PET/CT)		☑ Optional[c]	☑	☑

[a]Density on mammography, <35 years of age, multifocality/multicentricity suspicion, evaluation for neoadjuvant chemotherapy (i.e., if treatment change is considered)
[b]If a treatment change is considered in neoadjuvant chemotherapy evaluation
[c]Tumor biology (i.e., triple-negative breast cancer) or according to stage (stage II–III); PET-CT may be required in patients with suspicious findings in conventional imaging modalities

Non-Invasive Breast Cancer: In Situ Carcinoma

STAGE 0 (Tis, N0, M0) (diagnosis established pathologically with biopsy or surgical excision specimen) (Fig. 1.3)

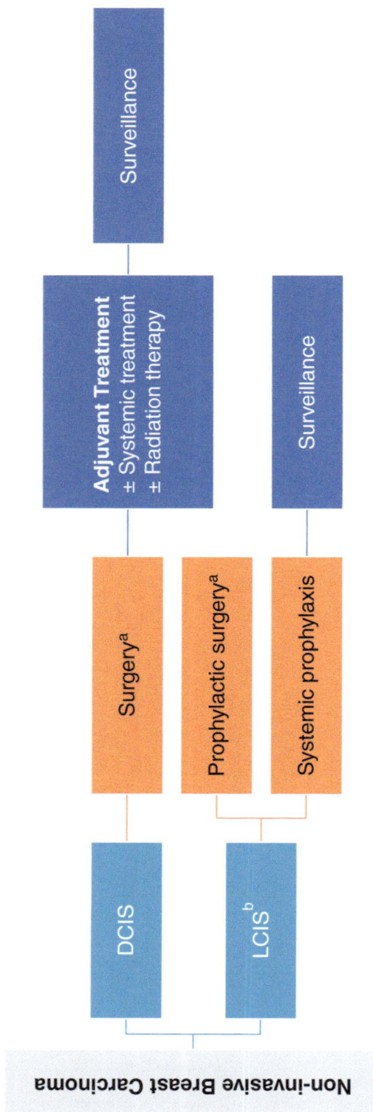

Fig. 1.3 Non-invasive breast cancer treatment. [a]Reconstruction is recommended if mastectomy is planned. [b]For the pleomorphic subtype of lobular carcinoma in situ (LCIS), ductal carcinoma in situ (DCIS) treatment alternatives should be administered. Surgical treatment is performed in high-risk patients or if there are familial risk factors for lobular carcinoma LCIS; chemoprevention is the choice in other patients. Patients with LCIS lesions detected by imaging methods are generally considered as higher-risk LCIS. DCIS treatment options should be applied in cases with the pleomorphic subtype of LCIS. Florid LCIS is a newly defined subtype that is suggested to be managed like pleomorphic LCIS. Multifocal LCIS (>4 terminal ductal lobular unit involvement) may be associated with higher risk for recurrence and invasive cancer. Tamoxifen, raloxifene or aromatase inhibitors may be preferred for chemoprevention

Non-Invasive Breast Cancer: In Situ Carcinoma: Ductal Carcinoma In Situ

Locoregional Therapy *(Fig. 1.4)*

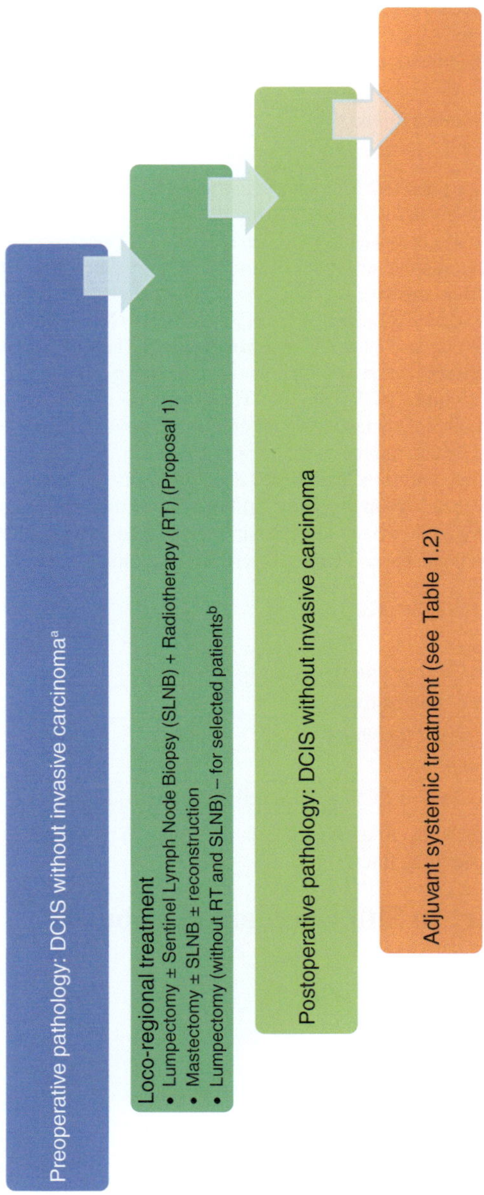

Fig. 1.4 Management of patient with ductal carcinoma in situ (DCIS). [a]Preoperative MR imaging is recommended in DCIS. The specimen should be evaluated with X-ray imaging. Radiation therapy (RT) after breast-conserving surgery is the standard treatment in DCIS. The disease-free surgical margin should be adequate (≥2 mm) [1–3]. At the St Gallen 2017 consensus meeting, a few researchers stated that "no ink on margin" may be considered sufficient in selected cases, whereas a surgical margin of 2 mm and above is considered safe in patients with DCIS undergoing breast-conserving surgery (BCS). In cases undergoing BCS, a surgical margin of 2 mm or above is considered safe only in those with DCIS. If the invasive tumor is <1 mm in DCIS, the surgical border safety is evaluated according to DCIS. If the invasive focus is >1 mm in DCIS, the surgical margin width should be evaluated according to the invasive cancer. A sufficient surgical margin should be decided together with clinical, radiological and pathological findings. The decision regarding the "sufficient surgical margin" should be made according to findings such as additional radiological foci (multiple foci, microcalcification), invasive lobular carcinoma, presence of more than one surgical margin and persistence of surgical marginal proximity in re-excision. [b]ER-positive, postmenopausal case, advanced age, low-grade tumors

Adjuvant Systemic Therapy (Table 1.2)

Table 1.2 Adjuvant systemic therapy of ductal carcinoma in situ

Risk reduction treatment for the ipsilateral breast after breast-conserving surgery
Tamoxifen for 5 years:
–For ER- or PgR-positive patients who have undergone breast-conserving surgery (BCS) and RT
–Benefit of tamoxifen is not definite for ER-negative patients
–Patients treated with excision only
Aromatase inhibitor for 5 years[a]:
–For ER-positive or PgR-positive postmenopausal (<60 years) patients who have undergone BCS and RT
Risk-mitigating treatment for the contralateral breast
Counseling for risk reduction (see Figs. 1.45, 1.46, and 1.47 and Table 1.9)

[a]The primary endpoint of NSABP B-35, a phase III trial comparing anastrozole to tamoxifen for DCIS after breast-conserving surgery, each given for 5 years, was breast cancer-free interval (BCFI), defined as the time from randomization to any breast cancer (BC) event including local, regional, or distant recurrence or contralateral disease, invasive or DCIS. Postmenopausal women with ER- or PgR-positive (by IHC analysis) DCIS and no invasive BC who had undergone a lumpectomy with clear resection margins were randomly assigned. Stratification was by age (<60 v ≥60). There were 198 BCFI events, 114 in the tamoxifen group and 84 in the anastrozole group (hazard ratio, 0.73; $p = 0.03$). There was a significant interaction between treatment and age group ($p = 0.04$); the benefit of anastrozole was observed only in women <60 years old. There were 63 cases of invasive breast cancer in the tamoxifen group and 39 in the anastrozole group (hazard ratio, 0.61; $p = 0.02$). There was a non-significant trend for a reduction in breast second primary cancers with anastrozole (hazard ratio, 0.68; $p = 0.07$). In conclusion, anastrozole provided a significant improvement compared to tamoxifen for BCFI, which was seen later in the study, primarily in women <60 years old [7]. In the IBIS-II DCIS trial, anastrozole was shown to reduce recurrence, similar to tamoxifen [8]. The non-inferiority of anastrozole was well-established but its superiority to tamoxifen was not

Monitoring and Follow-Up (Table 1.3)

Table 1.3 DCIS—monitoring and follow-up[a]

Medical history and physical examination
–Every 6 months for 5 years
–Once a year thereafter
Mammography
–Once a year (If BCS is performed, at months 6–12 following RT)

[a]If treated with tamoxifen monitor according to breast cancer risk mitigation guidelines

Non-Invasive Breast Cancer: In Situ Carcinoma: Lobular Carcinoma In Situ

Diagnosis and Management

Medical History
Physical Examination
Mammography

Pathology: Lobular carcinoma in situ (without DCIS or invasive carcinoma). For the pleomorphic subtype of lobular carcinoma in situ, DCIS treatment alternatives should be administered.

Counseling for risk-mitigating approaches (see Figs. 1.45, 1.46, and 1.47)

Follow-up

Invasive Breast Cancer (IBC)

Clinical Staging (Fig. 1.5)

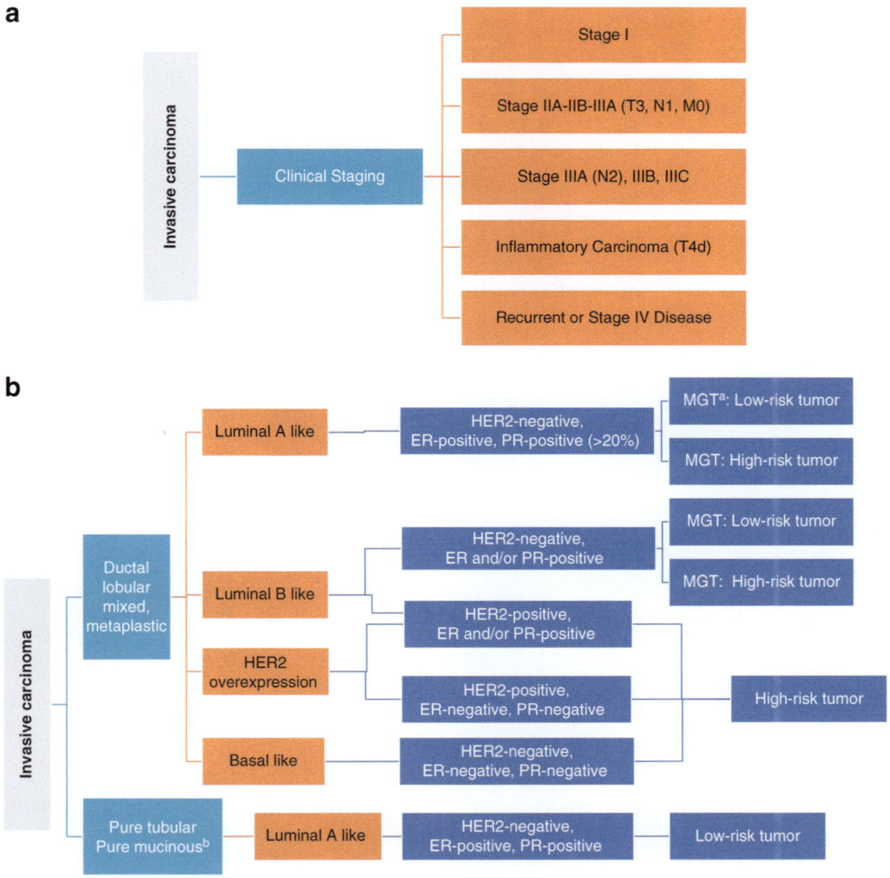

Fig. 1.5 (**a**) Clinical stages of invasive breast cancer. (**b**) Intrinsic subtype and clinicopathological surrogate definitions of invasive carcinoma. [a]*MGT* multigene tests. *Oncotype DX* (Genomic Health); *EndoPredict* (Sividon Diagnostics, Germany); *MammaPrint* (Agendia, Irvine, CA); *PAM50 ROR score* (Prosigna Breast Cancer Prognostic Gene Signature Assay; NanoString Technologies, Seattle, WA); *Breast Cancer Index* (Biotheranostics); *uPA and PAI-1*. [b]Very rarely (1%) mucinous invasive cancer can be a "non-luminal A" type

Invasive Breast Cancer: Clinical Stage I, II, IIIA (T3N1M0)

Axillary Evaluation (Fig. 1.6)

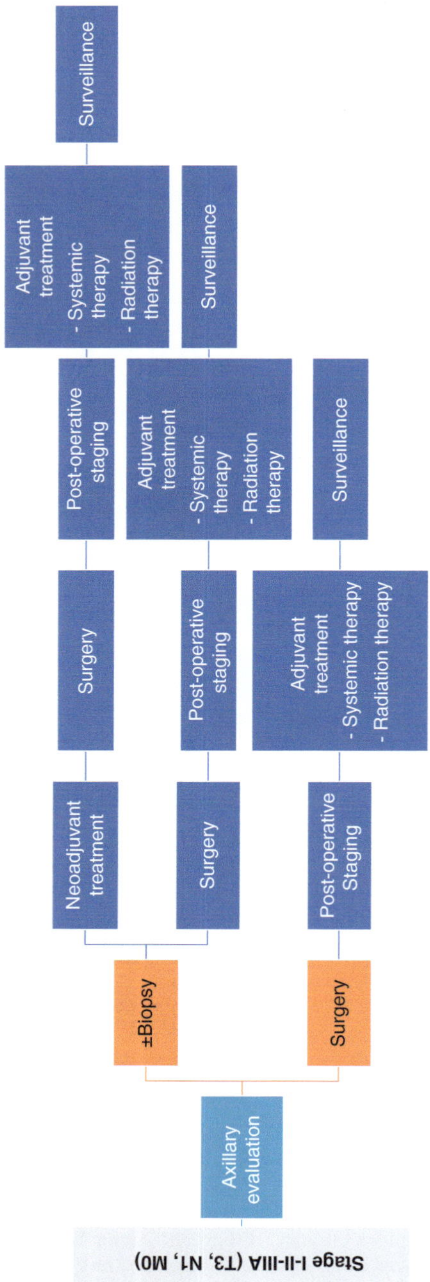

Fig. 1.6 Axillary evaluation and management of patients with clinical stages I, II or IIIA (T3, N1, M0)

Invasive Breast Cancer: Clinical Stage[1] I, II, IIIA (T3N1M0)

Surgical Axillary Staging and Management (*Fig. 1.7*)

[1] Stage I (T1, N0, M0); Stage IIA (T0, N1, M0; T1, N1, M0; T2, N0, M0); Stage IIB (T2, N1, M0; T3, N0, M0); Stage IIIA (T3, N1, M0).

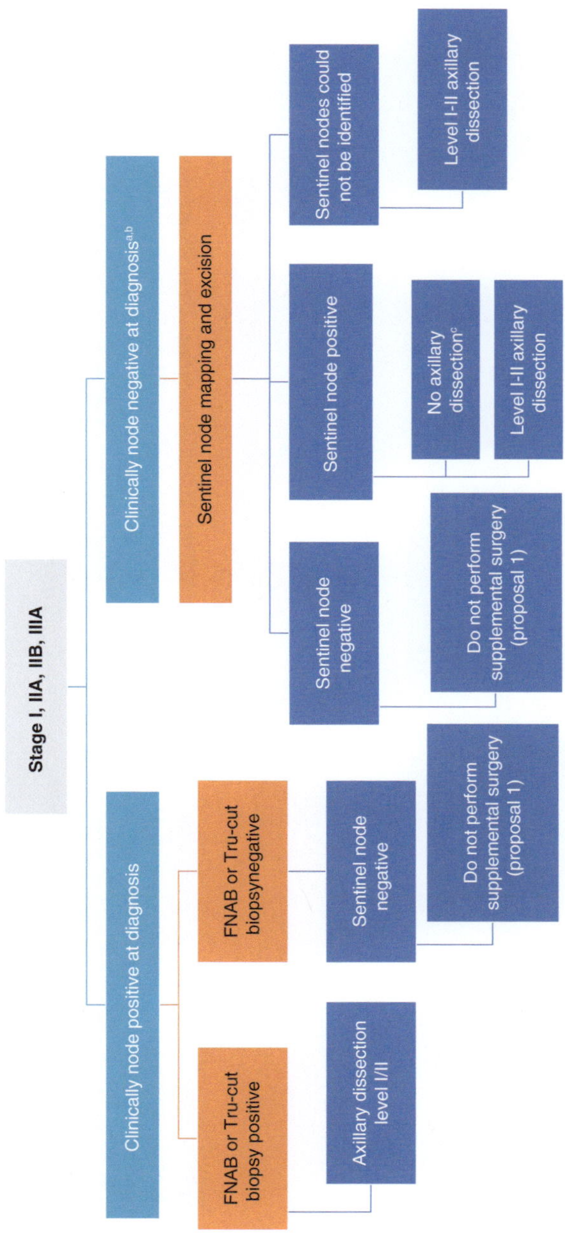

Fig. 1.7 Axillary management of patients with clinical stages I, II or IIIA (T3, N1, M0). *FNAB* fine-needle aspiration biopsy, *SLN* sentinel lymph node, *BCS* breast-conserving surgery. [a]For BCS: In patients with macrometastases in 1–2 sentinel lymph nodes, complete axillary dissection can be safely omitted when "conservative resection with RT" is performed [1, 3, 9–11]. [b]For mastectomy: In patients with macrometastases in 1–2 sentinel lymph nodes, complete axillary dissection must be performed when 'no adjuvant RT is planned'; however, in patients for whom RT is planned, no consensus exists for omitting axillary dissection [1, 3, 9]. [c]In patients with T1 or T2 tumors with BCS and 1–2 positive SLNs, if there is no neoadjuvant chemotherapy and whole-breast irradiation is planned, axillary dissection is not needed [1, 3, 9–17]. Axillary dissection is considered for SLN-positive patients with triple-negative breast cancer

Invasive Breast Cancer: Clinical Stage[2] II, IIIA (T3N1M0)

Axillary Management After Neoadjuvant Therapy (Fig. 1.8)

[2] Stage IIA (T0, N1, M0; T1, N1, M0; T2, N0, M0); Stage IIB (T2, N1, M0; T3, N0, M0); Stage IIIA (T3, N1, M0).

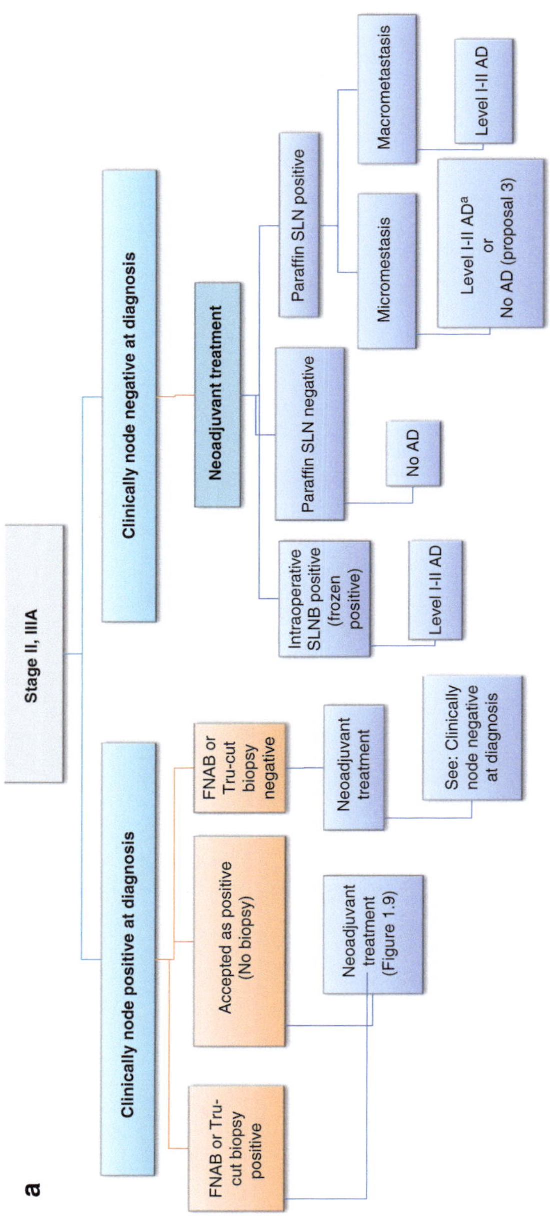

Fig. 1.8 Axillary management of patients with clinical stage II or IIIA (T3, N1, M0) invasive breast cancer. FNAB: fine-needle aspiration biopsy, *SLN* sentinel lymph node biopsy, *AD* axillary dissection. [a]Moo et al. examined the false-negative rate of frozen section after neoadjuvant chemotherapy (NAC) and the association between size of SLN metastasis and residual axillary disease at axillary dissection (ALND) [18]. A total of 702 patients underwent SLN biopsy after NAC. Overall, 17% patients with isolated tumor cells and 50% with micrometastases had additional nodal metastases at ALND. The authors concluded that low-volume disease in the SLN after NAC is not an indicator of a low risk of additional positive axillary nodes. These tumor cells are potentially drug resistant and are an indication of ALND, even when not detected on intraoperative frozen section

Invasive Breast Cancer: Clinical Stage[3] II, IIIA (T3N1M0)

Axillary Management After Neoadjuvant Therapy (*Fig. 1.9*)

[3] Stage IIA (T0, N1, M0; T1, N1, M0); Stage IIB (T2, N1, M0); Stage IIIA (T3, N1, M0).

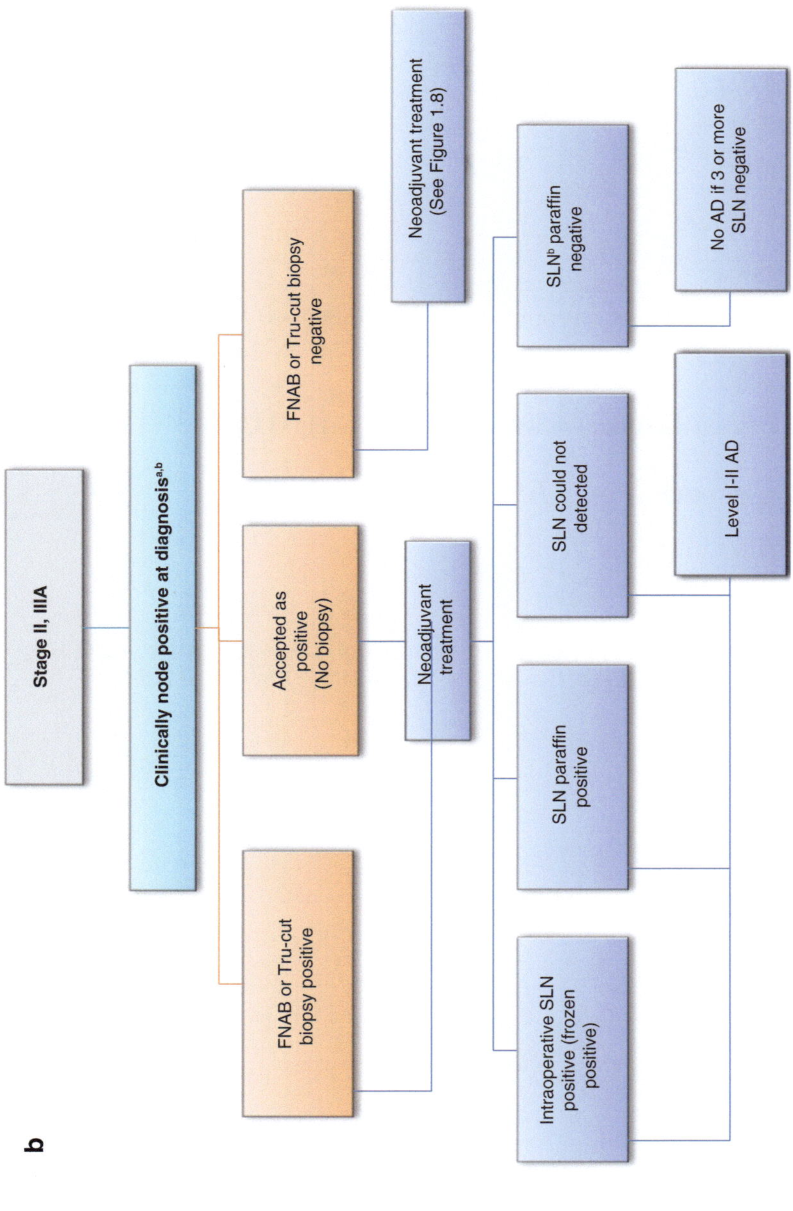

Fig. 1.9 Axillary management of patients with clinical node-positive stage II or IIIA (T3, N1, M0) invasive breast cancer. *FNAB* fine-needle aspiration biopsy, *SLN* sentinel lymph node biopsy, *AD* axillary dissection. [a]After neoadjuvant therapy, if the SLN is positive in frozen or paraffin sections, level I–II axillary dissection is recommended [1, 3, 9–17]. [b]At least 3 SLNs should be assessed in patients receiving neoadjuvant treatment

Invasive Breast Cancer: Clinical (T1–2N0M0) Disease

Box 1.1 Summary of approach to axilla—*no neoadjuvant treatment***—clinically node negative**

Clinical T1–T2N0 patients:

Paraffin block examination after primary surgery:

–SLN negative: Axillary dissection is NOT performed

–SLN positive:

Micrometastasis only:

Axillary dissection is NOT performed

If *all of the following* are present, axillary dissection is NOT performed:

T1–T2 tumour;

1 or 2 positive SLNs;

BCS;

RT is planned for the entire breast;

No preoperative treatment.

–Undetermined SLN: Perform level I–II axillary dissection

Invasive Breast Cancer: Clinical Stage[4] I, II, IIIA (T3N1M0)

Surgical Approach (Fig. 1.10)

[4] Stage IA (T1, N0, M0); Stage IB (T0, N1mi; M0; T1, N1mi, M0); Stage IIA (T0, N1, M0; T1, N1, M0; T2, N0, M0); Stage IIB (T2, N1, M0; T3, N0, M0); Stage IIIA (T3, N1, M0).

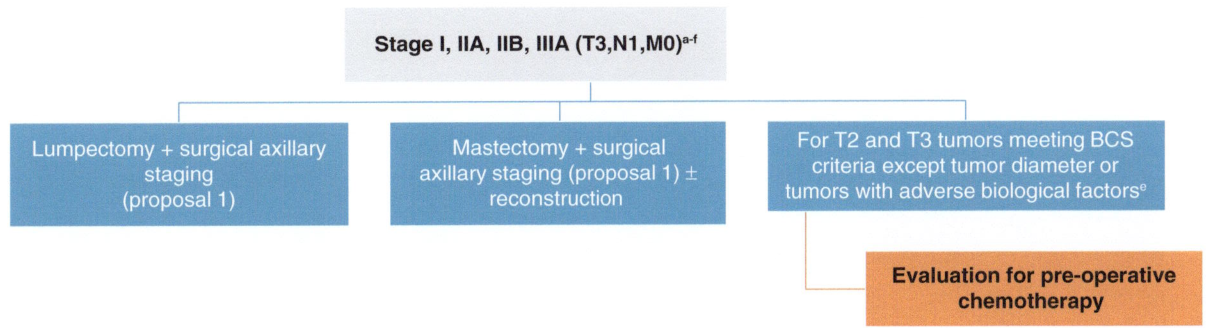

Fig. 1.10 Surgical treatment of patients with clinical stage I, II or IIIA (T3N1M0) disease[(a–f)]. [a]Absolute contraindications to breast-conserving surgery (BCS) include diffuse suspicious microcalcifications, multicentric tumors, widespread disease, and persistent positive pathological margins [1, 3, 12]. Relative contraindications include tumor size >5 cm, prior radiation therapy, active connective tissue disease, focally positive margins, and a known or suspected genetic predisposition to breast cancer. According to the St. Gallen 2017 consensus meeting, multifocal tumors can be treated with BCS "provided that the margins are clear and that whole breast radiotherapy (RT) is planned" [3]. A meta-analysis reported that the risk of local-regional recurrence after nipple-conserving surgery was very low [19]. At the consensus meeting, it was stated that nipple-conserving surgery can be performed in patients with hereditary BRCA1/2 mutations if the retroareolar tissue is determined to be clean by a pathologist [3]. [b]In women undergoing BCS for invasive BC and proceeding to standard RT and adjuvant systemic therapy, the minimum acceptable surgical margin is "no ink on invasive tumor" [1–3, 20]. Tumor biology or patient age (<40) does not change the minimum acceptable surgical margins. [c]For BCS: According to the ACOSOG Z-11 study, if adjuvant whole-breast RT and systemic treatment will be given to the patient with macrometastasis in 1–2 sentinel lymph nodes, complete axillary dissection may not be performed regardless of tumor biology [15]. According to the 2017 St Gallen consensus, "standard tangential" or "high tangential" RT can be given to these cases, and there is no special preference [3]. [d]For mastectomy: Complete axillary dissection should be performed in patients with macrometastases in 1–2 sentinel lymph nodes if adjuvant RT is not planned. However, there is no complete consensus regarding the omission of axillary dissection in patients for whom RT has been planned [3]. [e]In a multidisciplinary consensus panel, margin widths and ipsilateral breast tumor recurrence (IBTR) were reviewed in 33 studies including 28,162 patients [20]. Positive margins (ink on invasive carcinoma or ductal carcinoma in situ) were associated with a twofold increase in the risk of IBTR compared with negative margins. This increased

(continued)

Fig. 1.10 (continued)
risk was not mitigated by favorable biology, endocrine therapy, or a radiation boost. More widely clear margins than no ink on tumor do not significantly decrease the rate of IBTR compared with "no ink on tumor". No evidence indicates that more widely clear margins reduce IBTR in young patients or in those with unfavorable biology, lobular cancers, or cancers with an extensive intraductal component. The authors concluded that the use of "no ink on tumor" is the standard for adequate margins in invasive cancer but not in DCIS. During the operation, it is best to perform the incision macroscopically 1 cm around the tumor. Postoperative MR imaging is appropriate for patients with tumors in close proximity to the surgical margin. In cases undergoing BCS, a surgical margin of 2 mm or greater is considered safe only in those with DCIS. If the invasive tumor is <1 mm in DCIS, the surgical border safety is evaluated according to DCIS. If the invasive focus is >1 mm in DCIS, the surgical margin width should be evaluated according to the invasive cancer. An adequate surgical margin should be decided by clinical, radiological and pathological evaluation. A "sufficient surgical margin" should be decided according to findings such as radiological additional foci (multifocal disease, microcalcification), invasive lobular carcinoma, multiple surgical margin involvement and persistent proximity of surgical margins in re-excision [2, 20]. [f]Neoadjuvant chemotherapy is recommended for patients with axillary lymph node-positive T1–T3 tumors and axillary lymph node-negative T2–T3 tumors with triple-negative or HER2-positive tumors [1, 3, 5, 12]. In Luminal B tumors, chemotherapy can be considered a priority. Neoadjuvant hormone therapy alone may be considered to avoid mastectomy in node-negative select patients (i.e., patients with strong hormone receptor positivity, advanced age, or poor performance status). Neoadjuvant hormonotherapy should last for 6–8 months, as long as the patient responds. The addition of hormonal agents to neoadjuvant chemotherapy can be made with a low level of evidence. Importantly, the guidelines emphasize that addition of endocrine therapy is not based on direct evidence. Additionally, they provide no reason why endocrine therapy should be delayed until completion of cytotoxic treatment [1, 3, 6, 12]. Tamoxifen as endocrine therapy should not be given with chemotherapy. When neoadjuvant chemotherapy is given, the use of chemotherapy in high-risk patients with very strong hormone-receptor positivity, aromatase inhibitors in the postmenopausal stage, and medical oophorectomy in the premenopausal stage [± aromatase inhibitor, especially in HER2-positive patients] may be considered (proposal 3)

Invasive Breast Cancer: Pathological Evaluation

Histology, Hormone Receptor (HR) Status, HER2 Status, Intrinsic Subtype

Ductal, Lobular, Mixed, Metaplastic Histology

ER positive and/or PgR positive
HR-positive–HER2-positive disease treatment
HR-positive–HER2-negative disease treatment
ER negative and PgR negative
HR-negative–HER2-positive disease treatment
HR-negative–HER2-negative disease treatment

Pure Tubular, Pure Mucinous Histology

ER positive and/or PgR positive (if ER negative and PgR negative, repeat assessment of tumor ER/PgR status)

Intrinsic Subtype [21]

Intrinsic subtype	
Luminal A	Luminal A like
Luminal B	Luminal B like (HER-2 negative)
	Luminal B like (HER-2 positive)
c-ERB B2 overexpression	HER2 positive (non-luminal)
Basal-like	Triple negative

Intrinsic Subtype: Luminal A- and B-Like (Table 1.4)

Table 1.4 Recommendations for breast cancer depending on the intrinsic subtype and clinicopathological surrogate definitions [1, 3, 6, 12, 21]

Intrinsic subtype	Clinicopathological definition
Luminal A	*Luminal like*
	ER positive, PgR positive[a] and HER2 negative and Ki67 ≤14 to 19%[b] and Low recurrence risk with multigene tests or low grade
Luminal B	*Luminal B like (HER2 negative)*
	ER positive, HER2 negative, and Ki67 ≥20 to 29%[c] or PgR low (<20%)/negative or high recurrence risk according to multigene tests
	Luminal B like (HER2 positive)
	ER positive, HER2 overexpression or amplification Any Ki-67

[a]Greater than 20% positivity
[b]The minimum Ki-67 score for Luminal B like is 20–29%. The Ki-67 scores should be interpreted according to local laboratory values. For example, if a laboratory's median Ki-67 score is 20% in receptor-positive disease, scores of 30% and above are considered clearly high, and those of 10% and below are considered low [21]. The Ki-67 values differ between laboratories. Standardization is recommended. Ki-67 is expected to correlate with the nuclear grade but may not directly correlate with histological grade. Taking the core biopsy in 4–6 pieces facilitates evaluation. Routine reporting of tumor-infiltrating lymphocytes (TILs) is not suggested in the St Gallen 2017 consensus report [3]
[c]The minimum value of Ki67 required for "Luminal B like" is 20–29%. Ki-67 scores should be interpreted in light of local laboratory values; for example, if a laboratory has a median Ki-67 score in receptor-positive disease of 20%, values of 30% or above could be considered clearly high [21]

Intrinsic Subtype: Luminal A- and B-Like (Table 1.5)

Table 1.5 Intrinsic subtype and clinicopathological definitions [3, 5, 6, 12]

Subtype	Clinicopathological definition
ER positive, HER2 negative	*High receptor, low proliferation, low grade (Luminal A-like)*
	High ER/PgR and markedly low Ki-67 or histological grade 1 Multi-parameter molecular marker "good" (i.e., Oncotype DX recurrence score < 12)
	Intermediate
	Multi-parameter molecular marker "intermediate" (i.e., Oncotype DX recurrence score = 12–25)
	Low receptor, high proliferation, high grade (Luminal B-like)
	Multi-parameter molecular marker "bad" (i.e., Oncotype DX recurrence score >25) Low ER/PgR and markedly high Ki67 or histological grade 3

HER2 Testing (*Fig. 1.11*)

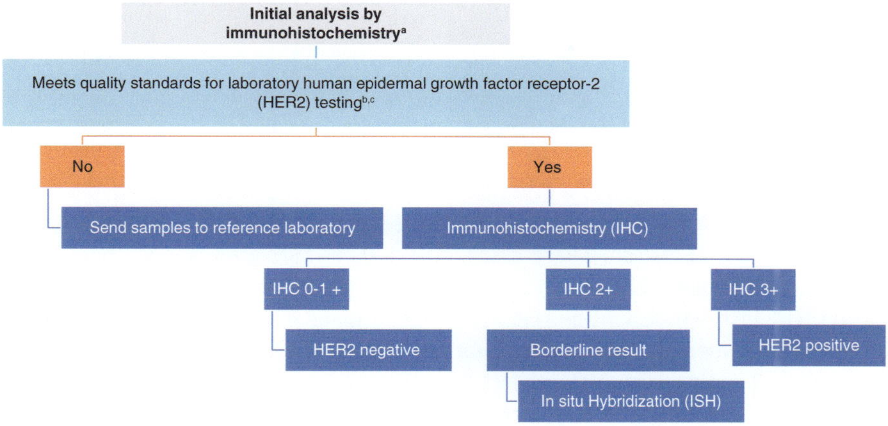

Fig. 1.11 Assessment of tumor HER-2 status. [a]Principles of HER 2 testing. The Update Committee of the American Society of Clinical Oncology and College of American Pathologists identified criteria and areas requiring clarification to improve the accuracy of HER2 testing by immunohistochemistry (IHC) or in situ hybridization (ISH) [22]. The Committee recommended that HER2 status (HER2 negative or positive) be determined in all patients with invasive (early-stage or recurrent) breast cancer based on one or more HER2 test results (negative, equivocal, or positive). Testing criteria define HER2-positive status if (upon observing an area of the tumor representing >10% contiguous and homogeneous tumor cells) there is evidence of protein overexpression (IHC) or gene amplification (HER2 copy number or HER2/CEP17 ratio by ISH based on counting at least 20 cells within the area). If the results are equivocal (revised criteria), reflex testing should be performed using an alternative assay (IHC or ISH). Repeat testing should be considered if the results appear to be discordant with other histopathological findings. Laboratories should demonstrate high concordance with a validated HER2 test on a sufficiently large and representative set of specimens. Testing must be performed in a laboratory accredited by CAP or another accrediting entity [1, 3, 5, 6, 12]. [b]In ASCO–CAP HER2 test guideline recommendations-2018 *HER2 IHC* scoring is reported as follows [22]: *Negative : Score 0*: No staining observed or membrane staining that is incomplete, faint/barely perceptible and in ≤10% of invasive tumor cells. *Score 1+*: Incomplete membrane staining that is faint/barely perceptible and in >10% of invasive tumor cells. *Equivocal (Score2+)*: Weak/moderate complete membrane staining in >10% of invasive tumor cells or complete and circumferential membrane staining that is intense and in ≤10% of invasive tumor cells. *Positive (Score3+)*: Circumferential membrane staining in >10% of invasive tumor cells that is complete and intense. Samples scored as 3+ are considered unequivocally positive, and those scoring 0/1+ are considered negative. Equivocal scores (2+) mandate further assessment using ISH. *Indeterminate*: The test should be reported as indeterminate if technical issues prevent one or both tests (IHC and ISH) from being reported as positive, negative or equivocal. Examples include inadequate specimen handling, artifacts (e.g., crushed or marked edge artifacts) that make interpretation difficult, analytical testing failure or controls that are not as expected. The test should be repeated if possible. [c]In ASCO–CAP HER2 test guideline recommendations-2018 *HER2 ISH* reporting is as follows [22]: *Positive*: Single-probe average HER2 copy number ≥6.0 signals/cell. [i,ii]Dual-probe HER2/CEP17 ratio ≥2.0 with an average HER2 copy number ≥4.0 signals per cell. *Negative*: Single-probe average HER2 copy number <4.0 signals/cell. Dual-probe HER2/CEP17 ratio <2.0 with an average HER2 copy number <4.0 signals/cell. [i]*Observed in a homogeneous and contiguous population and within >10% of the invasive tumor cells.*, [ii]*By counting at least 20 cells within the area.* *The 2018 Focused Update addresses uncommon clinical scenarios and improves clarity, particularly for infrequent HER2 test results that are of uncertain biologic or clinical significance [22]

Updated findings of note include [22]:

Revision of the definition of IHC 2+ (equivocal) to the original FDA-approved criteria.

Repeat HER2 testing on a surgical specimen if the initially tested core biopsy is negative is no longer stated as mandatory. A new HER2 test *may* (no longer *should*) be ordered on the excision specimen on the basis of some criteria (such as tumor grade 3).

A more rigorous interpretation criteria of the less common patterns that can be seen in about 5% of all cases when HER2 status in breast cancer is evaluated using a dual-probe ISH testing. These cases, described as ISH groups 2–4, should now be assessed using a diagnostic approach that includes a concomitant review of the IHC test, which will help the pathologist make a final determination of the tumor specimen as HER2 positive or negative. The update on recommendations for HER2 testing with ISH method cancelled an equivocal result. Instead, forced pathologists to make a judgement as positive or negative using combination of repeated IHC and dual-probe ISH method. According to final update, if the HER2/CEP 17 ratio $\geq$2.0 and average HER2 copy number is <4.0 the result should be negative after completion of a work-up. If the average HER2 copy number is $\geq$6.0 and the ratio is <2.0 the result should be positive after completion of a work-up.

The Expert Panel also preferentially recommends the use of dual-probe instead of single-probe ISH assays, but it recognizes that several single-probe ISH assays have regulatory approval in many parts of the world.

Invasive Breast Cancer: Adjuvant Systemic Therapy

Luminal A Like, Luminal B Like, HER-2 Positive, Triple Negative (*Table 1.6*)

Table 1.6 Recommendations for adjuvant treatment of breast cancer depending on intrinsic subtype and clinicopathological surrogate definitions [1, 3, 5, 6, 12, 21, 23–28]

Intrinsic subtype	Clinicopathological definition	Treatment	Special considerations[b–f]
Luminal A	*Luminal A like*		
	ER positive and PgR positive[a] and HER2-negative and Kİ 67 ≤ (14–19%)[b] and Recurrence risk low with multigene tests	Endocrine therapy	Cytotoxics administered if high gene recurrence score (RS) (with Oncotype DX, RS > 25)[d], grade 3 disease, extensive lymphovascular invasion,[c] ≥4 lymph node metastasis, young age (<35 years)[f]
Luminal B	*Luminal B like (HER2 negative)*		
	ER positive and HER2 negative and Ki67 ≥ (20–29%)[b] or, PgR low/negative or, Recurrence risk high with multigene tests	Endocrine therapy for all, cytotoxics for most	
	Luminal B like (HER2 positive)		
	HER2 overexpressed or amplified Any Ki-67	Cytotoxics and antiHER-2 and endocrine therapy	
HER-2 overexpression	*HER2 positive (non-luminal)*		
	HER2 overexpressed or amplified and ER and PgR absent	Cytotoxics and antiHER-2 therapy	
Basal-like	*Triple negative*		
	ER negative and PgR negative HER2 negative	Cytotoxics	80% overlap between triple-negative and basal-like subtypes

[a]More than 20% positivity [3, 5, 21]
[b]St. Gallen 2015: The minimum value of Ki67 required for "Luminal B like" is 20–29%. Ki-67 scores should be interpreted in the light of local laboratory values: as an example, if a laboratory has a median Ki-67 score in receptor-positive disease of 20%, values of 30% or above could be considered clearly high; values of 10% or less are clearly low [21]
[c]Lymphovascular invasion without any other poor prognostic factor is not an indication for cytotoxic chemotherapy [3, 5, 12, 21]
[d]In early-stage breast cancer, there are biomarkers that can be used to decide adjuvant systemic treatment [1, 3, 12, 25, 29–31]. The situations in which multigene tests may be specifically performed can be summarized as follows: *tumour* size between 1 and 3 cm *and* ER/PgR positive *and* HER2 negative *and* node negative or $N1_{mi}$ *and* Grade 2 *and* Ki-67 between 15% and 35% [3, 12,

(continued)

Table 1.6 (continued)

29–31]. *ER/PgR positive, HER2 negative (node negative): Oncotype DX* (Genomic Health Inc., Redwood City, CA); *EndoPredict* (Sividon Diagnostics, Germany); *MammaPrint* (Agendia, Irvine, CA); *PAM50 ROR score* (Prosigna Breast Cancer Prognostic Gene Signature Assay; NanoString Technologies, Seattle, WA, USA); *Breast Cancer Index* (bio Theranostics); *uPA and PAI-1*. *ER/PgR positive, HER2 negative (node positive)*: *MammaPrint* (Agendia, Irvine, CA): In cases with 1–3 positive lymph nodes and high clinical but low genomic risk group according to MINDACT categorization, do not administer adjuvant chemotherapy (patients should be informed about the possible additional benefit of chemotherapy in multiple LN positivity) [31]. For patients with hormone receptor-positive, HER2-negative, and lymph node-negative tumors, prognostic gene signatures (Oncotype DX, MammaPrint, Endopredict, BCI) with a low risk score regardless of T size place the tumor in the same prognostic category as T1a–T1b N0M0, and the tumor is staged using the AJCC prognostic stage group table as stage I (AJCC 8th edition). The recurrence score based on the 21-gene breast cancer assay predicts chemotherapy benefit if it is high and a low risk of recurrence in the absence of chemotherapy if it is low. In the TAILORx ClinicalTrial (ASCO Congress 2018), adjuvant endocrine therapy and chemoendocrine therapy had similar efficacy in women with hormone-receptor-positive, HER2-negative, axillary node-negative breast cancer who had a midrange 21-gene recurrence score. However, the chemotherapy benefit for invasive disease-free survival varied with the combination of recurrence score and age ($P = 0.004$), with some benefit of chemotherapy found in women 50 years of age or younger with a recurrence score of 16–25

[e]Multigene tests should not be used in low-risk patients (e.g., T1a/b, grade 1, ER high, N0) for whom endocrine therapy has definitely been planned or in patients who cannot undergo chemotherapy due to comorbidity. Multigene tests should not be used for indications for extended endocrine therapy (e.g., administration of tamoxifen for 10 years) [3, 21]

[f]In the St Gallen panel, participants voted 56% yes and 44% no in terms of being a relative indication for the addition of adjuvant cytotoxic treatment at young age (<35) in patients who were identified as at risk according to the immunohistochemistry results [3]

Ductal, Lobular, Mixed, Metaplastic Histology—Stage IA (T1N0M0) Disease

HR-Positive or HR-Negative and HER2-Positive Disease *(Fig. 1.12)*

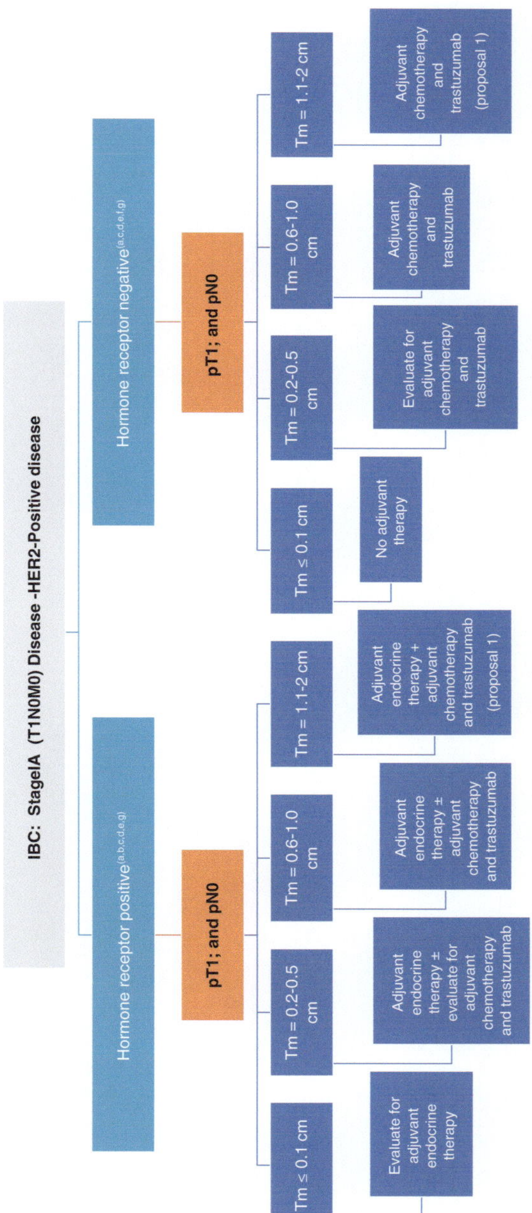

Fig. 1.12 Adjuvant systemic therapy for stage IA—hormone receptor-positive or—negative and HER2-positive disease. [a]There is no absolute age limit. Instead, treatment depends on the disease, the presence of comorbidities, the patient's life expectancy, and patient preferences. Treatment should be individualized for patients >70 years of age. [b]Chemotherapy and endocrine therapy as adjuvant therapy should be given sequentially, with endocrine therapy following chemotherapy. The available data suggest that sequential or concurrent endocrine therapy with radiation therapy is acceptable. [c]Assuming that HER2 positivity is determined according to the ASCO/CAP guidelines, most patients with T1b disease and all patients with T1c disease require anti-HER2 therapy [3, 12, 21, 32]. The chemotherapy regimen for these patients may contain anthracyclines. If provided in stage I and if the tumor diameter is <1 to 2 cm, the combination of paclitaxel and trastuzumab may be preferred regimen [32]. For patients in stage I with a tumor diameter >1 to 2 cm, anthracyclines fol-

(continued)

Fig. 1.12 (continued)

lowed by taxanes and trastuzumab may be preferred, although paclitaxel-trastuzumab may also be an option in select patients [3]. Trastuzumab or chemotherapy is not recommended for microinvasive disease (invasive tumor ≤1 mm). [d]A meta-analysis consisting of eight studies has shown that the HER2-positive phenotype is associated with a poorer outcome compared to HR-positive and HER2-negative groups in terms of disease-free survival (DFS; RR = 3.677, $P < 0.001$) and distant disease-free survival (DDFS; RR = 3.824, $P < 0.001$) [33]. However, there was no significant difference in terms of clinical endpoints between HER2-positive and triple-negative breast cancers. Moreover, the addition of trastuzumab in patients with pT1a-bN0M0 disease yielded a significant improvement in terms of DFS (RR = 0.323, $P < 0.001$). This meta-analysis showed that the intrinsic subtype may be a reliable marker for prognosis in patients with pT1a-bN0M0 breast cancer. Adjuvant trastuzumab may provide a significant survival benefit even in early-stage HER2-positive breast cancer patients [33]. [e]In an uncontrolled, single-group, multicenter study of adjuvant paclitaxel and trastuzumab, 406 patients with tumors measuring up to 3 cm in the greatest dimension were included [32]. Patients received weekly treatment with paclitaxel and trastuzumab for 12 weeks, followed by 9 months of trastuzumab monotherapy. The median follow-up period was 4.0 years. The 3-year rate of survival free from invasive disease was 98.7% (95% confidence interval [CI], 97.6–99.8). Among women with predominantly stage I HER2-positive breast cancer, treatment with adjuvant paclitaxel plus trastuzumab was associated with a risk of early recurrence of approximately 2%; 6% of patients withdrew from the study due to protocol-specified adverse events. [f]Fertility preservation (e.g., by ovarian tissue or oocyte conservation) should be offered to women <40 years of age. Ovarian function suppression with LHRHa during chemotherapy should be offered especially for hormone receptor-negative disease [1, 3, 34, 35]. [g]Consider adjuvant bisphosphonate therapy in postmenopausal (natural or induced) patients receiving adjuvant therapy

HR-Positive or HR-Negative and HER2-Negative Disease (Fig. 1.13)

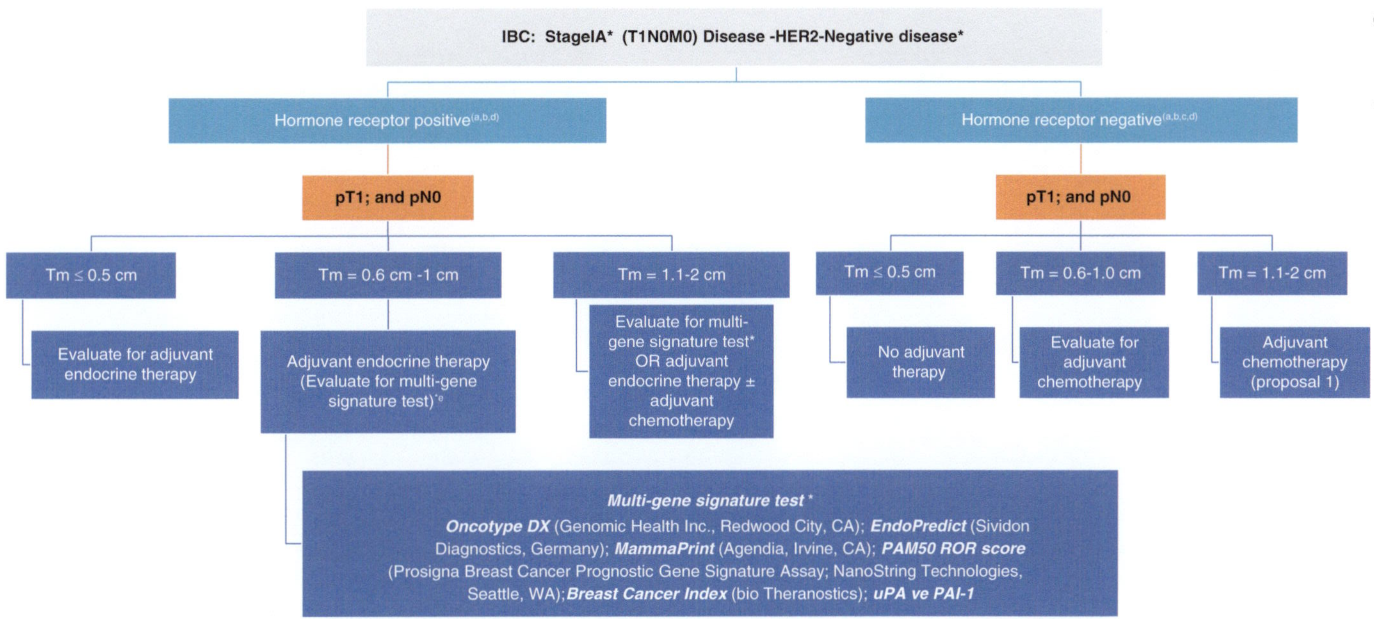

Fig. 1.13 Adjuvant systemic therapy for stage IA—hormone receptor-positive or-negative and HER2-negative disease. *In early-stage breast cancer, there are biomarkers that can be used to decide adjuvant systemic treatment administration [1, 3, 12, 21, 25, 28]. Based on multigene signature tests, chemotherapy may be omitted for patients with Luminal B-like (HER2 negative) disease with a low Oncotype Dx® score, MammaPrint® low-risk status, low PAM50 ROR score, or EndoPredict® low-risk status. The situations in which multigene tests may be particularly helpful can be summarized as follows: tumor size between 1 and 3 cm *and* ER/PR positive *and* HER2 negative *and* node negative or N_{mi} *and* Grade 2 *and* Ki-67 between 15% and

(continued)

Fig. 1.13 (continued)
35%. In hormone receptor-positive T1c N0 (1–2 cm) tumors, grade 3 disease with a high Ki-67 value (e.g., above 35%) and PgR <20% may be considered adequate for chemotherapy indication. In cases where multigene tests cannot be performed, the risk factors can be determined using web-based formulas, and an indication for chemotherapy administration can be established [1, 3, 5, 6, 12, 21, 26, 28]. For patients with hormone receptor-positive, HER2-negative, and lymph node-negative tumors, prognostic gene signatures (Oncotype DX, MammaPrint, Endopredict, BCI) with a low risk score regardless of T size place the tumor in the same prognostic category as T1a–T1b N0M0, and the tumor is staged using the AJCC prognostic stage group table as stage I (AJCC 8th edition). [a]There is no absolute age limit. Rather, treatment depends on the disease, the presence of comorbidities, the patient's life expectancy, and patient preferences. Treatment should be individualized for patients >70 years of age. [b]Chemotherapy and endocrine therapy as adjuvant therapy should be given sequentially, with endocrine therapy following chemotherapy. The available data suggest that sequential or concurrent endocrine therapy with radiation therapy is acceptable [1, 3, 12, 21]. [c]Fertility preservation (e.g., by ovarian tissue or oocyte conservation) should be offered to women <40 years of age. Ovarian function suppression with LHRHa during chemotherapy should be offered especially for HR-negative disease [3, 34, 35]. [d]Consider adjuvant bisphosphonate therapy in postmenopausal (natural or induced) patients receiving adjuvant therapy. [e]Evaluate for multi-gene signature test, especially for Luminal B-like, high Ki67, or grade III tumors [3, 12, 21]

Useful Biomarkers for the Decision of Adjuvant Systemic Treatment in Early-Stage Breast Cancer [25]

ER/PgR Positive, HER2 Negative (Node Negative)

Oncotype DX (Genomic Health Inc., Redwood City, CA)
EndoPredict (Sividon Diagnostics, Germany)
MammaPrint (Agendia, Irvine, CA)
PAM50 ROR score (Prosigna Breast Cancer Prognostic Gene Signature Assay; NanoString Technologies, Seattle, WA)
Breast Cancer Index (bio Theranostics)
uPA and PAI-1

ER/PgR Positive, HER2 Negative (Node Positive)

MammaPrint (Agendia, Irvine, CA) can be used to avoid adjuvant chemotherapy in cases with 1–3 positive lymph nodes if they are at high clinical risk group [31] according to MINDACT categorization. The patient with low genomic risk should be informed that there may be additional benefit of chemotherapy in cases with positivity of more than one LN.

Ductal, Lobular, Mixed, Metaplastic histology: STAGE I–II–IIIA (T3N1M0) Disease

HR-Positive and HER2-Positive Disease (*Fig. 1.14*)

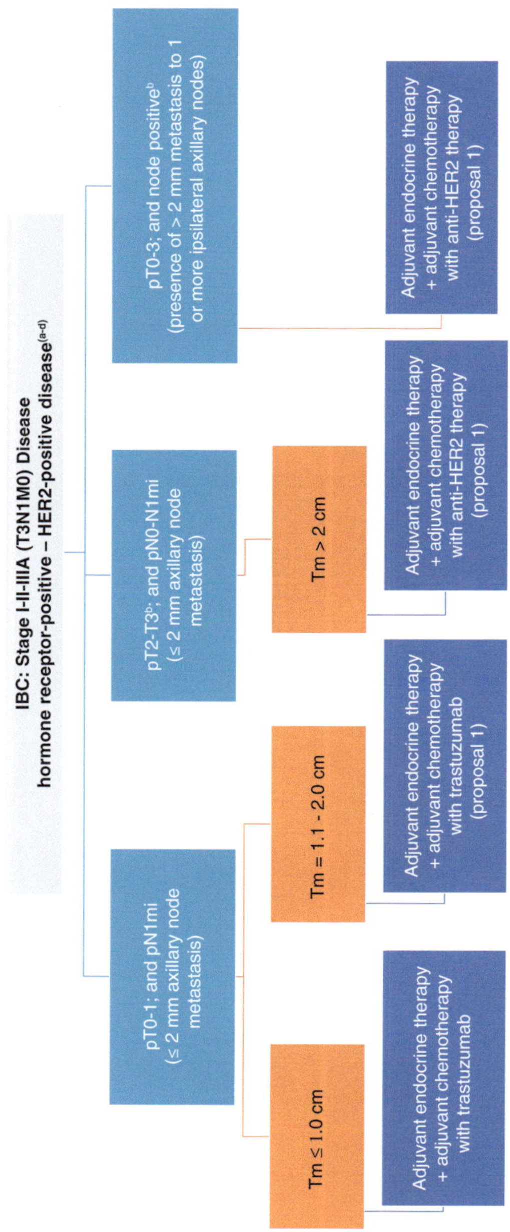

Fig. 1.14 Adjuvant systemic therapy for stage I, II, IIIA—hormone receptor-positive and HER2-positive disease. [a]There is no absolute age limit. Rather, treatment depends on the disease, the presence of comorbidities, the patient's life expectancy, and patient preferences. Treatment should be individualized for patients >70 years of age. [b]Neoadjuvant therapy is recommended in HER2-positive stage II and III patients [1, 3, 12, 21]. Trastuzumab and pertuzumab are recommended in neoadjuvant therapy [1, 3]. The version 1.0 2018 NCCN Guidelines recommend AC—paclitaxel and trastuzumab (± pertuzumab); TCH ± pertuzumab (pertuzumab given to patients with greater than or equal to T2 or greater than or equal to N1, HER2-positive early-stage breast cancer) [1, 24, 26]. The St Gallen panel did not support dual HER2 blockade with pertuzumab or lapatinib in the postoperative adjuvant treatment [3]. According to the APHINITY study, which published the early results, adjuvant trastuzumab + pertuzumab treatment prolonged disease-free survival in HER2-positive patients. This benefit was particularly evident in high-risk patients who were hormone receptor negative and node positive [24]. According to a randomized controlled trial, 1-year neratinib use after 1-year administration of trastuzumab reduced the recurrence rate [36]. This benefit was especially evident in ER-positive, Her-2-positive disease. However, diarrhea was an important adverse effect. The

St Gallen 2017 panel did not respond to the question regarding extended adjuvant neratinib administration [3]. However, after 1 year of trastuzumab administration in hormone receptor-positive patients, 1 year of neratinib can be used [26]. [c]In high-risk premenopausal patients, "LHRH-agonist + aromatase inhibitor" may be the preferred adjuvant endocrine therapy. In a randomized phase III study, a total of 3066 premenopausal women were stratified according to whether they previously received chemotherapy to receive 5 years of tamoxifen, tamoxifen plus ovarian suppression therapy, or exemestane plus ovarian suppression therapy [35]. After a median follow-up of 67 months, the estimated disease-free survival rate at 5 years was 86.6% in the tamoxifen-ovarian suppression group and 84.7% in the tamoxifen group (hazard ratio for disease recurrence, second invasive cancer, or death, 0.83; 95% confidence interval [CI], 0.66–1.04; P = 0.10). At 5 years, the rate of freedom from breast cancer was 85.7% in the exemestane-ovarian suppression group (hazard ratio for recurrence vs. tamoxifen, 0.65; 95% CI, 0.49–0.87) [35]. In high-risk postmenopausal patients, aromatase inhibitors may be preferred over tamoxifen [3, 12, 21, 23, 25, 27, 28]. [d]Chemotherapy and endocrine therapy as adjuvant therapy should be given sequentially, with endocrine therapy following chemotherapy. The available data suggest that sequential or concurrent endocrine therapy with radiation therapy is acceptable [1, 3, 12]

HR-Positive and HER2-Negative Disease (Fig. 1.15)

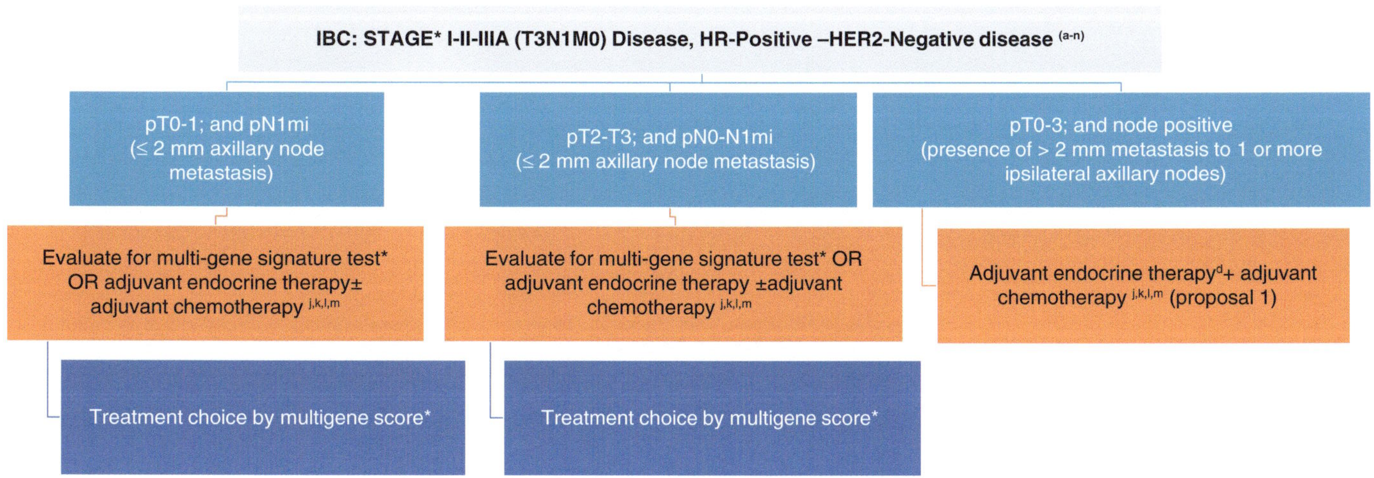

Fig. 1.15 Adjuvant systemic therapy for stage I, II, IIIA—hormone receptor-positive and HER2-negative disease [1, 3, 5, 6, 12, 25–28]. *By multi-gene signature tests: *Oncotype DX* (Genomic Health); *EndoPredict* (Sividon Diagnostics, Germany); *MammaPrint* (Agendia, Irvine, CA): If in the high clinical but low genomic risk group according to the MINDACT categorization, do not give adjuvant chemotherapy; *PAM50 ROR score* (Prosigna Breast Cancer Prognostic Gene Signature Assay; NanoString Technologies, Seattle, WA); *Breast Cancer Index* (bio Theranostics); *uPA and PAI-1*. Chemotherapy may be omitted for patients with Luminal B-like (HER2 negative) disease with a low Oncotype Dx® score (<25), MammaPrint® low-risk status [31], low PAM50 ROR score or EndoPredict® low-risk status). For patients with hormone receptor-positive, HER2-negative, and lymph node-negative tumors, prognostic gene signatures (Oncotype DX, MammaPrint, Endopredict, BCI) with a low risk score regardless of T size place the tumor in the same prognostic category as T1a–T1b N0 M0, and the tumor is staged using the AJCC prognostic stage group table as stage I (AJCC 8th edition). [a]There is no absolute age limit. The choice of treatment depends on disease, co-morbidities, life expectancy and patient preferences. In patients over 70 years of age, treatment should be individualized [3, 12]. A meta-analysis showed that dose-intensive treatment increased overall survival in hormone receptor-negative and hormone receptor-positive patients (EBTCG, San Antonio, 2017). [b]The following factors are indications for including ovarian

function suppression (OFS): age ≤35 years, premenopausal estrogen level following adjuvant chemotherapy, grade 3 disease, involvement of 4 or more nodes, and adverse multigene test results [3]. The ASCO Guideline recommends OFS in premenopausal patients with stage II and III disease who have chemotherapy indications; however, this is not recommended for stage I disease [27]. The optimal OFS duration is 5 years. [c]In high-risk premenopausal women, 'LHRH-agonist + aromatase inhibitor' may be the preferred adjuvant endocrine therapy [27, 35]. The following factors are indications for the use of OFS plus an aromatase inhibitor (AI) rather than OFS plus tamoxifen: age ≤35 years, grade 3 disease, involvement of 4 or more nodes, and adverse multigene test results [1, 3, 12, 27, 35]. [d]In patients with Luminal A-like tumors and 1–3 positive lymph nodes (with the evaluation of other factors such as grade, age, or multigene signature test results), "adjuvant endocrine therapy alone" may be an option [3, 5, 6, 12]. [e]Some patients may be adequately treated with tamoxifen alone. In high-risk postmenopausal patients, AIs may be preferred over tamoxifen [1, 3, 12, 27, 35]. The following factors support the inclusion of an AI at some point: lymph node involvement, grade 3 disease, high Ki67 proliferation index, or HER2 positivity. If an AI is used, it should be started upfront in patients at higher risk. The upfront AI can be switched to tamoxifen after 2 years in selected patients (e.g., those experiencing side effects of the AI) [1, 3, 12]. [f]After 5 years of adjuvant tamoxifen, continued AI (for postmenopausal estrogen levels at baseline or postmenopausal patients with premenopausal estrogen levels at baseline) or tamoxifen (for premenopausal or postmenopausal patients) for up to 10 years should be recommended to patients with node-positive disease, grade 3 disease, or high Ki-67 [1, 3, 5, 6, 12]. [g]After 5 years of adjuvant therapy involving a switch from tamoxifen to an AI (therefore assuming postmenopausal status at the 5-year time point and reasonable tolerance to endocrine therapy), patients may continue AI therapy for a cumulative total of 5 years [1, 3, 5, 6, 12]. [h]After 5 years of continuous AI adjuvant therapy, we do not (yet) know whether to provide 3–5 years of tamoxifen, 3–5 years of AI, or no further endocrine treatment [1, 3, 37]. AI can be considered for an additional 5 years. However, a randomized clinical trial failed to show a difference in survival between 2 and 5 years' use of additional AI (San Antonio BCS, 2017). [i]The optimal OFS duration is 5 years [1, 3, 6, 12]. [j]Factors that are relative indications for the inclusion of adjuvant cytotoxic chemotherapy include the following: histological grade 3 tumor, 4 or more positive nodes, high Ki67, extensive lymphovascular invasion, and low hormone receptor staining [1, 3, 5, 6, 12]. [k]The Luminal A phenotype is less responsive to chemotherapy. In node-negative disease, chemotherapy should not be added based on the T size. A combination of the biological properties of the tumor (such as Ki67, LVI, grade, and multigene signature) must be used to assess whether to provide chemotherapy [1, 3, 5, 6, 12, 25, 28]. Chemotherapy should be added in high-risk patients based on the involvement of 4 or more lymph nodes (Table 1.6). [l]Based on immunohistochemistry (IHC), in Luminal B-like (HER2-negative) tumors, chemotherapy may be omitted in some low-risk patients (based on combinations of certain prognostic factors such as low tumor mass, low grade, low Ki67, an absence of LVI, and older age) [1, 3, 5, 6, 12, 25, 28]. [m]Based on multigene signature tests, chemotherapy may be omitted for patients with Luminal B-like (HER2-negative) disease with a low Oncotype Dx® score, MammaPrint® low-risk status, low PAM50 ROR score or EndoPredict® low-risk status [1, 3, 12, 25]. MammaPrint can be used in node-positive patients [31]. MammaPrint (Agendia, Irvine, CA): In patients with 1–3 positive lymph nodes, tests can be performed to avoid adjuvant chemotherapy if the patient is at high clinical risk group in the MINDACT categorization (however, the patient should be informed that there may be an additional benefit of chemotherapy with multiple LN positivity). [n]For Luminal B-like (HER2-negative) tumors, the regimen, if given, should contain anthracyclines and taxanes. A high-risk group might exist for which dose-dense therapy with G-CSF may also be preferred [1, 3, 38]. The effect of dose-intensive treatment on disease recurrence has been investigated, and it has been shown that administration of 5-fluorouracil does not provide additional benefit [39, 40]

HR-Negative and HER2-Positive Disease (Fig. 1.16)

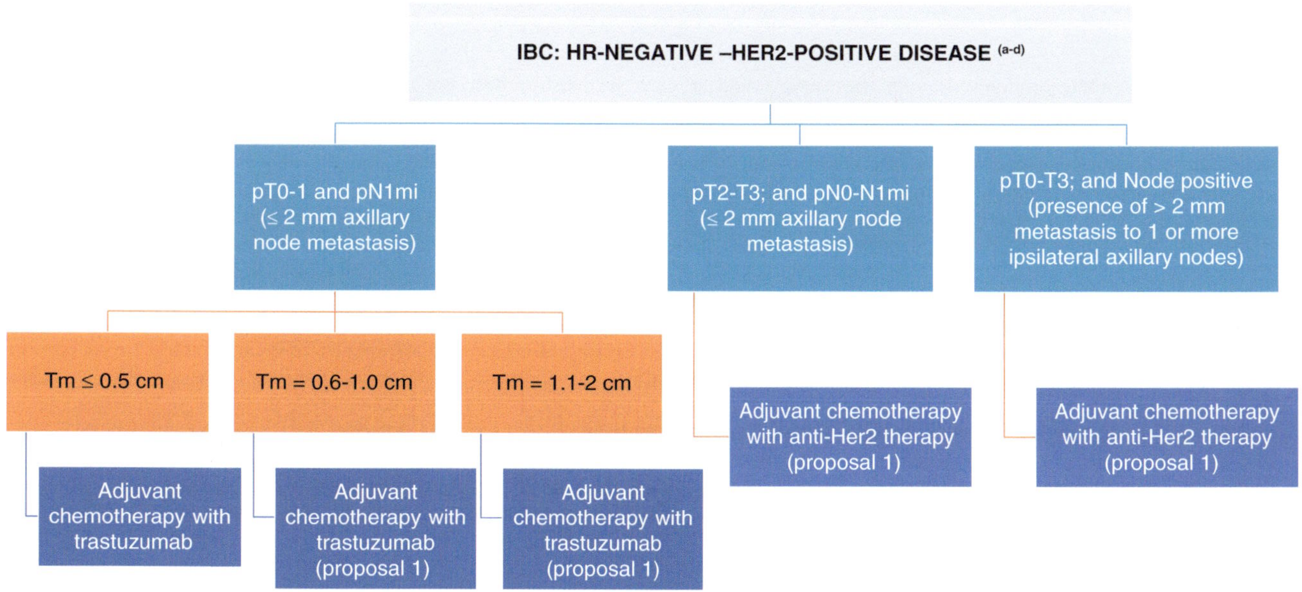

Fig. 1.16 Adjuvant systemic therapy for stage I, II, IIIA—hormone receptor-negative and HER2-positive disease. [a]There is no absolute age limit. The choice of treatment choice depends on disease, co-morbidities, life expectancy and patient preferences. In a meta-analysis, dose-intensive treatment was shown to improve overall survival in hormone receptor-negative and hormone receptor-positive patients (EBTCG, San Antonio BCS, 2017). For patients >70 years of age, treatment should be individualized [1, 3, 12]. [b]AC—paclitaxel and trastuzumab (± pertuzumab); TCH ± pertuzumab (pertuzumab given to patients with greater than or equal to T2 or greater than or equal to N1, HER2-positive, early-stage breast cancer) can be recommended [24, 26, 41]. According to the early results of the APHINITY study, the authors concluded that pertuzumab can be considered as adjuvant therapy in HR-negative patients with node-positive or locally advanced tumors [24]. [c]In patients with HER2-positive, stage 2 disease, chemotherapy should always be provided to patients who require anti-HER2 therapy. The chemotherapy regimen for these patients should preferably contain anthracyclines and taxanes. Anti-HER2 therapy should be initiated concurrently with taxane therapy. For tumors with a size of 1–2 cm or smaller, paclitaxel-trastuzumab can be used [3, 32, 33]. [d]Consider adjuvant bisphosphonate therapy in postmenopausal (natural or induced) patients receiving adjuvant therapy

HR-Negative and HER2-Negative Disease (Fig. 1.17)

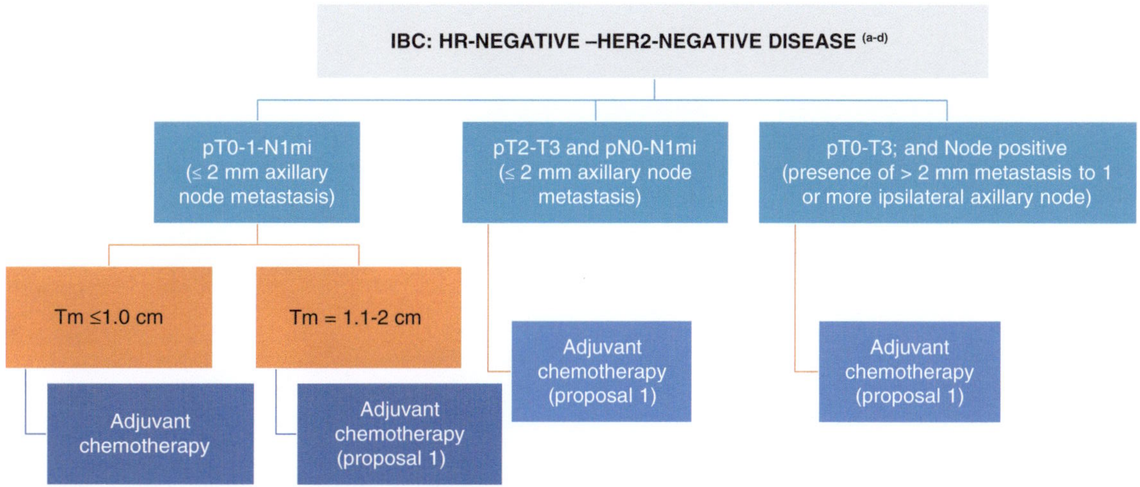

Fig. 1.17 Adjuvant systemic therapy for stage IB, II, IIIA—hormone receptor-negative and HER2-negative disease. [a]There is no absolute age limit. Rather, treatment depends on the disease, the presence of comorbidities, the patient's life expectancy, and patient preferences. For patients >70 years of age, treatment should be individualized. Regardless of the size of the invasive tumor, adjuvant chemotherapy may be recommended in the presence of $N1_{mi}$. [b]Fertility preservation (e.g., by ovarian tissue or oocyte conservation) should be offered to women <40 years of age. Ovarian function suppression with LHRHa during chemotherapy should be offered especially for receptor-negative disease [1, 3, 12, 21, 34]. [c]In triple-negative breast cancer (TNBC), the regimen should include anthracyclines and taxanes. Although the data are insufficient, a platinum-based regimen may be considered only when a BRCA mutation has been identified. Anthracyclines followed by taxanes represent an acceptable regimen for BRCA-mutant TNBC. Dose-dense chemotherapy requiring growth factor support may also be an option. The preference of dose-intensive treatment in these patients was not recommended in St. Gallen (37% yes, 55% no) [3]. However, a meta-analysis showed that dose-intensive treatment improved overall survival in hormone receptor-negative and hormone receptor-positive patients (EBTCG, San Antonio, 2017). Neoadjuvant treatment should be considered in triple-negative patients with stage II and III disease. Treatment with platinum or alkylating agents may be considered in neoadjuvant chemotherapy (71% yes, 15% no) [3, 38]. Provision of platinum-based treatment for all patients was voted as 10% 'yes' and 86% 'no' at St Gallen [3]. A platinum-based regimen may be recommended, particularly when a BRCA mutation is detected (voted as 47% 'yes' and 43% 'no' at St Gallen 2017) [3]. The administration of capecitabine after anthracycline and taxane treatment reduces recurrence in patients with TNBC [42]. Capecitabine reduces the recurrence rate in patients with residual tumors after neoadjuvant therapy [43]. [d]Consider adjuvant bisphosphonate therapy in postmenopausal (natural or induced) patients receiving adjuvant therapy

Pure Tubular and Pure Mucinous Carcinoma (Favorable Histologies): STAGE I–II–III Disease *(Fig. 1.18)*

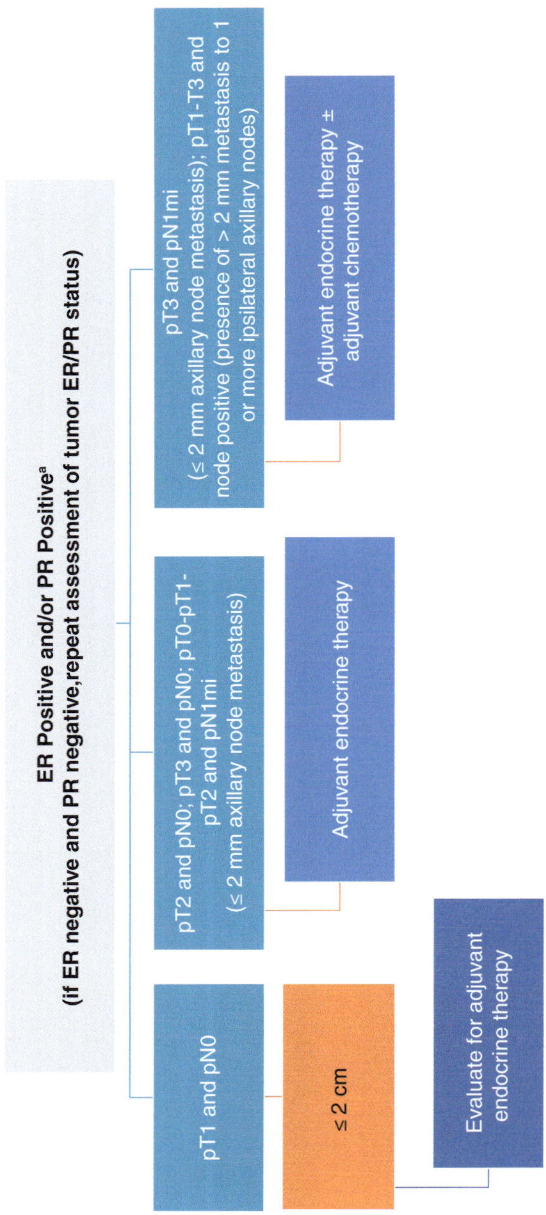

Fig. 1.18 Adjuvant systemic therapy for pure tubular and pure mucinous carcinoma [3, 5, 21]. [a]Consider adjuvant bisphosphonate therapy in postmenopausal (natural or induced) patients receiving adjuvant therapy. [b]If ER negative and PR negative treat as usual breast cancer histology

Invasive Breast Cancer: Adjuvant Endocrine Therapy

Premenopausal at Diagnosis (*Fig. 1.19*)

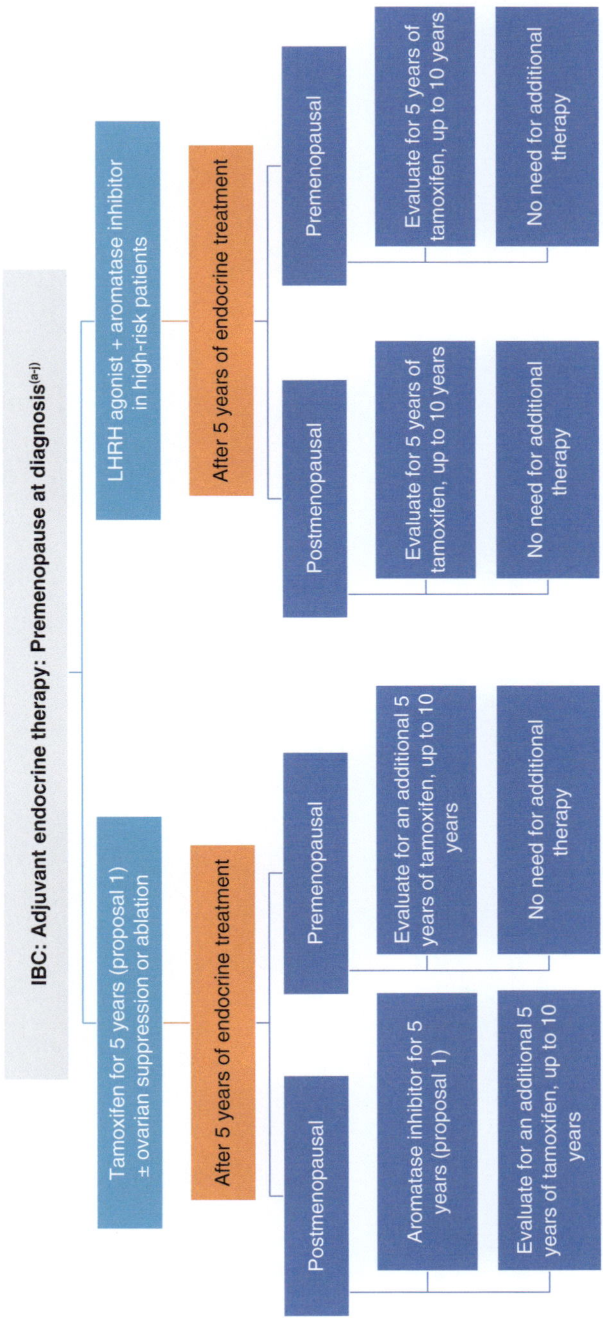

Fig. 1.19 Adjuvant endocrine therapy for premenopausal patients [3, 7–9, 12, 25]. [a]The following factors are indications for including ovarian function suppression (OFS): age ≤35 years, premenopausal estrogen levels following adjuvant chemotherapy, grade 3 disease, involvement of 4 or more nodes, and adverse multigene test results [3, 27, 35]. The ASCO Guideline recommends OFS for pre-menopausal patients with stage II and III disease for whom chemotherapy has been indicated. By contrast, OFS is not recommended in stage I disease [27]. [b]The optimal duration of OFS (with tamoxifen) may be 5 years. Its use for 5 years should be strongly recommended, especially in high-risk patients [1, 3, 27]. [c]In high-risk premenopausal patients, 5 years of "LHRH-agonist plus aromatase inhibitor (AI)" may be the preferred adjuvant endocrine therapy [35].

(continued)

Fig. 1.19 (continued)

Exemestane, letrozole or anastrozole can be used as an AI. The following factors are indications for the use of OFS plus AI rather than OFS plus tamoxifen: age ≤35 years, grade 3 disease, high Ki67, node positivity, lobular histology, HER-2 positivity, and adverse multigene test results [3, 35]. Serum estrogen, follicle-stimulating hormone (FSH) and luteinizing hormone (LH) levels should be measured in the evaluation of menopausal status for the use of an aromatase inhibitor in premenopausal patients who have received chemotherapy. Estradiol levels should be checked at certain intervals. [d]After 5 years of continuous "LHRH-agonist plus exemestane" adjuvant therapy, we do not (yet) know whether to provide further endocrine treatment [3, 35, 44]. [e]In patients with Luminal A-like tumors and 1–3 positive lymph nodes (with the evaluation of other factors such as grade, age or multigene signature test results), "adjuvant endocrine therapy alone" may be an option [3, 5, 6, 21, 25]. [f]Adjuvant endocrine therapy should be completed in 10 years in stage II and III patients, especially those with moderate to high recurrence risk, but is not recommended for stage I patients [1, 3, 23]. After 5 years of adjuvant tamoxifen, continued AI (for postmenopausal patients with premenopausal estrogen levels at baseline) or tamoxifen for up to 10 years should be recommended to patients with node-positive disease, grade 3 disease, or high Ki-67. [g]After 5 years of adjuvant therapy involving a switch from tamoxifen to an AI (therefore assuming postmenopausal status at the 5-year time point and reasonable tolerance to endocrine therapy), patients may continue AI therapy for a cumulative total of 5 years. This subject requires clarification [3]. There was no difference in survival between 2 years and 5 years of AI in a randomized clinical trial (San Antonio BCS, 2017). [h]By immunohistochemistry (IHC): In Luminal B-like (HER2-negative) tumors, chemotherapy may be omitted in some low-risk patients (based on combinations of certain prognostic factors such as low tumor mass, low grade, low Ki67, an absence of LVI, and older age) [3, 5, 6, 12, 21, 25, 28]. [i]By multigene signature tests: Chemotherapy may be omitted for patients with Luminal B-like (HER2- negative) disease with a low Oncotype Dx® score, MammaPrint® low-risk status, low PAM50 ROR score, or EndoPredict® low-risk status [1, 3, 12, 25, 28]. [j]Consider adjuvant bisphosphonate therapy in postmenopausal (natural or induced) patients receiving adjuvant therapy

Postmenopausal at Diagnosis *(Box 1.2) (Fig. 1.20)*

Box 1.2 The definition of menopause
Menopause can be defined as natural menopause (no menses for 12 months before starting chemotherapy or hormone therapy) or as menopause with ovarian ablation or suppression. Luteinizing hormone (LH), follicle-stimulating hormone (FSH), and serum estradiol (E2) levels should be at post-menopausal levels and should be measured before systemic treatment unless oophorectomy has been performed with hysterectomy in women aged 60 years or younger.

The definition of menopause: "Prior bilateral oophorectomy" OR "Age ≥60 years" OR "Age <60 years" and amenorrheic for 12 or more months in the absence of chemotherapy, tamoxifen, toremifene, or ovarian suppression and follicle-stimulating hormone (FSH) and estradiol in the postmenopausal range OR "If taking tamoxifen or toremifene, and age <60 years, then FSH and plasma estradiol levels in postmenopausal ranges".

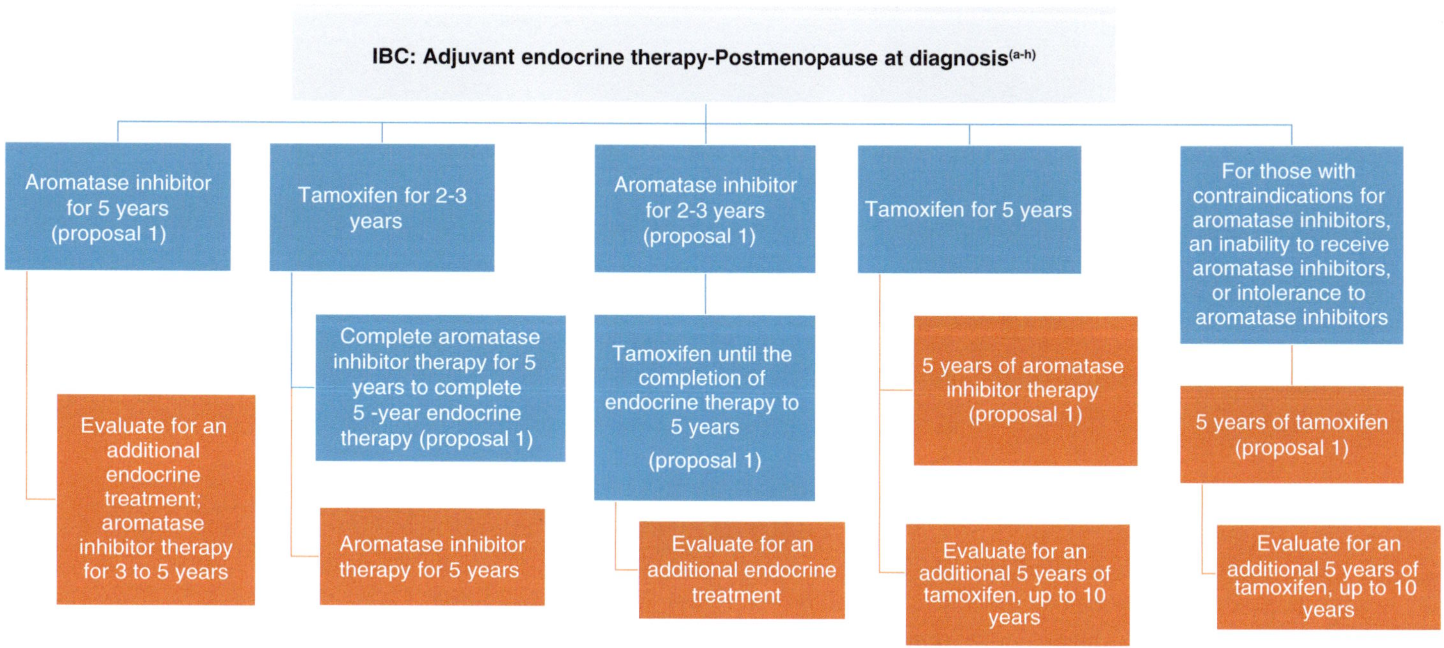

Fig. 1.20 Adjuvant endocrine therapy for postmenopausal patients. [a]In patients with Luminal A-like tumors and 1–3 positive lymph nodes (with the evaluation of other factors such as grade, age, or multigene signature test results), "adjuvant endocrine therapy alone" may be an option [3, 5, 6, 12]. [b]Some patients may be adequately treated with tamoxifen alone. In high-risk postmenopausal patients, aromatase inhibitors (AIs) may be preferred over tamoxifen [3]. The following factors argue for the inclusion of an AI at some point: lymph node involvement, grade 3 disease, high Ki67 proliferation index, or HER2 positivity. If an AI is used, it should be started upfront in patients at higher risk. The upfront AI can be switched to tamoxifen after 2 years in selected patients (e.g., those experiencing side effects of the AI) [3]. [c]After 5 years of adjuvant tamoxifen, continued AI or tamoxifen (for patients with intolerance to AI therapy) for up to 10 years should be recommended to patients with node-positive disease, grade 3 disease, or high Ki-67 [1, 3, 6, 12]. [d]After 5 years of adjuvant therapy involving a switch from tamoxifen to an AI (therefore assuming postmenopausal status at the 5-year time point and reasonable tolerance to endocrine therapy), patients may con-

tinue AI therapy for a cumulative total of 5 years. This subject requires clarification [3]. [e]After 5 years of continuous AI adjuvant therapy, extension of treatment with an aromatase inhibitor may be recommended for 3–5 years [1, 3, 23]. In a randomized study, no difference between the 2- and 5-year survival was observed (San Antonio BCS, 2017). In patients with moderate to high risk, adjuvant endocrine treatment should be increased to 10 years (in patients with stage II and III disease); this increase is not recommended for stage I patients [1, 3, 12, 23, 37]. [f]By multigene signature tests: chemotherapy may be omitted for patients with Luminal B-like (HER2-negative) disease with a low Oncotype Dx® score, MammaPrint® low-risk status, low PAM50 ROR score, or EndoPredict® low-risk status [1, 3, 12, 25]. [g]The definition of menopause is important and can include natural menopause (no menses for 12 months before starting chemotherapy or hormone therapy) or menopause with ovarian ablation or suppression. Luteinizing hormone (LH), follicle-stimulating hormone (FSH), and serum estradiol (E2) levels should be at postmenopausal levels and should be measured before systemic treatment unless oophorectomy has been performed with hysterectomy in women aged 60 years or younger (Box 1.2). [h]Consider adjuvant bisphosphonate therapy in postmenopausal (natural or induced) patients receiving adjuvant therapy

Invasive Breast Cancer: Adjuvant Radiotherapy

Pathologic Stage I, II, III (Fig. 1.21)

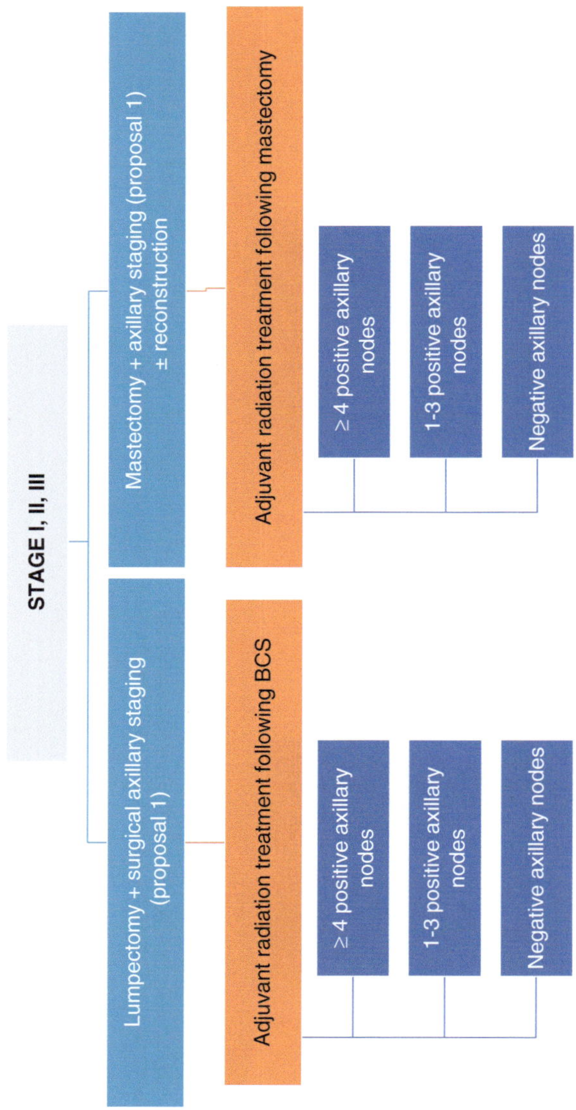

Fig. 1.21 Evaluation for adjuvant radiotherapy after breast-conserving surgery or mastectomy (see Figs. 1.22 and 1.23)

Invasive Breast Cancer: Adjuvant Radiotherapy After BCS

Pathologic Stage I, II, IIIA, IIIB, IIIC (Fig. 1.22)

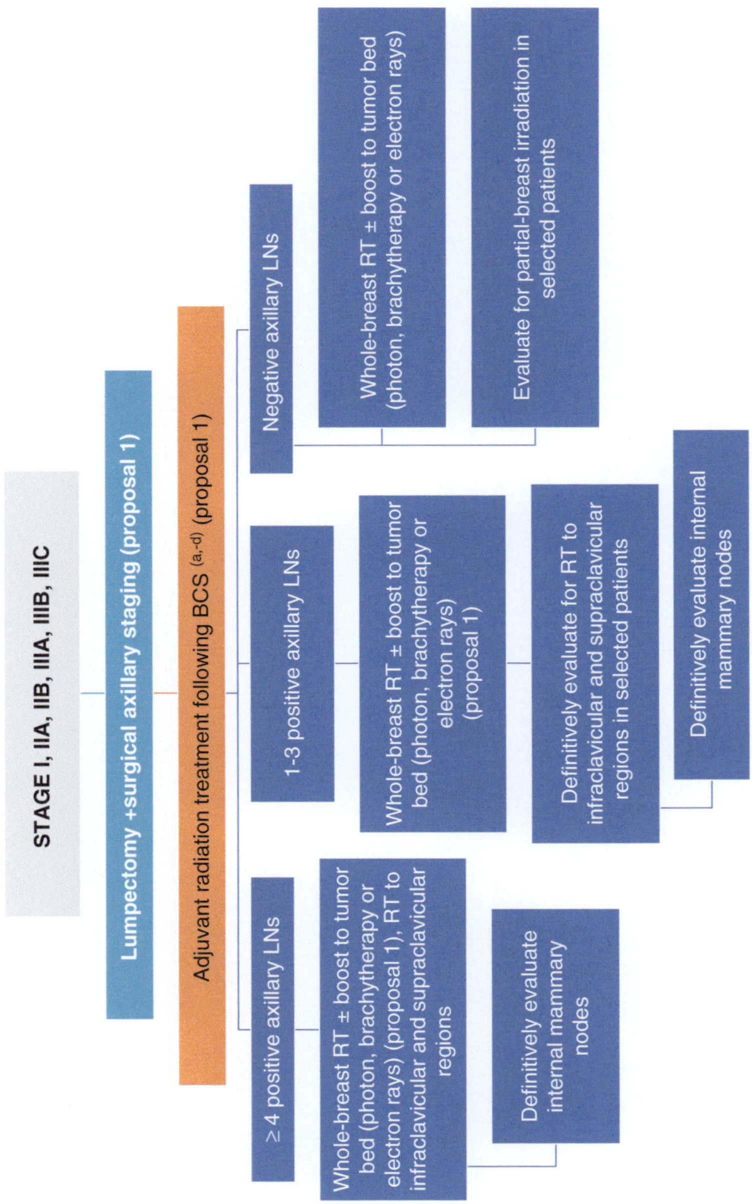

Fig. 1.22 Adjuvant radiotherapy after breast-conserving surgery [45–55]. [a]RT following chemotherapy if chemotherapy is indicated [3, 12, 21]. [b]Following BCS, hypofractionated whole-breast irradiation may be used in patients without prior chemotherapy or axil-

(continued)

Fig. 1.22 (continued)
lary lymph node involvement, in patients 50 years of age or older and in patients <50 years of age [3, 45, 49–52]. According to the results of a clinical trial that randomized low-risk early-stage breast cancer patients, accelerated partial-breast RT was not inferior to standard whole-breast RT [46]. Partial-breast RT can be performed in ASTRO/ESTRO "eligible" low-risk patients, although there are insufficient data in the literature (at St Gallen 2017 [3]: 67% yes, 24% no) [47]. Whole-breast RT should be performed in other patients. Boost therapy may not be performed in patients aged 60 years or older, patients with low-grade tumors having favorable tumor biology and/or patients who will receive adjuvant endocrine therapy [48, 54]. Regional node irradiation (RNI) prolongs disease-free survival in high-risk patients, but the risk of toxicity increases and may lead to complications during reconstruction surgery [45, 55]. At St. Gallen 2017, RNI was recommended in pN1 (1–3 positive lymph nodes) in the presence of unfavorable clinical features (40 years and younger, unfavorable tumor biology, low or negative estrogen-receptor status, high grade [grade 3], diffuse lymphovascular invasion, and positivity of more than 3 lymph nodes) [3]. According to the NCCN guidelines, axilla-negative patients should be evaluated for RNI for central/medial tumors or >2 cm tumors and the presence of other risk factors (young age or extensive lymphovascular invasion) [1]. [c]Bane et al. attempted to assess whether tumor grade, molecular subtype and hypoxia status could predict the response to hypofractionated versus standard RT following BCS for node-negative breast cancer in a randomized controlled trial (RCT) [49]. Review and tumor grade assessment using the Nottingham grading system was conducted. Tumors were classified by molecular subtype as Luminal A, Luminal B, HER2 enriched, basal like, or unclassified using a six-biomarker panel: ER, PgR, HER-2, Ki67, CK5/6, and EGFR. The median follow-up was 12 years. In the multivariable Cox model, molecular subtype was the only predictive factor for local recurrence; the 10-year cumulative incidence was 4.5% for Luminal A and basal-like, 7.9% for Luminal B, and 16.9% for HER2-enriched tumors ($p < 0.01$) [49]. [d]Studies are underway to evaluate the radiotherapy decision in patients with complete response after neoadjuvant chemotherapy. Patients must be evaluated individually. The decision for radiotherapy is determined according to the disease stage before neoadjuvant chemotherapy, but the disease stage may also be important for management after treatment. When the NSABP B-51 and Alliance A11202 studies are completed, they will provide information about the sufficiency of axillary staging and RT application after neoadjuvant chemotherapy

Invasive Breast Cancer: Adjuvant Radiotherapy After Mastectomy

Pathologic Stage I, II, IIIA, IIIB, IIIC (*Fig. 1.23*)

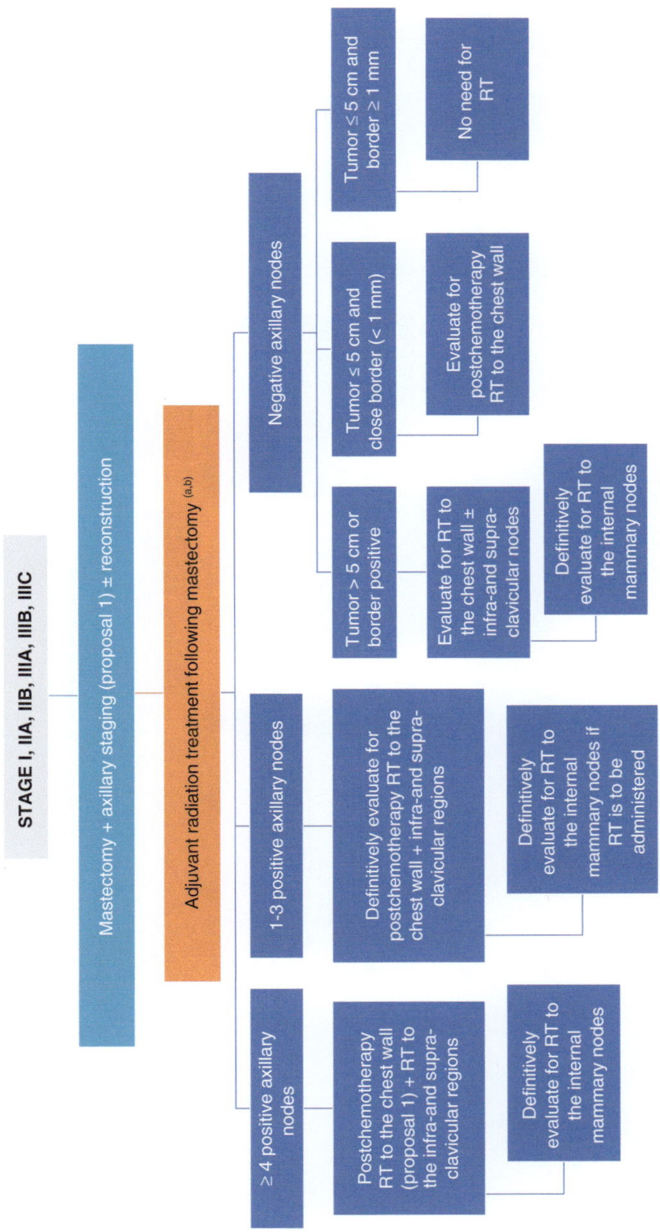

Fig. 1.23 Adjuvant radiotherapy after mastectomy [45–55]. [a]RT following chemotherapy if chemotherapy is indicated. [b]Post-mastectomy RT is standard for patients who meet the following criteria: T size ≥5 cm (node negative); 1–3 nodes with adverse pathology [this is not the sole criterion in patients of young age (<40)]; 4 or more positive axillary LNs; and positive sentinel lymph node biopsy with no axillary dissection [1, 3]. The tumor biology should be considered together with tumor size and stage in the decision for radiotherapy after mastectomy. For pN1 low-risk findings, RT should be performed after having considered the toxicity risks after mastectomy, and doing so is more important if the patient is to undergo breast reconstruction. Patients with pT1-pT2, pN1 [1–3] and favorable biological features should be evaluated for omitting radiotherapy after mastectomy

Invasive Breast Cancer: Neoadjuvant Systemic Therapy: Clinical Stage II–IIIA (T3N1M0) Disease

General Treatment Approach (*Fig. 1.24*)

Neoadjuvant chemotherapy should be administered to triple-negative and HER-2-positive patients.

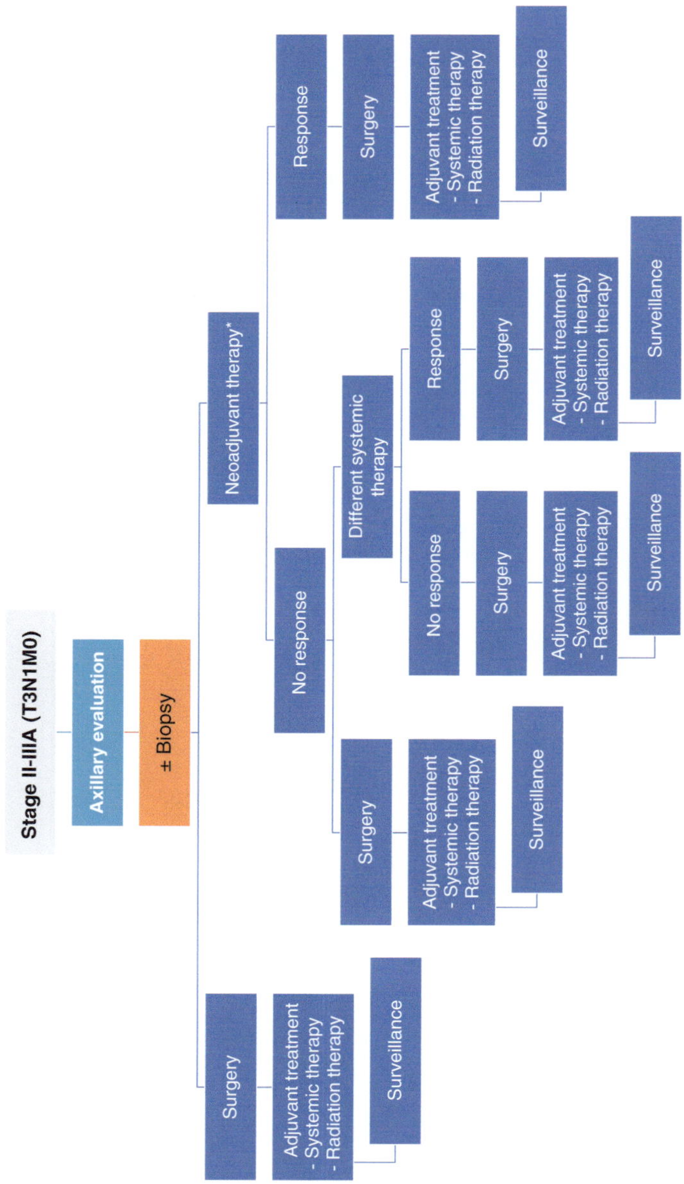

Fig. 1.24 Management of patients with neoadjuvant systemic therapy for stage II–IIIA (T3N1M0) breast cancer [3, 7, 8, 12, 30]. *T2 and T3 tumors (N0–N1) meeting BCS criteria except tumor diameter

Axillary Evaluation Before Neoadjuvant Therapy (*Fig. 1.25*)

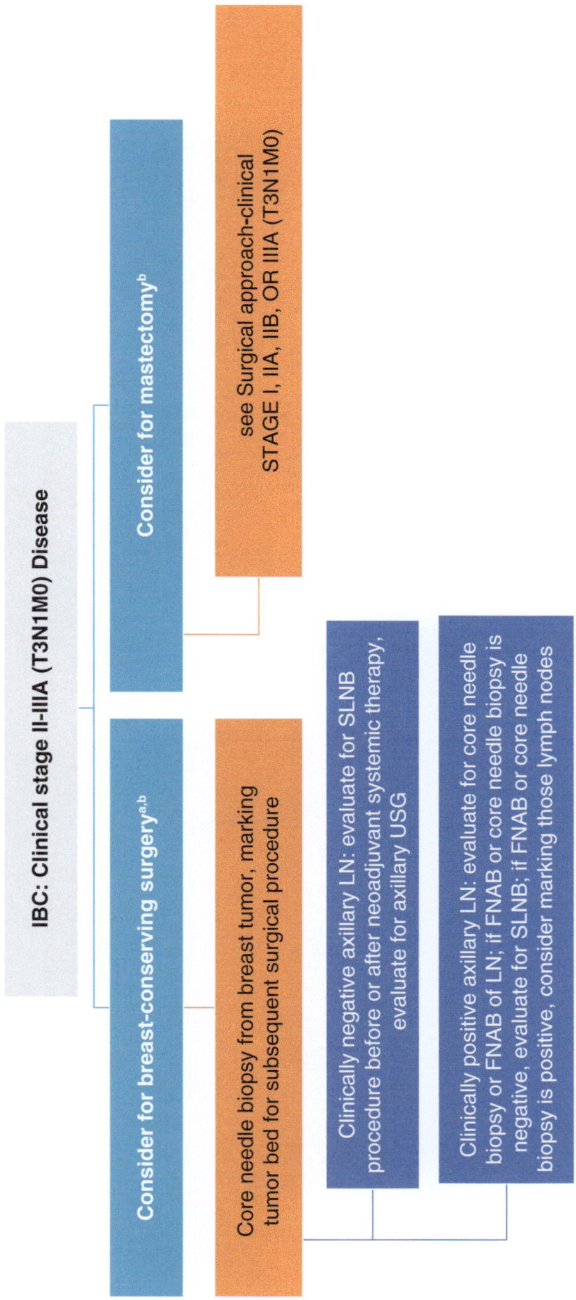

Fig. 1.25 Evaluation of axilla before neoadjuvant therapy [9–11, 13, 15–17]. [a]Clip placement is recommended on the tumor bed. In cases in which this cannot be performed, some surgeons recommend a topographic drawing of the mass before neoadjuvant treatment or a *tattoo* on the skin (Proposal 3). [b]MR imaging or PET-CT examinations may be performed as an adjunct to ultrasonography in axillary assessment

Axillary Management After Neoadjuvant Therapy (*Fig. 1.26*)

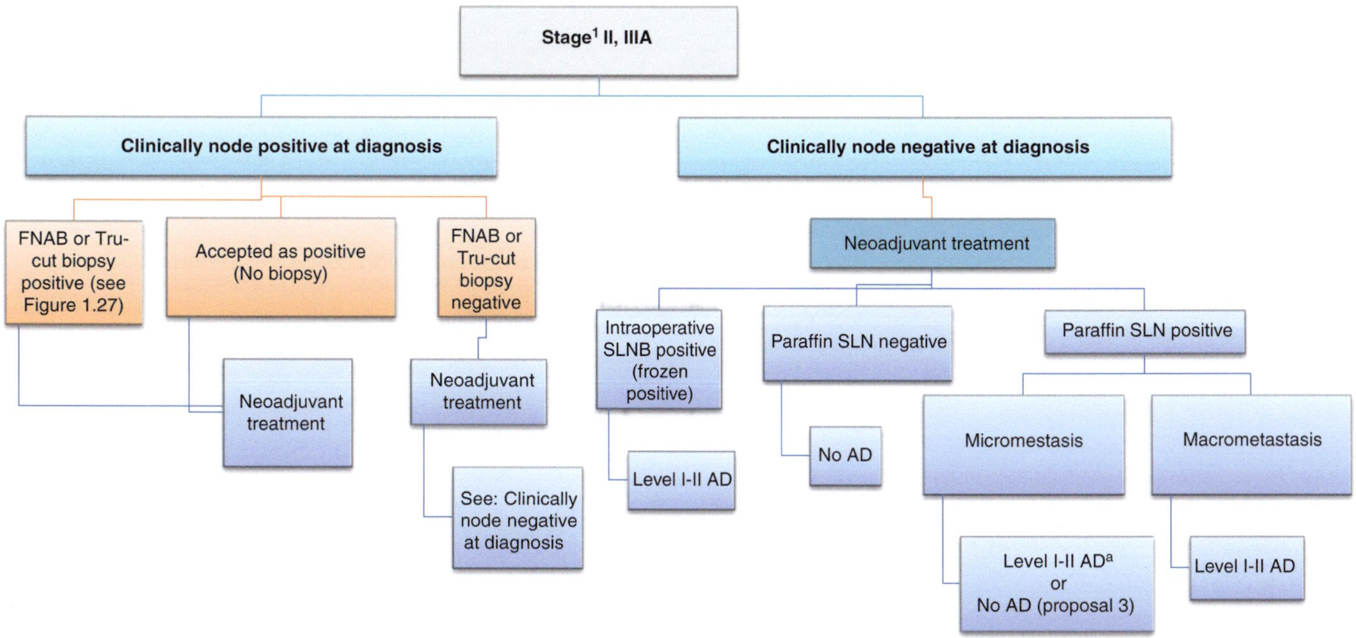

Fig. 1.26 Axillary management of clinical stage II or IIIA (T3, N1, M0) patients [9–11, 13, 15–17]. *FNAB* fine-needle aspiration biopsy, *SLN* sentinel lymph node, *SLNB* sentinel lymph node biopsy, *AD* axillary dissection. [1]STAGE IIA (T0, N1, M0; T1, N1, M0; T2, N0, M0); STAGE IIB (T2, N1, M0; T3, N0, M0); STAGE IIIA (T3, N1, M0). [a]Moo et al. examined the false-negative (FN) rate of frozen section (FS) after neoadjuvant chemotherapy (NAC) and the association between the size of SLN metastasis and residual axillary disease at axillary dissection (ALND) [18]. Overall, 17% patients with isolated tumour cells and 50% with micrometastases had additional nodal metastases at ALND. Moo et al. concluded that low-volume disease in the SLN after NAC is not an indicator of a low risk of additional positive axillary nodes. These tumor cells are potentially drug resistant and are an indication for ALND, even when they are not detected on an intraoperative frozen section

Axillary Management After Neoadjuvant Therapy (Fig. 1.27)

Box 1.3 Axillary management after neoadjuvant systemic treatment

- SLN Negative (At Least 3 SLNs should be examined after neoadjuvant treatment, in patients who are clinically node positive before neoadjuvant treatment): DO NOT perform axillary dissection
- SLN Paraffin Positive:
- Only micrometastases:
- Level I–II axillary dissection is Recommended
- Macrometastasis:
- Level I–II axillary dissection is Performed
- SLN Frozen Positive:
- Level I–II axillary dissection is Performed
- SLN Undetermined: Level I–II axillary dissection is Performed

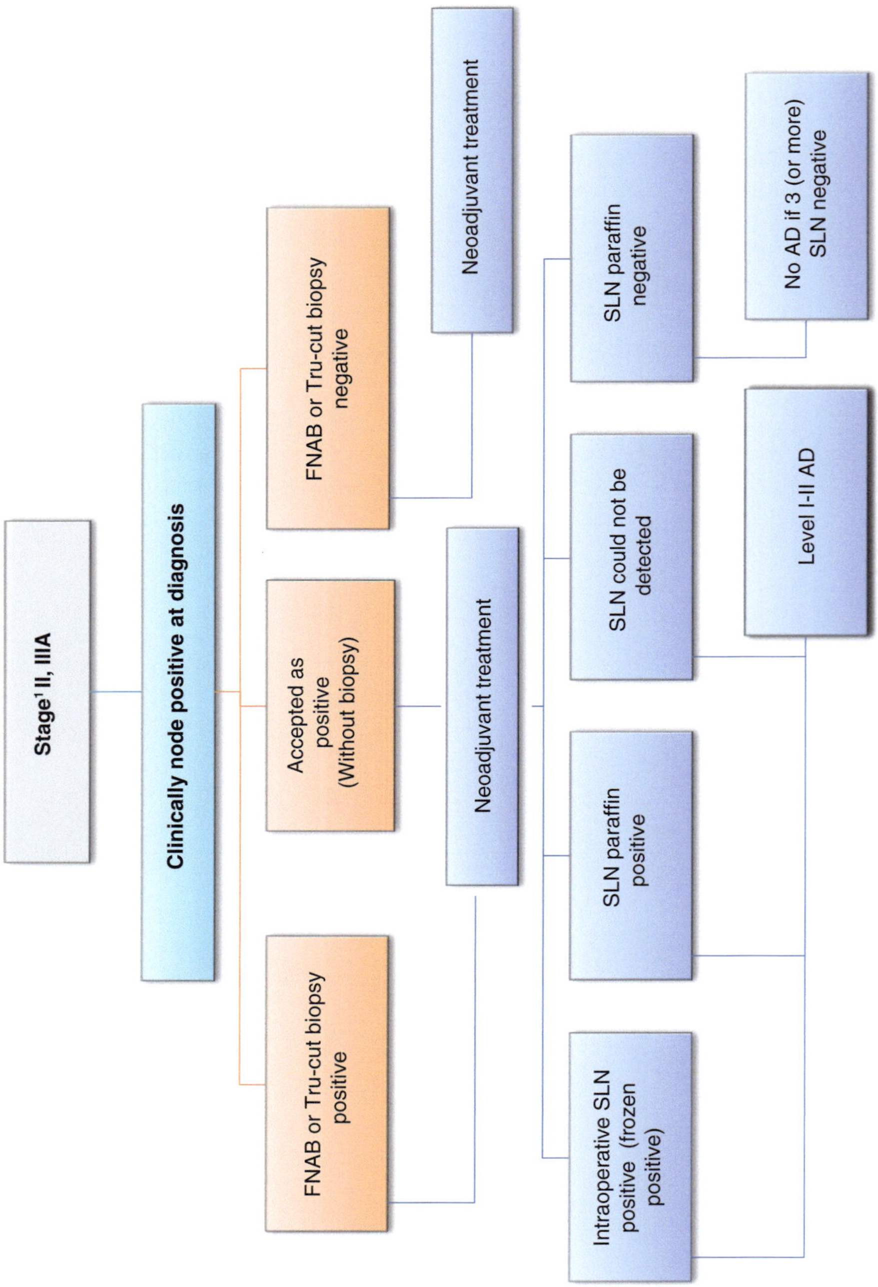
Stage[1] II, IIIA
Clinically node positive at diagnosis
FNAB or Tru-cut biopsy negative
Accepted as positive (Without biopsy)
FNAB or Tru-cut biopsy positive
Neoadjuvant treatment
Neoadjuvant treatment
SLN paraffin negative
SLN could not be detected
SLN paraffin positive
Intraoperative SLN positive (frozen positive)
No AD if 3 (or more) SLN negative
Level I-II AD

Fig. 1.27 Axillary management of node-positive patients with clinical stage II or IIIA (T3, N1, M0) [3, 9–11, 13, 15–17]. *FNAB* fine-needle aspiration biopsy, *SLN* sentinel lymph node, *SLNB* sentinel lymph node biopsy, *AD* axillary dissection. [1]STAGE IIA (N1) STAGE IIB (N1); STAGE IIIA (T3, N1, M0). [a]In SLNB, a combination of blue dye and lymphoscintigraphy should be preferred, and clinically palpable suspicious lymph node(s) should be removed [11, 13, 16, 17]. In prospective trials comparing SLNB and axillary dissection after neoadjuvant chemotherapy in node-positive patients, the false-negative rate of SLNB was greater than 10%. However, some studies suggest that SLNB may be performed. [b]There was no consensus regarding axillary evaluation after neoadjuvant therapy at the St Gallen 2017 meeting [3]. Axillary dissection may not be considered despite micrometastasis in SLNB in patients who are node positive before neoadjuvant treatment and considered clinically complete responders in post-treatment evaluation (physical examination, USG, MR imaging, optional PET-CT, intraoperative palpation) (should be determined individually for each patient in the multidisciplinary council) (Proposal 3)

Response Evaluation and Surgical Treatment (Fig. 1.28)

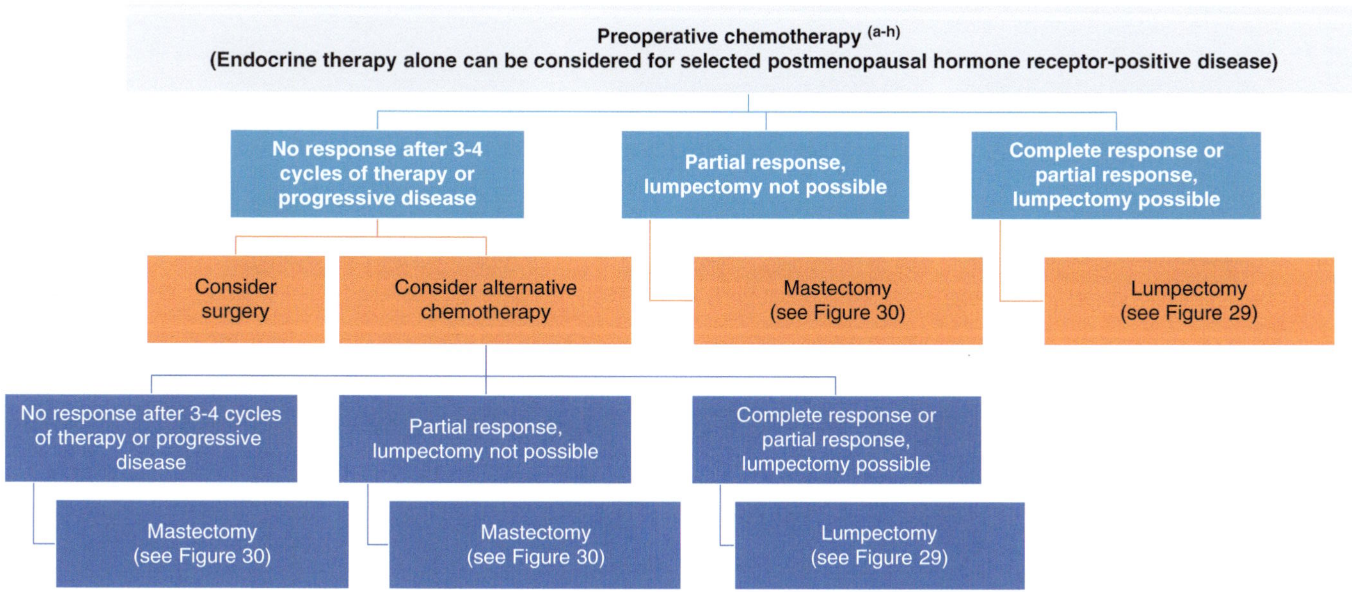

Fig. 1.28 Management of patients receiving neoadjuvant therapy for breast-conserving surgery (stage II or IIIA with N1). [a]HER2-targeted therapy: According to the version 1.0 2018 NCCN Guidelines, patients with HER2- positive disease should receive "pertuzumab + trastuzumab + chemotherapy" in the neoadjuvant setting [1, 26]. The St Gallen 2017 Consensus Panel supported dual anti-HER2 therapy as an acceptable regimen with neoadjuvant taxane, trastuzumab and pertuzumab in such patients and considered anthracycline-taxane and anti-HER2 treatments as the best options [3]. "Trastuzumab + pertuzumab" was recommended as anti-HER2 treatment in neoadjuvant therapy for stage II and III patients in the St Gallen 2017 consensus meeting [1, 3, 26]. In these patients, while the NCCN and ASCO guidelines considered double inhibition in postoperative adjuvant therapy feasible, the St Gallen consensus has indicated that there is no sufficient evidence yet. [b]Stage II–III triple-negative disease: If provided to patients with triple-negative tumors, the preferred regimen should include an anthracycline and a taxane [1, 3]. [c]Neoadjuvant cytotoxic therapy should be discussed as an option and provided frequently to patients with "Luminal A-like" tumors, only if conservative surgery would not otherwise be feasible [3]. [d]Neo-

adjuvant endocrine therapy without cytotoxics represents a reasonable option for some selected postmenopausal patients with endocrine-responsive disease. The duration of treatment must be at least 4 months, and treatment can be provided until a maximal response is reached [3]. [e]In triple-negative breast cancer (TNBC), the regimen should contain anthracyclines and taxanes. Although the available data are insufficient, a platinum-based regimen may be considered only in patients with a known BRCA mutation. Anthracyclines followed by taxanes is an acceptable regimen for BRCA-mutant TNBC. Dose-dense chemotherapy requiring growth factor support may also be an option [3]. [f]Sentinel lymph node biopsy (SLNB) is appropriate for patients who are clinically node positive on admission, respond well to chemotherapy and become clinically axillary negative. [g]Evaluation with MR imaging is recommended for patients who will undergo BCS after neoadjuvant therapy. After neoadjuvant chemotherapy, complete excision of the entire primary tumor area is not necessary (if there is shrinkage in the tumor). Clinical examination and radiological imaging modalities (USG, MMG, MR imaging) are used to evaluate the tissue to be excised (shrinking or patching). However, if the tumor response is patchy, the original tumor area should be removed with clean surgical margins [1, 3, 56]. If diffuse live tumor cells are observed in the excised lumpectomy specimen after neoadjuvant chemotherapy, re-excision should be performed even if there is no surgical margin involvement. Nipple-conserving surgery can be performed after neoadjuvant chemotherapy unless there is retroareolar tumor involvement [57]. [h]Consider adjuvant bisphosphonate therapy in postmenopausal (natural or induced) patients receiving adjuvant therapy

Adjuvant Therapy After Lumpectomy (Fig. 1.29)

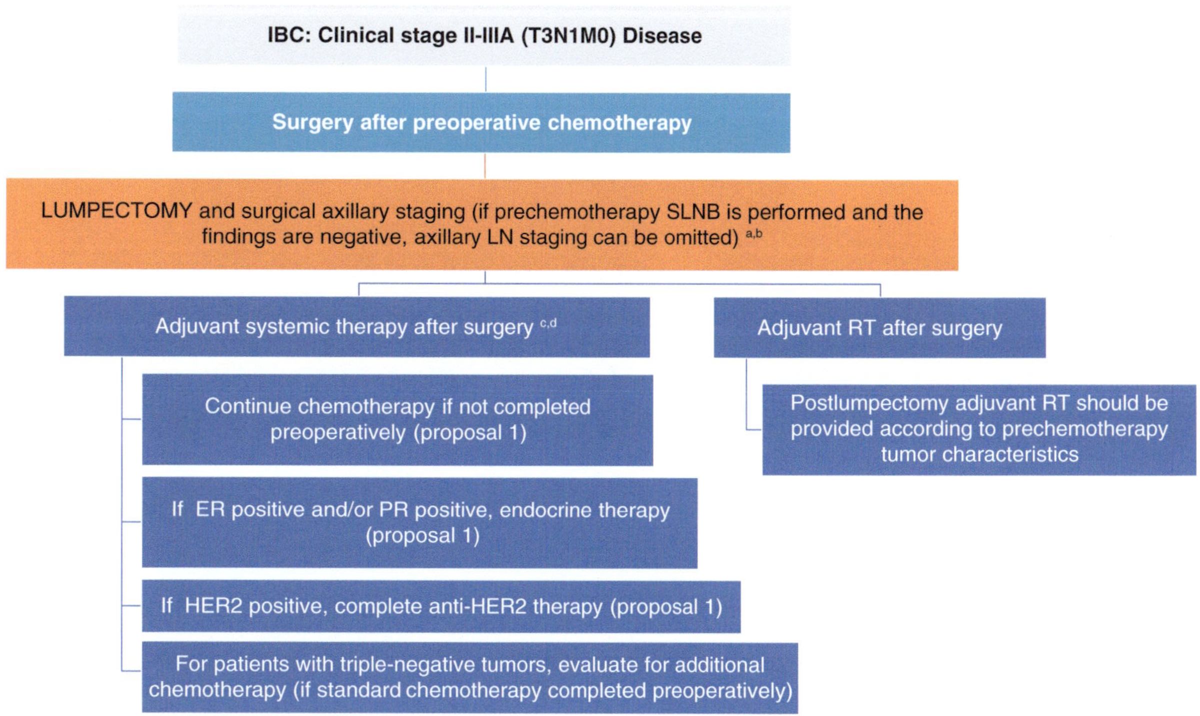

Fig. 1.29 Locoregional and adjuvant systemic treatment after neoadjuvant therapy: Lumpectomy. [a]In a patient who is clinically node positive at presentation and is downstaged after chemotherapy, sentinel lymph node (SLN) biopsy is appropriate. If SLN is positive, axillary lymph node dissection must be performed. After downstaging, resection of the entire area of the original primary tumor is not necessary (if there is shrinkage in the tumor). MR imaging is recommended in patients who will undergo BCS after neoadjuvant therapy. Clinical examination and radiological imaging modalities (USG, MMG, MR imaging) are used to evaluate the tissue to be excised (shrinking or patching). However, if the tumor response is patchy,

the original tumor area should be removed with clean surgical margins [1, 3, 56]. If diffuse live tumor cells are observed in the excised lumpectomy specimen after neoadjuvant chemotherapy, re-excision should be performed, even if there is no surgical margin involvement. [b]Consider adjuvant bisphosphonate therapy in postmenopausal (natural or induced) patients receiving adjuvant therapy [58–60]. [c]Additional adjuvant systemic chemotherapy may be given to patients who are considered to have an inadequate response according to postoperative pathology (adjuvant chemotherapy may be given if the pathological response to neoadjuvant taxane-anthracycline is inadequate in triple-negative tumors). In a randomized clinical trial, adjuvant capecitabine has been shown to be beneficial in triple-negative patients [43]. However, there is no other study confirming this suggestion. [d]HER2-targeted therapy: When indicated, trastuzumab can be administered with RT and together with endocrine therapy. According to the version 1.0 2018 NCCN and ASCO Guidelines, "pertuzumab + trastuzumab" should be used as anti-HER2 treatment in neoadjuvant treatment, and pertuzumab can be continued in adjuvant treatment in ≥T2 and ≥N1 HER2-positive patients [1, 26]. In the St. Gallen 2017 guidelines, since there is no evidence, only 6% of panelists accepted (69% voted 'no') the use of both trastuzumab and pertuzumab as postoperative adjuvant treatment in patients who had received neoadjuvant trastuzumab-pertuzumab treatment [3]. However, pertuzumab use in adjuvant therapy can be considered in node-positive, HR-negative patients according to APHINITY study results [24]. According to a randomized controlled trial, 1-year neratinib use after 1-year administration of trastuzumab reduced the recurrence rate [36]. This benefit was obvious especially in ER-positive, HER-2-positive disease. However, diarrhea is an important side effect [1, 3, 26]. No decision was made in the St Gallen consensus about neratinib use

Adjuvant Therapy After Mastectomy (Fig. 1.30)

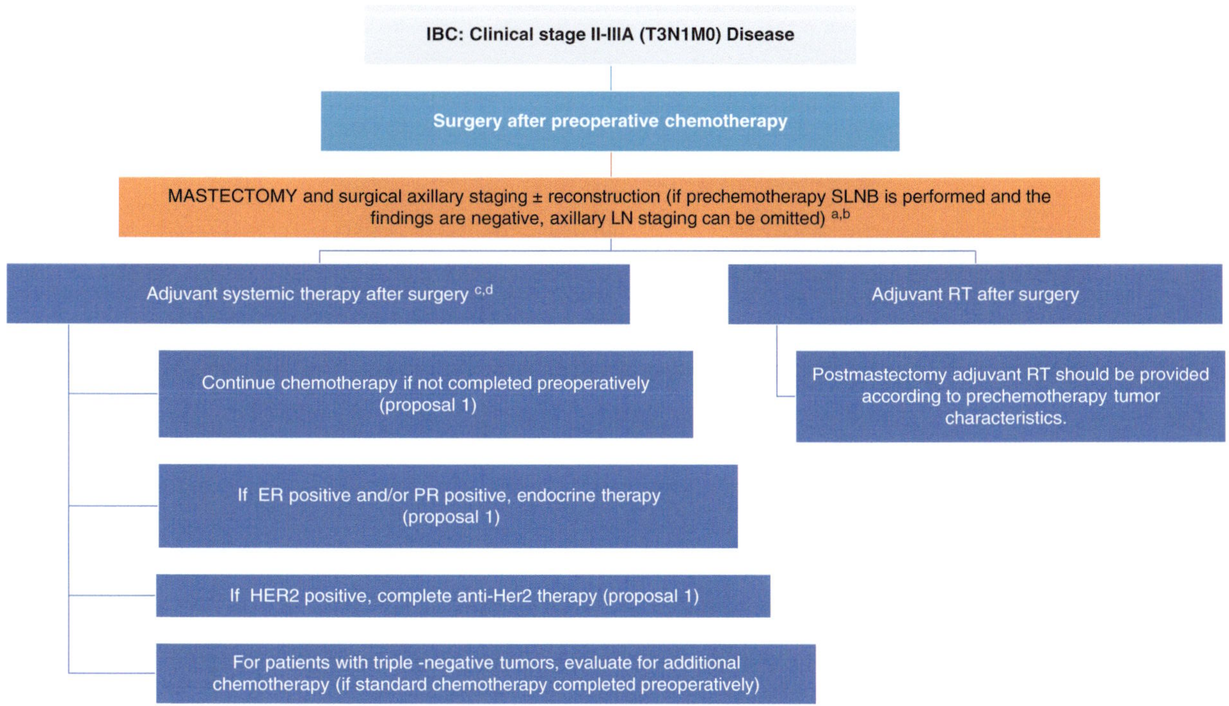

Fig. 1.30 Locoregional and adjuvant systemic treatment after neoadjuvant therapy: Mastectomy. [a]In a patient who is clinically node positive at presentation and is downstaged after chemotherapy, sentinel lymph node (SLN) biopsy is appropriate. If SLN is positive, axillar lymph node dissection must be performed [1, 3]. [b]Consider adjuvant bisphosphonate therapy in postmenopausal (natural or induced) patients receiving adjuvant therapy [58–60]. [c]Additional adjuvant systemic chemotherapy is controversial in triple-negative tumor patients, who are considered to have an inadequate response in postoperative pathology, and 31% of the panelists did not recommend additional treatment in the 2017 St. Gallen consensus meeting [3]. Furthermore, 49% of

the panelists recommended capecitabine, 7% recommended platinum, 9% recommended BRCA-positive platinum, and 4% recommended metronomic treatment [3, 43]. Additional adjuvant systemic chemotherapy may be given to patients who are considered to have an inadequate response according to postoperative pathology (adjuvant chemotherapy may be given if the pathological response to neoadjuvant taxane-anthracycline is inadequate in triple-negative tumors). In a randomized clinical trial, adjuvant capecitabine was shown to be beneficial in triple-negative patients [43]. However, there is no other study confirming this suggestion. [d]HER2-targeted therapy: When indicated, trastuzumab can be administered with RT and together with endocrine therapy. "Pertuzumab + trastuzumab" should be used as anti-HER2 treatment in neoadjuvant treatment, and pertuzumab can be continued in adjuvant treatment in ≥T2 and ≥N1 HER2-positive patients [1, 26]. In the St. Gallen 2017 guidelines, since there is no evidence, only 6% of panelists accepted (69% voted 'no') the use of both trastuzumab and pertuzumab as postoperative adjuvant treatment in patients who had received neoadjuvant trastuzumab-pertuzumab treatment [3]. However, pertuzumab use in adjuvant therapy can be considered in node-positive, HR-negative patients according to APHINITY study results [24]. According to the results of a randomized study, 1-year administration of trastuzumab after neratinib use for 1 year reduced the recurrence rate [36]. This benefit was obvious, especially in ER-positive, HER-2-positive disease. However, diarrhea is an important side effect [1, 3, 26]. Despite the recommendations of NCCN and ASCO, no decision was made in the St Gallen consensus about neratinib use

Invasive Breast Cancer: Neoadjuvant Systemic Therapy: Clinical Stage IIIA (N2M0) IIIB and IIIC (Non-Inflammatory)

General Treatment Approach (Fig. 1.31)

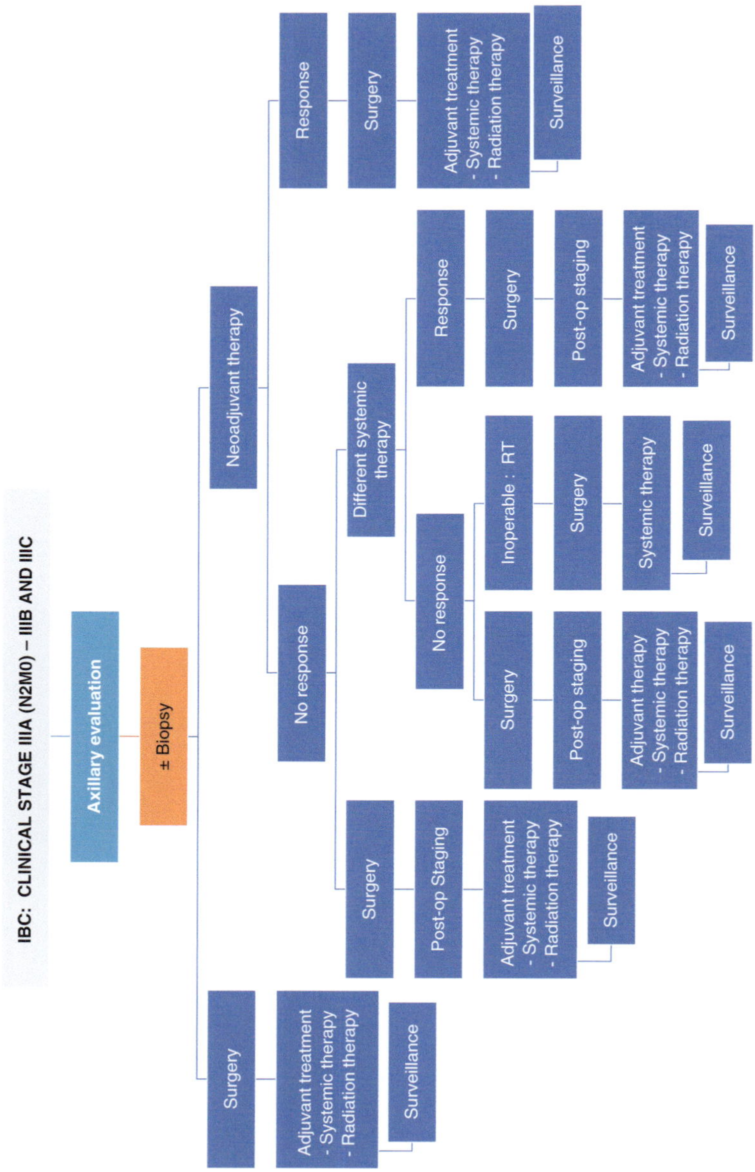

Fig. 1.31 Locoregional and adjuvant systemic treatment for clinical stage IIIA (N2M0)—IIIB and IIIC disease

Locoregional Treatment After Neoadjuvant Chemotherapy (Fig. 1.32)

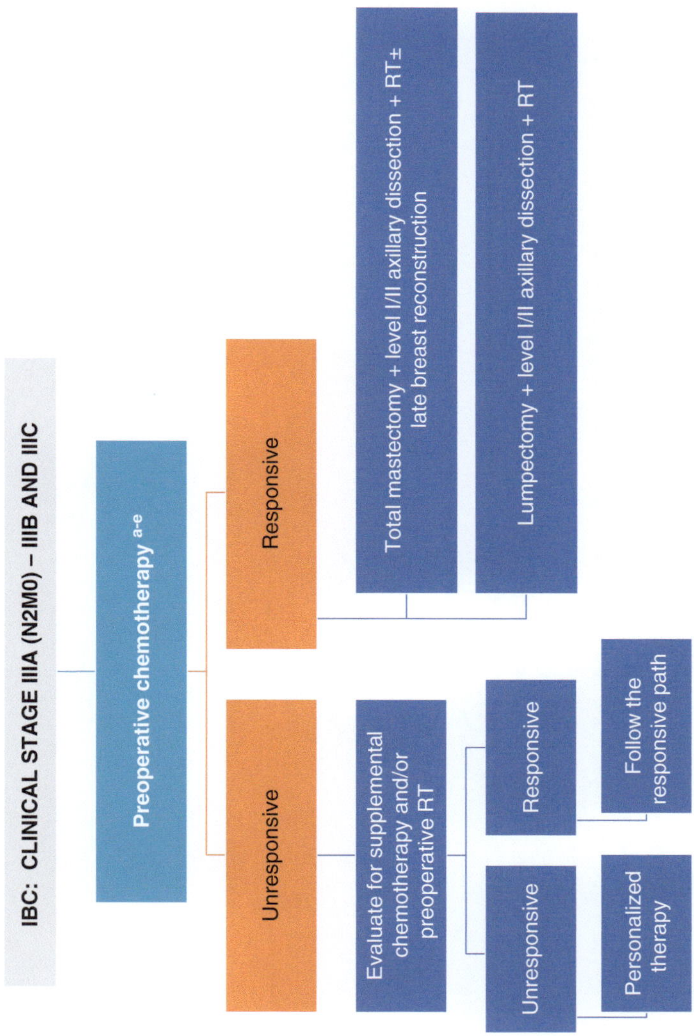

Fig. 1.32 Surgical approach after neoadjuvant systemic treatment for patients with clinical stage IIIA (N2M0)—IIIB and IIIC breast cancer. [a]HER2-targeted therapy: Patients with HER2- positive disease should receive anti-HER2 treatment plus chemotherapy in the neoadjuvant setting. "Pertuzumab + trastuzumab" should be used as anti-HER2 treatment in neoadjuvant treatment, and pertuzumab can be continued in adjuvant treatment in ≥T2

(continued)

Fig. 1.32 (continued)
and ≥N1 HER2-positive patients [1, 26]. In the St. Gallen 2017 guidelines, since there is no evidence, only 6% of the panelists accepted (69% voted 'no') the use of both trastuzumab and pertuzumab as postoperative adjuvant treatment in patients who had received neoadjuvant trastuzumab-pertuzumab treatment [3]. However, pertuzumab use in adjuvant therapy can be considered in node-positive, HR-negative patients with locally advanced tumors according to APHINITY study results [24]. According to the results of a randomized study, 1-year administration of trastuzumab after neratinib use for 1 year reduced the recurrence rate [36]. This benefit was obvious especially in ER-positive, HER-2-positive disease. However, diarrhea is an important side effect [1, 3, 26]. The rate of pCR is lower when neoadjuvant ado-trastuzumab emtansine (TDM-1) is given with pertuzumab than for chemotherapy-trastuzumab-pertuzumab (TCHP) treatment [3]. Adaptive therapy with the dual tyrosine kinase inhibitor neratinib increases the rate of pCR compared to trastuzumab-based therapy, but this needs to be confirmed [36]. [b]For triple-negative breast cancer (TNBC), the regimen should contain anthracyclines and taxanes. The addition of carboplatin to the treatment increases the rate of pathologic complete response (pCR), which prolongs disease-free survival [38]. Although the available data are insufficient, a platinum-based regimen may be considered only in patients with a known BRCA mutation. Anthracyclines followed by taxanes is an acceptable regimen for BRCA-mutant TNBC. In an adaptive study, the addition of veliparib and carboplatin to the treatment increased the rate of pCR [61]. Dose-dense chemotherapy requiring growth factor support may also be an option [1]. [c]Data regarding the use of nab-paclitaxel instead of paclitaxel in neoadjuvant chemotherapy, or metronomic therapy are inconsistent [62, 63]. [d]Neoadjuvant endocrine therapy shows high response rates in patients with low genomic scores [3]. The addition of cyclin-dependent kinase (CDK) 4/6 inhibitors to aromatase inhibitors significantly decreases tumor cell proliferation rates [64, 65]. [e]Consider adjuvant bisphosphonate therapy in postmenopausal (natural or induced) patients receiving adjuvant therapy [58–60]

Adjuvant Therapy After Surgical Treatment (Fig. 1.33)

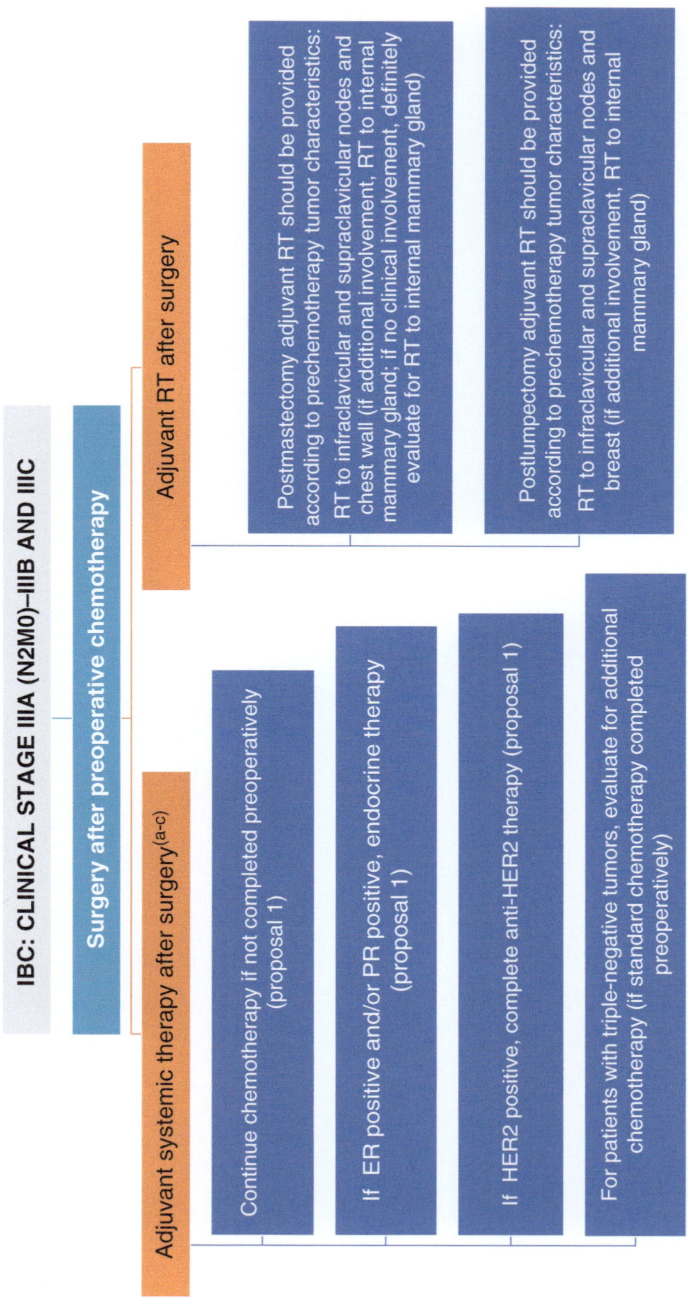

Fig. 1.33 Adjuvant treatment approach after neoadjuvant systemic treatment and surgery for patients with clinical stage IIIA (N2M0)—IIIB and IIIC breast cancer. [a]HER2-targeted therapy: When indicated, anti-HER2 therapy can be administered with RT and together with endocrine therapy. "Pertuzumab + trastuzumab" should be used as anti-HER2 treatment in neoadjuvant treatment, and pertuzumab can be continued in adjuvant treatment in ≥T2 and ≥N1 HER2-positive patients [1, 26]. In the St. Gallen 2017 guidelines, since there is no evidence, only 6% of the panelists accepted (69% voted 'no') the use of both trastuzumab and pertuzumab as postoperative adjuvant treatment in patients who had

(continued)

Fig. 1.33 (continued)
received neoadjuvant trastuzumab-pertuzumab treatment [3]. However, pertuzumab use in adjuvant therapy can be considered in node-positive, HR-negative patients with locally advanced tumors according to APHINITY study results [24]. According to the results of a randomized study, 1-year administration of neratinib after 1 year trastuzumab reduced the recurrence rate [36]. This benefit was obvious especially in ER-positive, HER-2-positive disease. However, diarrhea is an important side effect [1, 3, 26]. [b]For triple-negative breast cancer (TNBC), the regimen should contain anthracyclines and taxanes. Although available data are insufficient, the platinum-based regimen can be considered only when a BRCA mutation is determined. Anthracyclines followed by taxanes is an acceptable regimen for BRCA-mutant TNBC [1, 3, 12]. If an inadequate response to chemotherapy is considered at postoperative pathological examination, additional adjuvant chemotherapy can be considered (e.g., treatment including capecitabine or platinum in TNBC) despite completion of preoperative chemotherapy [43]. Clinical trials of post-neoadjuvant therapy are ongoing, namely, CDK 4/6 inhibitors, poly ADP ribose polymerase (PARP) inhibitors, platinums, ado-trastuzumab emtansine, and immunotherapeutic agents. The addition of cyclin-dependent kinase (CDK) 4/6 inhibitors to aromatase inhibitors significantly decreases tumor cell proliferation rates [3, 64, 65]. [c]Consider adjuvant bisphosphonate therapy in postmenopausal (natural or induced) patients receiving adjuvant therapy [58–60]

Invasive Breast Cancer: Post-Therapy Follow-Up (Table 1.7)

Table 1.7 Post-therapy follow-up of patients[a] [1, 3, 12]

–History and physical examination every 3–6 months in the first 3 years, every 6 months in the following 2 years, and then at 12-month intervals.
–Annual mammography (mammography can be performed in the sixth month in those undergoing RT after BCS).
–Women receiving tamoxifen: if the uterus is present, annual gynecological examination.
–Women receiving an aromatase inhibitor or developing treatment-induced ovarian failure should be monitored for bone health by bone mineral density measurements at baseline and periodically thereafter.
–Evaluate and encourage compliance with adjuvant endocrine therapy.
–Evidence suggests that maintaining an active lifestyle and reaching and maintaining an ideal body mass index (BMI 20–25) lead to optimal breast cancer outcomes. To reduce the risk of recurrence, an exercise regimen can be part of standard care. Weight loss and avoiding weight gain should be recommended.
–Pregnancy in breast cancer survivors: timing has no impact on prognosis. Considering pregnancy two years following completion of therapy is better to allow for adequate ovarian recovery and to bypass the period of high risk of recurrence. Pregnancy is safe irrespective of the ER status of the tumor. However, endocrine therapy should be discontinued when pregnancy is planned. In this case, the risk of disease recurrence should be evaluated together with the patient.

[a]Depending on the patient's local and systemic relapse risk, the follow-up intervals and screening tests may vary.

Invasive Breast Cancer: Inflammatory Breast Cancer: STAGE T4D, N0–N3, M0

General Treatment Approach (*Fig. 1.34*)

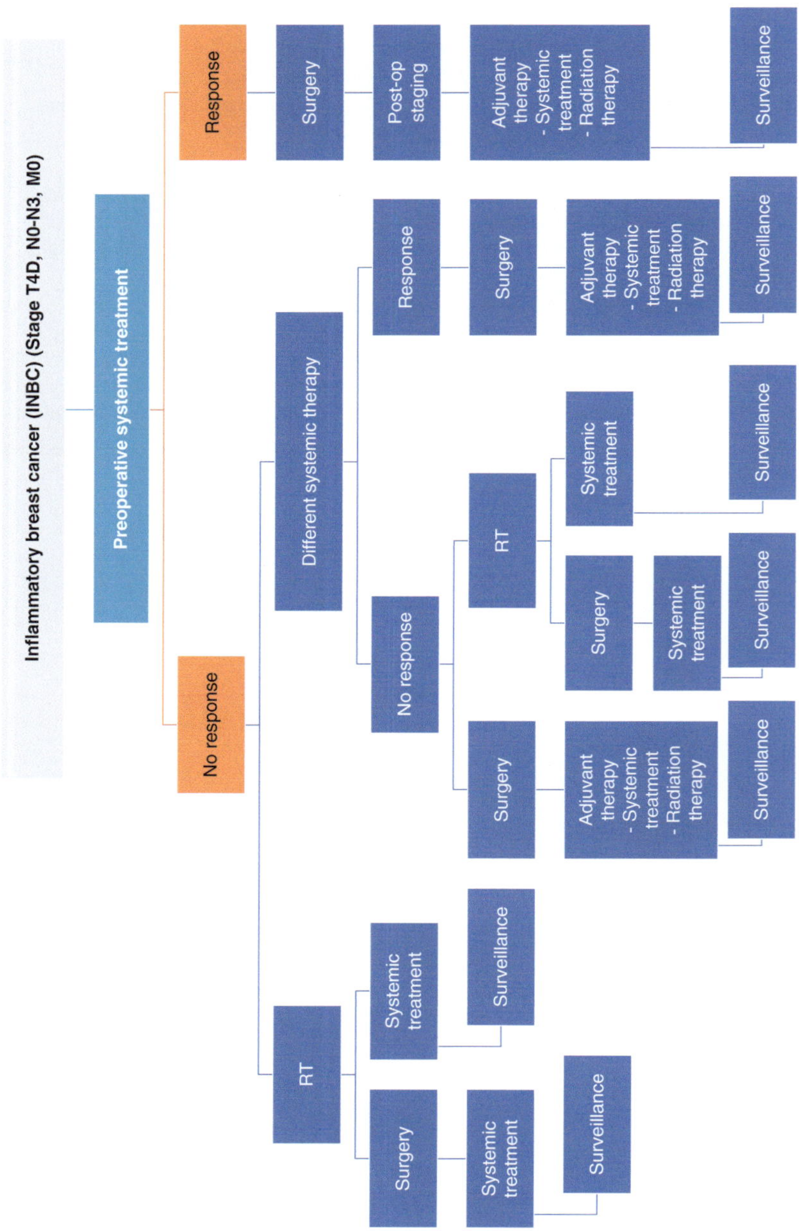

Fig. 1.34 Management of inflammatory breast cancer [3, 66]

Locoregional and Systemic Therapy (Fig. 1.35)

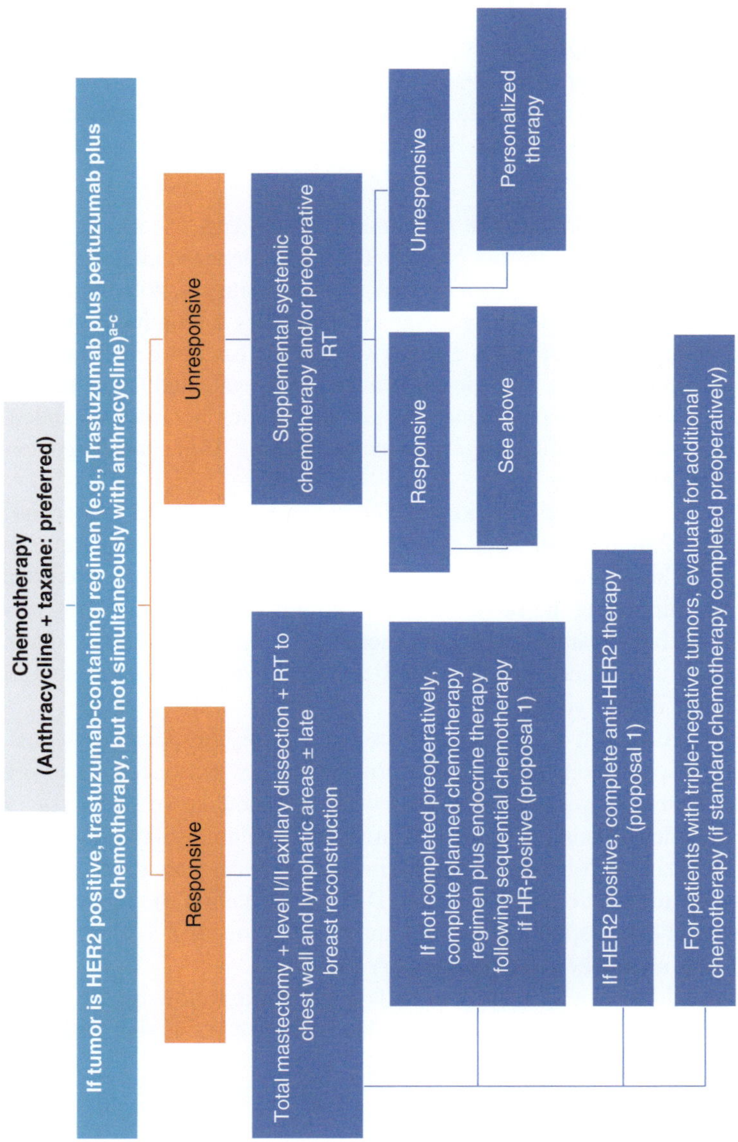

Fig. 1.35 Locoregional and systemic treatment of inflammatory breast cancer [3, 66]. [a]HER2-targeted therapy: Trastuzumab + chemotherapy should be administered to HER2-positive patients in neoadjuvant therapy [1, 3]. Pertuzumab can be added and can also be administered in addition to adjuvant treatment [26]. [b]If an inadequate response to chemotherapy is considered on postoperative pathological examination, additional adjuvant chemotherapy can be given (e.g., treatment including capecitabine or platinum in TNBC), despite the completion of preoperative chemotherapy. [c]Consider adjuvant bisphosphonate therapy in postmenopausal (natural or induced) patients receiving adjuvant therapy [58–60]

Invasive Breast Cancer: Adjuvant Bisphosphonates

Pathological Stage II, IIIA, IIIB, IIIC, Inflammatory

Bisphosphonates are recommended in adjuvant treatment for postmenopausal patients [58–60]. The potential benefits and risks should be discussed with patients before administration. Bisphosphonates are especially recommended in breast cancer patients with high recurrence risk. Patients should be evaluated for jaw osteonecrosis and renal insufficiency. Complete treatment for breast cancer should also be given. There are no data on its use in local recurrence after complete local resection.

1. Zoledronic acid and clodronate are recommended in breast cancer. However, clodronate has not been specifically investigated with aromatase inhibitors.
2. In patients who will receive adjuvant bisphosphonate treatment, zoledronic acid 4 mg is recommended intravenously for 15–30 min every 6 months for 5 years or oral clodronate 1600 mg/day for 3 years. Clodronate has not been evaluated for more than 3 years, and zoledronic acid has not been evaluated for more than 5 years in adjuvant treatment; hence longer use is not yet recommended. Treatment can be started after surgery or chemotherapy. Denosumab reduces bone health problems.
3. The definition of menopause is important. It can be seen as natural menopause (no menses for 12 months before starting chemotherapy or hormonotherapy) or as menopause with ovarian ablation or suppression. The luteinizing hormone (LH), follicle-stimulating hormone (FSH), and serum estradiol (E2) levels should be at postmenopausal levels and should be measured before systemic treatment unless oophorectomy has been performed with hysterectomy in women aged 60 years or younger.
4. Dental examination is important before treatment with bisphosphonates begins. Patients using bisphosphonate should be warned about jaw osteonecrosis before tooth extraction or invasive dental procedures. Patients should give the necessary information to their dentists. Serum calcium and creatinine levels should be checked before starting zoledronic acid and monitored during treatment. If there is no contraindication, calcium and vitamin D supplementation should be given. Calcium and oral bisphosphonates should not be taken together. For maximum absorption, there should be a minimum interval of 2 h.
5. Side effects should be closely monitored. It is important to follow-up patients in terms of jaw osteonecrosis, hypocalcemia, inflammatory eye findings, and renal dysfunction.

Invasive Breast Cancer: Recurrent or Stage IV Disease

Diagnostic Procedures

History and physical examination

Biopsy should be taken from the site of first disease recurrence. If not known, originally negative or not excessively expressed, tumor ER, PR, and HER2 status should be determined.

Blood tests, including tumor markers (CEA, Ca 153)

Thoracic diagnostic CT

Abdominopelvic diagnostic CT or MRI

If suspicious CNS symptoms, brain MRI

Bone scintigraphy or fluoride PET/CT

Radiologic examinations of symptomatic bones and of long and weight-bearing bones appearing abnormal in bone scintigraphy

FDG PET/CT scan

Genetic counseling if at high risk for hereditary breast cancer

Invasive Breast Cancer: Recurrent Disease: Local Recurrence Only

General Treatment Approach (*Fig. 1.36*)

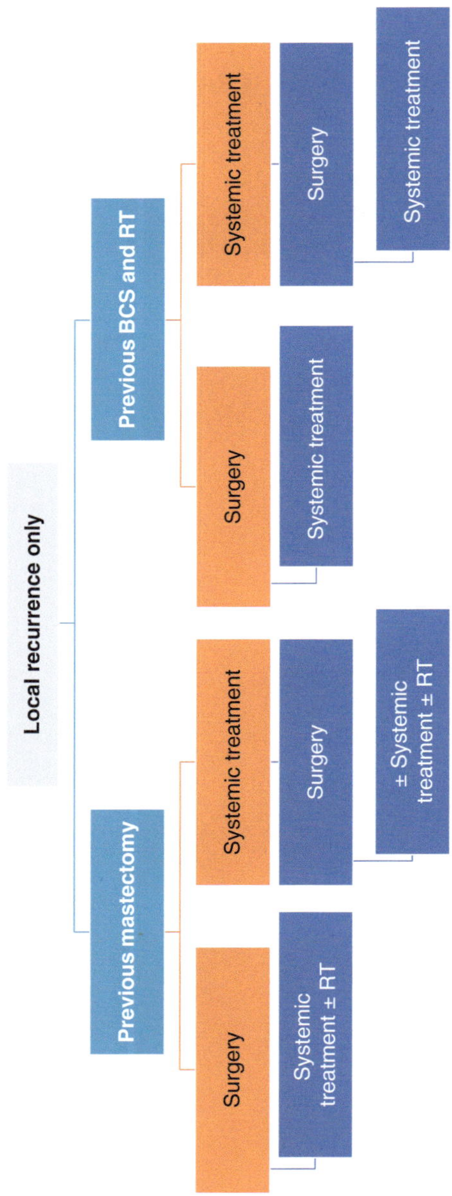

Fig. 1.36 Management of breast cancer patients with "local recurrence only"

Locoregional Treatment *(Fig. 1.37)*

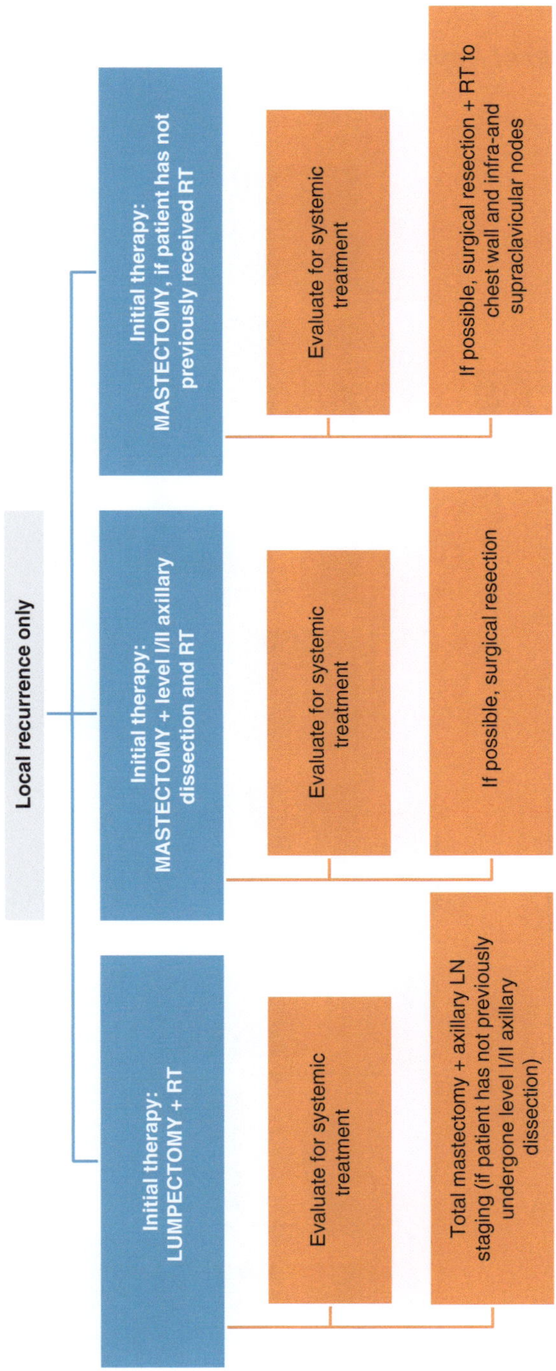

Fig. 1.37 Locoregional management of breast cancer patients with "local recurrence only"

Invasive Breast Cancer: Recurrent Disease: Locoregional Recurrence Only

General Treatment Approach (Fig. 1.38)

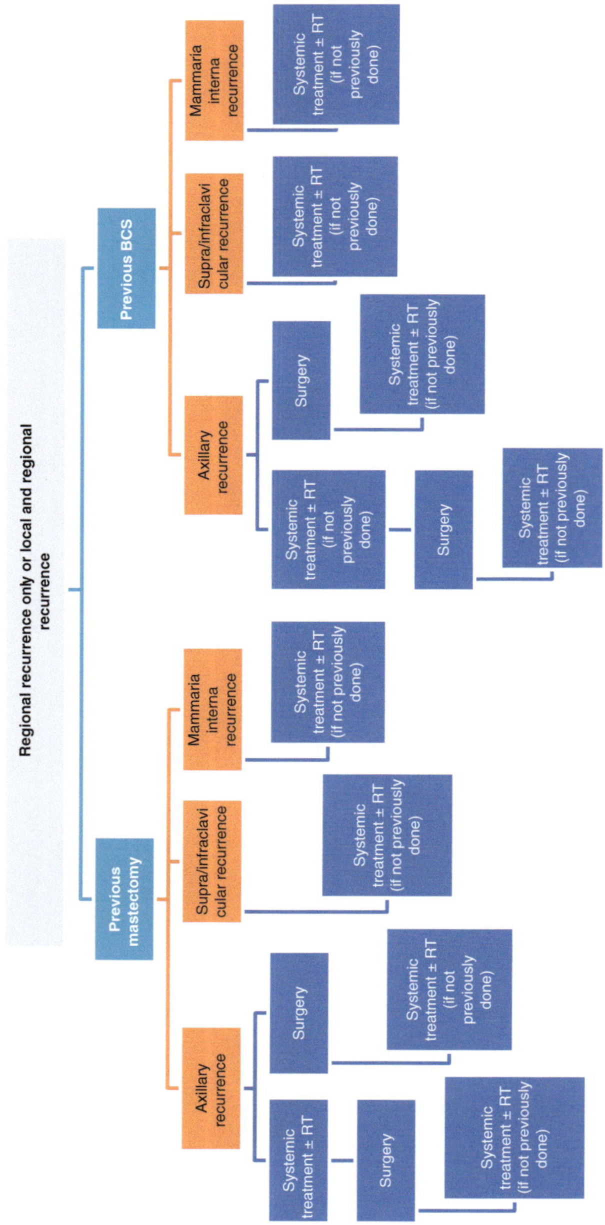

Fig. 1.38 Management of patients with "regional recurrence only" or "local and regional recurrence" [5, 67, 68]

Locoregional Treatment (Fig. 1.39)

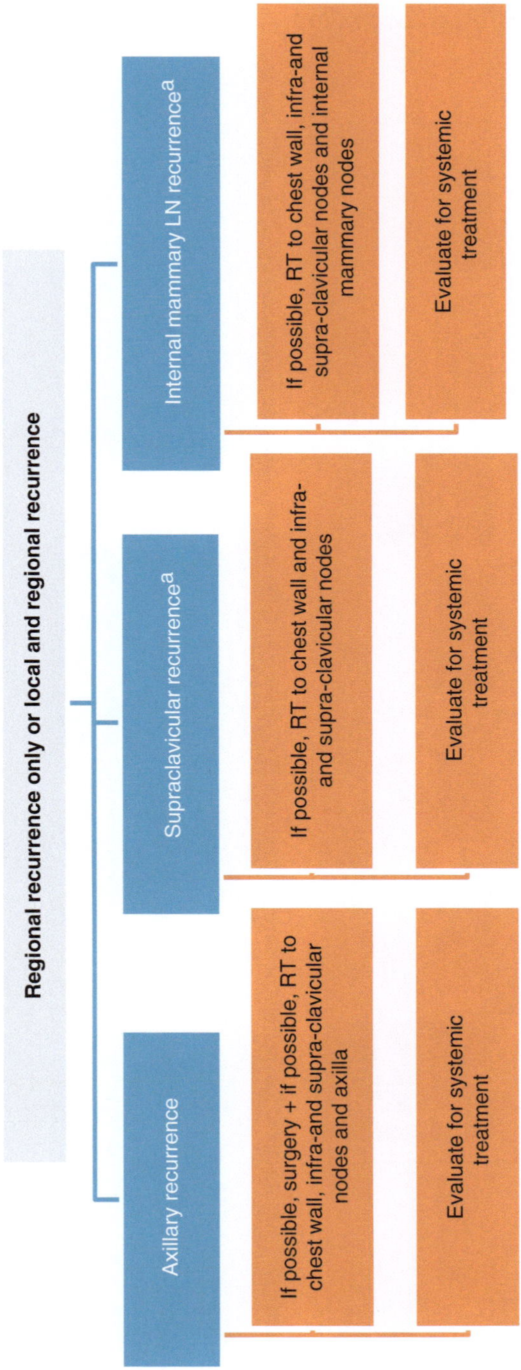

Fig. 1.39 Management of patients with regional recurrence [5, 67–69]. [a]Surgical treatment is not a good option, but surgical treatment can be considered in select patients (Proposal 3)

Invasive Breast Cancer: Recurrent or Stage IV Disease

General Treatment Approach (*Fig. 1.40*)

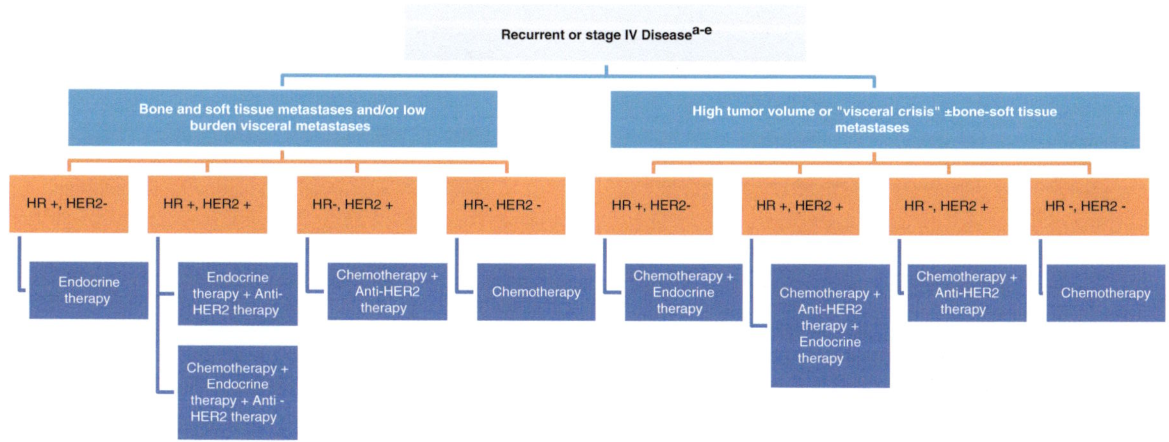

Fig. 1.40 Systemic treatment for recurrent or stage IV disease [5, 6, 67–83]. [a]If possible, a biopsy should be performed for pretreatment receptor assessment in relapse tumors. The benefit of palliative local breast surgery to women presenting with stage IV disease remains unclear. This local therapy should be considered only after a response to initial systemic therapy. Notably, some studies suggest that surgery is only valuable if performed with the same attention to detail (e.g., attaining clear margins and addressing disease in the axilla) as in patients with early-stage disease. If bone disease is present, add denosumab, zoledronic acid, ibandronic acid, or pamidronate. [b]"Anti-programmed death-1" (PD-1)/"Programmed death ligand" (PDL-1) antibodies were found to be effective alone or with taxanes in patients with triple-negative tumors [72]. [c]The addition of CDK4/6 inhibitors to the first- or second-choice endocrine treatment was found to be effective in randomized clinical trials [73, 74] (Table 1.8). [d]Anti-HER2 therapy must be added to HER2-positive patients. Administration of ado-trastuzumab emtansine and pertuzumab was not superior to treatment with chemotherapy + trastuzumab or ado-trastuzumab alone as the first-choice treatment in HER2-positive disease [75]. According to the PERTAIN trial, addition of pertuzumab to trastuzumab and endocrine treatment in the first choice prolonged progression-free survival. The addition of pertuzumab in the second line in patients who did not receive pertuzumab in the first line provided a minor clinical benefit [68]. [e]Retrospective studies suggest a potential survival benefit from complete excision of the primary tumor in select patients with metastatic breast cancer. Substantial selection biases exist in all of these studies and are likely to confound the study results. Two recent prospective, randomized studies assessed whether or not surgery on the primary tumor in the breast is necessary for women who are diagnosed with metastatic breast cancer. The results from both studies were similar and showed that surgical treatment of primary tumors in woman presenting with stage IV disease does not produce an increase in OS in general [76, 77]. However, a survival advantage for primary tumor excision was observed only in patients with solitary bone metastasis in the Turkish study [77]

Invasive Breast Cancer: Recurrent or Stage IV Disease: Systemic Treatment

HR-Positive; HER2-Positive or HER2-Negative (*Table 1.8*) (*Fig. 1.41*)

Table 1.8 Endocrine therapy in hormone receptor positive HER2-negative advanced breast cancer

Ovarian suppression (GnRH agonist) or ablation to all premenopausal patients			
Endocrine treatment naïve		*Previous endocrine treatment*	
No contraindication to CDK inhibitors	*Contraindication to CDK inhibitors*	*Under endocrine treatment or within 12 months after the end of adjuvant endocrine treatment*	*Disease recurrence at least one year after the end of adjuvant endocrine treatment*
CDK inhibitor[a] and aromatase inhibitors	Fulvestrant	CDK inhibitor and fulvestrant	Treat as patients who are endocrine treatment naïve
CDK inhibitor[b] and Fulvestrant	Aromatase inhibitors	CDK inhibitor and aromatase inhibitors	
Fulvestrant	Tamoxifen	Everolimus and exemestane OR tamoxifen OR fulvestrant	
		Abemeciclib and tamoxifen if not used previously	
		Abemaciclib	
		Fulvestrant if not used previously	
		If an aromatase inhibitor used previously, switch to other (steroidal to nonsteroidal or vice versa)	
		Tamoxifen	
		Progestins	
		Estrogens or androgens	

[a]Pablociclib, ribociclib, abemaciclib
[b]Ribociclib

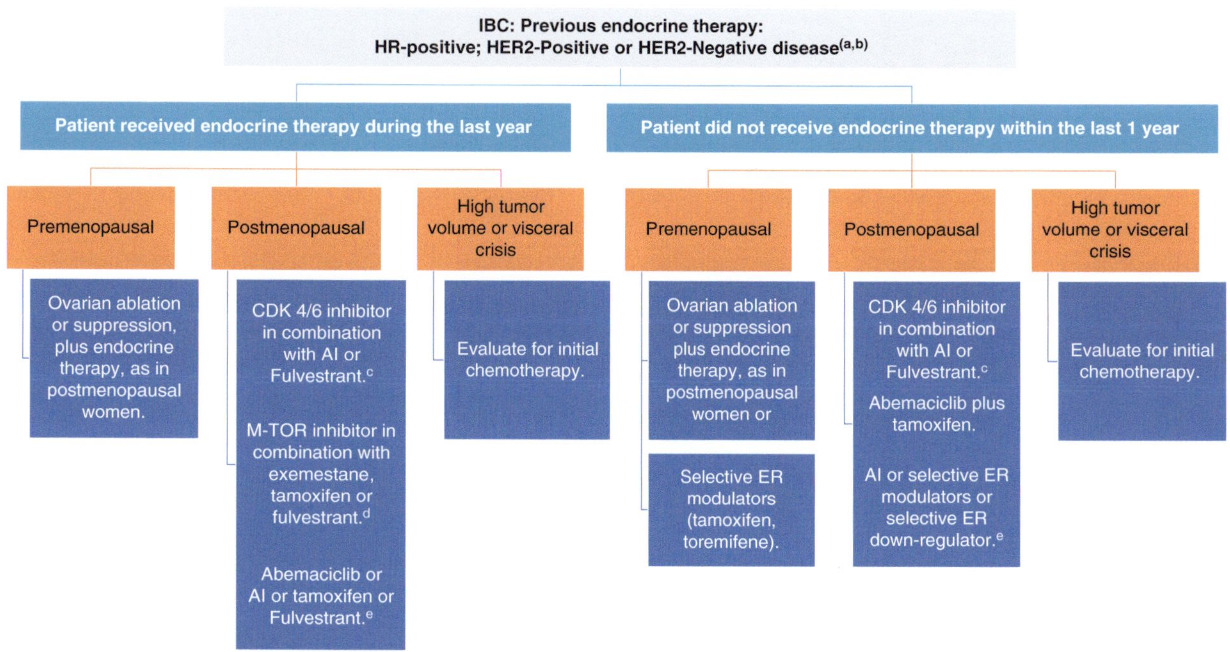

Fig. 1.41 Systemic treatment of recurrent stage IV hormone receptor-positive disease [1, 5, 6, 23, 24, 67–83]. [a]Anti-HER2 therapy must be added to HER2-positive patients [24, 68]. [b]If bone disease is present, add denosumab, zoledronic acid, ibandronic acid or pamidronate. [c]CDK 4/6 inhibitor in combination with AI or Fulvestrant may be considered as a treatment option for first-line therapy for postmenopausal patients with ER-positive, HER2-negative breast cancer [1, 69–71, 73, 74, 79–81]. [d]A combination of exemestane with everolimus (M-TOR inhibitor) can be considered for patients who meet the eligibility criteria for BOLERO-2 (progressed within 12 months, on a non-steroidal AI, or on tamoxifen at any time) [3, 5, 83]. [e]Fulvestrant (selective ER downregulator) can be used in the first choice in de novo metastatic disease that has never received any endocrine treatment. Fulvestrant was found to be superior to anastrozole in patients with bone metastases

Treatment of HER2-Overexpressing Metastatic Breast Cancer (Fig. 1.42)

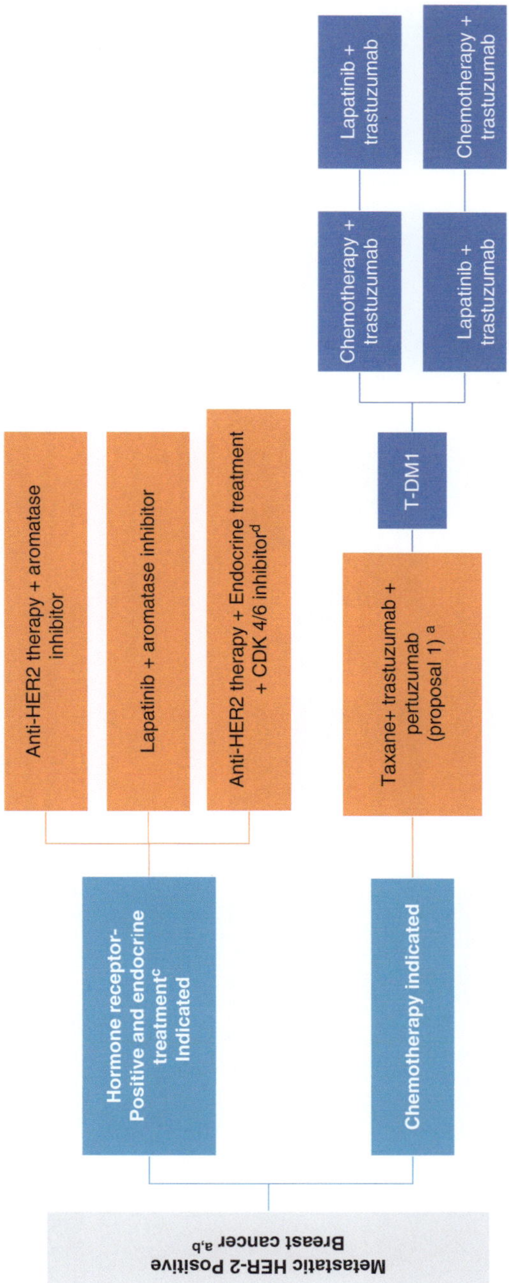

Fig. 1.42 Systemic treatment of recurrent or metastatic HER2-overexpressing breast cancer. [a]Administration of ado-trastuzumab emtansine and pertuzumab was not superior to treatment with chemotherapy + trastuzumab or ado-trastuzumab alone as the first choice treatment in HER2-positive disease [75]. According to the PERTAIN trial, addition of pertuzumab to trastuzumab and endocrine treatment in the first choice prolonged progression-free survival. The addition of pertuzumab in the second choice in patients who did not receive pertuzumab in the first choice provided a minor clinical benefit [1, 68]. [b]T-DM1 may be used as the front line therapy if the patient develops metastasis within 6 months of finishing adjuvant therapy with anti-HER2 treatment [1, 68]. [c]In premenopausal patients, medical or surgical oophorectomy must be performed. [d]Clinical trials are ongoing for anti-HER2 therapy + endocrine treatment + CDK 4/6 inhibitor

HER2-Negative, HR-Negative, or HR-Positive and Endocrine Refractory (Fig. 1.43)

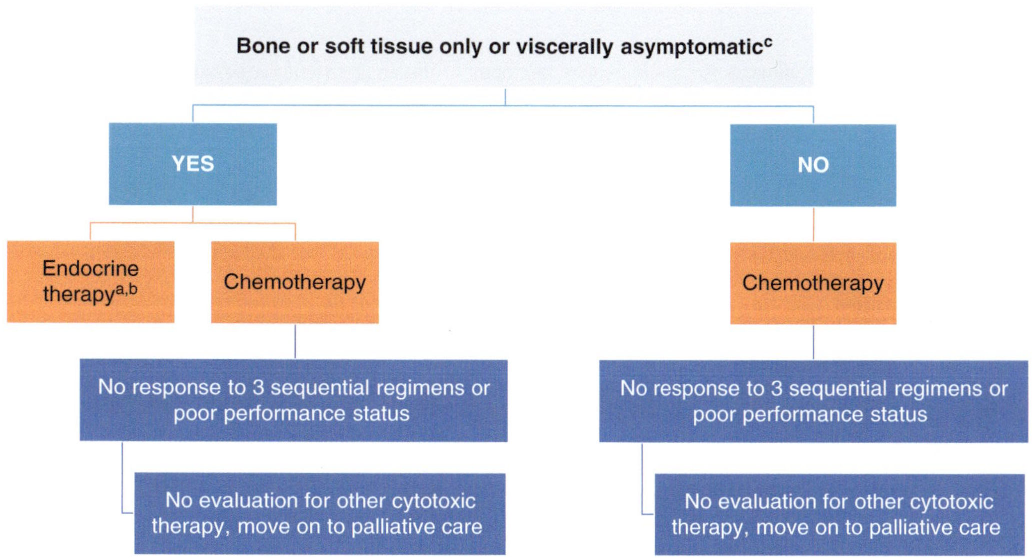

Fig. 1.43 Systemic therapy of patients with HER2-negative, HR-negative or HR-positive and endocrine refractory (see Table 1.8) disease [5, 6, 23, 24, 28, 69, 73, 78, 80–83]. [a]Among patients with hormone receptor-positive metastatic breast cancer who had progression of disease during prior endocrine therapy, a combination of exemestane with everolimus can be considered for patients who meet the eligibility criteria for BOLERO-2 (progressed within 12 months, on a non-steroidal AI, or on tamoxifen at any time) [3, 78]. AI or tamoxifen can be used alone, depending on the type and duration of previous endocrine treatment. Everolimus can be combined with exemestane, tamoxifen or fulvestrant. [b]Among patients with hormone receptor–positive metastatic breast cancer who had progression of disease during prior endocrine therapy, palbociclib combined with fulvestrant resulted in longer PFS than fulvestrant alone (premenopausal or perimenopausal women also received goserelin) [80]. CDK 4/6 inhibitor in combination with AI or Fulvestrant may be considered as a treatment option for postmenopausal patients with ER-positive, HER2-negative breast cancer [1, 5]. [c]If bone disease present, add denosumab, zoledronic acid, ibandronic acid, or pamidronate

HER2 Positive, HR Negative or HR Positive and Endocrine Refractory *(See Figs. 1.42 and 1.44)*

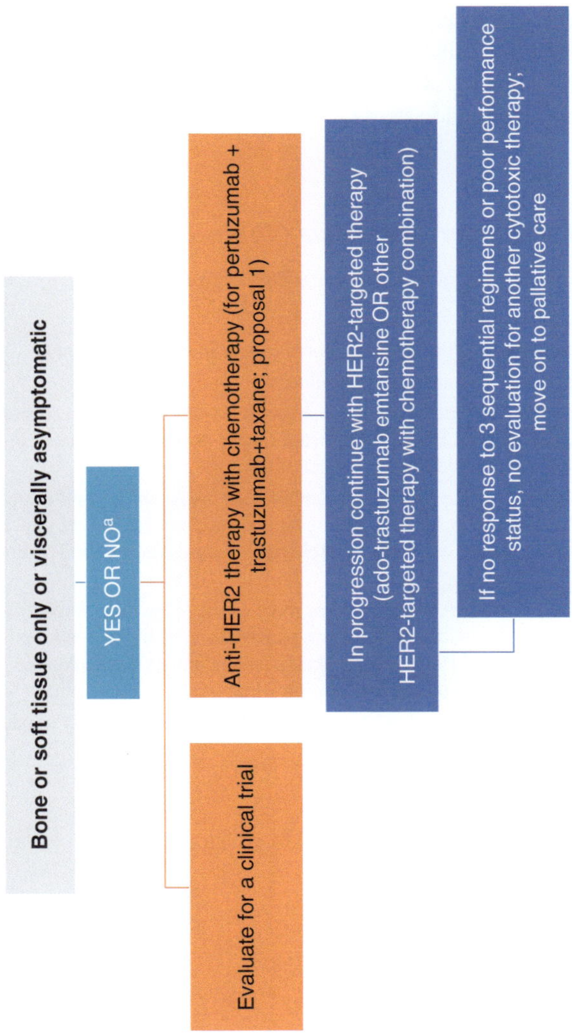

Fig. 1.44 Systemic therapy of patients with HER2-positive, HR-negative or HR-positive and endocrine refractory disease (see Fig. 1.42) [1, 5, 6, 68]. [a]If bone disease present, add denosumab, zoledronic acid, ibandronic acid, or pamidronate

Approach for High-Risk Patients: Genetic Risk Evaluation

At the St Gallen 2017 Consensus meeting, BRCA-1 and BRCA-2 tests were recommended, regardless of age, in patients with a strong history of breast cancer in relatives. These tests have been proposed regardless of the tumor subtype in patients with age ≤40–45 years and those with triple-negative tumors 60 years of age and younger. A germline multi-gene panel test can be performed based on a suspicion of hereditary cancer syndromes such as breast and ovarian cancer syndrome or Lynch syndrome, those with a history of premature breast cancer, or when BRCA1/2 cannot provide sufficient information [3, 84].

Individuals with a Cancer Diagnosis (*Table 1.9*)

Table 1.9 Genetic risk evaluation for an individual with a cancer diagnosis [1, 3, 5, 6]

–Early onset of female breast cancer (<45 years of age)
–Breast and ovarian/fallopian tube/primary peritoneal cancer in the same patient
–Two primary breast cancers (ipsilateral or contralateral)
-Breast cancer at any age and with at least one close blood relative with breast cancer at ≤50 years of age, ≥2 close blood relatives with breast cancer or pancreatic cancer at any age or ≥1 close blood relative with invasive ovarian cancer at any age
–The presence of one or more of the following together with breast cancer in the same side of the family: thyroid cancer, sarcoma, adrenocortical cancer, endometrial cancer, pancreatic cancer, brain tumor, diffuse gastric cancer, dermatological manifestations and leukemia/lymphoma
–A history of early-onset breast cancer and three or more of the following: thyroid cancer, sarcoma, adrenocortical cancer, endometrial cancer, pancreatic cancer, brain tumors, diffuse gastric cancer, dermatological manifestations, leukemia/lymphoma, prostate cancer (Gleason score ≥7), and hamartomatous polyps of the gastrointestinal tract
–A known mutation in one family member in one of the genes with a tendency to cause breast cancer
–Male breast cancer
–Ashkenazi Jew <60 years of age with breast cancer
–Triple-negative (ER−, PgR−, HER2−) breast cancer and ≤60 years of age

Approach for High-Risk Patients: Genetic Risk Evaluation

Individuals with Family History of Breast/Ovarian Cancer (Table 1.10)

Table 1.10 Genetic risk evaluation for individuals without cancer but with a family history of breast/ovarian cancer [1, 3, 5, 6]

–Male breast cancer
–First- or second-degree relative with breast cancer $\leq$45 years of age
–$\geq$2 individuals with primary breast cancer on the same side of the family
–$\geq$2 primary breast cancers in a single individual
–$\geq$1 primary invasive ovarian cancer
–History of early onset and three or more of the following: thyroid cancer, sarcoma, adrenocortical cancer, endometrial cancer, pancreatic cancer, brain tumors, diffuse gastric cancer, dermatological manifestations, leukemia/lymphoma, prostate cancer (Gleason score $\geq$ 7), and hamartomatous polyps of the gastrointestinal tract
–A known mutation in one family member in one of the genes with a tendency to cause breast cancer

Approach for High-Risk Patients

High-Risk Women Requesting Risk-Reducing Therapy (Fig. 1.45)

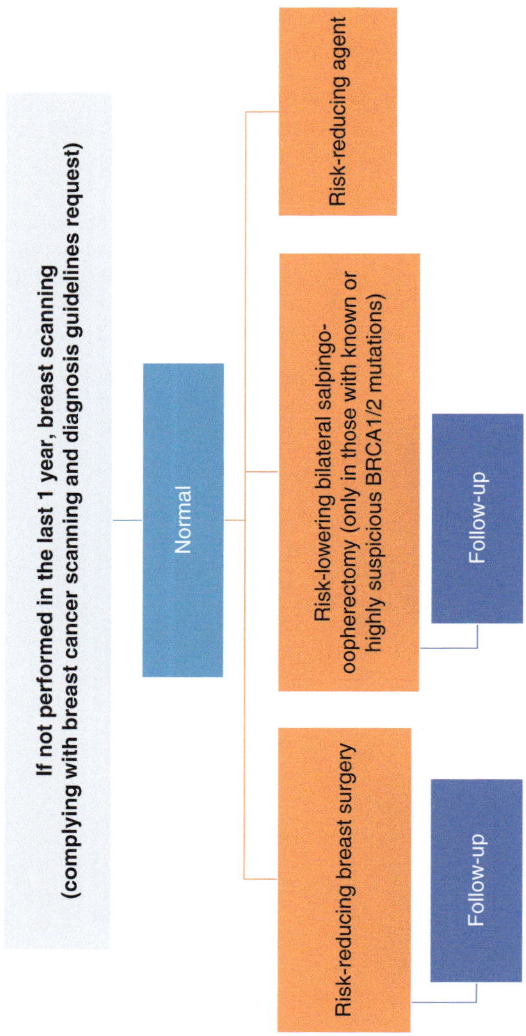

Fig. 1.45 Decision pathways for women requesting risk-reducing therapy [3, 4]

Risk-Reducing Agents *(Fig. 1.46)*

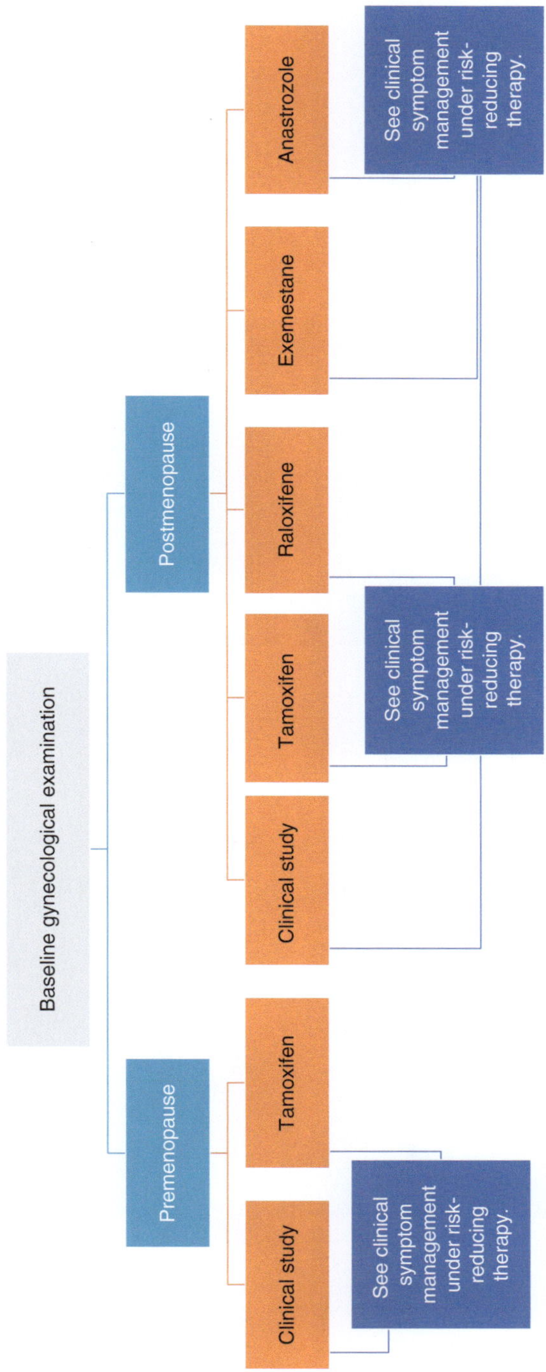

Fig. 1.46 Risk-reducing agents for premenopausal and postmenopausal women [1, 3, 4]

Clinical Symptom Management Under Risk-Reducing Therapy (Fig. 1.47)

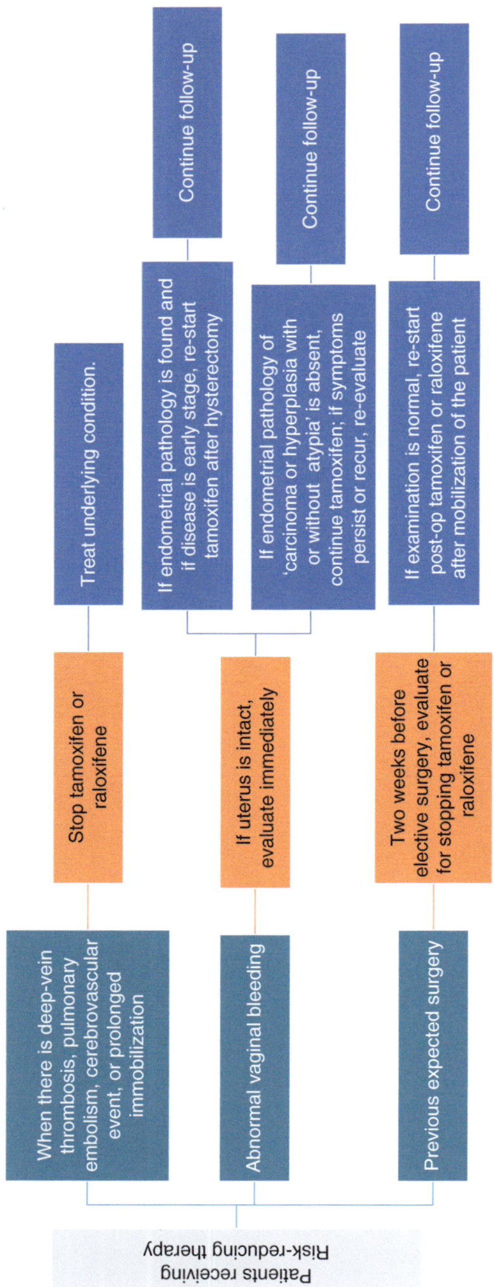

Fig. 1.47 Clinical symptom management of patients using risk-reducing therapy [1, 3–6]

Special Conditions

Phyllodes Tumor. [a]Phyllodes tumors, also termed phylloides tumors or cystosarcoma phyllodes, are rare fibroepithelial neoplasms of the breast that remain challenging for both surgeons and pathologists. The World Health Organization (WHO) established the name phyllodes tumor and the following histological types: benign, borderline, and malignant. Breast imaging studies may fail to distinguish a phyllodes tumor from a fibroadenoma. A core needle biopsy is preferable to fine-needle aspiration for tissue diagnosis. The common treatment for phyllodes tumors is wide local excision. Mastectomy is indicated for patients with a large lesion. The benefits of adjuvant chemotherapy and radiotherapy are controversial. [b]Borderline malignant phyllodes tumors should be treated with large surgical excision with a clean surgical margin of 1 cm or more. The width of the surgical margin for benign phyllodes tumors is controversial, and a negative surgical margin is sufficient [85, 86]

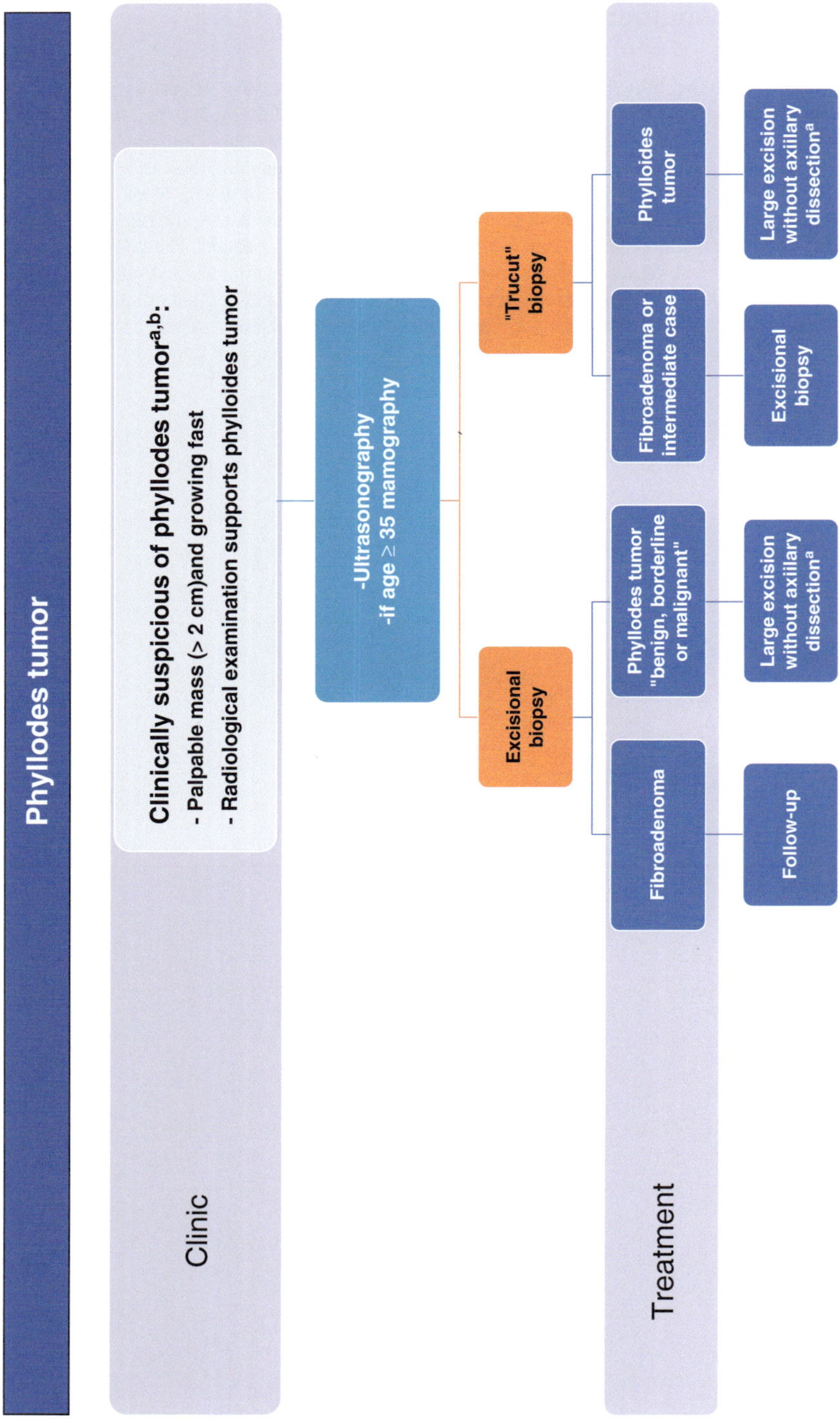
Phyllodes tumor
Clinic
Clinically suspicious of phyllodes tumor[a,b]:
- Palpable mass (> 2 cm)and growing fast
- Radiological examination supports phylloides tumor
-Ultrasonography
-if age ≥ 35 mamography
Excisional biopsy
"Trucut" biopsy
Treatment
Fibroadenoma
Phyllodes tumor "benign, borderline or malignant"
Fibroadenoma or intermediate case
Phylloides tumor
Follow-up
Large excision without axillary dissection[a]
Excisional biopsy
Large excision without axillary dissection[a]

Paget Disease. Paget's disease of the breast is characterized by eczema-form changes accompanied by erosion and ulceration of the nipple and areolar epidermis. This condition is primarily correlated with ductal carcinoma in situ (DCIS); additionally, it can be accompanied by invasive ductal carcinoma (IDC). The diagnosis is determined upon microscopic observation of Paget cells in a skin biopsy. The width of the lesion is evaluated via mammography and MRI in patients for whom breast-conserving surgery is planned. Depending on the extent of the lesion, SLNB and axillary curettage for those with axillary metastases are treatment alternatives to breast-preserving surgery or mastectomy [1, 3, 87]

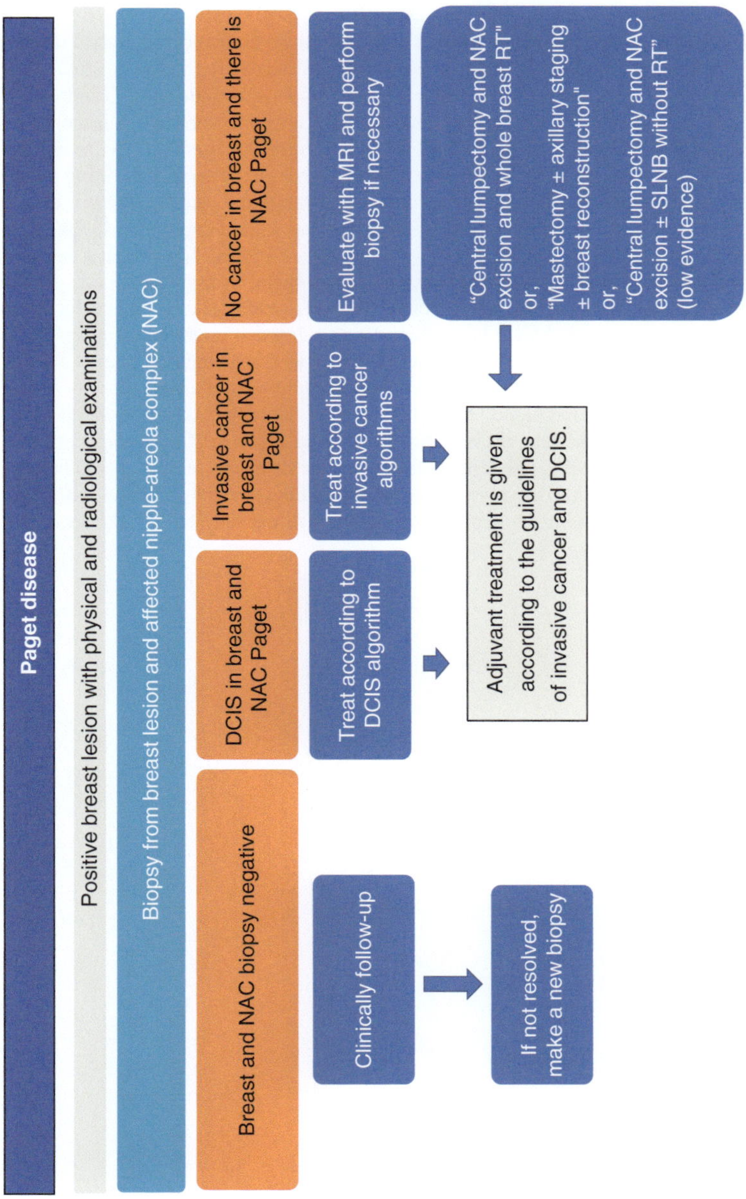

Breast Cancer During Pregnancy. [a]Pregnancy should be terminated in patients who become pregnant during tamoxifen treatment. The risk of malformation is high in the first trimester for tamoxifen use. Adjuvant trastuzumab is not recommended in pregnancy. However, the pregnancy can be continued by informing the patient because there are no sufficient data regarding the risk of malformation in women who become pregnant under trastuzumab treatment. Trastuzumab should be discontinued [1, 3, 5, 88]. [b]Premature delivery should be avoided. In patients receiving chemotherapy, the last chemotherapy cycle should not be given for a period of 1 month prior to the estimated date of birth (due to the risk of neutropenia in the baby). BCS can be performed in pregnancy, but the patient should be informed about the risk of local recurrence since RT will be performed after delivery (if RT cannot be started within 6 months after surgical operation). Blue dye is not used as the SLNB method. The radionuclide method in SLNB can be used as of the second trimester. Adjuvant RT, endocrine therapy and trastuzumab are administered after delivery when adjuvant therapy is indicated. Doxorubicin, 5-fluorouracil, and cyclophosphamide (FAC) can be used as chemotherapy (or AC). Ondansetron is preferred for nausea. Currently, there are no data encouraging safe administration of dose-dense AC with or without taxanes. A systematic review regarding taxane administration during pregnancy identified twenty-three publications describing a total of 40 women [89]. There were no spontaneous abortions or intrauterine deaths reported. In two cases exposed to paclitaxel, acute respiratory distress possibly was related to prematurity [90, 91]. The only malformation possibly related to taxanes was a case of pyloric stenosis in a neonate whom mother had received multiagent chemotherapy (doxorubicin, cyclophosphamide, paclitaxel, and docetaxel). Although there are no sufficient data yet, weekly paclitaxel can be given after the first trimester if there is a clinical indication (e.g., progression under neoadjuvant treatment with anthracycline). Since the safety of taxanes is less well documented than is that of anthracyclines, in some situations an additional cycle of anthracycline-based chemotherapy during pregnancy and completion of taxane-based chemotherapy after delivery can be considered [92]. According to the limited published data, the major cause of undesirable fetal outcome appears to be derived from premature delivery rather than from any direct effect of the chemotherapy. Follow-up of children with specialized assessment including detailed physiological and neurological functions is necessary. The timing for permitting pregnancy in women with breast cancer is a matter of research

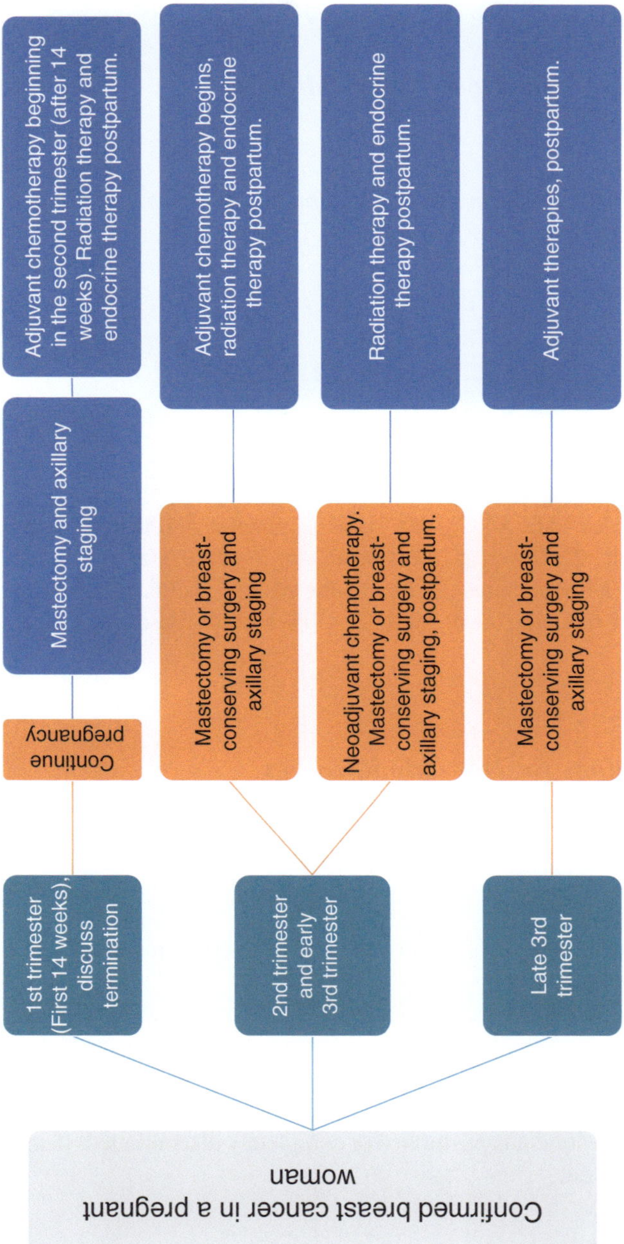
Confirmed breast cancer in a pregnant woman
1st trimester (First 14 weeks), discuss termination
2nd trimester and early 3rd trimester
Late 3rd trimester
Continue pregnancy
Mastectomy and axillary staging
Adjuvant chemotherapy beginning in the second trimester (after 14 weeks). Radiation therapy and endocrine therapy postpartum.
Mastectomy or breast-conserving surgery and axillary staging
Adjuvant chemotherapy begins, radiation therapy and endocrine therapy postpartum.
Neoadjuvant chemotherapy. Mastectomy or breast-conserving surgery and axillary staging, postpartum.
Radiation therapy and endocrine therapy postpartum.
Mastectomy or breast-conserving surgery and axillary staging
Adjuvant therapies, postpartum.

Basic Recommendations in Chemotherapy Dose Modification

Basic Recommendations for Dose Modification in Hematological Toxicity

New doses of chemotherapy according to the maximum toxicity in the previous chemotherapy:

The toxicity grade	Dose in the next cycle
ANC[a] < 0.5 (×10^9)/L for 5–7 days or febrile neutropenia	Reduce by 25%[b]
Thrombocyte < 25 (×10^9)/L or bleeding	Reduce by 25%

[a]ANC = Absolute neutrophil count = Neutrophils + number of rod cells
[b]Dosage may not be reduced by administering G-CSF in curative treatments

Chemotherapy is avoided until ANC $\geq 1.5 \times 10^9$/L, platelet $\geq 100 \times 10^9$/L and other toxicities are ≤ grade 2. However, if it is necessary to administer chemotherapy despite lower blood laboratory results due to the patient's clinical condition, treatment may be given by reducing the doses by 25–50% and administering G-CSF, if necessary.

Basic Recommendations for Dose Modification in Non-Hematological Toxicity

New doses of chemotherapy according to the maximum toxicity in the previous chemotherapy:

Toxicity Grade 1: The treatment is continued, and the symptoms are treated. There is no change in dosage.

Toxicity Grade 2: The treatment is continued, and the symptoms are treated. No dose changes or modifications can be made according to the treatment regimen applied.

Toxicity Grade 3: Treatment is postponed, and the symptoms are treated; 75% of the previous dose is given.

Toxicity Grade 4: The treatment is postponed or completely discontinued. If continued, the doses are modified.

Assessment of the Response to Treatment in Metastatic Disease

The response should be determined in treated patients. Here, tumor markers and radiological evaluations are used as objective parameters. The patient's clinical status, tumor markers and radiological evaluation provide more accurate results when they are considered together.

Sensitivity and Specificity in Clinical Tests

Diagnostic and follow-up methods are compared according to their sensitivity and specificity.

The following terminology is used:

1. True positive: The disease is present in the patient, and the test is positive.
2. False positive: The patient has no disease, but the test is positive.
3. True negative: There is no specified disease in the patient, and the test is negative.
4. False negative: The patient has the disease, but the test is negative.

Sensitivity = true positives/(true positives + false negatives)

75% Sensitivity = 75% of those with the disease are diagnosed with the test (true positive), but 25% of the patients cannot be recognized (false negative)

Specificity = true negatives/(true negatives + false positives)

75% specificity: The test finds 75% of the people without the disease (true negatives), but 25% of those without the disorder are found to be ill (false positives).

A first diagnostic method in cancer may have high sensitivity and low specificity. In this case, it can be concluded that many patients with false-positive results would be specified as disease-free by the second diagnostic method to be performed. Although it is not realistic to develop a 100% accurate diagnostic tool, it is possible to achieve the best diagnosis by using a first diagnostic method with high sensitivity-low specificity and a second method with low sensitivity-high specificity.

Positive predictive value (PPV) = True positives/(True positives + False Positives)

This expresses the 'probability that a person with a positive test result is really ill'.

Negative predictive value (NPV) = True negatives/(True negatives + False negatives)

This expresses the 'probability that a person with a negative test result is really disease-free'.

Radiological Findings

The most commonly used method in the response evaluation is *RECIST* (*R*esponse *E*valuation *C*riteria *in S*olid *T*umors). The patient is defined as "responsive" if the tumor regresses, "stable" if the tumor remains the same, and "progressive" if it worsens. The PET response criteria have been published as *PERCIST* (*PE*T *R*esponse *C*riteria *in S*olid *T*umors).

In RECIST, lesions are divided into four subgroups:

Measurable lesions: The tumor is ≥10 mm on CT or MR imaging, and the lymph node is ≥15 mm or ≥20 mm on chest X-ray.

Non-measurable lesions: Lesions smaller than those mentioned above or not suitable for direct measurement (such as sclerotic bone metastases, leptomeningeal disease, ascites, pleural/pericardial effusion)

Target lesions: They are measurable lesions used in the response evaluation.

Non-target lesions: Assessment of non-measurable tumors or findings

Summary of response evaluation according to RECIST 1.1

The smallest possible target lesion size	≥10 mm (CT + MRG) ≥15 mm lymph nodes ≥20 mm chest X-ray
Number of lesions measured	Maximum of 5, maximum of 2 per organ
Progressive disease according to measurable lesion	20% increase in total diameter (TD) + a net increase of at least 5 mm from the initial measurement of the tumor
Progressive disease according to non-target lesion	Progression if there is significant worsening or if the tumor burden has increased
PET-CT	Can be used to confirm progression

The following rules are applied for use of RECIST:

1. The longest diameter of the tumor is measured.
2. The non-tumor area is not included in the measurements.
3. There is no obligation to select the largest tumors in the measurement. Tumors that are best identifiable and that can be evaluated in the measurements in repeated examinations are selected.
4. Ensure that the imaging quality is good.
5. Radiological examinations with intravenous contrast provide the most accurate results among imaging modalities. This is especially important in clinical study participants (however, patients without adequate kidney function may require unenhanced CT).
6. The same tumors should be measured in all repeated evaluations to improve the reliability of comparisons.
7. In the measurement, large tumors with high measurement reliability are used.
8. Mild growth in non-target tumors other than the measured target tumors is not evidence of progression alone.
9. If the measured target lesions become discrete lesions, the longest diameter of each lesion is measured separately, and the sum is calculated to determine the total diameter (TD).
10. When the target lesions unite, the largest diameter of the final lesion is measured.
11. The hypervascular border area around the lesion is also measured (for example, in the brain tumor, the contrast agent appears as a bright ring around the tumor, and this area should be included in the measurement). The largest diameter is measured without taking the central necrosis into account.
12. The largest diameter is measured even if cavities and necrosis occur at the center of the target lesion. However, if the sum of the diameters is not compatible with the patient's clinical response, another assessment method may be required.

Special Rules for Radiological Evaluation

Lymph Nodes The longest diameter of the lymph node or nodal ligature is determined (e.g., 20 mm); then the longest short axis perpendicular to this line is measured (e.g., 13 mm). A lymph node with a short axis of 13 mm is considered pathological (>10 mm) but is not measurable (non-target). The diameter should be ≥15 mm for a measurable (target) lesion.

Lytic Bone Lesions The visible soft tissue component can be assessed by CT or MRI when present. The soft tissue component may be a "target" lesion if it is compatible with the measurable lesion rules. Blastic bone lesions are non-measurable lesions (non-target).

MRI This provides very good contrast, and good measurements can be achieved using different techniques. However, the MRI quality is very important. MRI is not used to measure lesions in the lung parenchyma. The measurement can be sagittal or coronal (oblique). The measurements should always be made in the same plane.

PET-CT In some cases, PET-CT may be required to determine progression.

Patients who initially had a negative PET-CT result: If the new PET-CT is positive, it is considered progression due to presence of the new lesion.

Patients not initially evaluated with PET-CT:

- In a positive PET result, 'progression' is perceived if the CT finding is in a new, previously unidentified location.
- If the finding in the positive PET is not identified as a new lesion in CT, the new lesion must be verified with CTs performed at specific time intervals to be considered 'progression'.
- It is not accepted as progression if the positive PET lesion is present in previous CTs and there is no anatomical growth.

References

1. NCCN guidelines for treatment of cancer by site. v.1.2018. Breast Cancer. www.nccn.org.
2. Morrow M, Van Zee KJ, Solin LJ, Houssami N, Chavez-MacGregor M, Harris JR, et al. Society of Surgical Oncology–American Society for Radiation Oncology–American Society of Clinical Oncology consensus guideline on margins for breast-conserving surgery with whole-breast irradiation in ductal carcinoma in situ. J Clin Oncol. 2016;34:4040–6.
3. Curigliano G, Burstein HJ, Winer EP, Gnant M, Dubsky P, Loibl S, et al. De-escalating and escalating treatments for early-stage breast cancer: the St. Gallen International Expert Consensus Conference on the Primary Therapy of Early Breast Cancer 2017. Ann Oncol. 2017;28(8):1700–12.
4. Visvanathan K, Hurley P, Bantug E, Brown P, Col NF, Cuzick J, et al. Use of pharmacologic interventions for breast cancer risk reduction: American Society of Clinical Oncology clinical practice guideline. J Clin Oncol. 2013;31:2942–62.

5. Aydiner A, Sen F, Karanlik H, Aslay I, Dincer M, İgci A. A review of local and systemic therapy in breast cancer. In: Aydiner A, İğci A, Soran A, editors. Breast disease, vol. II. Switzerland: Springer; 2016. p. 731–64.
6. Guidelines of the AGO breast committee. Version 17.1.0. https://www.ago-online.de/en/guidelines-mamma/april-2017/. April 2017.
7. Margolese RG, Cecchini RS, Julian TB, Ganz PA, Costantino JP, et al. Primary results, NRG Oncology/NSABP B-35: a clinical trial of anastrozole (A) versus tamoxifen (tam) in postmenopausal patients with DCIS undergoing lumpectomy plus radiotherapy. J Clin Oncol. 2015;33(Suppl):abstr LBA500.
8. Forbes JF, Sestak I, Howell A, Bonanni B, Bundred N, Levy C, et al. Anastrozole versus tamoxifen for the prevention of locoregional and contralateral breast cancer in postmenopausal women with locally excised ductal carcinoma in situ (IBIS-II DCIS): a double-blind, randomised controlled trial. Lancet. 2016;387(10021):866–73.
9. Lyman GH, Somerfield MR, Bosserman LD, Perkins CL, Weaver DL, Giuliano AE. Sentinel lymph node biopsy for patients with early-stage breast cancer: American Society of Clinical Oncology clinical practice guideline update. J Clin Oncol. 2016;35:561–4.
10. Giuliano AE, Mc Call LM, Beitsch PD, Whit PW, Morrow M, Blumencranz PW, et al. ACOSOGZ0011: a randomized trial of axillary node dissection in women with clinical T1-2 N0M0 breast cancer who have a positive sentinel node. J Clin Oncol. 2010;28(18):CRA 506.
11. Bouughey JC, Suman VJ, Mittendorf EA, Ahrendt GM, Wilke LG, Taback B, et al. Sentinel lymph node surgery after neoadjuvant chemotherapy in patients with node-positive breast cancer: the ACOSOG Z1071 (Alliance) clinical trial. JAMA. 2013;310:1455–61.
12. Senkus E, Kyriakides S, Ohno S, Penault-Llorca F, Poortmans P, Rutgers E, Zackrisson S, Cardoso F, et al. Primary breast cancer: ESMO Clinical Practice Guidelines for diagnosis, treatment and follow-up. Ann Oncol. 2015;26(Suppl 5):v8–v30.
13. Kuehn T, Bauerfeind I, Fehm T, Fleige B, Hausschild M, Helms G, et al. Sentinel-lymph-node biopsy in patients with breast cancer before and after neoadjuvant chemotherapy (SENTINA): a prospective, multicentre cohort study. Lancet. 2013;14:609–18.
14. Giuliano AE, Hunt KK, Ballman KV, Beitsch PD, Whitworth PW, Blumencranz PW, et al. Axillary dissection vs no axillary dissection in women with invasive breast cancer and sentinel node metastasis: a randomized clinical trial. JAMA. 2011;305(6):569–75.
15. Giuliano AE, Ballman KV, McCall L, Beitsch PD, Brennan MB, Kelemen PR, et al. Effect of axillary dissection vs no axillary dissection on 10-year overall survival among women with invasive breast cancer and sentinel node metastasis: the ACOSOG Z0011 (Alliance) randomized clinical trial. JAMA. 2017;318(10):918–26.
16. Boileau JF, Poirier B, Basik M, Holloway CM, Gaboury L, Sideris L, et al. Sentinel node biopsy after neoadjuvant chemotherapy in biopsy-proven node-positive breast cancer: the SN FNAC study. J Clin Oncol. 2015;33(3):258–64.
17. Mamtani A, Barrio AV, King TA, Van Zee KJ, Plitas G, Pilewskie M, et al. How often does neoadjuvant chemotherapy avoid axillary dissection in patients with histologically confirmed nodal metastases? Results of a prospective study. Ann Surg Oncol. 2016;23(11):3467–74.
18. Moo T, Edelweiss E, Hajiyeva S, Stempel M, Raiss M, Barrio AV. Is low-volume disease in the sentinel node after neoadjuvant chemotherapy an indication for axillary dissection. In: Society for Surgical Oncology (SSO) annual cancer symposium, Chicago; 2018(abstract 47).
19. De La Cruz L, Moody AM, Tappy EE, Blankenship SA, Hecht EM. Overall survival, disease-free survival, local recurrence, and nipple-areolar recurrence in the setting of nipple-sparing mastectomy: a meta-analysis and systematic review. Ann Surg Oncol. 2015;22(10):3241–9.
20. Moran MS, Schnitt SJ, Giuliano AE, Harris JR, Khan SA, Horton J, et al. Society of Surgical Oncology-American Society for Radiation Oncology consensus guideline on margins for breast-conserving surgery with whole-breast irradiation in stages I and II invasive breast cancer. Int J Radiat Oncol Biol Phys. 2014;88:553–64.
21. Coates AS, Winer EP, Goldhirsch A, Gelber RD, Gnant M, et al. Tailoring therapies—improving the management of early breast cancer: St Gallen International Expert Consensus on the Primary Therapy of Early Breast Cancer 2015. Ann Oncol. 2015;26:1533–46.

22. Wolff AC, Hammond MEH, Allison KH, Harvey BE, Mangu PB, Bartlett JMS, et al. Human epidermal growth factor receptor 2 testing in breast cancer: American Society of Clinical Oncology/College of American Pathologists clinical practice guideline focused update. J Clin Oncol. 2018. https://doi.org/10.1200/JCO.2018.77.8738.
23. Burstein HJ, Temin S, Anderson H, Buchholz TA, Davidson NE, Gelmon KE, et al. Adjuvant endocrine therapy for women with hormone receptor-positive breast cancer: American Society of Clinical Oncology clinical practice guideline focused update. J Clin Oncol. 2014;32(21):2255–69.
24. von Minckwitz G, Procter M, de Azambuja E, Zardavas D, Benyunes M, Viale G, et al. Adjuvant pertuzumab and trastuzumab in early HER2-positive breast cancer. N Engl J Med. 2017;377(2):122–31.
25. Krop I, Ismaila N, Andre F, Bast RC, Barlow W, Collyar DE, et al. Biomarkers to guide decisions on adjuvant systemic therapy for women with early stage invasive breast cancer: American Society of Clinical Oncology clinical practice guideline focused update. J Clin Oncol. 2017;35(24):2838–47.
26. Denduluri N, Chavez-MacGregor M, Telli ML, Eisen A, Graff SL, Hassett MJ, et al. Selection of optimal adjuvant chemotherapy and targeted therapy for early breast cancer: ASCO clinical practice guideline focused update. J Clin Oncol. 2018. https://doi.org/10.1200/JCO.2018.78.8604.
27. Burstein HJ, Lacchetti C, Anderson H, Buchholz TA, Davidson NE, Gelmon KE, et al. Adjuvant endocrine therapy for women with hormone receptor–positive breast cancer: American Society of Clinical Oncology clinical practice guideline update on ovarian suppression. J Clin Oncol. 2016;34:1689–701.
28. Henry NL, Somerfield MR, Abramson VG, Allison KH, Anders CK, Diana T, et al. Role of patient and disease factors in adjuvant systemic therapy decision making for early-stage, operable breast cancer: American Society of Clinical Oncology endorsement of cancer care ontario guideline recommendations. J Clin Oncol. 2016;34:2303–11.
29. Sparano JA, Gray RJ, Makower DF, Pritchard KI, Albain KS, Hayes DF, et al. Prospective validation of a 21-gene expression assay in breast cancer. N Engl J Med. 2015;373:2005–14.
30. Gluz O, Nitz UA, Christgen M, Kates RE, Shak S, Clemens M, et al. West German Study Group Phase III PlanB Trial: first prospective outcome data for the 21-gene recurrence score assay and concordance of prognostic markers by central and local pathology assessment. J Clin Oncol. 2016;34:2341–9.
31. Cardoso F, van 't Veer LJ, Bogaerts J, Slaets L, Viale G, Delaloge S, MINDACT Investigators. 70-gene signature as an aid to treatment decisions in early-stage breast cancer. N Engl J Med. 2016;375(8):717–29.
32. Tolaney SM, Barry WT, Dang CT, Yardley DA, Moy B, Marcom PK, et al. Adjuvant paclitaxel and trastuzumab for node-negative, HER2-positive breast cancer. N Engl J Med. 2015;372:134–41.
33. Zhou Q, Yin W, Du Y, Lu J. For or against adjuvant trastuzumab for pT1a-bN0M0 breast cancer patients with HER2-positive tumors: a meta-analysis of published literatures. PLoS One. 2014;9(1):e83646.
34. Gerber B, Ortmann O. Prevention of Early Menopause Study (POEMS): is it possible to preserve ovarian function by gonadotropin releasing hormone analogs (GnRHa)? Arch Gynecol Obstet. 2014;290:1051–3.
35. Francis PA, Regan MM, Fleming GF, Láng I, Ciruelos E, Bellet M, et al. Adjuvant ovarian suppression in premenopausal breast cancer. N Engl J Med. 2015;372:436–46.
36. Park JW, Liu MC, Yee D, Yau C, van 't Veer LJ, Symmans WF, I-SPY 2 Investigators, et al. Adaptive randomization of neratinib in early breast cancer. N Engl J Med. 2016;375(1):11–22.
37. Goss PE, Ingle JN, Pritchard KI, Robert NJ, Muss H, Gralow J, et al. Extending aromatase-inhibitor adjuvant therapy to 10 years. N Engl J Med. 2016;375(3):209–19.
38. Sikov WM, Berry DA, Perou CM, Singh B, Cirrincione CT, Tolaney SM, et al. Impact of the addition of carboplatin and/or bevacizumab to neoadjuvant once-per-week paclitaxel followed by dose-dense doxorubicin and cyclophosphamide on pathologic complete response

rates in stage II to III triple-negative breast cancer: CALGB 40603 (Alliance). J Clin Oncol. 2015;33(1):13–21.
39. Del Mastro L, De Placido S, Bruzzi P, De Laurentiis M, Boni C, Cavazzini G, et al. Fluorouracil and dose-dense chemotherapy in adjuvant treatment of patients with early-stage breast cancer: an open-label, 2×2 factorial, randomised phase 3 trial. Lancet. 2015;385(9980):1863–72.
40. Foukakis T, von Minckwitz G, Bengtsson NO, Brandberg Y, Wallberg B, Fornander T, et al. Effect of tailored dose-dense chemotherapy vs standard 3-weekly adjuvant chemotherapy on recurrence-free survival among women with high-risk early breast cancer: a randomized clinical trial. JAMA. 2016;316(18):1888–96.
41. Gianni L, Pienkowski T, Im YH, Tseng LM, Liu MC, Lluch A, et al. 5-year analysis of neoadjuvant pertuzumab and trastuzumab in patients with locally advanced, inflammatory, or early-stage HER2-positive breast cancer (NeoSphere): a multicentre, open-label, phase 2 randomised trial. Lancet Oncol. 2016;17(6):791–800.
42. Joensuu H, Kellokumpu-Lehtinen PL, Huovinen R, Jukkola-Vuorinen A, Tanner M, Kokko R, et al. Adjuvant capecitabine in combination with docetaxel, epirubicin, and cyclophosphamide for early breast cancer: the randomized clinical FinXX trial. JAMA Oncol. 2017;3(6):793–800.
43. Masuda N, Lee SJ, Ohtani S, Im YH, Lee ES, Yokota I, et al. Adjuvant capecitabine for breast cancer after preoperative chemotherapy. N Engl J Med. 2017;376(22):2147–59.
44. Pagani O, Regan MM, Francis PA, TEXT and SOFT Investigators, International Breast Cancer Study Group. Exemestane with ovarian suppression in premenopausal breast cancer. N Engl J Med. 2014;371(14):1358–9.
45. Whelan TJ, Olivotto IA, Parulekar WR, Ackerman I, Chua BH, Nabid A, et al. Regional nodal irradiation in early-stage breast cancer. N Engl J Med. 2015;373(4):307–1.
46. Strnad V, Ott OJ, Hildebrandt G, Kauer-Dorner D, Knauerhase H, Major T, Groupe Europe´en de Curiethe´rapie of European Society for Radiotherapy and Oncology (GEC-ESTRO), et al. 5-year results of accelerated partial breast irradiation using sole interstitial multicatheter brachytherapy versus whole-breast irradiation with boost after breast-conserving surgery for low-risk invasive and in-situ carcinoma of the female breast: a randomised, phase 3, non-inferiority trial. Lancet. 2016;387(10015):229–38.
47. Correa C, Harris EE, Leonardi MC, Smith BD, Taghian AG, Thompson AM, et al. Accelerated partial breast irradiation: executive summary for the update of an ASTRO evidence-based consensus statement. Pract Radiat Oncol. 2017;7:73–9.
48. Bartelink H, Maingon P, Poortmans P, Weltens C, Fourquet A, Jager J, et al. Whole-breast irradiation with or without a boost for patients treated with breast-conserving surgery for early breast cancer: 20-year follow-up of a randomised phase 3 trial. Lancet Oncol. 2015;16(1):47–56.
49. Bane AL, Whelan TJ, Pond GR, Parpia S, Gohla G, Fyles AW, et al. Tumor factors predictive of response to hypofractionated radiotherapy in a randomized trial following breast conserving therapy. Ann Oncol. 2014;25:992–8.
50. Marta GN, Macedo CR, Carvalho Hde A, Hanna SA, da Silva JL, Riera R. Accelerated partial irradiation for breast cancer: systematic review and meta-analysis of 8653 women in eight randomized trials. Radiother Oncol. 2015;114:42–9.
51. Budach W, Kammers K, Boelke E, Matuschek C. Adjuvant radiotherapy of regional lymph nodes in breast cancer—a meta-analysis of randomized trials. Radiat Oncol. 2013;8:267.
52. Bellon JR, Golshan M, Solin LJ. Controversies in radiation oncology for early-stage breast cancer. Ann Surg Oncol. 2015;22:3213.
53. Recht A, Comen EA, Fine RE, Fleming GF, Hardenbergh PH, Ho AY, et al. Postmastectomy radiotherapy: an American Society of Clinical Oncology, American Society for Radiation Oncology, and Society of surgical oncology focused guideline update. J Clin Oncol. 2016;34:4431–42.
54. Vrieling C, van Werkhoven E, Maingon P, Poortmans P, Weltens C, Fourquet A, et al. Prognostic factors for local control in breast cancer after long-term follow-up in the EORTC boost vs no boost trial: a randomized clinical trial. JAMA Oncol. 2017;3(1):42–8.

55. Poortmans PM, Collette S, Kirkove C, Van Limbergen E, Budach V, Struikmans H, et al. Internal mammary and medial supraclavicular irradiation in breast cancer. N Engl J Med. 2015;373(4):317–27.
56. Ataseven B, Lederer B, Blohmer JU, Denkert C, Gerber B, Heil J, et al. Impact of multifocal or multicentric disease on surgery and locoregional, distant and overall survival of 6,134 breast cancer patients treated with neoadjuvant chemotherapy. Ann Surg Oncol. 2015;22(4):1118–27.
57. Santoro S, Loreti A, Cavaliere F, Costarelli L, La Pinta M, Manna E, et al. Neoadjuvant chemotherapy is not a contraindication for nipple sparing mastectomy. Breast. 2015;24(5):661–6.
58. Gnant M, Pfeiler G, Dubsky PC, Hubalek M, Greil R, Jakesz R, et al. Adjuvant denosumab in breast cancer (ABCSG-18): a multicentre, randomised, double-blind, placebo-controlled trial. Lancet. 2015;386(9992):433–43.
59. Gnant M, Mlineritsch B, Schippinger W, Luschin-Ebengreuth G, Pöstlberger S, Menzel C, et al. Endocrine therapy plus zoledronic acid in premenopausal breast cancer. N Engl J Med. 2009;360(7):679–91.
60. Dhesy-Thind S, Fletcher GG, Blanchette PS, Clemons MJ, Dillmon MS, Frank ES, et al. Use of adjuvant bisphosphonates and other bone-modifying agents in breast cancer: a Cancer Care Ontario and American Society of Clinical Oncology clinical practice guideline. J Clin Oncol. 2017;35:2062–81.
61. Rugo HS, Olopade OI, DeMichele A, Yau C, van 't Veer LJ, Buxton MB, et al. Adaptive randomization of veliparib-carboplatin treatment in breast cancer. N Engl J Med. 2016;375(1):23–34.
62. Untch M, Jackisch C, Schneeweiss A, Conrad B, Aktas B, Denkert C, et al. Nab-paclitaxel versus solvent-based paclitaxel in neoadjuvant chemotherapy for early breast cancer (GeparSepto-GBG 69): a randomised, phase 3 trial. Lancet Oncol. 2016;17(3):345–56.
63. Colleoni M, Gray KP, Gelber S, Láng I, Thürlimann B, Gianni L, et al. Low-dose oral cyclophosphamide and methotrexate maintenance for hormone receptor-negative early breast cancer: International Breast Cancer Study Group Trial 22-00. J Clin Oncol. 2016;34(28):3400–8.
64. Curigliano G, Gómez Pardo P, Meric-Bernstam F, Conte P, Lolkema MP, Beck JT, et al. Ribociclib plus letrozole in early breast cancer: a presurgical, window-of-opportunity study. Breast. 2016;28:191–8.
65. Ma CX, Gao F, Luo J, Northfelt DW, Goetz M, Forero A, et al. NeoPalAna: neoadjuvant palbociclib, a cyclin-dependent kinase 4/6 inhibitor, and anastrozole for clinical stage 2 or 3 estrogen receptor-positive breast cancer. Clin Cancer Res. 2017;23(15):4055–65.
66. Dawood S, Merajver SD, Viens P, Vermeulen PB, Swain SM, Buchholz TA, et al. International expert panel on inflammatory breast cancer: consensus statement for standardized diagnosis and treatment. Ann Oncol. 2011;22:515–23.
67. Partridge AH, Rumble B, Carey LA, Come SE, Davidson NE, Leo AD, et al. Chemotherapy and targeted therapy for women with human epidermal growth factor receptor 2–negative (or unknown) advanced breast cancer: American Society of Clinical Oncology Clinical Practice Guideline. J Clin Oncol. 2014;32:3307–29.
68. Giordano SH, Temin S, Kirshner JJ, Chandarlapaty S, Crews JR, Davidson NE, et al. Systemic therapy for patients with advanced human epidermal growth factor receptor 2-positive breast cancer: ASCO clinical practice guideline update. J Clin Oncol. 2018;36 https://doi.org/10.1200/JCO.2018.79.2697.
69. Cardoso F, Costa A, Senkus E, Aapro M, André F, Barrios CH, et al. 3rd ESO-ESMO international consensus guidelines for advanced breast cancer (ABC 3). Ann Oncol. 2017;28(1):16–33.
70. Goetz MP, Toi M, Campone M, Sohn J, Paluch-Shimon S, Huober J, et al. MONARCH 3: abemaciclib as initial therapy for advanced breast cancer. J Clin Oncol. 2017;35(32):3638–46.
71. Slamon DJ, Neven P, Chia S, Fasching PA, De Laurentiis M, Im SA, et al. Phase III randomized study of ribociclib and fulvestrant in hormone receptor-positive, human epidermal growth factor receptor 2-negative advanced breast cancer: MONALEESA-3. J Clin Oncol. 2018;3:JCO2018789909. https://doi.org/10.1200/JCO.2018.78.9909. [Epub ahead of print]

72. Nanda R, Chow LQ, Dees EC, Berger R, Gupta S, Geva R, et al. Pembrolizumab in patients with advanced triple-negative breast cancer: phase Ib KEYNOTE-012 study. J Clin Oncol. 2016;34(21):2460–7.
73. Finn RS, Martin M, Rugo HS, Jones S, Im SA, Gelmon K, et al. Palbociclib and letrozole in advanced breast cancer. N Engl J Med. 2016;375(20):1925–36.
74. Hortobagyi GN, Stemmer SM, Burris HA, Yap YS, Sonke GS, Paluch-Shimon S, et al. Ribociclib as first-line therapy for HR-positive, advanced breast cancer. N Engl J Med. 2016;375(18):1738–48.
75. Perez EA, Barrios C, Eiermann W, Toi M, Im YH, Conte P, et al. Trastuzumab emtansine with or without pertuzumab versus trastuzumab plus taxane for human epidermal growth factor receptor 2-positive, advanced breast cancer: primary results from the phase III MARIANNE study. J Clin Oncol. 2017;35(2):141–8.
76. Badwe R, Hawaldar R, Nair N, Kaushik R, Parmar V, Siddique S, et al. Locoregional treatment versus no treatment of the primary tumour in metastatic breast cancer: an open-label randomised controlled trial. Lancet Oncol. 2015;16(13):1380–8.
77. Soran A, Ozmen V, Ozbas S, Karanlik H, Muslumanoglu M, Igci A, et al. Randomized trial comparing resection of primary tumor with no surgery in stage IV breast cancer at presentation: protocol MF07-01. Ann Surg Oncol. 2018. https://doi.org/10.1245/s10434-018-6494-6. [Epub ahead of print].
78. Piccart M, Hortobagyi GN, Campone M, Pritchard KI, Lebrun F, Ito Y, et al. Everolimus plus exemestane for hormone-receptor-positive, human epidermal growth factor receptor-2-negative advanced breast cancer: overall survival results from BOLERO-2†. Ann Oncol. 2014;25:2357–62.
79. Finn RS, Crown JP, Lang I, Boer K, Bondarenko IM, Kulyk SO, et al. The cyclin-dependent kinase 4/6 inhibitor palbociclib in combination with letrozole versus letrozole alone as first-line treatment of oestrogen receptor-positive, HER2-negative, advanced breast cancer (PALOMA-1/TRIO-18): a randomised phase 2 study. Lancet Oncol. 2015;16:25–35.
80. Cristofanilli M, Turner NC, Bondarenko I, Ro J, Im SA, Masuda N, et al. Fulvestrant plus palbociclib versus fulvestrant plus placebo for treatment of hormone-receptor-positive, HER2-negative metastatic breast cancer that progressed on previous endocrine therapy (PALOMA-3): final analysis of the multicentre, double-blind, phase 3 randomised controlled trial. Lancet Oncol. 2016;17(4):425–39.
81. Turner NC, Ro J, André F, Loi S, Verma S, Iwata H, et al. Palbociclib in hormone-receptor–positive advanced breast cancer. N Engl J Med. 2015. https://doi.org/10.1056/NEJMoa1505270.
82. Rugo HS, Rumble RB, Macrae E, Barton DL, Connolly HK, Dickler MN, et al. Endocrine therapy for hormone receptor–positive metastatic breast cancer: American Society of Clinical oncology guideline. J Clin Oncol. 2016;34:3069–103.
83. Jerusalem G, Mariani G, Ciruelos EM, Martin M, Tjan-Heijnen VC, Neven P, et al. Safety of everolimus plus exemestane in patients with hormone-receptor-positive, HER2-negative locally advanced or metastatic breast cancer progressing on prior non-steroidal aromatase inhibitors: primary results of a phase IIIb, open-label, single-arm, expanded-access multicenter trial (BALLET). Ann Oncol. 2016;27(9):1719–25.
84. Kurian AW, Hare EE, Mills MA, Kingham KE, McPherson L, Whittemore AS, et al. Clinical evaluation of a multiple-gene sequencing panel for hereditary cancer risk assessment. J Clin Oncol. 2014;32(19):2001–9.
85. Rageth CJ, O'Flynn EA, Comstock C, Kurtz C, Kubik R, Madjar H, et al. First International Consensus Conference on lesions of uncertain malignant potential in the breast (B3 lesions). Breast Cancer Res Treat. 2016;159:203–13.
86. Strode M, Khoury T, Mangieri C, Takabe K. Update on the diagnosis and management of malignant phyllodes tumors of the breast. Breast. 2017;33:91–6.

87. Li YJ, Huang XE, Zhou XD. Local breast cancer recurrence after mastectomy and breast-conserving surgery for Paget's disease: a meta-analysis. Breast Care. 2014;9(6):431–4.
88. Shafique MR, Lee MC, Han HS. Treatment of the pregnant patient with breast cancer. South Med J. 2017;110(10):627–31.
89. Mir O, Berveiller P, Goffinet F, Treluyer JM, Serreau R, Goldwasser F, et al. Taxanes for breast cancer during pregnancy: a systematic review. Ann Oncol. 2010;21:425–6.
90. Garcia-Gonzalez J, Cueva J, Lamas MJ, Curiel T, Graña B, López-López R. Paclitaxel and cisplatin in the treatment of metastatic non-small-cell lung cancer during pregnancy. Clin Transl Oncol. 2008;10:375–6.
91. Bader AA, Schlembach D, Tamussino KF, Pristauz G, Petru E. Anhydramnios associated with-administration of trastuzumab and paclitaxel for metastatic breast cancer during pregnancy. Lancet Oncol. 2007;8:79–81.
92. Amant F, Deckers S, Van Calsteren K, Loibl S, Halaska M, Brepoels L, et al. Breast cancer in pregnancy: recommendations of an international consensus meeting. Eur J Cancer. 2010;46:3158–68.

Chapter 2
Breast Cancer Staging

Neslihan Cabioglu, Ekrem Yavuz, and Adnan Aydiner

Introduction

The TNM staging system for breast cancer described by the American Joint Committee on Cancer (AJCC) applies to invasive and in situ carcinomas with or without microinvasion [1, 2]. This classification system was introduced to reflect the risk of recurrence and for use as a standard prognostic assessment tool for patients with newly diagnosed breast cancer. The improved understanding of prognostic and predictive biological markers, such as estrogen receptor (ER) and HER2 overexpression, has been used to predict the response to systemic therapies (antiestrogen, anti-HER2) [3, 4]. Therefore, rapid advances in both clinical and laboratory sciences along with translational research have raised questions about the feasibility of using the TNM staging as a guide to determine whether to apply systemic therapy based on anatomic prognosis. A recently reported validation study has emphasized that the prognostic stage provides more accurate prognostic information than does the anatomic stage alone, thus

N. Cabioglu
Department of General Surgery, Istanbul Medical Faculty, Istanbul University, Istanbul, Turkey

E. Yavuz
Department of Pathology, Istanbul Medical Faculty, Istanbul University, Istanbul, Turkey
e-mail: yavuze@istanbul.edu.tr

A. Aydiner (✉)
Internal Medicine, Medical Oncology, Istanbul Medical Faculty, Department of Medical Oncology, Institute of Oncology, Istanbul University, Istanbul, Turkey

A. Aydiner et al. (eds.), *Breast Cancer*, https://doi.org/10.1007/978-3-319-96947-3_2

supporting the use of prognostic stage in breast cancer staging [5]. Furthermore, breast cancer therapy has evolved with the increasing application of neoadjuvant therapy, so additional pretreatment and post-treatment staging have been incorporated into the TNM staging system to determine chemotherapy response and treatment efficacy.

Changes in Breast Cancer Staging

Due to advances in personalized medicine, the last update of AJCC Breast Cancer Staging incorporated more molecular gene assays and new prognostic and predictive markers [6–9]. Lobular carcinoma in situ was removed from TNM staging. An anatomic stage table, clinical prognostic stage table and pathological prognostic stage table were added in the 8th edition. The pathological stage table is based on clinical information, biomarker data, and findings from surgery and resected tissue. The largest contiguous tumor or tumor deposit is used for pT and pN; for the primary tumor, the sizes of multiple tumors or lymph node-adjacent satellite tumors are not added. The last edition clarified the post neoadjuvant therapy pathological T category (ypT), which is based on the largest contiguous focus of residual invasive cancer, if present. When multiple foci of a residual tumor are present, the (m) modifier is included. Although multi-gene expression assays may provide additional prognostic and predictive information beyond anatomic TNM staging and ER/PR and HER2 status, incorporating these biomarkers into the TNM system may be difficult. In the AJCC 8th edition, for patients with T1 and T2 hormone receptor-positive, HER-2 negative, and lymph node-negative tumors, a multigene panel is included in pathological prognostic staging. In the low-risk range, these tumors are placed in the same prognostic group category as T1a-T1bN0M0 regardless of T size (Tables 2.1, 2.2, 2.3, and 2.4).

Prognostic Breast Cancer Staging

Tumor Size

Tumor size should ideally be measured before fixation and should be checked with microscopic size. Many studies have shown that patients with smaller tumors have better long-term survival than do those with larger tumors [10–13]. Tumor size is based on the size of the invasive component of the tumor [14, 15]. In cases with an accompanying in situ component, the in situ area that is outside the invasive tumor is not included in the tumor size 'T'. However, if the in situ

Table 2.1 TNM primary tumor definitions

T: TNM primary tumor definitions[a]
Tx: Primary tumor cannot be assessed
T₀: No evidence of primary tumor
Tis: Carcinoma in situ
• Tis (DCIS)[b]: Ductal carcinoma in situ
• *Tis (LCIS): Lobular carcinoma* in situ *(LCIS is treated as a benign entity and was removed from TNM staging in the AJCC 8th edition)*
• Tis (Paget): Paget's disease of the nipple (without an invasive carcinoma and/or carcinoma in situ (DCIS) in the underlying parenchyma)
T1: T <2 cm
• T1mi: ≤0.1 cm (microinvasive tumor)
• Tla: > 0.1 cm, <0.5 cm (AJCC 8th edition: round any measurement >1.0–1.9 mm to 2 mm)
• Tlb: >0.5 cm, ≤1 cm
• Tlc: >1 cm, ≤2 cm
T2: >2 cm, ≤5 cm
T3: T > 5 cm
T4: Regardless of the size of the tumor: (a) involvement of the thoracic wall: *ribs, intercostal muscles and serratus muscles*; (b) skin involvement (ulceration or macroscopic nodules); invasion of the dermis alone does not qualify as T4b
• T4a: Extension to the chest wall including muscularis pectoralis major (invasion or adherence to pectoralis muscle in the absence of invasion of chest wall structures does not qualify as T4)
• T4b: Edema, peau d'orange, ulceration, macroscopic satellite skin nodules in the ipsilateral breast (not an inflammatory carcinoma)
• T4c: a + b
• T4d: Inflammatory breast cancer

[a]Small microscopic satellite foci of the tumor around the primary tumor do not appreciably alter tumor volume and are not added to the maximum size (AJCC 8th). The 8th edition specifically continues using only the maximum dimension of the largest tumor for cT and pT, and the sizes of multiple tumors are not added

[b]The assigned grade should be nuclear grade

component is intermingled with the invasive area, T includes these in situ areas. If there are multiple areas of invasion, the size of the largest invasive carcinoma is used in T staging.

Lymph Node Status

Lymph node staging should be based on histological evaluation of the excised lymph nodes since clinical evaluation is not sufficient for accurate staging. The dimension of the area containing several or multiple tumor deposits is not used

Table 2.2 Clinical classification of regional lymph nodes and distant metastases

Clinical classification of regional lymph nodes (cN)
cNx: Regional lymph nodes cannot be assessed (e.g., previously removed)
cN0: No regional lymph node metastases
c N1: Metastases movable ipsilateral level I, II axillary lymph nodes
• *cN1mi*[a]: >0.2–2 mm, approximately 200 cells
cN2
• *cN2a*: Metastases in the ipsilateral level I, II axillary lymph nodes fixed to one another or to other structures
• *cN2b*: Metastases only in imaging detected ipsilateral internal mammary nodes (excluding lymphoscintigraphy) in the absence of axillary metastases
cN3
• *cN3a*: Ipsilateral infraclavicular lymph node(s) (level III axillary) metastasis
• *cN3b*: Ipsilateral internal mammary lymph node metastasis with axillary lymph node(s) metastases
• *cN3c*: Ipsilateral supraclavicular lymph node metastases
Distant metastases (M)
Mx Distant metastasis unknown
M0 No clinical or radiological evidence of distant metastases
• cM0 (i+) No clinical or radiological evidence of distant metastases, but deposits of molecularly or microscopically detected tumor cells in circulating blood, bone marrow, or other non-regional nodal tissue that are not larger than 0.2 mm in a patient without symptoms or signs of metastases
cM1 Distant detectable metastases as determined by classic clinical and radiographic means and/or histologically proven larger than 0.2 mm

[a]In cases where sentinel lymph node biopsy is performed before tumor resection (before neoadjuvant therapy)

to determine the pN category. The largest contiguous tumor deposit is used for pN; adjacent satellite tumor deposits are not included.

Hormone Receptors

The ER is a nuclear transcription factor that is a regulator of cellular growth, proliferation, and differentiation in the breast epithelium. Progesterone receptor (PR) is an estrogen-regulated gene, and its expression therefore indicates a functioning ER pathway.

Immunohistochemical determination of these receptors is the standard tool in current pathology-oncology practice. A cutoff of 1% of tumor cells is recommended for a specimen to be considered positive for ER or PR because clinical data have indicated that these patients can respond to hormonal treatment [3].

Table 2.3 Pathological classification of regional lymph nodes

Pathological classification of regional lymph nodes (pN)[a]
pNx: Regional lymph nodes cannot be assessed (e.g., previously removed or not removed for pathologic study)
pN0: No regional lymph node metastasis identified histologically
• pN0 (i−): No regional lymph node metastases, immunohistochemistry (IHC) (−)
• pN0 (i+): Malignant cells in regional lymph nodes no greater than 0.2 mm [detected by H&E or IHC including isolated tumor cells (ITC)]
• pN0 (mol−): No regional lymph node metastases, negative molecular findings: RT-PCR (−)
• pN0 (mol+): Positive molecular findings by reverse transcriptase polymerase chain reaction (RT-PCR) (+); no ITCs detected
pN1
• pN1mic: Micrometastases >0.2 mm and/or >200 cells, ≤2 mm
• pN1a: Metastases in 1–3 axillary lymph nodes, at least one metastasis greater than 2 mm
• pN1b: Metastases in ipsilateral internal mammary nodes (excluding ITCs), with micrometastasis or macrometastases detected by sentinel lymph node biopsy but not clinically or by imaging
• pN1c Metastases in 1–3 axillary lymph nodes and metastases in internal mammary nodes with micrometastasis or macrometastases detected by sentinel lymph node biopsy but not clinically or by imaging (pN1a and pN1b combined)
pN2
• pN2a: Metastases in 4–9 axillary lymph nodes (at least one tumor deposit >2.0 mm)
• pN2b: Metastases in clinically/radiologically detected internal mammary lymph node metastases (except lymphoscintigraphy) with or without microscopic confirmation in the absence of axillary lymph node metastases
pN3
• pN3a: 10 or more axillary lymph nodes (at least one tumor deposit >2.0 mm) or metastases to the infraclavicular (level 3 axillary) lymph nodes
• pN3b: Metastases in clinically/radiologically detected (except lymphoscintigraphy) ipsilateral internal mammary lymph nodes plus at least one axillary lymph node metastasis, or metastases in more than 3 axillary lymph nodes and internal mammary lymph node micro- or macrometastases detected by SLNB (not clinically/radiologically)
• pN3c: Metastases in ipsilateral supraclavicular lymph nodes
pM1 Any histologically proven metastases in distant organs or, if in non-regional nodes, metastases greater than 0.2 mm

[a]The largest contiguous tumor deposit is used for pN; adjacent satellite tumor deposits are not included in the 8th edition

HER-2 Test

The most commonly used methods to evaluate HER2/neu in breast cancer are immunohistochemistry (IHC) and in situ hybridization (ISH). ISH determines the number of HER2 copies using a DNA probe coupled to a fluorescent (FISH), chromogenic (CISH) or silver (SISH) detection system.

Table 2.4 Postneoadjuvant therapy staging

Postneoadjuvant therapy (yc or ypTNM)
• In the setting of patients who received neoadjuvant therapy, pretreatment clinical T (cT) should be based on clinical or imaging findings. Clinical nodal (cN) status is defined by clinical and radiographic findings (with or without histologic examination)
• Postneoadjuvant therapy T should be based on clinical or imaging (ycT) or pathologic findings (ypT)
• A subscript is added to the clinical *N* for both node-negative and node-positive patients to indicate whether the *N* was derived from clinical examination, fine needle aspiration, core needle biopsy, or sentinel lymph node biopsy. The "sn" modifier is used if sentinel lymph node evaluation without axillary dissection was performed after neoadjuvant treatment
• The post-treatment ypT is defined as the largest contiguous focus of invasive cancer as defined histopathologically with a subscript to indicate the presence of multiple tumor foci. The "m" modifier indicates multiple foci of residual tumor. Note: The definition of post-treatment ypT remains controversial and an area in transition
• Post-treatment nodal metastases no greater than 0.2 mm are classified as ypN0(i+) as in patients who have not received neoadjuvant systemic therapy. However, patients with this status are not considered to have pathologic complete response (pCR)
• A description of the degree of response to neoadjuvant therapy (complete, partial, no response) is collected by the registrar with the post-treatment ypTNM. The registrars are requested to describe how they defined response [by physical examination, imaging techniques (mammogram, ultrasound, magnetic resonance imaging (MRI)), or pathologically]
• If a patient presents with inflammatory disease (cT4d) before neoadjuvant chemotherapy, the cancer is still classified as inflammatory breast cancer after therapy, regardless of the response to neoadjuvant therapy. The post-treatment pathological classification (yPT) should reflect the identified residual disease, e.g., ypT1a(m)
• If a patient presents with Ml prior to systemic therapy, they are considered stage IV and remain stage IV, regardless of the response to neoadjuvant therapy[a]
• Post-neoadjuvant therapy is designated with the "yc" or "yp" prefix. Of note, no stage group is assigned if there is a complete pathologic response (CR) to neoadjuvant therapy, e.g., ypT0ypN0Cm0
• When the only residual cancer in the breast is intralymphatic or intravascular (LVI), the case cannot be classified as pCR, but the ypT0 category is assigned. The presence of in situ cancer after treatment in the absence of residual invasive disease constitutes pCR
• Patients with axillary nodal tumor deposits of any size, including isolated tumor foci less than 0.2 mm, are not classified as having pCR

[a]The stage designation may be changed if postsurgical imaging studies reveal the presence of distant metastases, provided that the studies are conducted within 4 months of diagnosis in the absence of disease progression and that the patient has not received neoadjuvant therapy

In 2013 and 2018 updates of the American Society of Clinical Oncology/College of American Pathologists (ASCO/CAP) guidelines were published [4, 16]. In 2015, a short comment on upcoming modifications was released [17].

HER2 IHC scoring is reported as follows:

Negative Score 0: No staining observed or membrane staining is incomplete, faint/barely perceptible, and within ≤10% of the invasive tumor cells.

Score 1+: Incomplete membrane staining that is faint/barely perceptible and within >10% of the invasive tumor cells.

Equivocal (Score 2+): Weak/moderate complete membrane staining in >10% of the invasive tumor cells or complete and circumferential membrane staining that is intense and within ≤10% of the invasive tumor cells.

Positive (Score3+): Circumferential membrane staining in >10% of invasive tumor cells that is complete and intense.

Samples scoring 3+ are considered unequivocally positive, and those scoring 0/1+ are negative. Equivocal scores (2+) mandate further assessment using ISH. Repeat HER2 testing on a surgical specimen if the initially tested core biopsy is negative is no longer stated as mandatory. A new HER2 test *may* (no longer *should*) be ordered on the excision specimen on the basis of some criteria (such as tumor grade 3) (Table 2.5).

Table 2.5 In situ hybridization (ISH) reporting

ISH reporting
Positive
• Single-probe average HER2 copy number ≥6.0 signals/cell • Dual-probe HER2/CEP17 ratio ≥2.0 with an average HER2 copy number ≥4.0 signals per cell
Negative
• Single-probe average HER2 copy number <4.0 signals/cell • Dual-probe HER2/CEP17 ratio <2.0 with an average HER2 copy number <6.0 signals/cell
Indeterminate
• This category was added in the 2013 update. The test should be reported as indeterminate if technical issues prevent one or both tests (IHC and ISH) from being reported as positive, negative or equivocal. Examples include inadequate specimen handling, artifacts (e.g., crushing or marked edge artifacts) that make interpretation difficult, analytical testing failure or controls that are not as expected. The test should be repeated if possible
2018 Update
• The 2018 update on recommendations for HER2 testing with ISH method cancelled an equivocal result [16]. Instead, forced pathologists to make a judgement as positive or negative using combination of repeated IHC and dual-probe ISH method. According to final update, if the HER2/CEP 17 ratio ≥2.0 and average HER2 copy number is <4.0 the result should be negative after completion of a work-up. If the average HER2 copy number is ≥6.0 and the ratio is <2.0 the result should be positive after completion of a work-up

Grade (G)

Histologic Grade

The Nottingham (Elston-Ellis) modification of the Scarff-Bloom-Richardson (SBR) grading system, also known as the Nottingham Grading System (NGS) [18], is the grading system recommended by professional organizations such as the World Health Organization (WHO) [16], American Joint Committee on Cancer [AJCC], the Royal College of Pathologists (UK RCPath), and CAP [4, 15, 16] (Table 2.6).

NGS is based on the evaluation of three morphological features [14, 18, 19]:

(a) Degree of tubule or gland formation,
(b) Nuclear pleomorphism, and
(c) Mitotic count (found in 10 consecutive high-power fields (HPFs) in the most mitotically active part of the tumor).

Table 2.6 Histologic grade scoring and definition

Feature	NGS[a] score
Tubule formation	
• Majority of tumor (>75%)	1
• Moderate degree (10–75%)	2
• Little or none (<10%)	3
Nuclear pleomorphism	
• Small, regular uniform cells	1
• Moderate increase in size and variability	2
• Marked variation	3
Mitotic counts	
• Dependent on microscopic field area	1–3
G	Grade definition
GX	Grade cannot be assessed
G1	Well-differentiated/favorable; low combined histologic grade: NGS score of 3–5 points
G2	Moderately differentiated/moderately favorable; intermediate combined histologic grade: NGS score of 6–7 points
G3	Poorly differentiated/unfavorable; high combined histologic grade: NGS score of 8–9 points

[a]*NGS* Nottingham Grading System

Table 2.7 DCIS nuclear grade definition

G	Grade definition
GX	Grade cannot be assessed
G1	Low nuclear grade
G2	Intermediate nuclear grade
G3	High nuclear grade

Ductal Carcinoma In Situ (DCIS) Grade (Nuclear Grade)

Most cases of DCIS are positive for ER. Positivity (defined as $\geq$1% of tumor cells) is observed in 70–85% of cases [10]. Expression correlates with the grade of DCIS. Almost all cases of ER-negative DCIS are of high nuclear grade (Table 2.7). PR expression is lower than ER expression.

Gene Expression Tests

Several gene expression profiling assays have been developed in an attempt to predict the survival and response of breast cancer patients to therapies. These are based on the identification of prognostic gene signatures by using microarrays. Many groups have attempted to develop genomic tests based on genomic profiling with the expectation that such tests might better predict clinical outcome than the standard pathological and clinical markers [20–24].

The Expert Panel of AJCC considered incorporating results from multi-gene genomic profile assays into Pathological Prognostic Stage [2]. The *Oncotype DX test (Genomic Health, Redwood, CA, USA)* is a quantitative reverse transcriptase–polymerase chain reaction (RT–PCR) assay. It measures a panel of 21 genes, including 16 cancer-related (prognostic) genes and five reference genes, and generates a recurrence score (RS) that classifies patients as low (RS < 18), intermediate (RS 18–30), or high (RS $\geq$ 31) risk of recurrence [20]. The 10-year distant recurrence rates of each category are 6.8%, 14.3%, and 30.5%, respectively. The Trial Assigning Individualized Options for Treatment (Rx) (TAILORx) study demonstrated that a group of TAILORx trial participants with low 21-gene recurrence score (Oncotype DX® Recurrence Score®) of *10 or less* who received hormonal therapy alone without chemotherapy had a less than 1% chance of distant recurrence at 5 years [21, 23, 24]. In the TAILORx ClinicalTrial, adjuvant endocrine therapy and chemoendocrine therapy had similar efficacy in women with hormone-receptor-positive, HER2-negative, axillary node-negative breast cancer who had a midrange 21-gene recurrence score [23]. However, the chemotherapy benefit for invasive disease-free survival varied with the combination of recurrence score and age ($p = 0.004$), with some benefit of chemotherapy found in women 50 years of age or younger with a recurrence score of 16–25. For patients with T1 and T2 hormone receptor-positive, HER-2 negative, and lymph node-negative tumors in the low risk range, these tumors are placed into the same prognostic group category, T1a-T1bN0M0, regardless of T size.

Conclusion

Due to advances in personalized medicine, the last update of AJCC Breast Cancer Staging incorporated more molecular gene assays and new prognostic and predictive markers (Tables 2.8, 2.9, 2.10, 2.11, 2.12, 2.13, 2.14, 2.15, 2.16, 2.17, 2.18, and 2.19). Clinical and pathological stage tables were incorporated in addition to the traditional anatomical prognostic stage tables. The pathological stage table is based on clinical information, biomarker data, and findings from surgery and resected tissue. It is anticipated that updates will be made on a more frequent basis than the 6- to 8-year cycle of TNM revisions, when relevant validated information is available.

Table 2.8 Clinical prognostic stage: HER2-Positive, ER-Positive, PR-Positive

	T0		T1mi		T1		T2		T3		T4	
AJCC 7th												
N0			IA		IA		IIA		IIB		IIIB	IIIB
N1mi	IB		IB		IB		IIB		IIIA	IIIA	IIIB	IIIB
N1	IIA		IIA		IIA		IIB		IIIA	IIIA	IIIB	IIIB
N2	IIIA	IIIA	IIIA	IIIA	IIIA	IIIA	IIIA	IIIA	IIIA	IIIA	IIIB	IIIB
N3	IIIC	IIIC	IIIC	IIIC	IIIC	IIIC	IIIC	IIIC	IIIC	IIIC	IIIC	IIIC
G[a]	1,2	3	1,2	3	1,2	3	1,2	3	1,2	3	1,2	3
AJCC 8th												
N0			IA		IA		IB		IB		IIIA	IIIB
N1mi	IA		IA		IA		IB		IIA	IIB	IIIA	IIIB
N1	IB		IB		IB		IB		IIA	IIB	IIIA	IIIB
N2	IIA	IIB	IIA	IIB	IIA	IIB	IIA	IIB	IIA	IIB	IIIA	IIIB
N3	IIIA	IIIB	IIIA	IIIB	IIIA	IIIB	IIIA	IIIB	IIIA	IIIB	IIIA	IIIB
G	1,2	3	1,2	3	1,2	3	1,2	3	1,2	3	1,2	3
Differences between AJCC 7 and AJCC 8												
AJCC 7th												
N0							IIA		IIB		IIIB	
N1mi	IB		IB		IB		IIB		IIIA	IIIA	IIIB	
N1	IIA		IIA		IIA		IIB		IIIA	IIIA	IIIB	
N2	IIIA	IIIA	IIIA	IIIA	IIIA	IIIA	IIIA	IIIA	IIIA	IIIA	IIIB	
N3	IIIC	IIIC	IIIC	IIIC	IIIC	IIIC	IIIC	IIIC	IIIC	IIIC	IIIC	IIIC
G	1,2	3	1,2	3	1,2	3	1,2	3	1,2	3	1,2	3
AJCC 8th												
N0							IB		IB		IIIA	
N1mi	IA		IA		IB		IB		IIA	IIB	IIIA	
N1	IB		IB		IB		IB		IIA	IIB	IIIA	
N2	IIA	IIB	IIA	IIB	IIA	IIB	IIA	IIB	IIA	IIB	IIIA	
N3	IIIA	IIIB	IIIA	IIIB	IIIA	IIIB	IIIA	IIIB	IIIA	IIIB	IIIA	IIIB
G	1,2	3	1,2	3	1,2	3	1,2	3	1,2	3	1,2	3

[a]*G* histologic grade

Table 2.9 Clinical prognostic stage: HER2-Positive, ER or PR-Positive

	T0	T1mi	T1	T2		T3		T4
AJCC 7th								
N0		IA	IA	IIA		IIB	IIB	IIIB
N1mi	IB	IB	IB	IIB	IIB	IIIA		IIIB
N1	IIA	IIA	IIA	IIB	IIB	IIIA		IIIB
N2	IIIA	IIIA	IIIA	IIIA		IIIA		IIIB
N3	IIIC	IIIC	IIIC	IIIC		IIIC		IIIC
G	1,2,3	1,2,3	1,2,3	1,2	3	1,2	3	1,2,3
AJCC 8th								
N0		IA	IA	IIA		IIA	IIB	IIIB
N1mi	IA	IA	IA	IIA	IIB	IIIA		IIIB
N1	IIA	IIA	IIA	IIA	IIB	IIIA		IIIB
N2	IIIA	IIIA	IIIA	IIIA		IIIA		IIIB
N3	IIIB	IIIB	IIIB	IIIB		IIIB		IIIB
G	1,2,3	1,2,3	1,2,3	1,2	3	1,2	3	1,2,3
Differences between AJCC 7 and AJCC 8								
AJCC 7th								
N0						IIB		
N1mi	IB	IB	IB	IIB				
N1				IIB				
N2								
N3	IIIC	IIIC	IIIC	IIIC		IIIC		IIIC
G	1,2,3	1,2,3	1,2,3	1,2	3	1,2	3	1,2,3
AJCC 8th								
N0						IIA		
N1mi	IA	IA	IA	IIA				
N1				IIA				
N2								
N3	IIIB	IIIB	IIIB	IIIB		IIIB		IIIB
G	1,2,3	1,2,3	1,2,3	1,2	3	1,2	3	1,2,3

Table 2.10 Clinical prognostic stage: HER2-Positive, ER-Negative, PR-Negative

	T0	T1mi	T1	T2	T3	T4
AJCC 7th						
N0		IA	IA	IIA	IIB	IIIB
N1mi	IB	IB	IB	IIB	IIIA	IIIB
N1	IIA	IIA	IIA	IIB	IIIA	IIIB
N2	IIIA	IIIA	IIIA	IIIA	IIIA	IIIB
N3	IIIC	IIIC	IIIC	IIIC	IIIC	IIIC
G	1,2,3	1,2,3	1,2,3	1,2,3	1,2,3	1,2,3
AJCC 8th						
N0		IA	IA	IIA	IIB	IIIB
N1mi	IA	IA	IA	IIB	IIIA	IIIB

(continued)

Table 2.10 (continued)

	T0	T1mi	T1	T2	T3	T4
N1	IIA	IIA	IIA	IIB	IIIA	IIIB
N2	IIIA	IIIA	IIIA	IIIA	IIIA	IIIB
N3	IIIB	IIIB	IIIB	IIIB	IIIB	IIIB
G	1,2,3	1,2,3	1,2,3	1,2,3	1,2,3	1,2,3
Differences between AJCC 7 and AJCC 8						
AJCC 7th						
N0						
N1mi	IB	IB	IB			
N1						
N2						
N3	IIIC	IIIC	IIIC	IIIC	IIIC	IIIC
G	1,2,3	1,2,3	1,2,3	1,2,3	1,2,3	1,2,3
AJCC 8th						
N0						
N1mi	IA	IA	IA			
N1						
N2						
N3	IIIB	IIIB	IIIB	IIIB	IIIB	IIIB
G	1,2,3	1,2,3	1,2,3	1,2,3	1,2,3	1,2,3

Table 2.11 Clinical prognostic stage: HER2-Negative, ER-Negative, PR-Negative

	T0			T1mi			T1			T2			T3			T4
AJCC 7th																
N0				IA			IA			IIA	IIA		IIB	IIB		IIIB
N1mi	IB			IB			IB			IIB	IIB		IIIA		IIIA	IIIB
N1	IIA	IIA		IIA	IIA		IIA	IIA		IIB	IIB	IIB	IIIA		IIIA	IIIB
N2	IIIA		IIIA	IIIA		IIIA	IIIA		IIIA	IIIA		IIIA	IIIA		IIIA	IIIB
N3	IIIC			IIIC			IIIC			IIIC			IIIC			IIIC
G	1	2	3	1	2	3	1	2	3	1	2	3	1	2	3	1,2,3
AJCC 8th																
N0				IB			IB			IIA	IIB		IIB	IIIB		IIIC
N1mi	IB			IB			IB			IIB	IIIB		IIIB		IIIC	IIIC
N1	IIA	IIB		IIA	IIB		IIA	IIB		IIB	IIIB	IIIB	IIIB		IIIC	IIIC
N2	IIIB		IIIC	IIIB		IIIC	IIIB		IIIC	IIIB		IIIC	IIIB		IIIC	IIIC
N3	IIIC			IIIC			IIIC			IIIC			IIIC			IIIC
G	1	2	3	1	2	3	1	2	3	1	2	3	1	2	3	1,2,3
Differences between AJCC 7 and AJCC 8																
AJCC 7th																
N0				IA			IA				IIA			IIB		IIIB
N1mi											IIB		IIIA		IIIA	IIIB

Table 2.11 (continued)

	T0			T1mi			T1			T2			T3			T4
N1		IIA			IIA			IIA			IIB	IIB	IIIA		IIIA	IIIB
N2	IIIA		IIIA	IIIA		IIIA	IIIA		IIIA	IIIA		IIIA	IIIA		IIIA	IIIB
N3																
G	1	2	3	1	2	3	1	2	3	1	2	3	1	2	3	1,2,3
AJCC 8th																
N0				IB			IB				IIB			IIIB		IIIC
N1mi											IIIB		IIIB		IIIC	IIIC
N1		IIB			IIB			IIB			IIIB	IIIB	IIIB		IIIC	IIIC
N2	IIIB		IIIC	IIIB		IIIC	IIIB		IIIC	IIIB		IIIC	IIIB		IIIC	IIIC
N3																
G	1	2	3	1	2	3	1	2	3	1	2	3	1	2	3	1,2,3

Table 2.12 Clinical prognostic stage: HER2-Negative, ER-Positive, PR-Positive

	T0		T1mi		T1		T2		T3		T4
AJCC 7th											
N0			IA		IA		IIA	IIA	IIB	IIB	IIIB
N1mi	IB		IB		IB		IIB	IIB	IIIA	IIIA	IIIB
N1	IIA	IIA	IIA	IIA	IIA	IIA	IIB	IIB	IIIA	IIIA	IIIB
N2	IIIA	IIIA	IIIA	IIIA	IIIA	IIIA	IIIA	IIIA	IIIA	IIIA	IIIB
N3	IIIC		IIIC		IIIC		IIIC		IIIC		IIIC
G	1,2	3	1,2	3	1,2	3	1,2	3	1,2	3	1,2,3
AJCC 8th											
N0			IA		IA		IB	IIA	IIA	IIB	IIIB
N1mi	IA		IA		IA		IIA	IIB	IIA	IIIA	IIIB
N1	IB	IIA	IB	IIA	IB	IIA	IIA	IIB	IIA	IIIA	IIIB
N2	IIA	IIIA	IIA	IIIA	IIA	IIIA	IIA	IIIA	IIA	IIIA	IIIB
N3	IIIB		IIIB		IIIB		IIIB		IIIB		IIIB
G	1,2	3	1,2	3	1,2	3	1,2	3	1,2	3	1,2,3
Differences between AJCC 7 and AJCC 8											
AJCC 7th											
N0							IIA		IIB		
N1mi	IB		IB		IB		IIB		IIIA		
N1	IIA		IIA		IIA		IIB		IIIA		
N2	IIIA		IIIA		IIIA		IIIA		IIIA		
N3	IIIC		IIIC		IIIC		IIIC		IIIC		IIIC
G	1,2	3	1,2	3	1,2	3	1,2	3	1,2	3	1,2,3
AJCC 8th											
N0							IB		IIA		
N1mi	IA		IA		IA		IIA		IIA		
N1	IB		IB		IB		IIA		IIA		
N2	IIA		IIA		IIA		IIA		IIA		
N3	IIIB		IIIB		IIIB		IIIB		IIIB		IIIB
G	1,2	3	1,2	3	1,2	3	1,2	3	1,2	3	1,2,3

Table 2.13 Clinical prognostic stage: HER2-Negative, ER or PR-Positive

	T0		T1mi		T1		T2		T3		T4	
AJCC 7th												
N0			IA	IA	IA	IA	IIA	IIA	IIB	IIB	IIIB	IIIB
N1mi	IB	IB	IB	IB	IB	IB	IIB	IIB	IIIA	IIIA	IIIB	IIIB
N1	IIA	IIA	IIA	IIA	IIA	IIA	IIB	IIB	IIIA	IIIA	IIIB	IIIB
N2	IIIA	IIIA	IIIA	IIIA	IIIA	IIIA	IIIA	IIIA	IIIA	IIIA	IIIB	IIIB
N3	IIIC	IIIC	IIIC	IIIC	IIIC	IIIC	IIIC	IIIC	IIIC	IIIC	IIIC	IIIC
G	1,2	3	1,2	3	1,2	3	1,2	3	1,2	3	1,2	3
AJCC 8th												
N0			IA	IB	IA	IB	IIA	IIB	IIB	IIIA	IIIB	IIIC
N1mi	IA	IB	IA	IB	IA	IB	IIB	IIIA	IIIA	IIIB	IIIB	IIIC
N1	IIA	IIB	IIA	IIB	IIA	IIB	IIB	IIIA	IIIA	IIIB	IIIB	IIIC
N2	IIIA	IIIB	IIIA	IIIB	IIIA	IIIB	IIIA	IIIB	IIIA	IIIB	IIIB	IIIC
N3	IIIB	IIIC	IIIB	IIIC	IIIB	IIIC	IIIB	IIIC	IIIB	IIIC	IIIB	IIIC
G	1,2	3	1,2	3	1,2	3	1,2	3	1,2	3	1,2	3
Differences between AJCC 7 and AJCC 8												
AJCC 7th												
N0				IA		IA		IIA		IIB		IIIB
N1mi	IB		IB		IB			IIB		IIIA		IIIB
N1		IIA		IIA		IIA		IIB		IIIA		IIIB
N2		IIIA		IIIA		IIIA		IIIA		IIIA		IIIB
N3	IIIC		IIIC		IIIC		IIIC		IIIC		IIIC	
G	1,2	3	1,2	3	1,2	3	1,2	3	1,2	3	1,2	3
AJCC 8th												
N0				IB		IB		IIB		IIIA		IIIC
N1mi	IA		IA		IA			IIIA		IIIB		IIIC
N1		IIB		IIB		IIB		IIIA		IIIB		IIIC
N2		IIIB		IIIB		IIIB		IIIB		IIIB		IIIC
N3	IIIB		IIIB		IIIB		IIIB		IIIB		IIIB	
G	1,2	3	1,2	3	1,2	3	1,2	3	1,2	3	1,2	3

Table 2.14 Pathological prognostic stage: HER2-Positive, ER-Positive, PR-Positive

	T0		T1mi		T1		T2			T3			T4	
AJCC 7th														
N0			IA		IA		IIA			IIB	IIB		IIIB	IIIB
N1mi	IB		IB		IB		IIB	IIB		IIIA		IIIA	IIIB	IIIB
N1	IIA		IIA		IIA		IIB	IIB		IIIA		IIIA	IIIB	IIIB
N2	IIIA	IIIA	IIIA	IIIA	IIIA	IIIA	IIIA		IIIA	IIIA		IIIA	IIIB	IIIB
N3	IIIC	IIIC	IIIC	IIIC	IIIC	IIIC	IIIC		IIIC	IIIC		IIIC	IIIC	IIIC
G	1,2	3	1,2	3	1,2	3	1	2	3	1	2	3	1,2	3
AJCC 8th														
N0			IA		IA		IA			IA	IB		IIIA	IIIB
N1mi	IA		IA		IA		IA	IB		IB		IIA	IIIA	IIIB
N1	IA		IA		IA		IA	IB		IB		IIA	IIIA	IIIB
N2	IB	IIA	IB	IIA	IB	IIA	IB		IIA	IB		IIA	IIIA	IIIB
N3	IIIA	IIIB	IIIA	IIIB	IIIA	IIIB	IIIA		IIIB	IIIA		IIIB	IIIA	IIIB
G	1,2	3	1,2	3	1,2	3	1	2	3	1	2	3	1,2	3
Differences between AJCC 7 and AJCC 8														
AJCC 7th														
N0							IIA			IIB	IIB		IIIB	
N1mi	IB		IB		IB		IIB	IIB		IIIA		IIIA	IIIB	
N1	IIA		IIA		IIA		IIB	IIB		IIIA		IIIA	IIIB	
N2	IIIA	IIIA	IIIA	IIIA	IIIA	IIIA	IIIA		IIIA	IIIA		IIIA	IIIB	
N3	IIIC	IIIC	IIIC	IIIC	IIIC	IIIC	IIIC		IIIC	IIIC		IIIC	IIIC	IIIC
G	1,2	3	1,2	3	1,2	3	1	2	3	1	2	3	1,2	3
AJCC 8th														
N0							IA			IA	IB		IIIA	
N1mi	IA		IA		IA		IA	IB		IB		IIA	IIIA	
N1	IA		IA		IA		IA	IB		IB		IIA	IIIA	
N2	IB	IIA	IB	IIA	IB	IIA	IB		IIA	IB		IIA	IIIA	
N3	IIIA	IIIB	IIIA	IIIB	IIIA	IIIB	IIIA		IIIB	IIIA		IIIB	IIIA	IIIB
G	1,2	3	1,2	3	1,2	3	1	2	3	1	2	3	1,2	3

Table 2.15 Pathological prognostic stage: HER2-Positive, ER or PR-Positive

	T0		T1mi		T1		T2		T3	T4
AJCC 7th										
N0			IA		IA		IIA	IIA	IIB	IIIB
N1mi	IB		IB		IB		IIB		IIIA	IIIB
N1	IIA	IIA	IIA	IIA	IIA	IIA	IIB		IIIA	IIIB
N2	IIIA		IIIA		IIIA		IIIA		IIIA	IIIB
N3	IIIC		IIIC		IIIC		IIIC		IIIC	IIIC
G	1,2	3	1,2	3	1,2	3	1,2	3	1,2,3	1,2,3
AJCC 8th										
N0			IA		IA		IB	IIA	IIB	IIIB
N1mi	IA		IA		IA		IIB		IIIA	IIIB
N1	IB	IIA	IB	IIA	IB	IIA	IIB		IIIA	IIIB
N2	IIIA		IIIA		IIIA		IIIA		IIIA	IIIB
N3	IIIB		IIIB		IIIB		IIIB		IIIB	IIIB
G	1,2	3	1,2	3	1,2	3	1,2	3	1,2,3	1,2,3
Differences between AJCC 7 and AJCC 8										
AJCC 7th										
N0							IIA			
N1mi	IB		IB		IB					
N1	IIA		IIA		IIA					
N2										
N3	IIIC		IIIC		IIIC		IIIC		IIIC	IIIC
G	1,2	3	1,2	3	1,2	3	1,2	3	1,2,3	1,2,3
AJCC 8th										
N0							IB			
N1mi	IA		IA		IA					
N1	IB		IB		IB					
N2										
N3	IIIB		IIIB		IIIB		IIIB		IIIB	IIIB
G	1,2	3	1,2	3	1,2	3	1,2	3	1,2,3	1,2,3

Table 2.16 Pathological prognostic stage: HER2-Positive, ER-Negative, PR-Negative

	T0	T1mi	T1	T2	T3	T4
AJCC 7th						
N0		IA	IA	IIA	IIB	IIIB
N1mi	IB	IB	IB	IIB	IIIA	IIIB
N1	IIA	IIA	IIA	IIB	IIIA	IIIB
N2	IIIA	IIIA	IIIA	IIIA	IIIA	IIIB
N3	IIIC	IIIC	IIIC	IIIC	IIIC	IIIC
G	1,2,3	1,2,3	1,2,3	1,2,3	1,2,3	1,2,3
AJCC 8th						
N0		IA	IA	IIA	IIB	IIIB
N1mi	IA	IA	IA	IIB	IIIA	IIIB
N1	IIA	IIA	IIA	IIB	IIIA	IIIB
N2	IIIA	IIIA	IIIA	IIIA	IIIA	IIIB
N3	IIIB	IIIB	IIIB	IIIB	IIIB	IIIB
G	1,2,3	1,2,3	1,2,3	1,2,3	1,2,3	1,2,3
Differences between AJCC 7 and AJCC 8						
AJCC 7th						
N0						
N1mi	IB	IB	IB			
N1						
N2						
N3	IIIC	IIIC	IIIC	IIIC	IIIC	IIIC
G	1,2,3	1,2,3	1,2,3	1,2,3	1,2,3	1,2,3
AJCC 8th						
N0						
N1mi	IA	IA	IA			
N1						
N2						
N3	IIIB	IIIB	IIIB	IIIB	IIIB	IIIB
G	1,2,3	1,2,3	1,2,3	1,2,3	1,2,3	1,2,3

Table 2.17 Pathological prognostic stage: HER2-Negative, ER-Negative, PR-Negative

	T0			T1mi			T1			T2			T3			T4	
AJCC 7th																	
N0				IA	IA		IA	IA		IIA			IIB	IIB	IIB	IIIB	IIIB
N1mi	IB	IB		IB	IB		IB	IB		IIB		IIB	IIIA	IIIA	IIIA	IIIB	IIIB
N1	IIA			IIA			IIA			IIB		IIB	IIIA	IIIA	IIIA	IIIB	IIIB
N2	IIIA	IIIA	IIIA	IIIA	IIIA	IIIA	IIIA	IIIA	IIIA	IIIA	IIIA	IIIA	IIIA	IIIA	IIIA	IIIB	IIIB
N3	IIIC	IIIC		IIIC	IIIC		IIIC	IIIC		IIIC	IIIC		IIIC	IIIC		IIIC	IIIC
G	1	2	3	1	2	3	1	2	3	1	2	3	1	2	3	1	2,3
AJCC 8th																	
N0				IA	IB		IA	IB		IIA			IIB	IIB	IIIA	IIIB	IIIC
N1mi	IA	IB	IB	IA	IB	IB	IA	IB		IIB		IIIA	IIIA	IIIB	IIIC	IIIB	IIIC
N1	IIA			IIA			IIA			IIB		IIIA	IIIA	IIIB	IIIC	IIIB	IIIC
N2	IIIA	IIIB	IIIC	IIIA	IIIB	IIIC	IIIA	IIIB	IIIC	IIIA	IIIB	IIIC	IIIA	IIIB	IIIC	IIIB	IIIC
N3	IIIB	IIIC		IIIB	IIIC		IIIB	IIIC		IIIB	IIIC		IIIB	IIIC		IIIB	IIIC
G	1	2	3	1	2	3	1	2	3	1	2	3	1	2	3	1	2,3
Differences between AJCC 7 and AJCC 8																	
AJCC 7th																	
N0					IA			IA							IIB		IIIB
N1mi	IB			IB			IB					IIB		IIIA	IIIA		IIIB
N1												IIB		IIIA	IIIA		IIIB
N2		IIIA	IIIA		IIIA	IIIA		IIIA	IIIA		IIIA	IIIA		IIIA	IIIA		IIIB
N3	IIIC			IIIC			IIIC			IIIC			IIIC			IIIC	
G	1	2	3	1	2	3	1	2	3	1	2	3	1	2	3	1	2,3

AJCC 8th																	
N0					IB			IB							IIIA		IIIC
N1mi	IA			IA			IA					IIIA		IIIB	IIIC		IIIC
N1												IIIA		IIIB	IIIC		IIIC
N2		IIIB	IIIC		IIIB	IIIC		IIIB	IIIC		IIIB	IIIC		IIIB	IIIC		IIIC
N3	IIIB			IIIB			IIIB			IIIB			IIIB			IIIB	
G	1	2	3	1	2	3	1	2	3	1	2	3	1	2	3	1	2,3

Table 2.18 Pathological prognostic stage: HER2-Negative, ER-Positive, PR-Positive

	T0		T1mi		T1		T2			T3			T4	
AJCC 7th														
N0			IA		IA		IIA	IIA	IIA	IIB	IIB	IIB	IIIB	IIIB
N1mi	IB		IB		IB		IIB	IIB	IIB	IIIA	IIIA	IIIA	IIIB	IIIB
N1	IIA	IIA	IIA	IIA	IIA	IIA	IIB	IIB	IIB	IIIA	IIIA	IIIA	IIIB	IIIB
N2	IIIA	IIIA	IIIA	IIIA	IIIA	IIIA	IIIA	IIIA	IIIA	IIIA	IIIA	IIIA	IIIB	IIIB
N3	IIIC	IIIC	IIIC	IIIC	IIIC	IIIC	IIIC	IIIC	IIIC	IIIC	IIIC	IIIC	IIIC	IIIC
G	1,2	3	1,2	3	1,2	3	1	2	3	1	2	3	1,2	3
AJCC 8th														
N0			IA		IA		IA	IA	IB[a]	IA	IB	IIA	IIIA	IIIB
N1mi	IA		IA		IA		IA	IB	IIA	IB	IB	IIB	IIIA	IIIB
N1	IA	IB	IA	IB	IA	IB	IA	IB	IIA	IB	IB	IIB	IIIA	IIIB
N2	IB	IIB	IB	IIB	IB	IIB	IB	IB	IIB	IB	IB	IIB	IIIA	IIIB
N3	IIIA	IIIB	IIIA	IIIB	IIIA	IIIB	IIIA	IIIA	IIIB	IIIA	IIIA	IIIB	IIIA	IIIB
G	1,2	3	1,2	3	1,2	3	1	2	3	1	2	3	1,2	3
Differences between AJCC 7 and AJCC 8														
AJCC 7th														
N0							IIA	IIA	IIA	IIB	IIB	IIB	IIIB	
N1mi	IB		IB		IB		IIB	IIB	IIB	IIIA	IIIA	IIIA	IIIB	
N1	IIA	IIA	IIA	IIA	IIA	IIA	IIB	IIB	IIB	IIIA	IIIA	IIIA	IIIB	
N2	IIIA	IIIA	IIIA	IIIA	IIIA	IIIA	IIIA	IIIA	IIIA	IIIA	IIIA	IIIA	IIIB	
N3	IIIC	IIIC	IIIC	IIIC	IIIC	IIIC	IIIC	IIIC	IIIC	IIIC	IIIC	IIIC	IIIC	IIIC
G	1,2	3	1,2	3	1,2	3	1	2	3	1	2	3	1,2	3

AJCC 8th

N0							IA	IA	IB[a]	IA	IB	IIA	IIIA	
N1mi	IA		IA		IA		IA	IB	IIA	IB	IB	IIB	IIIA	
N1	IA	IB	IA	IB	IA	IB	IA	IB	IIA	IB	IB	IIB	IIIA	
N2	IB	IIB	IB	IIB	IB	IIB	IB	IB	IIB	IB	IB	IIB	IIIA	
N3	IIIA	IIIB	IIIA	IIIB	IIIA	IIIB	IIIA	IIIA	IIIB	IIIA	IIIA	IIIB	IIIA	IIIB
G	1,2	3	1,2	3	1,2	3	1	2	3	1	2	3	1,2	3

[a]When the Oncotype Dx test result is less than 11 (Level 1 evidence) or a multigene panel, genomic profile, and signature score are in the low-risk category, the case should be assigned as IA

Table 2.19 Pathological prognostic stage: HER2-Negative, ER or PR-Positive

	T0			T1mi			T1			T2			T3			T4	
AJCC 7th																	
N0				IA			IA			IIA	IIA		IIB			IIIB	IIIB
N1mi	IB			IB			IB			IIB			IIIA			IIIB	IIIB
N1	IIA	IIA		IIA	IIA		IIA	IIA		IIB			IIIA			IIIB	IIIB
N2	IIIA			IIIA			IIIA			IIIA			IIIA			IIIB	IIIB
N3	IIIC		IIIC	IIIC		IIIC	IIIC		IIIC	IIIC		IIIC	IIIC		IIIC	IIIC	IIIC
G	1	2	3	1	2	3	1	2	3	1	2	3	1	2	3	1,2	3
AJCC 8th																	
N0				IA			IA			IB[a]	IIA[a]		IIB			IIIB	IIIC
N1mi	IA			IA			IA			IIB			IIIA			IIIB	IIIC
N1	IB	IIA		IB	IIA		IB	IIA		IIB			IIIA			IIIB	IIIC
N2	IIIA			IIIA			IIIA			IIIA			IIIA			IIIB	IIIC
N3	IIIB		IIIC	IIIB		IIIC	IIIB		IIIC	IIIB		IIIC	IIIB		IIIC	IIIB	IIIC
G	1	2	3	1	2	3	1	2	3	1	2	3	1	2	3	1,2	3
Differences between AJCC 7 and AJCC 8																	
AJCC 7th																	
N0										IIA	IIA						IIIB
N1mi	IB			IB			IB										IIIB
N1	IIA			IIA			IIA										IIIB
N2																	IIIB
N3	IIIC			IIIC			IIIC			IIIC			IIIC			IIIC	
G	1	2	3	1	2	3	1	2	3	1	2	3	1	2	3	1,2	3
AJCC 8																	
N0										IB[a]	IIA[a]						IIIC
N1mi	IA			IA			IA										IIIC
N1	IB			IB			IB										IIIC
N2																	IIIC
N3	IIIB			IIIB			IIIB			IIIB			IIIB			IIIB	
G	1	2	3	1	2	3	1	2	3	1	2	3	1	2	3	1,2	3

[a]When the Oncotype Dx test result is less than 11 (Level 1 evidence) or a multigene panel, genomic profile, and signature score are in the low-risk category, the case should be assigned as IA

References

1. AJCC. In: Edge SB, Byrd DR, Compton CC, Fritz AG, Greene FL, Trotti A, editors. Cancer staging handbook. From the AJCC cancer staging manual. 7th ed. New York: Springer; 2010.
2. AJCC: American College of Surgeons. In: Amin MB, et al., editors. AJCC cancer staging manual. 8th ed. Basel: Springer; 2017. p. 588–636. https://doi.org/10.1007/978-3-319-40618-3_48.
3. Hammond ME, Hayes DF, Dowsett M, Allred DC, Hagerty KL, Badve S, et al. American Society of Clinical Oncology/College of American Pathologists guideline recommendations for immunohistochemical testing of estrogen and progesterone receptors in breast cancer. J Clin Oncol. 2010;28:2784–95.
4. Wolff AC, Hammond ME, Hicks DG, Dowsett M, McShane LM, Allison KH, American Society of Clinical Oncology, College of American Pathologists, et al. Recommendations for human epidermal growth factor receptor 2 testing in breast cancer: American Society of

Clinical Oncology/College of American Pathologists clinical practice guideline update. J Clin Oncol. 2013;31:3997–40133.
5. Weiss A, Chavez-MacGregor M, Lichtensztajn DY, Yi M, Tadros A, Hortobagyi GN, et al. Validation study of the American Joint Committee on Cancer eighth edition prognostic stage compared with the anatomic stage in breast cancer. JAMA Oncol. 2018;4(2):203–9.
6. Mittendorf EA, Vila J, Tucker SL, Chavez-MacGregor M, Smith BD, Symmans WF, et al. The neo-bioscore update for staging breast cancer treated with neoadjuvant chemotherapy: incorporation of prognostic biologic factors into staging after treatment. JAMA Oncol. 2016;2(7):929–36.
7. Giuliano AE, Connolly JL, Edge SB, Mittendorf EA, Rugo HS, Solin LJ, et al. Breast cancer- major changes in the American Joint Committee on Cancer eighth edition cancer staging manual. CA Cancer J Clin. 2017;67(4):290–303.
8. Chavez-MacGregor M, Mittendorf EA, Clarke CA, Lichtensztajn DY, Hunt KK, Giordano SH. Incorporating tumor characteristics to the American Joint Committee on Cancer breast cancer staging system. Oncologist. 2017;22(11):1292–300.
9. Mittendorf EA, Chavez-MacGregor M, Vila J, Yi M, Lichtensztajn DY, Clarke CA, et al. A staging system for breast cancer patients that reflects the prognostic significance of underlying tumor biology. Ann Surg Oncol. 2017;24(12):3502–9.
10. Elston CW, Gresham GA, Rao GS, Zebro T, Haybittle JL, Houghton J, et al. The cancer research campaign (Kings/Cambridge) trial for early breast cancer- pathological aspects. Br J Cancer. 1982;45:655–69.
11. Fisher ER, Sass R, Fisher B. Pathologic findings from the national surgical adjuvant project for breast cancer (protocol no 4). Discrimination for tenth year treatment failure. Cancer. 1984;53:712–23.
12. Carter GL, Allen C, Henson DE. Relation of tumour size, lymph node status, and survival in 24,740 breast cancer cases. Cancer. 1989;63:181–7.
13. Neville AM, Bettelheim R, Gelber RD, Säve-Söderbergh J, Davis BW, Reed R, et al. Factors predicting treatment responsiveness and prognosis in node-negative breast cancer. J Clin Oncol. 1992;10:696–705.
14. Lakhani S, Ellis IO, Tan PH, van de Vijver MJ, editors. World health organization classification of tumors, WHO classification of tumors of the breast. 2nd ed. Lyon: IARC; 2012.
15. Lester SC, Bose S, Chen YY, Connolly JL, de Baca ME, Fitzgibbons PL, Members of the Cancer Committee, College of American Pathologists, et al. Protocol for the examination of specimens from patients with invasive carcinoma of the breast. Arch Pathol Lab Med. 2009;133(10):1515–38.
16. Wolff AC, Hammond MEH, Allison KH, Harvey BE, Mangu PB, Bartlett JMS, et al. Human epidermal growth factor receptor 2 testing in breast cancer: American Society of Clinical Oncology/College of American Pathologists Clinical Practice guideline focused update. J Clin Oncol 2018. https://doi.org/10.1200/JCO.2018.77.8738.
17. Wolff AC, Hammond ME, Hicks DG. American Society of Clinical Oncology/College of American Pathologists clinical practice guideline upcoming modifications. Proof the clinical practice guidelines are living documents. Arch Pathol Lab Med. 2015;139(8):970–1.
18. Elston CW, Ellis IO. Pathological prognostic factors in breast cancer I. The value of histological grade in breast cancer: experience from a large study with long-term follow-up. Histopathology. 1991;19:403–10.
19. Pathology reporting of breast disease: a joint document incorporating the third edition of the NHS breast screening programme's guidelines for pathology reporting in breast cancer screening and the second edition of the Royal College of Pathologists' minimum dataset for breast cancer histopathology. Sheffield: NHS Cancer Screening Programmes and The Royal College of Pathologists; 2005.
20. Paik S, Shak S, Tang G, Kim C, Baker J, Cronin M, et al. A multigene assay to predict recurrence of tamoxifen-treated, node-negative breast cancer. N Engl J Med. 2004;351(27):2817–26.
21. Sparano JA, Gray RJ, Makowe DF, Pritchard KI, Albain KS, Hayes DF, et al. Prospective validation of a 21-gene expression assay in breast cancer. N Engl J Med. 2015;373:2005–14.

22. Krop I, Ismaila N, Andre F, Bast RC, Barlow W, Collyar DE, et al. Biomarkers to guide decisions on adjuvant systemic therapy for women with early stage invasive breast cancer: American Society of Clinical Oncology clinical practice guideline focused update. J Clin Oncol. 2017;35(24):2838–47.
23. Sparano JA, Gray RJ, Makower DF, Pritchard KI, Albain KS, Hayes DF, et al. Adjuvant chemotherapy guided by a 21-gene expression assay in breast cancer. N Engl J Med. 2018;379(2):111–21. https://doi.org/10.1056/NEJMoa1804710.
24. Stemmer SM, Steiner M, Rizel S, Soussan-Gutman L, Ben-Baruch N, Bareket-Samish A, et al. Clinical outcomes in patients with node-negative breast cancer treated based on the recurrence score results: evidence from a large prospectively designed registry. NPJ Breast Cancer. 2017;3:33. https://doi.org/10.1038/s41523-017-0034-6.

Part II
Pathology of Breast Cancer

Chapter 3
Pathology of Breast Cancer

Sitki Tuzlali and Ekrem Yavuz

Introduction

Histopathologically, breast carcinoma can be simply divided into two major categories depending on involvement of the ductal-lobular system of the breast: *in situ* and *invasive*. In situ carcinoma is divided into ductal carcinoma in situ (DCIS) or lobular carcinoma in situ (LCIS). DCIS is characterized by the neoplastic proliferation of epithelial cells confined to the ductal-lobular system of the breast without evidence of invasion through the basement membrane into the surrounding stroma. Invasive carcinomas can broadly be divided into two categories: invasive carcinoma of no special type (NST) and special subtypes. NST is the most common type of invasive breast cancer.

Carcinoma In Situ

Ductal carcinoma in situ.
Lobular carcinoma in situ.

S. Tuzlali (✉)
Tuzlali Private Pathology Laboratory, Istanbul, Turkey

Istanbul University, Istanbul Medical Faculty, Department of Pathology, Istanbul, Turkey

E. Yavuz
Istanbul University, Istanbul Medical Faculty, Department of Pathology, Istanbul, Turkey
e-mail: yavuze@istanbul.edu.tr

A. Aydiner et al. (eds.), *Breast Cancer*, https://doi.org/10.1007/978-3-319-96947-3_3

Ductal Carcinoma In Situ (DCIS)

DCIS is characterized by the neoplastic proliferation of epithelial cells confined to the ductal-lobular system of the breast without evidence of invasion through the basement membrane into the surrounding stroma. DCIS encompasses a heterogeneous group of lesions that differ with regard to their presentation, histopathological features, biological markers, and risk for progression to invasive cancer [1]. Approximately 10–20% of DCIS cases are bilateral.

The non-comedo subtype is further subdivided into the solid, cribriform (Fig. 3.1), micropapillary, and papillary types.

Recent grading systems use the nuclear grade alone or in combination with comedo necrosis [2]. DCIS is generally divided into three grades according to the nuclear features [3, 4]:

High-Nuclear-Grade DCIS The tumor is composed of large, pleomorphic cells, often with prominent nucleoli. The nuclei are more than 2.5 times the diameter of red blood cells. Chromatin is coarse and clumped, and its distribution is irregular. Comedo necrosis is frequent but not necessary. Polarization toward the luminal surface is usually lost. Mitoses may be frequent.

Low-Nuclear-Grade DCIS The cells are small, monotonous cells that form arcades, micropapillae, and cribriform and solid patterns. Their nuclei are uniform and 1.5–2.5 times the size of normal red blood cells. Nuclei are usually small [1]. The chromatin is finely dispersed. Nucleoli are inconspicuous. Mitoses are sparse, and cell polarization is protected.

Intermediate-Nuclear-Grade DCIS When the lesion cannot be assigned easily to the high- or low-grade DCIS categories, it is diagnosed as intermediate grade.

In the presence of foci of different grades, the case should be graded according to the highest grade.

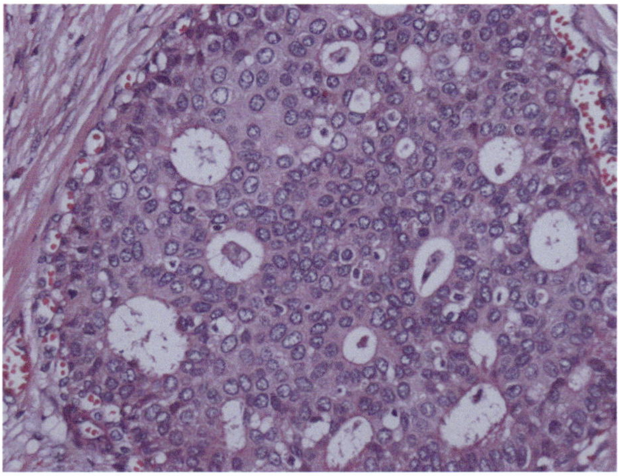

Fig. 3.1 DCIS of cribriform type. Atypical cells filling and distending the duct with formation of a secondary lumina

Pathology Reporting for DCIS

A pathology report for DCIS should include the following [2–5]:

- *Size/extent of the lesion*: Precisely measuring the extent of DCIS is often not possible. The volume of the breast tissue that is involved in DCIS is estimated by the pathologist based on the preferred sampling method. Mammographic correlation is also necessary, and this information should be provided by the clinician.
- *Nuclear grade*
- *The presence or absence of necrosis and its type*: The type of necrosis can be classified as punctate or comedo. Comedo necrosis is associated with mammographic microcalcifications. Punctate necrosis presents small foci or single-cell necrosis that is indistinct at low magnification.
- *Architectural pattern(s)*: Comedo, solid, cribriform, micropapillary and papillary patterns are considered in the traditional classification schemes.
- *Cell polarization*: The presence or loss of polarization toward the luminal surfaces is considered in some grading Schemes [6].
- *Location of microcalcifications*: When microcalcifications are present, their localization should be reported (in DCIS alone, in benign breast tissue, or in both). This information provides the correlation with mammographic findings.
- *Surgical margin status*: The surgeon provides the orientation using sutures or clips. In the presence of microcalcifications, specimen mammography should be provided. The specimen should be inked by the pathologist, and sampling is performed using any of several methods, depending on the pathologist's choice.

Necrosis and polarization appear to have secondary importance compared with the nuclear grade. Sampling the whole lesion is mandatory to exclude any minute foci of invasion before giving a diagnosis of DCIS.

Differential Diagnosis

- *Lobular carcinoma in situ (LCIS) versus DCIS*: DCIS with a solid pattern must sometimes be distinguished from LCIS. This distinction may be difficult. The presence of E-cadherin in immunohistochemical examination may be helpful in categorizing the case in favor of DCIS.
- *Usual ductal hyperplasia (UDH) and atypical ductal hyperplasia (ADH) versus low-grade DCIS*: ADH and low-grade DCIS differ in the extent of the involvement of the duct system. Page and Tavassoli propose that for a lesion to be described as low-grade DCIS, complete involvement should include at least two spaces or be larger than 2 mm [7, 8]. Lesions occupying fewer than two spaces or a total area smaller than 2 mm are called ADH. This distinction is imperfect, and the levels of concordance and consistency in their diagnosis are low [1].
- *Foci of microinvasion*: DCIS extending into a terminal ductal-lobular unit (TDLU) or an adjacent benign proliferative lesion such as sclerosing adenosis (SA) or a radial scar may create the impression of microinvasion. The absence of invasive foci can be confirmed by immunohistochemistry demonstrating the

presence of myoepithelial cells (using antibodies against smooth muscle actin, p63, CD10, calponin, etc.) or basement membrane (using antibodies against collagen type IV or laminin).

Receptor Status

Most cases of DCIS are positive for estrogen receptor (ER). Positivity (defined as $\geq$1% of tumor cells) is observed in 70–85% of cases [2, 3]. Expression correlates with the grade of DCIS. Almost all cases of ER-negative DCIS are of high nuclear grade. Progesterone receptor (PR) expression is lower than ER expression.

Columnar Cell Lesions and Flat Epithelial Atypia

Lesions lacking intraluminal proliferation have long been recognized and have been given a variety of names with regard to cell morphology and the presence or absence of atypia.

A simplified terminology combining the architecture and nuclear atypia under the term flat epithelial atypia (FEA) is now widely used [2, 9]:

- Columnar cell change (CCC)
- Columnar cell hyperplasia (CCH)
- Flat epithelial atypia (FEA)

CCC and CCH are lesions in the TDLU that are characterized by enlarged, variably dilated acini lined by columnar epithelial cells [2]. These lesions are microscopic in size and are increasingly detected as mammographic microcalcifications. The cells have ovoid nuclei that are oriented perpendicularly to the basement membrane, evenly dispersed, fine chromatin, and inconspicuous nucleoli. The lesions are frequently associated with intraluminal secretion and microcalcification. Lesions in which the epithelial lining is composed of one or two cell layers are categorized as CCC. If there is a cellular stratification of more than two layers and a piling up of several layers, the term CCH is used.

Columnar cell lesions are associated with a very low risk for subsequent development of invasive breast cancer, and these lesions do not increase this risk independent of concurrent proliferative changes [10].

FEA: Lesions exhibiting cellular atypia in addition to the architectural patterns described for CCC and CCH are categorized as FEA. FEA is characterized by the replacement of native epithelial cells with one to several layers of monotonous, cuboidal to columnar cells with low-grade cytologic atypia. The cells often have apical snouts. Well-developed bridges or arcades are absent.

A lesion with low-grade nuclear features that has well-developed bridges, arcades, or bulbous micropapillae should be diagnosed as ADH or low-grade DCIS depending on the size of the lesion (see above). The risk of subsequent invasive breast cancer in FEA is low and is substantially lower than the risk associated with established forms of ADH [2]. FEA is often associated with ADH, low-grade DCIS, lobular neoplasia (LN), and tubular carcinoma (TC).

In contrast to the normal breast and UDH, where ER and PR immunostaining is heterogeneous and limited to approximately 10–15% of cells, CCL and FEA present diffuse and homogenous staining in all lesional cells. Most cells show immunostaining for low-molecular-weight cytokeratins and are negative for CK5/6.

Lobular Neoplasia

Lobular Carcinoma In Situ (LCIS) The entire spectrum of atypical epithelial lesions originating in the TDLU of the breast, characterized by the proliferation of generally small, dyscohesive cells, is called LN. Proliferating cells are cuboidal or polygonal monotonous and poorly cohesive cells with clear or light cytoplasm. When more than half of the acini of a lobular unit are distended and distorted, the lesion is called LCIS (Fig. 3.2). Less involvement with cells showing the same characteristics is called ALH [7].

Pleomorphic LCIS The cells are markedly pleomorphic with large nuclei. Central necrosis and microcalcifications may be present [11].

The morphological distinction from solid-type DCIS is discussed above. LN is almost uniformly positive for ER and PR and negative for E-cadherin. Classical LCIS and LCIS with comedo necrosis are negative for HER2 and p53 and have a low Ki-67 index. However, pleomorphic LCIS may have HER2 and p53 overexpression and moderate to high Ki-67 [12].

LN is classically accepted as a risk indicator of breast cancer development for both breasts; however, recent, carefully conducted cohort studies suggest that the risk is higher in the ipsilateral breast (68% versus 24%) [13]. The available clinical and

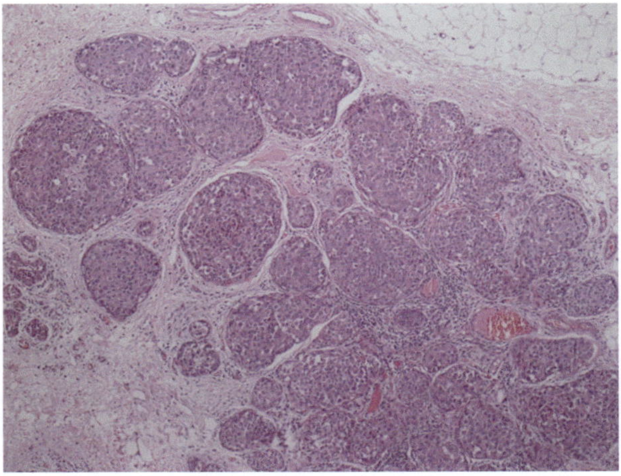

Fig. 3.2 Lobular carcinoma in situ. The breast terminal ductal-lobular unit (TDLU) is distended by atypical, homogenous-appearing cells

molecular evidence suggests that ALH and LCIS are clonal and neoplastic and that these lesions are both risk indicators and non-obligate precursors of breast cancer [14]. **Florid LCIS:** This is a growth pattern of LCIS in which neoplastic cells expand the ducts in a solid architectural pattern similar to solid pattern of DCIS, without having the degree of atypia of pleomprhic LCIS. The florid form of LCIS is more frequently associated with an invasive component than the nonflorid form (87% versus 73%, respectively). The invasive component is lobular in 100% of florid LCIS lesions but only 82% of nonflorid LCIS lesions [15]. Recent evidence also suggests that the florid form of LCIS is genetically more advanced compared with the indolent phenotype of classic LCIS. This difference may explain the higher frequency of concurrent invasive carcinoma in florid LCIS compared with classic LCIS [16].

Microinvasive Carcinoma

This tumor is characterized by one or more clearly separate microscopic foci of infiltration of tumor cells into the mammary stroma, each less than or equal to 1 mm in size, and is most commonly seen in a background of high-grade DCIS [2, 17]. The tumor is accompanied by stromal edema and desmoplasia and inflammatory infiltration [2]. This entity is commonly overdiagnosed. Central consultation usually downgrades the lesion [18].

The prognosis is not clearly different from patients with DCIS of equivalent grade (Figs. 3.1 and 3.2).

Invasive Carcinomas

Invasive carcinomas can broadly be divided into two categories, invasive carcinoma of no special type (NST) and special subtypes [2].

Invasive carcinoma NST and invasive lobular carcinoma (ILC) constitute the major types of breast carcinoma. The cytoarchitectural and spread patterns of some carcinomas are sufficiently distinctive to be recognized as special subtypes, especially when associated with a particular behavior [19].

According to the recent WHO classification, invasive breast carcinomas are classified as indicated in Table 3.1 [2].

Invasive Carcinoma of No Special Type (NST)

This carcinoma is the most common type of invasive breast cancer and represents up to 75% of cases in published series. Terms such as infiltrating ductal carcinoma and invasive ductal carcinoma, not otherwise specified (NOS), are also used.

Table 3.1 WHO classification of breast cancer

Invasive carcinoma of no special type
Pleomorphic carcinoma
Carcinoma with osteoclast-like stromal giant cells
Carcinoma with choriocarcinomatous features
Carcinoma with melanocytic features
Special types
Invasive lobular carcinoma
Classical lobular carcinoma
Solid lobular carcinoma
Alveolar lobular carcinoma
Pleomorphic lobular carcinoma
Tubulolobular carcinoma
Mixed lobular carcinoma
Tubular carcinoma
Cribriform carcinoma
Mucinous carcinoma
Carcinoma with medullary features
Medullary carcinoma
Atypical medullary carcinoma
Invasive carcinoma NST with medullary features
Carcinoma with apocrine differentiation
Carcinoma with signet ring cell differentiation
Invasive micropapillary carcinoma
Metaplastic carcinoma of no special type
Low-grade adenosquamous carcinoma
Fibromatosis-like metaplastic carcinoma
Squamous cell carcinoma
Spindle cell carcinoma
Metaplastic carcinoma with mesenchymal differentiation
Chondroid differentiation
Osseous differentiation
Other types of mesenchymal differentiation
Mixed metaplastic carcinoma
Myoepithelial carcinoma
Epithelial-myoepithelial tumors
Adenomyoepithelioma with carcinoma
Adenoid cystic carcinoma
Rare types
Carcinoma with neuroendocrine features
Neuroendocrine tumor, well differentiated
Neuroendocrine carcinoma, poorly differentiated (small-cell carcinoma)
Carcinoma with neuroendocrine differentiation

(continued)

Table 3.1 (continued)

Secretory carcinoma
Invasive papillary carcinoma
Acinic cell carcinoma
Mucoepidermoid carcinoma
Polymorphous carcinoma
Oncocytic carcinoma
Lipid-rich carcinoma
Glycogen-rich clear cell carcinoma
Sebaceous carcinoma

Modified from Lakhani et al. [2]

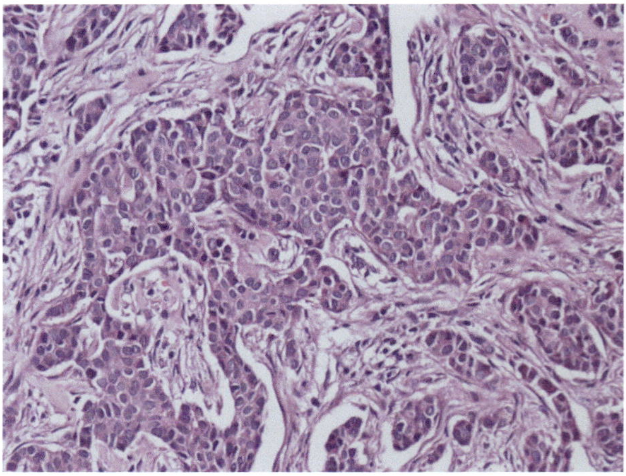

Fig. 3.3 Invasive ductal carcinoma of no special type (NST). Islands are formed by cohesive cells with discernible cytoplasmic borders

A tumor should be called invasive ductal carcinoma (IDC) NST if it cannot be categorized as one of the special or rare types.

Gross Features IDC NST has no specific gross features. It also shows a great variation in size, ranging from a few millimeters to huge masses. In typical cases, these tumors have irregular, stellate borders. They have a firm consistency, and their cut surface is generally gray-white with a gritty sensation. Less frequently, the tumor may have a nodular configuration with a softer consistency.

Microscopic Features The tumor cells are arranged in sheets, clusters, cords, trabeculae, and glands/tubules or sometimes in a solid pattern with no or little intervening stroma (Fig. 3.3). Cellular features also show great variability. Nuclei may be uniform and regular or highly pleomorphic with very prominent and multiple nucleoli. Mitotic activity is also highly variable.

IDC NST may have histopathological characteristics of special types. In IDC NST, at least 50% of the tumor should be composed of a nonspecialized type. The tumor stroma may be abundant. When a proportion of specialized histopathological forms accompany the IDC NST, these carcinomas are described as “mixed type” [2].

Pleomorphic carcinoma, carcinoma with osteoclast-like stromal giant cells, carcinoma with choriocarcinomatous features, and carcinoma with melanocytic features are not recognized as distinct special types but as variants of IDC NST [2]. The latter two are exceptionally rare.

Pleomorphic Carcinoma

Pleomorphic carcinoma is characterized by the proliferation of bizarre, highly anaplastic, and sometimes multinucleated cells. Approximately one-third of cases have a metaplastic spindle cell component [20, 21]. This prognostically unfavorable tumor represents the extreme end of the morphological spectrum of grade III infiltrating ductal carcinoma [20].

Carcinoma with Osteoclast-Like Stromal Giant Cells

The distinctive feature is the presence of osteoclastic giant cells (OGCs). Grossly, they have a striking red-brown cut section with a hemorrhagic appearance. The stroma is hypervascular with recent and old hemorrhages. The associated carcinomas are mostly well to moderately differentiated, showing a relatively more common cribriform pattern. OGCs are positive for CD 68, acid phosphatase, and lysozyme but negative for cytokeratin and alkaline phosphatase [22–25].

The immunohistochemical profile, along with the absence of any epithelial features in ultrastructural examination, supports the histiocytic origin of these cells [24]. They also express osteoclast markers and appear to form in response to the specific hypervascular stroma, which secretes matrix-metalloproteinase-12 (MMP-12) and cytokines such as vascular endothelial growth factor (VEGF) [26].

Axillary lymph node involvement has been reported in one third of cases [23, 24]. The 5-year survival rate is approximately 70%, which is similar to or slightly better than in patients with ordinary invasive ductal carcinoma [2].

Invasive Lobular Carcinoma

ILC is a carcinoma composed of non-cohesive cells that are individually dispersed or arranged in a single-file linear pattern in a fibrous stroma [2]. ILC represents 5–15% of invasive breast carcinomas [2]. In most series, its incidence is approximately 10% [24]. Lobular differentiation accompanying IDC NST is observed in approximately 5% of invasive breast cancers [2].

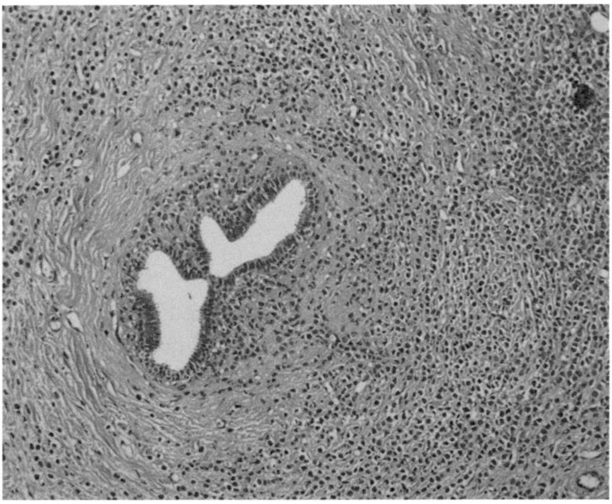

Fig. 3.4 Invasive lobular carcinoma. Single, uniform, small, non-cohesive cells around a duct space

ILC frequently presents as a mass with irregular borders that sometimes cannot be defined macroscopically, and the breast tissue appears normal with only a firm consistency by palpation [23]. The size ranges from occult, microscopic lesions to tumors that diffusely involve the entire breast [23]. Occasionally ILC forms numerous, fine, hard nodules that grossly and microscopically mimic sclerosing adenosis grossly and microscopically. The incidence of synchronous or metachronous bilateral carcinoma in ILCs is almost twice that observed in IDCs [27, 28].

Classical ILC

ILC is characterized by the proliferation of small, uniform cells that lack cohesion and are dispersed individually in a fibrous stroma or arranged in linear cords (Fig. 3.4). These cords usually present a concentric pattern around nonneoplastic ducts, forming a "targetoid pattern". The tumor cells are bland or monotonous and have round to ovoid nuclei. Mitoses are uncommon.

ILC has some histological variants: solid, alveolar, tubulolobular and pleomorphic [29].

Pleomorphic Variant

Pleomorphic ILC exhibits the growth pattern of classical ILC but a greater degree of cellular atypia and pleomorphism and a higher mitotic rate than classical ILC. These cells retain their lobular characteristics with a single-file and/or targetoid arrangement and non-cohesive appearance. LCIS is present in 45–60% of cases [11, 30, 31] and is frequently of the pleomorphic type [31]. Pleomorphic ILC may show apocrine [11] or histiocytoid [32, 33] differentiation and may be composed of signet ring cells [2].

Mixed Type

These cases exhibit mixtures of the abovementioned variants; Dixon [27] noted that "none of these patterns are prominent."

ILC is almost invariably ER positive. PR positivity is present in approximately 70–80% of cases. Her-2 positivity is very rare and is generally limited to pleomorphic ILC. Immunohistochemically, E-cadherin is absent or reduced in ILC compared with IDC. However, a subset of ILCs express E-cadherin, ranging from 10 to 16% of ILCs [34, 35], and this subset is described as aberrant without any significance or any correlation with known prognostic parameters [35, 36].

Most ILCs also show a loss of membrane-specific catenin immunoreactivity in parallel to E-cadherin loss [34] and mislocalization of catenin p120 in the cytoplasm [37].

In general, ILCs have more favorable prognostic features than IDC NST. A higher frequency of ILC was placed in the good Nottingham Prognostic Index group (40% compared with 21% for IDC) [38] and has a better or similar outcome in the short-term period (first 6–10 years). However, the long-term outcome for ILC is worse than that for IDC NST [38, 39]. A more favorable outcome is reported for the classical type than the pleomorphic type [23]. Differences in outcomes between variant forms and classical ILC are not statistically significant [23]. Rakha et al. found that survival in patients with pleomorphic lobular carcinoma was associated with mitotic score but not nuclear pleomorphism [40].

Distinctive patterns of metastases are associated with ILC. ILC shows a higher frequency of metastases in the intra-abdominal serosal surfaces and retroperitoneum, leptomeninges, gastrointestinal tract, and gynecological organs and a lower frequency of pulmonary metastases [2, 22–24].

Tubular Carcinoma

Tubular carcinoma (TC) is a low-grade (grade I) carcinoma with a particularly favorable prognosis. It is composed of well-differentiated tubular structures lined by a single layer of cells and has open lumina. Pure TC accounts for approximately 2% of invasive breast cancers. Its frequency is higher in populations where screening mammography is used. TC is more likely to be smaller lesions with less frequent nodal involvement and a better outcome than IDC NST.

TC often presents as an ill-defined, gray-white, firm to hard, stellate mass with an average size of 1.3 cm (0.2–5 cm). The cut surfaces frequently show elastotic, yellow streaks. Microscopically, the tubules are haphazardly arranged in a typical desmoplastic stroma. The lumina of the tubules are oval or rounded with angulated ends (Fig. 3.5). The single cells lining these tubules have mild nuclear pleomorphism with inconspicuous nucleoli, and they exhibit very few mitoses. The myoepithelial cell layer and basal membrane are lacking in contrast to nonneoplastic proliferations. TC occurs in association with FEA and low-grade DCIS.

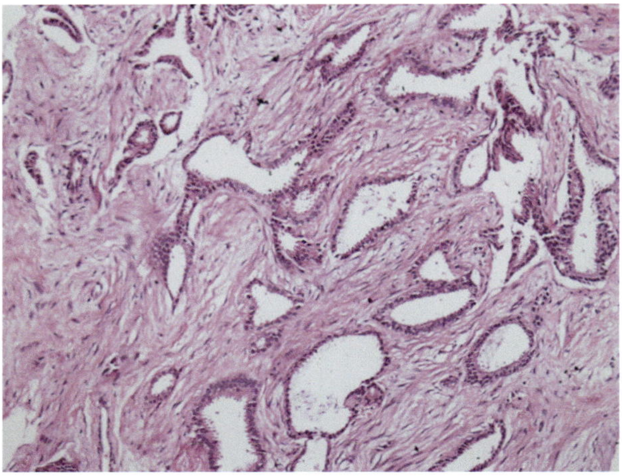

Fig. 3.5 Tubular carcinoma. Well-differentiated tubular structures lined by a single layer of cells

A carcinoma is a pure tubular carcinoma when 90% or more of the tumor consists of tubules [41]. Patients diagnosed with TC with this cut-off and small lesions have the same overall survival as the age-matched general population [41, 42].

Tubule formation in less than 90% of the tumor should be regarded as mixed type. One exception that should be considered is the cribriform pattern. In the presence of invasive cribriform carcinoma (ICC) intermingled with TC, these areas are also regarded as tubule formation.

Differential Diagnosis Microglandular adenosis (MGA): Glands in MGA are more rounded and regular and contain secretory material [2, 24]. The myoepithelium is lacking in both types of lesions, and immunostaining reveals no staining for calponin, p63, CD10, or cytokeratin 5. The basement membrane is lacking in TC, which can be demonstrated around the glands of MGA by periodic acid-Schiff (PAS) staining and immunostaining for collagen IV and laminin [2, 22–24]. Epithelial membrane antigen (EMA), which is present in TC, is absent in MGA [24].

- Sclerosing adenosis (SA): SA is a lobulocentric proliferation containing myoepithelial cells and basement membrane. TC does not have a lobulocentric growth pattern and does not contain myoepithelial cells or a basement membrane.
- Complex sclerosing lesion (CSL) (radial scar): The central fibroelastotic core of this lesion may have a few, distorted, entrapped, pseudoinfiltrative glands, creating diagnostic difficulty through its resemblance to TC. The glands at the periphery of the core are hyperplastic and dilated. This zoning phenomenon is lacking in TC. The glands in CSL also contain myoepithelial cells and a basement membrane.

Women with "pure" TC have an excellent prognosis. The frequency of axillary lymph node metastasis is approximately 10%. TC has a better prognosis than do grade I IDC or tubular mixed carcinomas, independent of other prognostic factors [41, 42]. In a follow-up of 127 months (4–217 months), recurrent disease was found in 13.2% of patients with TCs, with no cancer-specific deaths, compared with patients with grade I IDCs, in which the recurrent disease rate was 29.4% and the cancer-specific death rate was 9% [41].

Invasive Cribriform Carcinoma

ICC is a low-grade carcinoma with excellent prognosis in which the majority of the invasive component shows a cribriform pattern of growth. Pure ICC consists of an invasive cribriform pattern in more than 90% of the tumor [43, 44].

Differential Diagnosis

Adenoid cystic carcinoma (ACC) ICC most closely resembles ACC. ICC is composed of one cell type and lacks the basal-myoepithelial type. Tumor cells are diffusely positive for ER. In ACC, there are two cell types, basal-myoepithelial and luminal; ACC also shows a triple-negative immunoprofile.

Cribriform DCIS ICC has a more irregular and angular cribriform pattern with a more haphazard distribution compared with cribriform DCIS. Cribriform DCIS has a myoepithelial cell layer around the cribriform structures.

In invasive cribriform carcinomas, 100% of cases are ER positive, 69% of cases are PR positive [45], and HER2 expression is absent [24]. The prognosis of ICC is favorable [44] and similar to that of TC [43]. The 10-year overall survival is 90–100% [44, 45].

Carcinoma with Medullary Features

These tumors exhibit some or all of the following features:

- a circumscribed or pushing border,
- syncytial growth pattern,
- cells with high-grade nuclei, and

- prominent lymphoid infiltration.

In the recent WHO classification, these tumors are categorized into three groups under the heading "Carcinomas with medullary features" as follows [2]:

- Medullary carcinoma (MC)
- Atypical MC
- IDC NST with medullary features

The criteria that distinguish these groups are vague and have poor interobserver reproducibility.

Distinguishing between the last two groups is particularly difficult. In our institutional practice, we prefer to reserve the term MC for tumors that exhibit all of the features described above using very strict criteria and to call the tumors that exhibit some of these features atypical MC.

Despite having poor clinicopathological features, patients with medullary histology demonstrate favorable long-term distant relapse-free survival compared with patients with IDC NST. The local control rates of MC and IDC are comparable [46].

In a retrospective study of 165 cases of basal-like carcinomas, the Nottingham group found that prominent inflammation and anastomosing sheets in at least 30% of the tumor were associated with better prognosis in a univariate analysis [47]. The combination of these two features was present in 17% of tumors and was an independent prognostic factor in a multivariate analysis. They also proposed a simplified definition of medullary-like type based on these two features [47].

Mucinous Carcinoma

Mucinous carcinoma is characterized by the production of extracellular and/or intracellular mucinous material. A lesion is called pure mucinous carcinoma if the mucinous component constitutes more than 90% of the lesion [48]. Mucinous carcinoma is also observed as part of a mixed carcinoma with IDC NST. The axillary lymph nodes are rarely involved. Gross examination of mucinous carcinomas reveals a circumscribed, gelatinous mass with pushing margins and soft consistency. The cut surface has a glistening appearance. Confluent hemorrhagic areas are frequent [24].

The tumor size ranges from 0.5 to 20 cm. Despite these large diameters, axillary nodal involvement is infrequent. Microscopically, there are clusters of tumor cells floating in mucin lakes separated by delicate fibrovascular septae. The clusters are variable in size. Mucinous carcinoma can be divided into two categories: types A and B [49]:

Type A mucinous carcinoma: This is the classical or non-endocrine variant and is characterized by larger quantities of mucin. Mucin is always extracellular [24].

Type B mucinous carcinoma: This type is more cellular with large clusters and has frequent neuroendocrine differentiation. Intracytoplasmic mucin is abundant in this type.

Mucinous carcinoma is usually positive for ER and PR and negative for HER2.

The most important entity in the differential diagnosis is the "mucocele-like lesion" [48]. Mucinous carcinoma should also be distinguished from myxoid fibroadenomas, especially in fine-needle aspiration biopsies. Mucinous carcinomas have a favorable outcome [42]. In a follow-up series of 11,400 cases of pure mucinous carcinoma, the 5-, 10-, 15-, and 20-year survival rates were 94, 89, 85, and 81%, respectively [50]. Nodal involvement was associated with significant disease-free survival and overall survival [42]. The separation of cases as types A and B has no clinical significance.

Carcinomas with Signet Ring Cell Differentiation

Cells with signet ring cell differentiation have abundant mucin in their cytoplasm, which pushes the nucleus to one side, creating the typical signet ring cell appearance (Fig. 3.6). This is generally seen as a focal differentiation. Prominent signet ring cell differentiation is most common in ILC. Occasionally, these cases should be differentiated from gastrointestinal metastasis. The presence of an in situ component is a sign in favor of primary breast cancer. In difficult cases, steroid receptor expression and antibodies specific to breast carcinoma such as GCDFP, mammaglobin or GATA-3 are helpful. The prognostic importance of signet ring cell differentiation is uncertain [2].

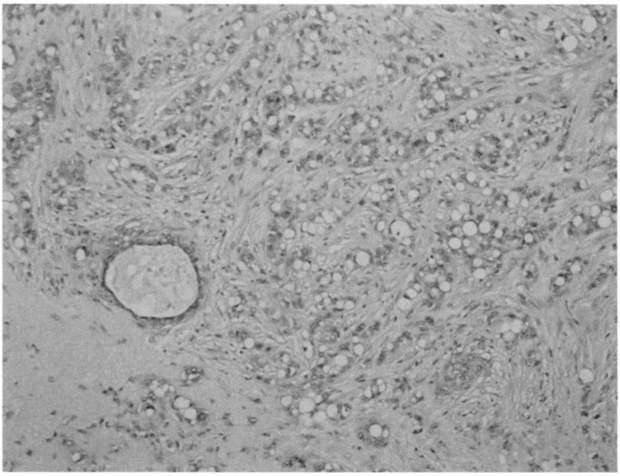

Fig. 3.6 Carcinoma with signet ring cell differentiation. Infiltration of tumor cells with vacuolated cytoplasm resembling a signet ring

Carcinoma with Apocrine Differentiation

This type includes any invasive carcinoma having cells with cytological features of apocrine differentiation. These cells have abundant, eosinophilic, granular cytoplasm and large nuclei with prominent nucleoli. Focal apocrine differentiation is not very rare. ER and PR expression is usually negative. Androgen receptor (AR) positivity is encountered in more than 70% of apocrine carcinomas. GCDFP-15 is characteristic but not specific for apocrine cells [24, 51]. From a practical perspective, we do not call tumors pure apocrine carcinoma if there is ER or PR expression. AR expression in ER-/PR-/HER2+ tumors, which commonly show apocrine differentiation, and a subset of triple-negative apocrine tumors suggests that these tumors together form a molecular apocrine group [52].

A recent study with long-term follow-up revealed that patients with pure apocrine carcinomas (negative for ER and PR and positive for AR) have shorter disease-free survival than patients with IDC NST and apocrine-like IDC (ER or PR positive and AR negative) [53].

Invasive Micropapillary Carcinoma (IMPC)

IMPC accounts for 0.9–1.7% of all invasive breast carcinomas, when occurring in pure form, and up to 7.6%, when admixed with other types of mammary carcinoma [54, 55]. Most patients present with a palpable mass [55]. The tumor is composed of small, hollow, or morula-like clusters of tumor cells that lack fibrovascular cores and are surrounded by clear stromal spaces. The presence of an in situ component is helpful in excluding rare cases of metastatic ovarian serous papillary carcinoma to the breast.

Most cases are grade 2 or 3 carcinomas, and the majority are ER and PR positive. HER2 overexpression is present in less than 10–35% of cases [2]. IMPCs present more frequently with lymphovascular invasion and lymph node metastasis when compared with the IDC NST [56]. However, the association of this histology with survival remains unclear. In a recent series of 49 patients, IMPC histology did not add any independent information to the risk of locoregional or distant relapse or to overall survival [57]. Meng et al. [58] found prostate stem cell antigen (PSCA) gene amplification in 45.2% (14/31) and PSCA protein expression in 58.9% (33/56) of cases of IMPC. These percentages are significantly high compared with IDC NST and may be used as a molecular marker of worse prognosis. In a recent study, we found that the loss of ARID1A expression and Her-2 positivity have significant adverse effects for clinical outcomes of IMPC patients [59].

Metaplastic Carcinoma

Metaplastic carcinoma encompasses a group of neoplasms that are characterized by the differentiation of the neoplastic epithelium into squamous and/or mesenchymal-looking elements, including but not restricted to spindle, chondroid, osseous, and rhabdomyoid cells [2]. The tumor may be entirely composed of metaplastic elements or may include a mixture of carcinoma and metaplastic elements. Its incidence is less than 1% [60, 61]. The mean size is 3.4–4.4 cm [60].

These tumors can present either as a circumscribed nodule or as a mass with indistinct borders. Cystic changes can occur, especially in cases that are accompanied by squamous cell carcinoma (SCC).

The recent WHO classification [2] categorizes metaplastic carcinomas in a descriptive manner:

- Low-Grade Adenosquamous Carcinoma (LGASC)

  This tumor is similar to the infiltrating syringomatous tumors of the salivary glands and microcystic adnexal carcinomas of the skin of the lip [62]. Patients present with a palpable mass [63], and grossly, the tumors are smaller than other forms of metaplastic carcinoma [23]. They have a hard consistency and ill-defined borders [63]. Squamous differentiation may be extensive, with large keratinizing cyst formations. In our experience, this rare tumor is an underdiagnosed entity and therefore may be left untreated; during their long evolution, they recur and metastasize.
- Fibromatosis-Like Metaplastic Carcinoma

  This tumor is characterized by bland spindle cells having slender nuclei with tapered ends. Nuclear atypia is mild or absent. Focal squamous differentiation is observed. Because of the bland appearance of tumor cells, this tumor may be underdiagnosed as benign. The tumor is always positive for keratins [64] and p63 [2]. In a recent study, Takano et al. [65] demonstrated that these tumors are characterized by low genomic instability and share no copy number aberrations with other metaplastic carcinomas. Local recurrence can occur after local excision, and distant metastases occur occasionally.
- Squamous Cell Carcinoma

  Grossly, squamous cell carcinoma is often a cystic lesion [2]. The cavity is lined by squamous cells, often with bland nuclear features. The infiltrating squamous cells form sheets and nests with varying degrees of differentiation. Combinations of patterns with transition to spindle cells or to less differentiated forms may occur. An origin from the overlying skin should be excluded. SCC may be mixed with IDC NST. Focal squamous differentiation can also be found in IDC NST and may accompany carcinomas with medullary features.

- Spindle Cell Carcinoma

  This tumor is characterized by the pseudosarcomatous growth pattern of its neoplastic spindle cells. The distinction between spindle cell carcinoma and primary sarcomas of the breast, including fibrosarcoma and malignant fibrous histiocytoma, may be problematic. Epithelial differentiation can be demonstrated by immunohistochemistry using a panel of antibodies (high-molecular-weight cytokeratins). P63 staining is also very common [66].
- Metaplastic Carcinoma with Mesenchymal Differentiation

  These tumors display an admixture of carcinomatous and mesenchymal elements. Mesenchymal components include chondroid, osseous, and rhabdomyoid elements with varying degrees of differentiation. Metaplastic carcinomas often contain a mixture of different elements.
- Matrix-Producing Carcinoma

  This is a subgroup of metaplastic carcinomas that show an abrupt transition from epithelial to mesenchymal elements without intervening spindle cells.

  More than 90% of metaplastic carcinomas are triple-negative cancers and express keratin 5/6/14 and EGFR [2]. Immunohistochemically, they show a basal-like phenotype, regardless of the types of metaplastic elements. They also overexpress EGFR in more than half of cases [67, 68]. Gene expression profiling has demonstrated that metaplastic carcinomas are part of the spectrum of basal-like breast carcinomas and display a myoepithelial and epithelial-to-mesenchymal transition-like molecular composition [69, 70]. However, there is no consistent immunophenotype, and no individual marker is positive in 100% of cases. Antibodies to a broad spectrum of cytokeratins (AE1/AE3 and MNF116) are most frequently positive (approximately 80%) [71].

  MBCs are genetically complex and heterogeneous, and mutations in PI3K/AKT/mTOR pathway-related and canonical Wnt pathway-related genes are significantly more common than triple-negative IDC NST [72].

Lymph node metastases are less frequent in metaplastic carcinomas than in IDC NST. However, distant metastasis can occur in the absence of lymph node metastasis, as observed in other triple-negative breast cancers [2].

Carcinomas with Neuroendocrine Features

These carcinomas exhibit morphological and immunohistochemical features of endocrine tumors, similar to those observed in the gastrointestinal tract and lung. In the recent WHO classification [2], neuroendocrine breast carcinomas are categorized as follows:

- Neuroendocrine tumor, well-differentiated
- Neuroendocrine carcinoma, poorly differentiated/small-cell carcinoma
- Invasive breast carcinoma with neuroendocrine differentiation

Invasive cancers of NST and other special types may show endocrine differentiation. These tumors do not have any specific clinical presentation.

- Well-Differentiated Neuroendocrine Tumor
  The tumor consists of densely cellular, solid nests and trabeculae of cells separated by a thin fibrovascular stroma [73]. These tumors are of low or intermediate grade (2). There is chromogranin positivity in more than 50% of cases [74]. Other endocrine markers, such as synaptophysin and CD 56, are also positive. These tumors are typically positive for ER and PR and negative for HER2.
- Neuroendocrine Carcinoma
  The tumor is composed of highly atypical cells with hyperchromatic nuclei and scant cytoplasm. Mitotic figures are frequent, and necrosis may accompany the lesion. The tumor should be distinguished from metastatic small-cell carcinoma of the lung; this distinction cannot be made on the sole basis of morphology. The presence of an in situ component supports the diagnosis of the breast as the primary cancer. Monoclonal NSE is positive in all cases of small-cell carcinomas, and other neuroendocrine markers are positive in approximately 50% of cases [2]. ER and PR expression may also be observed in more than 50% of cases and is generally correlated with the degree of differentiation. Small-cell carcinoma is negative for HER2 expression [74, 75].
- Invasive Breast Carcinoma with Neuroendocrine Differentiation
  Mucinous carcinoma of type B and solid papillary carcinoma (SPC) are the most frequent examples of this category [2, 75].

Secretory Carvcinoma

Secretory carcinoma presents as a well-circumscribed mobile mass. The median age of presentation is 25 years. Microscopically, the characteristic finding is the presence of intracellular and extracellular secretory material showing positive staining with PAS. ER, PR, and HER2 are absent. EMA, alpha-lactalbumin, and S-100 protein are frequently present. There is a high expression rate of basal-like markers (CK5/6 or epidermal growth factor receptor) in secretory carcinomas [75]. Tognon et al. [76] showed that 12 of 13 of their cases of secretory breast carcinoma expressed the ETV6-NTRK3 gene fusion. Secretory carcinoma has an indolent clinical behavior, especially in children and young adults [75].

Papillary Lesions

These lesions, especially from the clinical perspective, are often confused with each other. For this reason, all of them will be discussed consecutively under the title "papillary lesions."

- Intraductal Papillary Carcinoma (IDPC)

  IDPC is a malignant, noninvasive neoplastic epithelial proliferation with papillary architectural features that occurs in the lumen of the ductal-lobular system [2]. Two types of IDPC exist:

  - Central, solitary: Presentation may include nipple discharge.
  - Peripheral, multifocal: Presentation may be as a mass.

  Microscopically, ducts or the TDLU is filled with slender, branching fibrovascular stalks, lined by a single layer or several layers of monomorphic epithelial cells. High-grade nuclear features are rare. Solid, cribriform, and micropapillary patterns also exist. There is complete or near-complete (90%) absence of myoepithelial cells in the fibrovascular cores. However, there are myoepithelial cells at the periphery of the involved duct [77, 78].
- Encapsulated Papillary Carcinoma (EPC)

  This lesion has a fibrous capsule, and its size ranges between 0.5 and 8 cm [79]. It is also called intracystic papillary carcinoma. All papillary intraductal carcinomas arise in a background of a variably cystically dilated duct. EPC lacks myoepithelial cells both in the fibrovascular cores and at the periphery [78, 79]. The absence of these cells and reported cases of metastatic tumors raise the possibility that these tumors represent low-grade invasive carcinomas with an expansile growth pattern [80]. However, the presence of continuous and intense collagen IV expression at the periphery is considered highly suggestive of a noninvasive carcinoma that is confined within an intact basement membrane [80]. EPC without an adjacent DCIS or any invasive component has a very favorable prognosis with adequate local therapy. The presence of associated DCIS confers a higher risk of local recurrence.
- Solid Papillary Carcinoma

  SPC is a variant of papillary carcinoma that is characterized by compact cellular growth within multiple nodules representing dilated ducts [55]. It presents in older women [77]. SPC is homogenous and does not form papillary or cribriform patterns. Neuroendocrine differentiation is frequent. Mucin production is common, and invasive mucinous carcinoma may coexist. Other types of invasive carcinoma may also be observed [81]. The distinction between in situ and invasive disease in SPC is difficult. Some authors regard this entity to be an expansile variant of invasive carcinoma [81, 82]. SPC has an indolent clinical course, even in cases with obvious invasion [81].

  In the papillary lesions mentioned above, the lesion is called in situ if there is any doubt about the invasion. If there is obvious invasion, the staging should be conducted according to the measurement of the invasive component [83].
- Invasive Papillary Carcinoma

  Invasive papillary carcinoma (IPC) is a carcinoma with a predominantly papillary morphology in its "invasive" component. This is a rare lesion, and there are no specific clinical and macroscopic features of this tumor. It should be distinguished from invasive carcinomas arising from EPC and SPC. Many older series may have included such cases in this category [55].

Adenoid Cystic Carcinoma

ACC is a carcinoma of low-grade malignant potential that is histologically similar to its counterpart in the salivary gland. This is a rare tumor. Approximately half of the cases arise from the subareolar region [84]. ACC is usually a circumscribed tumor. Histologically, the tumor has the following basic patterns: tubular, cribriform, trabecular, and solid [85]. The neoplastic cells, which are epithelial and myoepithelial (basal), are arranged to form glandular spaces and pseudolumina [24]. With occasional exceptions, ACC is triple negative [24]. Breast ACC rarely involves the axillary lymph nodes, and survival is excellent [84, 86]. A solid variant with basaloid features has a higher frequency of axillary lymph node metastasis [87].

Glycogen–Rich Clear Cell Carcinoma

This is a carcinoma in which 90% or more of the tumor cells have abundant clear cytoplasm containing glycogen [2]. It accounts for 1–3% of breast carcinomas. The clear or finely granular cytoplasm contains PAS-positive diastase-labile glycogen. ER is present in 50% of cases, and PR is absent [23]. This tumor should be distinguished from lipid-rich carcinoma, histiocytoid carcinoma, and metastatic renal cell carcinoma [24]. There are conflicting reports regarding the prognosis of these tumors [88, 89].

Inflammatory Carcinoma

Inflammatory carcinoma (IC) is an aggressive form of breast carcinoma with distinct clinical features. Clinically, there is rapid breast enlargement with edema and erythema of the skin (orange peel skin). Currently, there are no definitive molecular or pathological diagnostic criteria for IC. Therefore, the diagnosis is based on the clinical findings described above [90]. Signs and symptoms required for a diagnosis of IC include erythema occupation of at least one-third of the breast, edema and/or peau d'orange of the breast, and/or a warm breast, without an underlying palpable mass in the majority of cases [90, 91]. IC is not considered a specific histological subtype of breast carcinoma, and there are no special pathological diagnostic criteria for IC [90, 91]. The underlying carcinoma is most often IDC NST of high grade; there may or may not be a distinct mass. The pathognomonic histopathological finding in IC is the presence of many lymphovascular tumor emboli in the papillary and reticular dermis overlying the breast. Approximately 55% of cases are negative for ER and PR, 45% are HER2 positive, and 33% are triple negative [92]. Survival is worse than in patients with locally advanced breast cancer without IC [2].

Mucoepidermoid carcinoma, polymorphous carcinoma, oncocytic carcinoma, sebaceous carcinoma, lipid-rich carcinoma, and acinic cell carcinoma are very rare tumors and beyond the scope of this chapter.

References

1. Ellis IO. Intraductal proliferative lesions of the breast: morphology, associated risk and molecular biology. Mod Pathol. 2010;23(Suppl 2):S1–7.
2. Lakhani S, Ellis IO, Tan PH, van de Vijver MJ, editors. World Health Organization classification of tumors, WHO classification of tumors of the breast. 2nd ed. Lyon: IARC; 2012.
3. Lester SC, Bose S, Chen YY, Connolly JL, de Baca ME, Fitzgibbons PL, Members of the Cancer Committee, College of American Pathologists, et al. Protocol for the examination of specimens from patients with ductal carcinoma in situ of the breast. Arch Pathol Lab Med. 2009;133(1):15–25.
4. Consensus conference on the classification of ductal carcinoma in situ. Hum Pathol. 1997;28:1221–5.
5. Schwartz GF, Solin LJ, Olivotto IA, Ernster VL, Pressman P. Breast. 2000;9:177–86.
6. Holland R, Peterse JL, Millis RR, Eusebi V, Faverly D, van de Vijver MJ, Zafrani B. Ductal carcinoma in situ: a proposal for a new classification. Semin Diagn Pathol. 1994;11(3):167–80.
7. Page DL, Dupont WD, Rogers LW, Rados MS. Atypical hyperplastic lesions of the female breast. A long-term follow-up study. Cancer. 1985;55:2698–708.
8. Tavassoli FA, Norris HJ. A comparison of the results of long-term follow-up for atypical intraductal hyperplasia and intraductal hyperplasia of the breast. Cancer. 1990;165(3):518–29.
9. Schnitt SJ. Clinging carcinoma: an American perspective. Semin Diagn Pathol. 2010;27(1):31–6.
10. Aroner SA, Collins LC, Schnitt SJ, Connolly JL, Colditz GA, Tamimi RM. Columnar cell lesions and subsequent breast cancer risk: a nested case-control study. Breast Cancer Res. 2010;12(4):R61.
11. Eusebi V, Magalhaes F, Azzopardi JG. Pleomorphic lobular carcinoma of the breast: an aggressive tumor showing apocrine differentiation. Hum Pathol. 1992;23:655–62.
12. O'Malley FP. Lobular neoplasia: morphology, biological potential and management in core biopsies. Mod Pathol. 2010;23:S14–25.
13. Page DL, Schuyler PA, Dupont WD, Jensen RA, Plummer WD Jr, Simpson JF. Atypical lobular hyperplasia as a unilateral predictor of breast cancer risk: a retrospective cohort study. Lancet. 2003;361:125–9.
14. Lopez-Garcia MA, Geyer FC, Lacroix-Triki M, Marchió C, Reis-Filho JS. Breast cancer precursors revisited: molecular features and progression pathways. Histopathology. 2010;57(2):171–92.
15. Bagaria SP, Shamonki J, Kinnaird M, Ray PS, Giuliano AE. The florid subtype of lobular carcinoma in situ: marker or precursor for invasive lobular carcinoma? Ann Surg Oncol. 2011;18(7):1845–51.
16. Shin SJ, Lal A, De Vries S, Suzuki J, Roy R, Hwang ES, et al. Florid lobular carcinoma in situ: molecular profiling and comparison to classic lobular carcinoma in situ and pleomorphic lobular carcinoma in situ. Hum Pathol. 2013;44(10):1998–2009.
17. Edge SB, Byrd DR, Compton CC, Fritz AG, Greene FL, Trotti H (eds). American Joint Committee on Cancer (AJCC) cancer staging manual 7th ed. New York, Springer, 2009.
18. Prasad ML, Osborne MP, Giri DD, Hoda SA. Microinvasive carcinoma (T1mic) of the breast: clinicopathologic profile of 21 cases. Am J Surg Pathol. 2000;24(3):422–8.
19. Rosai J. Breast. In: Rosai and Ackerman's surgical pathology. 9th ed. New York: Mosby; 2004. p. 1763–876.

20. Silver SA, Tavassoli FA. Pleomorphic carcinoma of the breast: clinicopathological analysis of 26 cases of an unusual high-grade phenotype of ductal carcinoma. Histopathology. 2000;36(6):505–14.
21. Nguyen CV, Falcón-Escobedo R, Hunt KK, Nayeemuddin KM, Lester TR, Harrell RK, et al. Pleomorphic ductal carcinoma of the breast: predictors of decreased overall survival. Am J Surg Pathol. 2010;34(4):486–93.
22. Tavassoli FA, Norris HJ. Breast carcinoma with osteoclastlike giant cells. Arch Pathol Lab Med. 1986;110(7):636–9.
23. Rosen PP. Rosen's breast pathology. 3rd ed. Philadelphia: Lippincott Williams & Wolters Kluwer Business; 2009.
24. Tavassoli FA, Eusebi V, editors. Tumors of the mammary gland. AFIP atlas of tumor pathology. Fourth series; fasc 10. Washington DC: American Registry of Pathology in Collaboration with the Armed Institute of Pathology; 2009.
25. Athanasou NA, Wells CA, Quinn J, Ferguson DP, Heryet A, McGee JO. The origin and nature of stromal osteoclast-like multinucleated giant cells in breast carcinoma: implications for tumour osteolysis and macrophage biology. Br J Cancer. 1989;59(4):491–8.
26. Shishido-Hara Y, Kurata A, Fujiwara M, Itoh H, Imoto S, Kamma H. Two cases of breast carcinoma with osteoclastic giant cells: are the osteoclastic giant cells pro-tumoural differentiation of macrophages? Diagn Pathol. 2010;5:55–61.
27. Dixon JM, Anderson TJ, Page DL, Lee D, Duffy SW. Infiltrating lobular carcinoma of the breast. Histopathology. 1982;6(2):149–61.
28. Tavassoli FA. Pathology of the breast. 2nd ed. New York: Appleton & Lange; 1999.
29. Fechner RE. Histologic variants of infiltrating lobular carcinoma of the breast. Hum Pathol. 1975;6(3):373–8.
30. Weidner N, Semple JP. Pleomorphic variant of invasive lobular carcinoma of the breast. Hum Pathol. 1992;23(10):1167–71.
31. Middleton LP, Palacios DM, Bryant BR, Krebs P, Otis CN, Merino MJ. Pleomorphic lobular carcinoma: morphology, immunohistochemistry, and molecular analysis. Am J Surg Pathol. 2000;24(12):1650–6.
32. Walford N, ten Velden J. Histiocytoid breast carcinoma: an apocrine variant of lobular carcinoma. Histopathology. 1989;14(5):515–22.
33. Eusebi V, Foschini MP, Bussolati G, Rosen PP. Myoblastomatoid (histiocytoid) carcinoma of the breast. A type of apocrine carcinoma. Am J Surg Pathol. 1995;19(5):553–62.
34. Rakha EA, Patel A, Powe DG, Benhasouna A, Green AR, Lambros MB, et al. Clinical and biological significance of E-cadherin protein expression in invasive lobular carcinoma of the breast. Am J Surg Pathol. 2010;34(10):1472–9.
35. Qureshi HS, Linden MD, Divine G, Raju UB. E-cadherin status in breast cancer correlates with histologic type but does not correlate with established prognostic parameters. Am J Clin Pathol. 2006;125(3):377–85.
36. Da Silva L, Parry S, Reid L, Keith P, Waddell N, Kossai M, et al. Aberrant expression of E-cadherin in lobular carcinomas of the breast. Am J Surg Pathol. 2008;32(5):773–83.
37. Sarrió D, Pérez-Mies B, Hardisson D, Moreno-Bueno G, Suárez A, Cano A, et al. Cytoplasmic localization of p120ctn and E-cadherin loss characterize lobular breast carcinoma from preinvasive to metastatic lesions. Oncogene. 2004;23(19):3272–83.
38. Rakha EA, El-Sayed ME, Powe DG, Green AR, Habashy H, Grainge MJ, et al. Invasive lobular carcinoma of the breast: response to hormonal therapy and outcomes. Eur J Cancer. 2008;44(1):73–83.
39. Pestalozzi BC, Zahrieh D, Mallon E, Gusterson BA, Price KN, Gelber RD, et al. International breast cancer study group. Distinct clinical and prognostic features of infiltrating lobular carcinoma of the breast: combined results of 15 international breast cancer study group clinical trials. Eur J Cancer. 2008;44(1):73–83.
40. Rakha EA, van Deurzen CH, Paish EC, Macmillan RD, Ellis IO, Lee AH. Pleomorphic lobular carcinoma of the breast: is it a prognostically significant pathological subtype independent of histological grade? Mod Pathol. 2013;26(4):496–501.

41. Rakha EA, Lee AHS, Evans AJ, Menon S, Assad NY, Hodi Z, et al. Tubular carcinoma of the breast: further evidence to support its excellent prognosis. J Clin Oncol. 2010;28(1):99–104.
42. Diab SG, Clark GM, Osborne CK, Libby A, Allred DC, Elledge RM. Tumor characteristics and clinical outcome of tubular and mucinous breast carcinomas. J Clin Oncol. 1999;17(5):1442–8.
43. Page DL, Dixon JM, Anderson TJ, et al. Invasive cribriform carcinoma of the breast. Histopathology. 1983;7(4):525–36.
44. Ellis IO, Galea M, Broughton N, Locker A, Blamer RW, Elston CW. Pathological prognostic factors in breast cancer. II. Histological type. Relationship with survival in a large study with long term of follow up. Histopathology. 1992;20:479–89.
45. Venable JG, Schwartz AM, Silverberg SG. Infiltrating cribriform carcinoma of the breast: a distinctive clinicopathologic entity. Hum Pathol. 1990;21(3):333–8.
46. Vu-Nishino H, Tavassoli FA, Ahrens WA, Haffty BG. Clinicopathologic features and long-term outcome of patients with medullary breast carcinoma managed with breast-conserving therapy (BCT). Int J Radiat Oncol Biol Phys. 2005;62(4):1040–7.
47. Marginean F, Rakha EA, Ho BC, Ellis IO, Lee AH. Histological features of medullary carcinoma and prognosis in triple-negative basal-like carcinomas of the breast. Mod Pathol. 2010;23(10):1357–63.
48. Tan PH, Tse GM, Bay BH. Mucinous breast lesions: diagnostic challenges. J Clin Pathol. 2008;61(1):11–9.
49. Capella C, Eusebi V, Mann B, Azzopardi JG. Endocrine differentiation in mucoid carcinoma of the breast. Histopathology. 1980;4(6):613–30.
50. Di Saverio S, Gutierrez J, Avisar E. A retrospective review with long term follow up of 11,400 cases of pure mucinous breast carcinoma. Breast Cancer Res Treat. 2008;111(3):541–7.
51. Tavassoli FA, Purcell CA, Bratthauer GL, Man YG. Androgen receptor positivity along with loss of bcl-2, ER, and PR expression in benign and malignant apocrine lesions of the breast. Implications for therapy. Breast J. 1996;2:1–10.
52. Niemeier LA, Dabbs DJ, Beriwal S, Striebel JM, Bhargava R. Androgen receptor in breast cancer: expression in estrogen receptor-positive tumors and in estrogen receptor-negative tumors with apocrine differentiation. Mod Pathol. 2010;23(2):205–12.
53. Dellapasqua S, Maisonneuve P, Viale G, Pruneri G, Mazzarol G, Ghisini R, et al. Immunohistochemically defined subtypes and outcome of apocrine breast cancer. Clin Breast Cancer. 2013;13(2):95–102.
54. Siriaunkgul S, Tavassoli FA. Invasive micropapillary carcinoma of the breast. Mod Pathol. 1993;6(6):660–2.
55. Ueng SH, Mezzetti T, Tavassoli FA. Papillary neoplasms of the breast: a review. Arch Pathol Lab Med. 2009;133:893–907.
56. Zekioglu O, Erhan Y, Ciris M, Bayramoglu H, Ozdemir N. Invasive micropapillary carcinoma of the breast: high incidence of lymph node metastasis with extranodal extension and its immunohistochemical profile compared with invasive ductal carcinoma. Histopathology. 2004;44(1):18–23.
57. Vingiani A, Maisonneuve P, Dell'orto P, Farante G, Rotmensz N, Lissidini G, et al. The clinical relevance of micropapillary carcinoma of the breast: a case-control study. Histopathology. 2013;63(2):217–24.
58. Meng F, Liu B, Xie G, Song Y, Zheng X, Qian X, et al. Amplification and overexpression of PSCA at 8q24 in invasive micropapillary carcinoma of breast. Breast Cancer Res Treat. 2017;166(2):383–92.
59. Onder S, Fayda M, Karanlık H, Bayram A, Şen F, Cabioglu N, et al. Loss of ARID1A expression is associated with poor prognosis in invasive micropapillary carcinomas of the breast: a clinicopathologic and immunohistochemical study with long-term survival analysis. Breast J. 2017;23(6):638–46.
60. Luini A, Aguilar M, Gatti G, Fasani R, Botteri E, Brito JA, et al. Metaplastic carcinoma of the breast, an unusual disease with worse prognosis: the experience of the European institute of oncology and review of the literature. Breast Cancer Res Treat. 2007;101(3):349–53.

61. Tavassoli FA. Classification of metaplastic carcinomas of the breast. Pathol Annu. 1992;27(Pt 2):89–119.
62. Foschini MP, Eusebi V. Carcinomas of the breast showing myoepithelial cell differentiation. A review of the literature. Virchows Arch. 1998;432(4):303–10.
63. Van Hoeven KH, Drudis T, Cranor ML, Erlandson RA, Rosen PP. Low-grade adenosquamous carcinoma of the breast. A clinocopathologic study of 32 cases with ultrastructural analysis. Am J Surg Pathol. 1993;17(3):248–58.
64. Sneige N, Yaziji H, Mandavilli SR, Perez ER, Ordonez NG, Gown AM, Ayala A. Low-grade (fibromatosis-like) spindle cell carcinoma of the breast. Am J Surg Pathol. 2001;25(8):1009–16.
65. Takano EA, Hunter SM, Campbell IG, Fox SB. Low-grade fibromatosis-like spindle cell carcinomas of the breast are molecularly exiguous. J Clin Pathol. 2015;68(5):362–7.
66. Reis-Filho JS, Milanezi F, Paredes J, Silva P, Pereira EM, Maeda SA, et al. Novel and classic myoepithelial/stem cell markers in metaplastic carcinomas of the breast. Appl Immunohistochem Mol Morphol. 2003;11(1):1–8.
67. Reis-Filho JS, Schmitt FC. p63 expression in sarcomatoid/metaplastic carcinomas of the breast. Histopathology. 2003;42(1):94–5.
68. Reis-Filho JS, Milanezi F, Steele D, Savage K, Simpson PT, Nesland JM, et al. Metaplastic breast carcinomas are basal-like tumours. Histopathology. 2006;49(1):10–21.
69. Weigelt B, Kreike B, Reis-Filho JS. Metaplastic breast carcinomas are basal-like breast cancers: a genomic profiling analysis. Breast Cancer Res Treat. 2009;117(2):273–80.
70. Rakha EA, Coimbra ND, Hodi Z, Juneinah E, Ellis IO, Lee AH. Immunoprofile of metaplastic carcinomas of the breast. Histopathology. 2017;70(6):975–85.
71. Ng CKY, Piscuoglio S, Geyer FC, Burke KA, Pareja F, et al. The landscape of somatic genetic alterations in metaplastic breast carcinomas. Clin Cancer Res. 2017;23(14):3859–70.
72. Righi L, Sapino A, Marchiò C, Papotti M, Bussolati G. Neuroendocrine differentiation in breast cancer: established facts and unresolved problems. Semin Diagn Pathol. 2010;27(1):69–76.
73. Sapino A, Righi L, Cassoni P, Papotti M, Pietribiasi F, Bussolati G. Expression of the neuroendocrine phenotype in carcinomas of the breast. Semin Diagn Pathol. 2000;17(2):127–37.
74. Shin SJ, Delellis RA, Ying L, Rosen PP. Small cell carcinoma of the breast: a clinicopathologic and immunohistochemical study of nine patients. Am J Surg Pathol. 2000;24(9):1231–8.
75. Li D, Xiao X, Yang W, Shui R, Tu X, Lu H, Shi D. Secretory breast carcinoma: a clinicopathological and immunophenotypic study of 15 cases with a review of the literature. Mod Pathol. 2012;25(4):567–75.
76. Tognon C, Knezevich SR, Huntsman D, Roskelley CD, Melnyk N, Mathers JA, et al. Expression of the ETV6-NTRK3 gene fusion as a primary event in human secretory breast carcinoma. Cancer Cell. 2002;2:367–37.
77. Collins LC, Schnitt SJ. Papillary lesions of the breast: selected diagnostic and management issues. Histopathology. 2008;52(1):20–9.
78. Collins LC, Carlo VP, Hwang H, Barry TS, Gown AM, Schnitt SJ. Intracystic papillary carcinomas of the breast: a reevaluation using a panel of myoepithelial cell markers. Am J Surg Pathol. 2006;30(8):1002–7.
79. Esposito NN, Dabbs DJ, Bhargava R. Are encapsulated papillary carcinomas of the breast in situ or invasive? A basement membrane study of 27 cases. Am J Clin Pathol. 2009;131(2):228–42.
80. Mulligan AM, O'Malley FP. Metastatic potential of encapsulated (intracystic) papillary carcinoma of the breast: a report of 2 cases with axillary lymph node micrometastases. Int J Surg Pathol. 2007;15:143–7.
81. Nassar H, Qureshi H, Adsay NV, Visscher D. Clinicopathologic analysis of solid papillary carcinoma of the breast and associated invasive carcinomas. Am J Surg Pathol. 2006;30(4):501–7.
82. Nicolas MM, Wu Y, Middleton LP, Gilcrease MZ. Loss of myoepithelium is variable in solid papillary carcinoma of the breast. Histopathology. 2007;51(5):657–65.
83. Rakha EA, Badve S, Eusebi V, Reis-Filho JS, Fox SB, Dabbs DJ, et al. Breast lesions of uncertain malignant nature and limited metastatic potential: proposals to improve their recognition and clinical management. Histopathology. 2016;68(1):45–56.

84. Ghabach B, Anderson WF, Curtis RE, Huycke MM, Lavigne JA, Dores GM. Adenoid cystic carcinoma of the breast in the United States (1977 to 2006): a population-based cohort study. Breast Cancer Res. 2010;12(4):R54.
85. Marchiò C, Weigelt B, Reis-Filho JS. Adenoid cystic carcinomas of the breast and salivary glands (or 'The strange case of Dr Jekyll and Mr Hyde' of exocrine gland carcinomas). J Clin Pathol. 2010;63(3):220–8.
86. Kulkarni N, Pezzi CM, Greif JM, Suzanne Klimberg V, Bailey L, Korourian S, Zuraek M. Rare breast cancer: 933 adenoid cystic carcinomas from the National Cancer Data Base. Ann Surg Oncol. 2013;20(7):2236–41.
87. Shin SJ, Rosen PP. Solid variant of mammary adenoid cystic carcinoma with basaloid features: a study of nine cases. Am J Surg Pathol. 2002;26(4):413–20.
88. Hayes MM, Seidman JD, Ashton MA. Glycogen-rich clear cell carcinoma of the breast. A clinicopathologic study of 21 cases. Am J Surg Pathol. 2002;19(8):904–11.
89. Kuroda H, Sakamoto G, Ohnisi K, Itoyama S. Clinical and pathological features of glycogen-rich clear cell carcinoma of the breast. Breast Cancer. 2005;12(3):189–95.
90. Yamauchi H, Woodward WA, Valero V, Alvarez RH, Lucci A, Buchholz TA, et al. Inflammatory breast cancer: what we know and what we need to learn. Oncologist. 2012;17(7):891–9.
91. Robertson FM, Bondy M, Yang W, Yamauchi H, Wiggins S, Kamrudin S, et al. Inflammatory breast cancer: the disease, the biology, the treatment. CA Cancer J Clin. 2010;60(6):351–75.

Chapter 4
Mesenchymal and Fibroepithelial Tumors of the Breast

Ekrem Yavuz and Sitki Tuzlali

Introduction

A variety of neoplastic and nonneoplastic mesenchymal lesions exist in the breast. In this chapter, relatively frequent lesions and those of importance in differential diagnosis are discussed. Fibroepithelial tumors are biphasic neoplasms characterized by a proliferation of both epithelial and mesenchymal elements. Fibroadenoma and phyllodes tumors constitute the major entities.

Mesenchymal Tumors of the Breast

Benign mesenchymal tumors that occur elsewhere in the body have been described in the breast, including lipoma, angiolipoma, leiomyoma, neurofibroma and schwannoma [1].

Malignant mesenchymal tumors of the breast other than angiosarcomas are extremely rare. However, any type of sarcoma may occur in the breast as a primary lesion, including liposarcoma, leiomyosarcoma, rhabdomyosarcoma, malignant peripheral nerve sheath tumor, and osteosarcoma [1]. Their histological features are similar to their counterparts occurring elsewhere. A surgical pathologist is frequently confronted with the difficulty of differentiating these lesions from "metaplastic carcinoma of the breast" (MBC) and "sarcomatous overgrowth in malignant phyllodes tumor" (MPT), which is more important than their subclassification as a primary sarcoma.

E. Yavuz (✉)
Istanbul University, Istanbul Medical Faculty, Department of Pathology, Istanbul, Turkey
e-mail: yavuze@istanbul.edu.tr

S. Tuzlali
Istanbul University, Istanbul Medical Faculty, Department of Pathology, Istanbul, Turkey

Tuzlali Private Pathology Laboratory, Istanbul, Turkey

A. Aydiner et al. (eds.), *Breast Cancer*, https://doi.org/10.1007/978-3-319-96947-3_4

Cases composed of malignant spindle cells without any morphological evidence of epithelial differentiation are often challenging, even in surgical specimens [2]. In the absence of in situ carcinoma or small cohesive epithelial foci, the absence of immunohistochemical expression of epithelial differentiation markers and the absence of the characteristic leaf-like architecture of malignant phyllodes tumors helps rule out the diagnosis of MBC or MPT. A primary sarcoma of the breast can then be diagnosed. Other entities such as malignant melanoma and metastatic sarcomatoid tumors should also be considered in differential diagnosis.

Nodular Fasciitis

Nodular fasciitis ((NF) is a self-limited, mass-forming fibroblastic-myofibroblastic proliferation that is clonal [1]. NF of the breast is a rare, rapidly growing lesion that may be painful. Unexcised lesions regress spontaneously within a couple of months [3]. NF mostly arises in the subcutis as a well-circumscribed nodule that may have cystic changes. Parenchymal involvement is less frequent. Microscopically, NF is a well-circumscribed proliferation of plump, spindle cells arranged in short fascicles. Mitoses are usually frequent. Immunohistochemically, these cells are negative for keratin, CD34 and S100 and typically positive for smooth muscle actin (SMA). Although these lesions regress spontaneously, they are very frequently excised to obtain a definite diagnosis.

Differential diagnosis: Fibromatosis, fibromatosis-like spindle cell metaplastic carcinoma and postoperative spindle cell nodules are the entities that should be considered in differential diagnosis [4, 5].

Hemangioma

Hemangioma is a benign proliferation of mature blood vessels [1]. Hemangiomas may arise in the skin and within the breast tissue. Hemangiomas of the breast parenchyma are incidental findings, and palpable and mammographic lesions are rare and should be distinguished from angiosarcomas [6].

Microscopic minute hemangiomas that are smaller than 2 mm can be located anywhere in the breast stroma and are called "perilobular hemangioma" [7, 8].

The importance of these lesions is that they should be distinguished from well-differentiated angiosarcomas.

Atypical Vascular Lesions

Atypical vascular lesion (AVL) is a term that refers to a continuum of cutaneous lesions that have some but not all features of angiosarcoma [9]. These angioformative proliferations develop in the skin of patients with a history of breast-conserving surgery and radiation therapy. The lesions develop within the radiation field 1–12 years (median 6.0 years) after therapy [9]. AVLs present as one or more flesh-colored, brown or erythematous patches and papules ranging from 0.1 to 6 cm [1, 10] but are generally less than 1 cm.

AVLs can be categorized as lymphatic and vascular types.

Recent studies have shown that MYC expression is detected by IHC and/or gene amplification is detected by FISH in 54–100% of secondary angiosarcomas, in contrast to AVL and primary angiosarcomas of the breast [11, 12].

Recurrent or additional AVLs may occur. In a series of 30 patients from the European Institute of Oncology, Milan, the lesion showed benign behavior in 93.3%, one patient developed local recurrence of AVL, and two patients progressed to angiosarcoma at the previous AVL site. Venous-type AVLs were found to have a higher risk of progression to AS compared to the lymphatic-type lesions [12]. Further studies are needed to better understand the clinical behavior of AVLs. Complete excision with free surgical margins and close follow-up is recommended [12].

Angiosarcoma

These tumors can be subdivided as follows [1]:

1. *Primary (de novo)*: Arising in the breast parenchyma.
2. Secondary: Developing in the skin, chest wall or breast parenchyma subsequent to surgery and postoperative radiation for breast cancer.

Primary angiosarcomas are located deep in the breast parenchyma as a mass averaging 5–7 cm. Skin involvement causes a bluish-red discoloration on the overlying skin. They are ill-defined lesions with a spongy appearance.

Low-grade (Grade I) (well-differentiated) tumors are characterized by interanastomosing and dissecting vascular channels that are filled with erythrocytes. They often involve and disrupt the breast ducts and lobules. The endothelial cells show nuclear hyperchromasia. Mitoses are scarce, and necrosis and papillary and solid areas are absent. The lesions have a benign-looking appearance and are often multifocal.

Intermediate-grade (Grade II) lesions have focally increased cellularity, and these solid areas are scattered throughout the tumor [6]. There is endothelial tufting, which is not a feature of grade I tumors (Figs. 4.1 and 4.2).

High-grade (Grade III) (poorly differentiated) angiosarcomas are easily recognized by the presence of solid spindle cell areas with a high mitotic index. Necrosis and hemorrhage are frequent.

CD31 and CD34 are used to prove endothelial differentiation in these tumors. High histological grade and early metastasis (within 12 months after diagnosis) are associated with poor prognosis [13]. However, a large series of 49 cases revealed that grade had no prognostic effect in primary angiosarcomas of the breast, and the risk of metastasis is at least 50% in tumors of any grade [14]. Radiation therapy is ineffective, and chemotherapy is of little benefit. Mastectomy is the treatment of

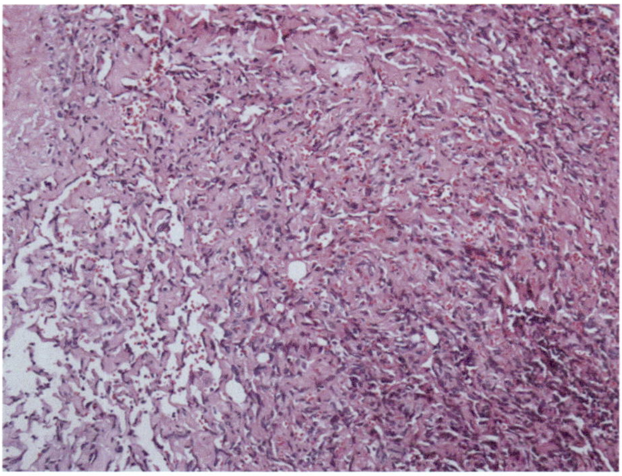

Fig. 4.1 Angiosarcoma. Interanastomosing vascular channels lined by atypical cells

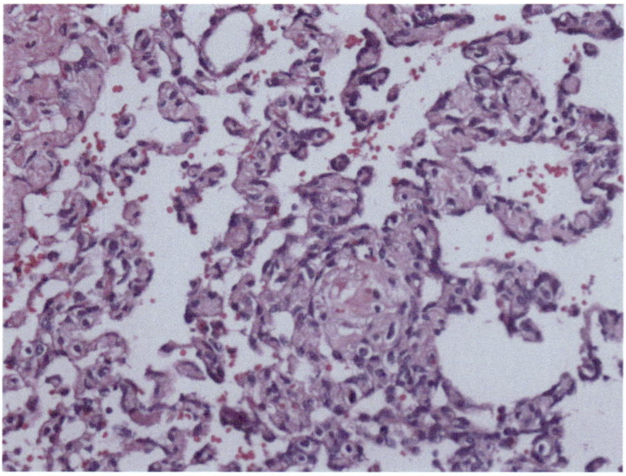

Fig. 4.2 Vascular channels with endothelial tufting

choice, irrespective of grade. The most common sites of metastases are the lung, liver, bone, skin. At presentation, the contralateral breast has metastatic deposits in 21% of cases [15].

Fibromatosis

Fibromatosis is a clonal proliferation of fibroblasts/myofibroblasts that has a propensity for local recurrence. These lesions are categorized as extra-abdominal deep fibromatoses (desmoids). They frequently arise from the connective tissue of the pectoralis muscle or the overlying fascia [6]. Primary fibromatosis of the breast is uncommon. The age range for primary fibromatosis is 13–80 years, but it most commonly affects females in the third to fifth decades. Sporadic cases may appear after trauma or augmentation with implants. It may also occur as part of familial adenomatous polyposis (FAP) or hereditary desmoid syndrome and Gardner's syndrome.

The size of the lesion varies from 0.7 to 10 cm, with an average size of 2.5 cm, which is notably smaller than other extra-abdominal desmoid tumors [6, 16, 17]. Grossly, the lesion presents as an ill-defined, firm nodule, but cases with a stellate appearance are not rare [6]. Clinical suspicion for carcinoma is common.

The lesion is composed of elongated, spindle cells with a bland appearance, which form long sweeping fascicles. Entrapped parenchymal elements are usually seen at the periphery of the lesion. The mitotic rate is variable but usually low. The amount of collagen and the cellularity of the lesion vary considerably. A zoning phenomenon with a tendency for central hyalinization and increased cellularity at the periphery is observed.

The spindle cells stain for vimentin and smooth muscle actin. Desmin and S-100 positivity are observed in a small percentage of cases. Nuclear positivity for beta catenin, which is observed in 70–75% of the lesions, is supportive but not definitive for diagnosis. Beta catenin positivity is observed in other myofibroblastic tumors, such as solitary fibrous tumors [18].

Differential diagnosis: Scars, nodular fasciitis, sarcomas and fibromatosis-like metaplastic breast carcinomas.

Recurrences are observed in up to 27% of cases [17], especially in cases with inadequate excision margins [19]. Wide local excision is recommended for treating these cases.

Myofibroblastoma

Myofibroblastoma of the breast is an uncommon, benign, nonrecurring tumor. It occurs over a wide age range (25–78) but most often in the sixth to eighth decades [20]. The frequency of occurrence is equal in both sexes [20]. It presents as a solitary, mobile, slow-growing lesion with an average diameter of 2 cm [20–22].

The proliferating spindle cells are arranged in short fascicles that are separated by hyalinized collagen bands. In a classical case, the lesion is well-circumscribed, and the compressed breast parenchyma forms a pseudocapsule. Occasionally, the margins of the lesion are infiltrative. Mast cells are always present. There is little or no nuclear pleomorphism. Mitoses are infrequent [20–22].

In the majority of these lesions, the spindle cells are positive for desmin and CD34. Positivity for smooth muscle actin is variable.

Inflammatory Myofibroblastic Tumor

Inflammatory myofibroblastic tumor (IMT) is a low-grade neoplasm consisting of myofibroblastic spindle cells mixed with prominent inflammatory cells, usually plasma cells. IMT is very rare in the breast [1].

IMT in the breast presents as a painless, circumscribed firm mass. The majority of lesions are benign with a local recurrence rate of 10–25%. Fewer than 5% of cases of IMT arising at any site metastasize, and metastasis from IMT arising in the breast has not been reported [1].

Granular Cell Tumor

Granular cell tumors (GCTs) are tumors with eosinophilic cytoplasm derived from Schwann cells of peripheral nerves. They may simulate an invasive carcinoma clinically, radiologically and microscopically. They can cause skin dimpling or nipple retraction. They are usually unifocal lesions. Grossly, they usually present as a well-circumscribed mass [1]. Microscopically they have an infiltrative growth pattern with sheets, nests and clusters of round to polygonal cells. The cells have PAS-positive diastase-resistant granules in their cytoplasm and strong and diffuse positivity for S-100 protein and CD68. Patients with GCT are treated by wide local excision. The tumor has little long-term risk for recurrence, even when excised with positive margins [23].

A large tumor size (over 5 cm), pleomorphism, increased mitotic activity and presence of necrosis are features suggestive of malignancy [1].

Pseudoangiomatous Stromal Hyperplasia

Pseudoangiomatous stromal hyperplasia (PASH) is a benign myofibroblastic proliferation with the appearance of anastomosing slit-like spaces lined by spindle-shaped cells [1]. It occurs most commonly in premenopausal women.

The widely accepted hypothesis is that the stromal hyperplasia in PASH results from an exaggerated, aberrant response of mammary myofibroblasts to endogenous or exogenous hormonal stimuli. The main hormone implicated in stimulating the myofibroblasts is progesterone [24]. PASH can occur as an isolated mass or may coexist with any breast lesion ranging from benign to malignant. When it presents as a palpable mass and a radiological lesion mimicking fibroadenoma, the term "tumorous or nodular PASH" is used.

The size of tumorous PASH ranges from 0.6 to 12 cm. Gross examination reveals a well-circumscribed, round or oval, non-encapsulated, rubbery, homogenous, lobulated nodular mass.

Microscopically, PASH is characterized by complex anastomosing, slit-like spaces in a dense fibrous stroma. These spaces are lined by a layer of flat, benign spindle cells resembling endothelial cells. Mitosis or nuclear atypia is lacking (Fig. 4.3). The stromal hyperplasia may involve perilobular and intralobular stroma. Rarely, the proliferating myofibroblasts form bundles and fascicles in a background of conventional PASH, which may pose diagnostic difficulty.

Myofibroblasts of PASH are positive for CD34 and progesterone receptor with variable staining for smooth muscle actin and desmin [2]. They are negative for endothelial cell markers, cytokeratin, and S100.

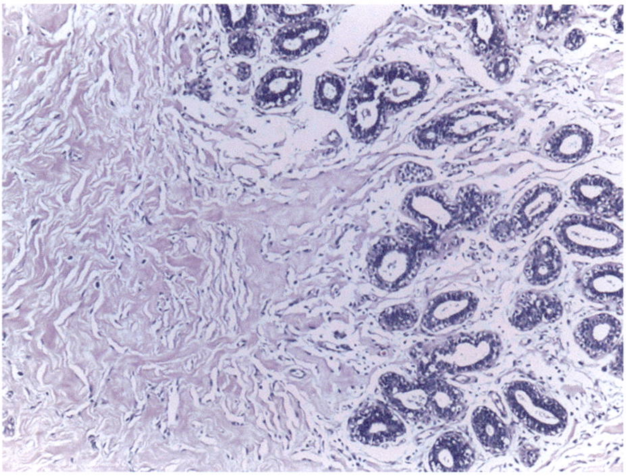

Fig. 4.3 Pseudoangiomatous stromal hyperplasia (PASH). Slit-like spaces lined by a layer of flat, benign spindle cells resembling endothelial cells in continuous with the breast lobule in the right

The differential diagnoses of PASH include low-grade angiosarcoma and myofibroblastoma. Angiosarcoma is an infiltrative lesion and has positive staining with endothelial cell markers. The fascicular form of PASH may be difficult to distinguish from myofibroblastoma, which is believed to have a common histogenetic origin with PASH. Vimentin, CD34 and actin are positive in both lesions. The presence of more typical areas of PASH, positivity for progesterone receptor in PASH, and positivity for androgen receptor in myofibroblastoma are helpful clues in the differential diagnosis of these lesions.

PASH is a benign lesion that is adequately treated by local excision, although rates of recurrence varying from 13% to 26% have been reported. Recurrence is more likely if the lesion is not completely excised [1, 25].

Fibroepithelial Tumors

Fibroepithelial tumors are biphasic neoplasms characterized by the proliferation of both epithelial and mesenchymal elements. Fibroadenoma and phyllodes tumors constitute the major entities.

Fibroadenoma

Fibroadenoma is a very common benign breast tumor occurring in women of childbearing age, i.e., 20–30 years of age, but it may be encountered at any age [1]. It is the most common lesion among women younger than 25 years of age [6]. Fibroadenomas originate from the terminal duct lobular unit [26].

Fibroadenomas typically present as a slow-growing, well-circumscribed, firm, painless, mobile mass that is generally less than 3 cm in size. Less frequently, particularly for the juvenile variant, they may present as a very large mass. The cut

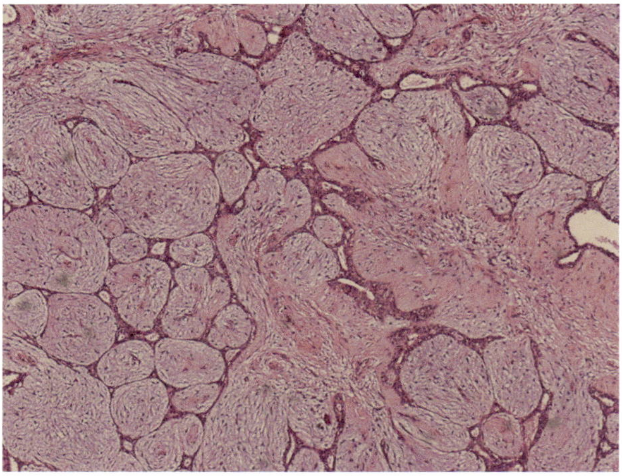

Fig. 4.4 Fibroadenoma intracanalicular type

surface is gray-white, solid, and rubbery with a lobulated appearance and slit-like spaces [1, 27].

It is believed that fibroadenomas develop as a result of unopposed estrogenic influences [6].

Microscopically, fibroadenomas consist of an admixture of stromal and epithelial elements. Two growth patterns are recognized:

- The intracanalicular pattern is characterized by the proliferation of stromal cells around compressed ducts that resemble clefts (Fig. 4.4).
- The pericanalicular pattern is characterized by the proliferation of stroma around glandular structures with open lumina that resemble tubules.

These patterns often coexist and are thought to have no clinical significance.

The epithelial and mesenchymal elements may undergo some metaplastic and proliferative changes. Stroma may occasionally exhibit focal or diffuse cellularity, extensive myxoid changes, hyalinization with dystrophic calcification or even ossification.

Lipomatous, smooth muscle and osteochondromatous metaplasia may occur in fibroadenomas.

Fibroadenomas that have cystic spaces, sclerosing adenosis, and apocrine hyperplasia are called "complex fibroadenomas".

Fibroadenomas with a prominent cellular stroma are called "cellular fibroadenomas".

"Juvenile fibroadenomas" are characterized by stromal hypercellularity and epithelial hyperplasia. They are most commonly seen in patients younger than 20 years of age [27].

Phyllodes Tumor

Phyllodes tumors (PTs) are regarded as deriving de novo from periductal and specialized lobular stroma.

They may occur at any age, with a median age of approximately 45, approximately 20 years older than the median age of fibroadenomas [27]. There are no specific clinical features that distinguish these tumors from fibroadenomas. However, in the presence of a history of rapid growth, diagnosis of PT may be favored [27].

The classical histological appearance has two features:

- an exaggerated intracanalicular pattern with leaf-like fronds protruding into cystically dilated spaces;
- stromal hypercellularity.

PTs are classified as benign, borderline and malignant on the basis of some pathological features [1].

The distinction between benign PT and cellular FA is problematic in core needle biopsies. However, definitive distinction between them may not be crucial in light of the similar reported recurrence rates.

PT Versus Cellular FA Benign PT shows mildly increased stromal cellularity compared with fibroadenomas, has minimal nuclear atypia, pushing borders, and mitoses in less than five mitotic figures per ten high-power fields (HPFs). Stromal overgrowth is not present [28].

Malignant PT A fibroepithelial lesion is called malignant PT when there are marked stromal hypercellularity, nuclear atypia, increased mitoses in more than ten mitotic figures per ten HPFs, permeative tumor borders, and stromal overgrowth that can be easily identified. The presence of a malignant heterologous component such as liposarcoma or chondrosarcoma places the tumor in the malignant category regardless of other histological features [28].

Borderline PT Phyllodes tumors with intermediate features are categorized as borderline PT.

A practical approach is to grade a phyllodes tumor as malignant when it shows all histological changes of malignancy and as borderline when not all malignant characteristics are present [28].

The problem in these lesions is that the degrees of stromal cellularity and cellular atypia are subjective. The issue becomes more problematic in an individual case when intratumoral heterogeneity is present, which is not an uncommon finding in PTs.

From a clinical standpoint, we may state the following:

- Benign PTs have the potential to recur.
- Borderline PTs have the potential to recur, with a very low risk of metastasis.
- Malignant PTs have the highest risk of metastatic behavior, which may eventually prove fatal.
- Malignant PTs are associated with a recurrence rate of 29.6% [29], with metastasis and death observed in 22% [1] of cases.

Although the literature often refers to a margin width of at least 10 mm, a robust evidence base to support this approach is lacking. Therefore, an ideal margin width remains to be determined and may need to be considered in relation to factors such as tumor size and cosmesis. Axillary dissection is not recommended because of the rarity of lymph node metastasis [28].

A multivariate analysis study revealed that stromal nuclear atypia, stromal overgrowth and status of surgical margins are independent predictive parameters of clinical behavior [29].

References

1. Lakhani S, Ellis IO, Tan PH, van de Vijver MJ, editors. World Health Organization classification of tumors, WHO classification of tumors of the breast. 2nd ed. Lyon: IARC; 2012.
2. Rakha EA, Aleskandarany MA, Lee AHS, Ellis IO. An approach to the diagnosis of spindle cell lesions of the breast. Histopathology. 2016;68:33–44.
3. Stanley MW, Skoog L, Tani EM, Horwitz CA. Nodular fasciitis: spontaneous resolution following diagnosis by fine-needle aspiration. Diagn Cytopathol. 1993;9(3):322–4.
4. Gobbi H, Simpson JF, Borowsky A, Jensen RA, Page DL. Metaplastic breast tumors with a dominant fibromatosis-like phenotype have a high risk of local recurrence. Cancer. 1999;85(10):2170–82.
5. Garijo MF, Val-Bernal JF, Vega A, Val D. Postoperative spindle cell nodule of the breast: Pseudosarcomatous myofibroblastic proliferation following endo-surgery. Pathol Int. 2008;58(12):787–91.
6. Tavassoli FA, Eusebi V, editors. Tumors of the mammary gland. AFIP atlas of tumor pathology. Fourth series; fasc 10. Washington DC: American Registry of Pathology in Collaboration with the Armed Institute of Pathology; 2009.
7. Rosen PP, Ridolfi RL. The perilobular hemangioma. A benign microscopic vascular lesion of the breast. Am J Clin Pathol. 1977;68(1):21–3.
8. Tavassoli FA. Pathology of the breast. 2nd ed. New York: Appleton & Lange; 1999.
9. Goldblum JR, Weiss SW, Folpe A. Enzinger and Weiss's soft tissue tumors. 6th ed. Philadelphia: Elsevier Saunders; 2014.
10. Patton KT, Deyrup AT, Weiss SW. Atypical vascular lesions after surgery and radiation of the breast: a clinicopathologic study of 32 cases analyzing histologic heterogeneity and association with angiosarcoma. Am J Surg Pathol. 2008;32(6):943–50.
11. Cornejo KM, Deng A, Wu H, Cosar EF, Khan A, St Cyr M, et al. The utility of MYC and FLT4 in the diagnosis and treatment of postradiation atypical vascular lesion and angiosarcoma of the breast. Hum Pathol. 2015;46(6):868–75.
12. Fraga-Guedes C, Gobbi H, Mastropasqua MG, Rocha RM, Botteri E, Toesca A, Viale G. Clinicopathological and immunohistochemical study of 30 cases of post-radiation atypical vascular lesion of the breast. Breast Cancer Res Treat. 2014;146(2):347–54.
13. Pandey M, Sutton GR, Giri S, Martin MG. Grade and prognosis in localized primary angiosarcoma. Clin Breast Cancer. 2015;15(4):266–9.
14. Nascimento AF, Raut CP, Fletcher CD. Primary angiosarcoma of the breast: clinicopathologic analysis of 49 cases, suggesting that grade is not prognostic. Am J Surg Pathol. 2008;32(12):1896–904.
15. Chen KT, Kirkegaard DD, Bocian JJ. Angiosarcoma of the breast. Cancer. 1980;46:268–71.
16. McMenamin ME, Deschryver K, Fletcher CD. Fibrous lesions of the breast: A review. Int J Surg Pathol. 2000;8(2):99–108.

17. Rosen PP, Ernsberger D. Mammary fibromatosis. A benign spindle-cell tumor with significant risk for local recurrence. Cancer. 1989;63(7):1363–9.
18. Carlson JW, Fletcher CD. Immunohistochemistry for beta-catenin in the differential diagnosis of spindle cell lesions: analysis of a series and review of the literature. Histopathology. 2007;51(4):509–14.
19. Wargotz ES, Norris HJ, Austin RM, Enzinger FM. Fibromatosis of the breast. A clinical and pathological study of 28 cases. Am J Surg Pathol. 1987;11(1):38–45.
20. McMenamin ME, Fletcher CD. Mammary-type myofibroblastoma of soft tissue: a tumor closely related to spindle cell lipoma. Am J Surg Pathol. 2001;25(8):1022–9.
21. Wargotz ES, Weiss SW, Norris HJ. Myofibroblastoma of the breast. Sixteen cases of a distinctive benign mesenchymal tumor. Am J Surg Pathol. 1987;11(7):493–502.
22. Magro G, Bisceglia M, Michal M, Eusebi V. Spindle cell lipoma-like tumor, solitary fibrous tumor and myofibroblastoma of the breast: a clinico-pathological analysis of 13 cases in favor of a unifying histogenetic concept. Virhows Arch. 2002;440:249–60.
23. Papalas JA, Wylie JD, Dash RC. Recurrence risk and margin status in granular cell tumors of the breast: a clinicopathologic study of 13 patients. Arch Pathol Lab Med. 2011;135:890–5.
24. Powell CM, Cranor ML, Rosen PP. Pseudoangiomatous stromal hyperplasia (PASH): a mammary stromal tumor with myofibroblastic differentiation. Am J Surg Pathol. 1995;19(3):270–7.
25. Virk RK, Khan A. Pseudoangiomatous stromal hyperplasia: An overview. Arch Pathol Lab Med. 2010;134:1070–4.
26. Wellings SR, Jensen HM, Marcum RG. An atlas of subgross pathology of the human breast with special reference to possible precancerous lesions. J Natl Cancer Inst. 1975;55(2):231–73.
27. Hoda S, Brogi E, Koerner FC, Rosen PP. Rosen's breast pathology. 4th ed. Philedelphia: Wolters Kluwer Health; 2014.
28. Tan BY, Acs G, Apple SK, Badve S, Bleiweiss IJ, Brogi E, et al. Phyllodes tumours of the breast: a consensus review. Histopathology. 2016;68(1):5–21.
29. Tan PH, Thike AA, Tan WJ, Thu MM, Busmanis I, Li H, et al. Predicting clinical behaviour of breast phyllodes tumours: a nomogram based on histological criteria and surgical margins. J Clin Pathol. 2012;65:69–76.

Chapter 5
Intraoperative Pathological Examination of Breast Lesions

Ekrem Yavuz and Sitki Tuzlali

Introduction

Intraoperative pathological examination (IPE) of the breast tissue may be performed for rapid diagnosis of a malignancy and assessment of surgical margins, sentinel lymph nodes, and, occasionally, tissue adequacy. Depending on the pathologist's experience and conditions, the method is usually either frozen section (FS) or cytology in addition to gross examination, although some molecular techniques have recently been developed for IPE.

Intraoperative Pathological Diagnosis of Breast Lesions

Although FS may be used for the rapid diagnosis of breast lesions in the operating room with high accuracy, specificity, and sensitivity [1, 2], it is rarely performed because the majority of breast malignancies are diagnosed with preoperative core or fine needle aspiration biopsies. Nevertheless, rapid FS diagnosis is subject to certain requirements. A possibly benign or grossly undetectable lesion or a lesion smaller than 1 cm is not appropriate for rapid FS diagnosis. Because rapid FS diagnosis is rarely requested, pathologists should be aware of the potential pitfalls, including benign lesions mimicking malignancy or vice versa. Although a correct intraoperative

---

E. Yavuz
Istanbul University, Istanbul Medical Faculty, Department of Pathology, Istanbul, Turkey
e-mail: yavuze@istanbul.edu.tr

S. Tuzlali (✉)
Istanbul University, Istanbul Medical Faculty, Department of Pathology, Istanbul, Turkey

Tuzlali Private Pathology Laboratory, Istanbul, Turkey

A. Aydiner et al. (eds.), *Breast Cancer*, https://doi.org/10.1007/978-3-319-96947-3_5

diagnosis should be reached by using only gross examination and cytology [3–5], many pathologists are reluctant to use only cytological methods in the operating room.

Intraoperative Pathological Assessment of Surgical Margins

The most important parameter for local recurrence after breast-conserving surgery (BCS) for the treatment of breast cancer is surgical margin negativity [6]. Hence, intraoperative assessment of the surgical margins (IASM) of breast excisions is usually requested. However, many factors can decrease the accuracy of IASM. Adipose tissue may be easily broken off during surgery, causing defects on the surface of the excision. The excised tissue may flatten after removal (pancake phenomenon), thus decreasing the distance between the tumor and the margin [7].

The success of IASM is also related to collaboration between surgeons and pathologists. The surgeon should inform the pathologist about the size, extent, and number of possibly malignant breast lesions and should send an intact specimen bearing orientation sutures. First, the pathologist should stain the surface of the specimen with India ink or another stain that is resistant to solutions used in processing. After slicing the specimen to a thickness of 0.5 cm, the distances to all surgical margins can be detected grossly. However, there may be microscopic satellite foci of invasive or in situ carcinoma around the gross tumor, and the true distance to the margin may be smaller than expected. Hence, FS may be performed if a tumor is close to the margin grossly (Figs. 5.1 and 5.2). FS may be performed using samples taken either perpendicular or parallel to the surface of the specimen. We prefer to take perpendicular samples to accurately detect the true distance. If parallel (en face) sections are used and no tumor is detected in microscopic examination of FS, than at least a 2-mm-free distance between the tumor and the margin

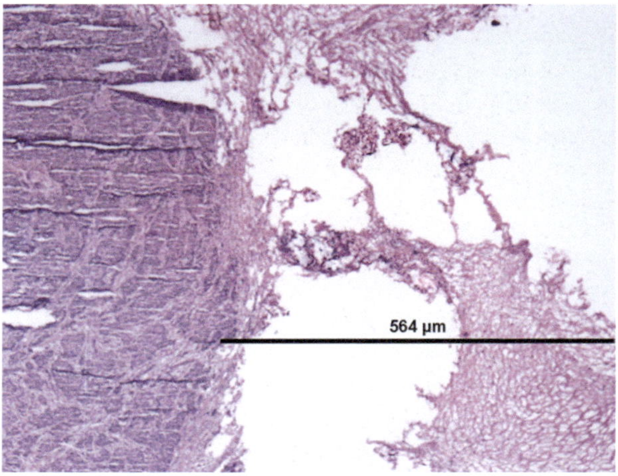

Fig. 5.1 Frozen section appearance of an invasive breast cancer. This section shows that the distance to the surgical margin is nearly 0.5 mm, although the fatty part of the tumor-free tissue could not observed due to the limitation of frozen sectioning (HE ×10 original magnification)

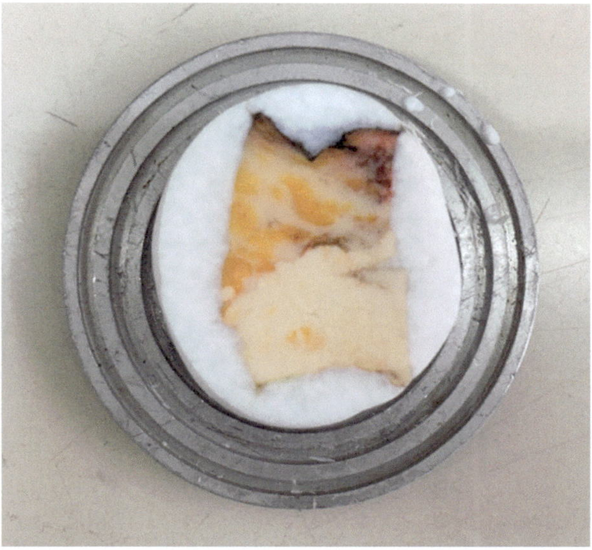

Fig. 5.2 The gross appearance of frozen sectioned tissue may also facilitate margin assessment because freezing usually highlights the tumor

may be anticipated. Some surgeons may perform re-excisions by shaving the cavity, and these re-excisions may be analyzed by FS as well [8, 9].

Even if immediate cavity margin shaving is performed after a lumpectomy with tumor-free margins, there may still exist microscopic foci of carcinoma in the breast at rates ranging from 9% to 39% [10, 11]. Invasive lobular carcinomas (Fig. 5.3) and invasive carcinomas with an extensive intraductal component and extensive lymphovascular invasion are more likely to show multifocality and result in false-negative margins. The impact of FS on margin assessment has been demonstrated in retrospective analyses, which reported immediate re-excision in 24–27% of cases and second re-excision due to definitive histopathological examination in 5–9% of cases [12–14].

Margin status may also be assessed using cytology intraoperatively. Although some authors have reported high rates of specificity and sensitivity of cytological methods in IASM [15, 16], experience with this method in breast cytology is required. Furthermore, success rates would decrease in cancers with low nuclear grade, such as invasive lobular carcinoma [17].

There are also methods for IASM that do not require microscopy, including intraoperative ultrasonography, specimen radiography for lesions with microcalcifications, and physical methods such as radiofrequency spectroscopy, optical coherence tomography, Raman spectroscopy, diffuse reflectance imaging, and multispectral photoacoustic tomography. The emerging physical methods need to compete with the diagnostic accuracy of existing techniques while offering advantages in terms of speed, cost, and reliability [18].

When reporting margin status, “positive” should be stated if tumor cells were detected on the inked surface; otherwise, the distance to the margin should be given. We do not recommend using the term “close to margin” due to its ambiguity.

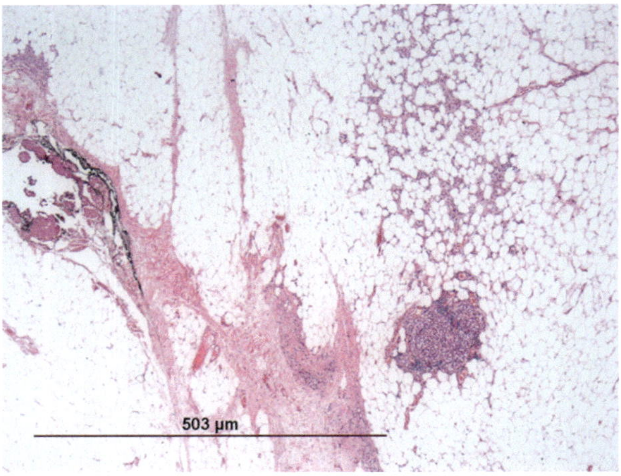

Fig. 5.3 A microscopic satellite focus in a case of invasive lobular carcinoma reveals that the surgical margin is closer than grossly expected (HE ×10 original magnification)

Pathological Examination of Sentinel Lymph Nodes

Intraoperative Pathological Examination of Sentinel Lymph Nodes

The frequency of intraoperative examination of sentinel lymph nodes (SLN) in breast cancer patients who will undergo BCS and radiotherapy has decreased since a randomized study showed that completion of axillary lymph node dissection was not superior to SLN biopsy alone regarding disease-free and overall survival [19, 20]. However, there are some clinical settings in which the pathologist will continue to perform intraoperative SLN examination.

Intraoperative pathological examination of SLN may be performed using either FS or cytological methods. Each method has some advantages and disadvantages. Imprint or scrape cytology is easy, rapid and preserves the tissue for subsequent paraffin-block examination. However, it requires experience, and the detected metastasis cannot be measured properly. The use of both methods has been found to be satisfactory in some meta-analyses. However, the use of both methods intraoperatively would not increase the success rate of detecting micrometastases (MIM) [21, 22].

Intraoperative rapid immunohistochemistry with cytokeratin and molecular techniques such as one-step nucleic acid amplification (OSNA) have shown satisfactory results in accurately detecting even MIMs [23, 24]. However, the American Society of Clinical Oncology has recommended that molecular techniques in intraoperative SLN examination remain investigational and that tissue for permanent pathological examination be preserved [25].

Permanent Pathological Analysis of Sentinel Lymph Nodes

Gross Examination

All SLNs should be measured and sliced in 2-mm thicknesses after dissection of fatty tissue. The slicing may be either in the longitudinal or transverse direction. If a dye was used in the surgical procedure, the afferent lymphatic can be observed. Pathological examination may be more successful if the section can be made where the afferent lymphatic is connected to the SLN. Partial involvement of the SLN by the metastatic tumor can be easily observed in the surface of the slice based on the sharp contrast between the tumor and lymphoid tissue. However, permeative metastases may be difficult to observe grossly.

Sectioning

The majority of metastases can easily be detected with standard examination of HE-stained slides [26, 27]. Superficial serial sectioning, which limits the observation to the upper parts of the tissue in the paraffin block, enables the detection of all macrometastases (MAM) [28, 29]. However, the majority of even MIMs can be detected if multiple-step serial sectioning is performed [30–32]. Furthermore, if the step serial sectioning is performed at 0.2-mm intervals, all MIMs can be detected [33], but an excessive number of slides will be generated.

Use of Immunohistochemistry

The use of immunohistochemistry to evaluate SLNs is not recommended by major organizations [26, 34, 35]. However, immunostaining with antibodies against cytokeratin is very helpful in the detection of dyscohesive cells of invasive lobular carcinoma that are dispersed through the sinuses of SLNs (Fig. 5.4).

Histopathology

MAMs usually replace the lymphoid tissue and can easily be observed. Lobular carcinomas may diffusely infiltrate the lymph node parenchyma with isolated cells or small clusters. MAM is the term used for a metastasis measuring more than 2 mm. “Isolated tumor cells/submicrometastasis” (ITC) is the term used for a metastatic focus measuring less than 0.2 mm. Another definition for ITC that is essential for lobular carcinoma is less than 200 neoplastic cells in a cross section of the

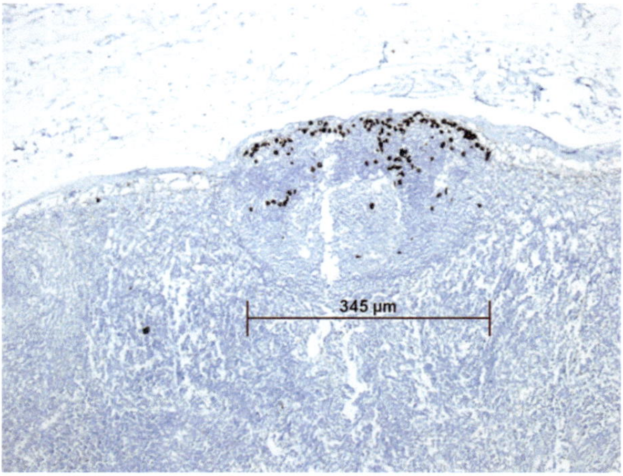

Fig. 5.4 Immunohistochemical staining using anti-cytokeratin antibody highlights the dispersed neoplastic cells of invasive lobular carcinoma within the subcapsular sinus and lymphoid parenchyma of the sentinel lymph node (anti-cytokeratin-Mayer's hematoxylin counterstaining ×10 original magnification)

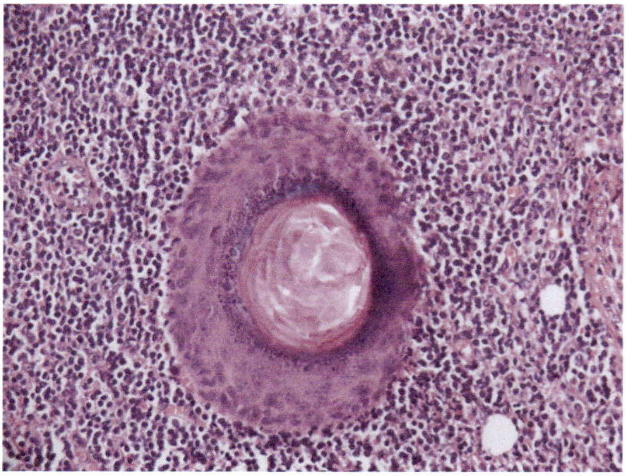

Fig. 5.5 A benign epithelial inclusion formed by squamous cells in the lymphoid parenchyma of the sentinel lymph node (HE ×40 original magnification)

SLN. MIM is the term used for a metastasis measuring less than 2 mm and more than 0.2 mm in size or the presence of 200 neoplastic cells in a cross section of the SLN [36]. MIMs and ITCs are usually detected in subcapsular sinuses of the SLN, and careful observation of these sites is crucial. Differential diagnosis of MIMs includes MAMs and ITCs and should be made according to the abovementioned measurements. Multiple MIMs can be detected and should not be diagnosed as a MAM. Other lesions included in the differential diagnosis of MIMs are mechanical transportation of breast epithelium, nevus cell aggregates, benign epithelial inclusions (Fig. 5.5), and extramedullary hematopoiesis; differential diagnosis of these lesions usually necessitates experience in this field and immunohistochemical techniques.

References

1. Fessia L, Ghiringhello B, Arisio R, Botta G, Aimone V. Accuracy of frozen section diagnosis in breast cancer detection: a review 4436 biopsies and comparison with cytodiagnosis. Pathol Res Pract. 1984;179:61–6.
2. Kaufman Z, Lew S, Griffel B, Dinbar A. Frozen-section diagnosis in surgical pathology. A prospective analysis of 526 frozen sections. Cancer. 1986;57:377–9.
3. Esteban JM, Zaloudek C, Silverberg SG. Intraoperative diagnosis of breast lesions. Comparison of cytologic with frozen section technics. Am J Clin Pathol. 1987;88:681–8.
4. De Rosa G, Boschi R, Boscaino A, Petrella G, Vetrani A, Palombini R, et al. Intraoperative cytology in breast cancer diagnosis: comparison between cytologic and frozen section techniques. Diagn Cytopathol. 1993;9:623–31.
5. Veneti S, Ioannidou-Mouzaka L, Toufexi H, Xenitides J, Anastasiadis P. Imprint cytology. A rapid, reliable method of diagnosing breast malignancy. Acta Cytol. 1996;40:649–52.
6. Spivack B, Khanna MM, Tafra L, Juillard G, Giuliano AE. Margin status and local recurrence after breast-conserving surgery. Arch Surg. 1994;138:1371–4.
7. Graham RA, Homer MJ, Katz J, Rothschild J, Safaii H, Supran S. The pancake phenomenon contributes to inaccuracy of margin assessment in patients with breast cancer. Am J Surg. 2002;184:89–93.
8. Barthelmes L, Al Awa A, Crawford DJ. Effects of cavity margin shavings to ensure completeness of excision on local recurrence rates following breast conserving therapy. Eur J Surg Oncol. 2003;29:644–8.
9. Cao D, Lin C, Woo SH, Vang R, Tsangaris TN, Argani P. Separate cavity margin sampling at the time of initial breast lumpectomy significantly reduces the need for reexcisions. Am J Surg Pathol. 2005;29:1625–32.
10. Guidi AJ, Connoly JL, Harris JR, Schnitt SJ. The relationship between shaved margin and inked margin status in breast excision specimens. Cancer. 1997;70:1568–73.
11. Rubin P, O'Honlon D, Browell D, Callanan K, Shrimankar J, Scott D, et al. Tumour bed biopsy detects the presence of multifocal disease in patients undergoing breast conservation therapy for primary breast carcinoma. Eur J Surg Oncol. 1996;22:23–6.
12. Riedl O, Fitzal F, Mader N, Dubsky P, Rudas M, Mittlboeck M, et al. Intraoperative frozen section analysis for breast-conserving therapy in 1016 patients with breast cancer. Eur J Surg Oncol. 2009;35:264–70.
13. Olson TP, Harter J, Munoz A, Mahvi DM, Breslin T. Frozen section analysis for intraoperative margin assessment during breast-conserving surgery results in low rates of re-excision and local recurrence. Ann Surg Oncol. 2007;14:2953–60.
14. Camp ER, McAuliffe PF, Gilroy JS, Morris CG, Lind DS, Mendenhall NP, et al. Minimizing local recurrence after breast conserving therapy using intraoperative shaved margins to determine pathologic tumor clearance. J Am Coll Surg. 2005;201:855–61.
15. Bakhshandeh M, Tutuncuoglu SO, Fischer G, Masood S. Use of imprint cytology for assessment of surgical margins in lumpectomy specimens of breast cancer patients. Diagn Cytopathol. 2007;35:656–9.
16. Klimberg VS, Westbrook KC, Korourian S. Use of touch preps for diagnosis and evaluation of surgical margins in breast cancer. Ann Surg Oncol. 1998;5:220–6.
17. Valdes EK, Boolbol SK, Ali I, Feldman SM, Cohen JM. Intraperative touch preparation cytology for margin assessment in breast-conservation surgery: does it work for lobular carcinoma? Ann Surg Oncol. 2007;14:2940–5.
18. St John ER, Al-Khudairi R, Ashrafian H, Athanasiou T, Takats Z, Hadjiminas DJ, et al. Diagnostic accuracy of intraoperative techniques for margin assessment in breast cancer surgery: a meta-analysis. Ann Surg. 2017;265:300–10.

19. Giuliano AE, Hunt KK, Ballman KV, Beitsch PD, Whitworth PW, Blumencranz PW, et al. Axillary dissection vs no axillary dissection in women with invasive breast cancer and sentinel node metastasis. A randomized clinical trial. JAMA. 2011;305:569–75.
20. Giuliano AE, Ballman KV, McCall L, Beitsch PD, Brennan MB, Kelemen PR, et al. Effect of axillary dissection vs no axillary dissection on 10-year overall survival among women with invasive breast cancer and sentinel node metastasis: the ACOSOG Z0011 (Alliance) randomized clinical trial. JAMA. 2017;318:918–26.
21. Tew K, Irwig L, Matthews A, Crowe P, Macaskill P. Metaanalysis of sentinel lypmh node cytology in breast cancer. Br J Surg. 2005;92:1068–80.
22. Liu LC, Lang JE, Lu Y, Roe D, Hwang SE, Ewing CA, et al. Intraoperative frozen section analysis of sentinel lymph nodes in breast cancer patients. A meta-analysis and single-institution experience. Cancer. 2011;117:250–8.
23. Fung V, Kohlhardt S, Vergani P, Zardin GJ, Williams NR. Intraoperative prediction of the two axillary lymph node macrometastases threshold in patients with breast cancer using a one-step nucleic acid cytokeratin-19 amplification assay. Mol Clin Oncol. 2017;7:755–62.
24. Shigematsu H, Ozaki S, Yasui D, Zaitsu J, Taniyama D, Saitou A, et al. Comparison of CK-IHC assay on serial frozen sections, the OSNA assay, and in combination for intraoperative evaluation of SLN metastases in breast cancer. Breast Cancer. 2017;25(2):191–7. https://doi.org/10.1007/s12282-017-0811-y.
25. Lyman GH, Giuliano AE, Somerfield MR, Benson AB, Bodurka DC, Burstein HJ, et al. American Society of Clinical Oncology guideline recommendations for sentinel lymph node biopsy in early-stage breast cancer. J Clin Oncol. 2005;23:7703–20.
26. Fitzgibbons PL, Page DL, Weaver D, Thor AD, Allred DC, Clark GM, et al. Prognostic factors in breast cancer: College of American Pathologists Consensus Statement 1999. Arch Pathol Lab Med. 2000;124:966–78.
27. Association of Directors of Anatomic and Surgical Pathology. Recommendations for processing and reporting of lymph node specimens submitted for evaluation of metastatic disease. Am J Clin Pathol. 2001;115:799–801.
28. Turner RR. Histopathologic processing of the sentinel lymph node. Semin Breast Dis. 2002;5:35–40.
29. Weaver DL, Krag DN, Ashikaga T, Harlow SP, O'Connell M. Pathologic analysis of sentinel and nonsentinel lymph nodes in breast carcinoma: a multicenter study. Cancer. 2000;88:1099–107.
30. Cserni G. Metastases in axillary sentinel lymph nodes in breast cancer as detected by intensive histopathological work up. J Clin Pathol. 1999;52:922–4.
31. Turner RR, Ollila DW, Stern S, Giuliano AE. Optimal histopathologic examination of the sentinel lymph node for breast carcinoma staging. Am J Surg Pathol. 1999;23:263–7.
32. Zhang PJ, Reisner RM, Nangia R, Edge SB, Brooks JJ. Effectiveness of multiple-level sectioning in detecting axillary nodal micrometastasis in breast cancer: a retrospective study with immunohistochemical analysis. Arch Pathol Lab Med. 1998;122:687–90.
33. Weaver DL, Le UP, Dupuis SL, Weaver KA, Harlow SP, Ashikaga T, et al. Metastasis detection in sentinel lymph nodes: comparison of a limited widely spaced (NSABP Protocol B-32) and a comprehensive narrowly spaced paraffin block sectioning strategy. Am J Surg Pathol. 2009;33:1583–9.
34. Kollias J, Gil PG, Chatterton B, Raymond W, Collins PJ. Sentinel node biopsy in breast cancer: recommendations for surgeons, pathologists, nuclear physicians and radiologists in Australia and New Zeeland. Aust N Z J Surg. 2000;70:132–6.
35. Cserni G, Amendoeira I, Apostolikas N, Bellocq JP, Bianchi S, Boecker W, et al. Discrepansies in current practice of pathological evaluation of sentinel lymph nodes in breast cancer. Results of a questionnaire-based survey by the European Working Group for Breast Screening Pathology. J Clin Pathol. 2004;57:695–701.
36. Green FL, Page DL, Fleming ID, Fritz AG, Balch CM, Haller DG, et al. AJCC Cancer staging manual. 6th ed. New York: Springer; 2002.

Chapter 6
Prognostic and Predictive Factors

Sitki Tuzlali and Ekrem Yavuz

Introduction

A variety of pathological parameters are used to assess the prognosis and predict the therapeutic response of breast cancer patients. These parameters include tumor size, axillary lymph node status, histological features (especially histological type, grade and lymphovascular invasion), hormone receptor status, HER2 status and proliferative capacity of the tumor. Considering these factors in combination is of greater clinical value than viewing each in isolation, and the combined approach forms the basis of a number of schema used to group patients into various risk categories, such as the St Gallen criteria, the NIH consensus criteria, the Nottingham Prognostic Index, and Adjuvant! Online (www.adjuvantonline.com) [1].

Prognostic and Predictive Factors

Tumor size and axillary lymph node status are the components of the TNM tumor staging system published by the American Joint Committee on Cancer (AJCC)/ Union for International Cancer Control (UICC) [2].

S. Tuzlali
Tuzlali Private Pathology Laboratory, Istanbul, Turkey

Istanbul University, Istanbul Medical Faculty, Department of Pathology, Istanbul, Turkey

E. Yavuz (✉)
Istanbul University, Istanbul Medical Faculty, Department of Pathology, Istanbul, Turkey
e-mail: yavuze@istanbul.edu.tr

A. Aydiner et al. (eds.), *Breast Cancer*, https://doi.org/10.1007/978-3-319-96947-3_6

Tumor Size

For the maximum correlation with prognosis, the size of tumors should only be assessed on pathological specimens because clinical evaluation is inaccurate. Tumor size should ideally be measured before fixation and confirmed microscopically. Many studies have shown that patients with smaller tumors have better long-term survival than do those with larger tumors [3–6]. Tumor size is based on the size of the invasive component of the tumor [7, 8]. In cases with an accompanying in situ component, the in situ area that is outside the invasive tumor is not included in the tumor size 'T'. However, if the in situ component is intermingled with the invasive areas, T will include these in situ areas. If there are multiple areas of invasion, the size of the largest invasive carcinoma is used in the T staging. Occasionally, multiple invasive foci occur in close proximity to each other, creating difficulty in determining the invasive tumor size. Correlation of radiological and gross findings with the microscopic appearance may be necessary. The choice of T staging may depend on the pathologist's own judgement. In cases when the tumor is transected by a previous biopsy, the sizes of the tumors in the separate specimens should not be added, and an estimation should be performed with the aid of imaging studies [8].

Lymph Node Status

The status of the axillary lymph nodes is the most important single prognostic parameter in breast carcinomas. Lymph node staging should be based on histological evaluation of the excised lymph nodes since clinical evaluation is not sufficient for an accurate staging. Numerous studies have shown that patients with histologically confirmed axillary lymph node involvement have a significantly poorer prognosis than those without nodal involvement. The extent of axillary invasion by level also has strong prognostic significance, and the involvement of higher levels of the axilla has a worse prognosis [9]. Surgical removal of positive nodes does not appear to have a major role in survival but is required for accurate staging and local control [10].

Sentinel lymph node biopsy and the importance of low-volume metastases are described in detail in other chapters.

Although basal-like carcinomas belong to a poor prognostic group, they are the least likely to exhibit extensive nodal involvement. For these patients, other prognostic markers will be more important than nodal staging [7]

Grading

The Nottingham (Elston-Ellis) modification of the Scarff-Bloom-Richardson grading system, also known as the Nottingham Grading System (NGS) [11], is the grading system recommended by various professional organizations, such as the World

Health Organization [7], American Joint Committee on Cancer [AJCC], the Royal College of Pathologists (UK RCPath), and College of American Pathologists (CAP) [8]. NGS provides a simple, inexpensive, and routinely applicable overview of the intrinsic biological characteristics and clinical behavior of tumors [12]. In NGS, the subjectivity of previous grading systems is reduced by strict definitions of the evaluation criteria.

Multiple independent studies have shown that NGS has prognostic value that is equivalent to that of LN status and greater than that of tumor size [12, 13].

NGS refers to the semi-quantitative evaluation of some morphological characteristics on an adequately prepared hematoxylin-eosin-stained tumor tissue section. This assessment should be performed by an appropriately trained pathologist using a standard protocol.

NGS is based on the evaluation of three morphological features [7, 11, 14]:

(a) degree of tubule or gland formation,
(b) nuclear pleomorphism, and
(c) mitotic count (found in 10 consecutive high-power fields (HPFs) in the most mitotically active part of the tumor).

Feature	Score
Tubule formation	
Majority of tumor (>75%)	1
Moderate degree (10–75%)	2
Little or none (<10%)	3
Nuclear pleomorphism	
Small, regular uniform cells	1
Moderate increase in size and variability	2
Marked variation	3
Mitotic counts	
Dependent on microscope field area	1–3
Final grading	
Add scores for tubule formation, nuclear pleomorphism and mitotic count	
Grade 1—well differentiated	3–5 points
Grade 2—moderately differentiated	6–7 points
Grade 3—poorly differentiated	8–9 points

Histological grade has been incorporated in multiple, validated, prognostic algorithms to determine breast cancer therapy, such as the Nottingham Prognostic Index and Adjuvant! Online.

Although grade identifies prognostic subgroups among special types of breast cancer, medullary carcinomas, which are, by definition, of high histological grade, have a relatively good prognosis. This favorable prognosis may be related to the prominent lymphoplasmacytic infiltrate in the tumor stroma [7].

Histological Type

The favorable prognosis of certain histological types of invasive carcinoma of the breast is well established. Tubular carcinoma, mucinous carcinoma, and invasive cribriform carcinoma have all been reported to have a favorable prognosis [15]. Other special types of breast cancer carrying an unfavorable prognosis are metaplastic carcinomas and invasive micropapillary carcinomas.

Lymphovascular Invasion

Lymphovascular invasion (LVI) is the finding of carcinoma in the small vessels outside the main tumor mass. It is strongly associated with lymph node status and is also an independent prognostic indicator of both local and distant recurrences and survival [16, 17]. The presence of both LVI and nodal metastases confers a worse prognosis than either alone [7].

Tumor emboli are usually identified within thin-walled vascular channels. It is not possible to determine whether these spaces are lymphatic, capillaries or venules, and the broad term 'lymphovascular invasion' is used.

Vascular invasion should only be assessed in the breast tissue surrounding the tumor and not within the tumor. The most common area to find LVI is within 0.1 cm of the edge of the carcinoma.

Suboptimal fixation is the major reason for misinterpretation of both ductal carcinoma in situ and shrinkage artifacts as LVI. With optimal fixation, processing and sectioning, LVI can be reliably identified in hematoxylin and eosin sections. Immunohistochemistry is not necessary.

Hormone Receptors

The estrogen receptor (ER) is a nuclear transcription factor that is a regulator of cellular growth, proliferation, and differentiation in the breast epithelium. In addition to its prognostic value, ER is the most important biological marker of clinical response to hormonal therapies such as tamoxifen. The progesterone receptor (PR) is an estrogen-regulated gene, and its expression therefore indicates a functioning ER pathway.

The best response is seen in patients whose tumors express both ER and PR [18]. Immunohistochemical determination of these receptors is the standard tool in current pathology-oncology practice. By immunohistochemistry (IHC), nuclear expression of ER protein is detected in approximately 80% of breast cancers (Fig. 6.1). Approximately 40% of ER-positive tumors are PR-negative. A lack of PR expression in ER-positive tumors may be a surrogate marker of aberrant growth factor signaling that could contribute to tamoxifen resistance [19].

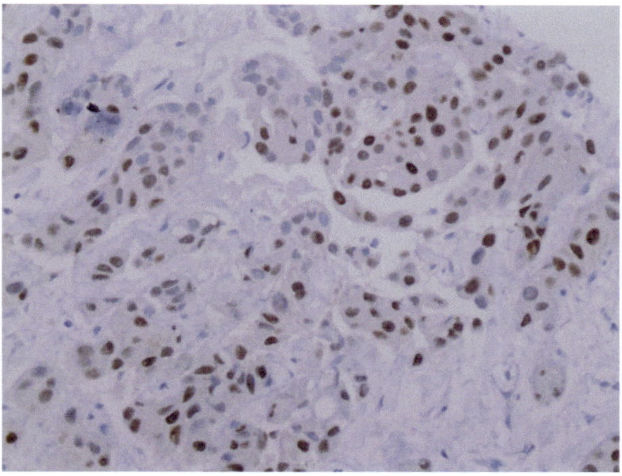

Fig. 6.1 Immunohistochemical determination of estrogen receptor in breast cancer. The brown-stained nuclei are positive for estrogen receptor. The other nuclei with bluish staining lack estrogen receptor

A cutoff of 1% of tumor cells is recommended for a specimen to be considered positive for ER/PR because clinical data have indicated that these patients can respond to hormonal treatment [20].

ASCO/CAP guidelines recommend the use of only 10% neutral buffered formalin as the fixative for breast cancer specimens. The fixation time should not be less than 6 h and not more than 72 h before processing [20, 21].

All tumor-containing areas on a given slide should be evaluated, and the percentage of tumor cells with positive staining should be recorded and reported. Only nuclear staining is considered positive. The intensity of staining is also recorded as weak, moderate, or strong; this measurement represents an estimate of the average staining intensity of the positively stained tumor cells in comparison with the positive control section [20].

Validated antibodies demonstrating good correlation with patient outcomes in published reports should be chosen for accurate results. The ASCO/CAP panel recommends [20] clones 1D5, 6F11, SP1, and 1D5 + ER.2.123 (cocktail) for ER and clones 1294, 312 and 1A6 for PR.

HER2

The HER2 (ERBB2) gene is located on chromosome 17 and encodes the protein p185, which is a growth factor receptor on the surface of normal breast epithelium. Studies have revealed that this gene is amplified in approximately 15–20% of breast cancers with consequent elevation of protein expression. Overexpression of HER2 is associated with aggressive histological features and poor prognosis.

More important is the use of the HER2/neu oncoprotein as a target for therapy. Trastuzumab (Herceptin) is a humanized monoclonal antibody that targets the extracellular domain of the HER2 receptor. Several randomized clinical trials have demonstrated substantial survival benefits in patients with

HER2-positive breast cancer treated with anti-HER2 targeted therapy, such as trastuzumab [22].

The most commonly used methods to evaluate HER2/neu in breast cancer are IHC and in situ hybridization (ISH). ISH determines the number of HER2 copies using a DNA probe coupled to a fluorescent (FISH), chromogenic (CISH) or silver (SISH) detection system.

In clinical practice, accurate assessment of HER2 is essential in selecting patients that are candidates for anti-HER2 treatment. Relatively low and unacceptable concordance rates between local and central laboratories in determining the presence of HER2 protein necessitated the refinement of test performance parameters [23]. The interpretation of equivocal immunohistochemistry and borderline FISH cases is difficult even for highly experienced and validated laboratories [24]. This difficulty is also one of the major reasons for the need for quality-control procedures. Many trials have also revealed that there is significant variation in HER2 testing, resulting in considerable false-negative and false-positive rates [25]. To overcome these difficulties, ASCO and CAP collaborated to develop HER2 testing guidelines to standardize preanalytical and analytical procedures and quality assurance measures. The adoption of the ASCO/CAP guidelines in 2007 led to the following outcomes [26]:

The concordance with FISH improved, and the number of FISH-inconclusive cases decreased from 10.8% to 3.4% (a 64% reduction) [27], resulting in a lower incidence of false-positive IHC results [28].

In 2013, an update of the ASCO/CAP guidelines was published [29]. In 2015, a short comment on upcoming modifications was also released [30].

The 2018 Focused Update addresses uncommon clinical scenarios and improves clarity, particularly for infrequent HER2 test results that are of uncertain biologic or clinical significance. Updated findings of note include [31]:

- Revision of the definition of IHC 2+ (equivocal) to the original FDA-approved criteria.
- Repeat HER2 testing on a surgical specimen if the initially tested core biopsy is negative is no longer stated as mandatory. A new HER2 test *may* (no longer *should*) be ordered on the excision specimen on the basis of some criteria (such as tumor grade 3).
- A more rigorous interpretation criteria of the less common patterns that can be seen in about 5% of all cases when HER2 status in breast cancer is evaluated using a dual-probe ISH testing. These cases, described as ISH groups 2–4, should now be assessed using a diagnostic approach that includes a concomitant review of the IHC test, which will help the pathologist make a final determination of the tumor specimen as HER2 positive or negative.
- The Expert Panel also preferentially recommends the use of dual-probe instead of single-probe ISH assays, but it recognizes that several single-probe ISH assays have regulatory approval in many parts of the world.

The current guidelines are as follows [31]:

HER2 IHC scoring is reported as follows:

Negative

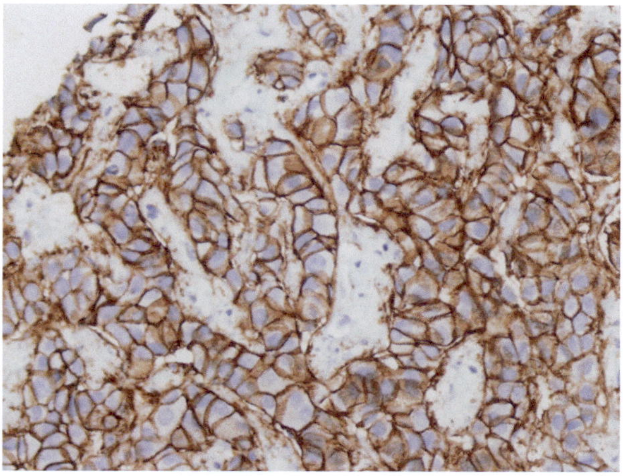

Fig. 6.2 Immunohistochemical score 3+ staining for c-erbB2. Strong, complete membranous staining with a chicken-wire appearance

- *Score 0:* No staining observed or membrane staining that is incomplete, faint/barely perceptible and in ≤10% of invasive tumor cells.
- *Score 1+:* Incomplete membrane staining that is faint/barely perceptible and in >10% of invasive tumor cells.
- *Equivocal (Score2+):* Weak/moderate complete membrane staining in >10% of invasive tumor cells or complete and circumferential membrane staining that is intense and in ≤10% of invasive tumor cells.
- *Positive (Score3+):* Circumferential membrane staining in >10% of invasive tumor cells that is complete and intense (Fig. 6.2).
- Samples scored as 3+ are considered unequivocally positive, and those scoring 0/1+ are considered negative. Equivocal scores (2+) mandate further assessment using ISH.
- *Indeterminate:* This category was added in the 2013 update. The test should be reported as indeterminate if technical issues prevent one or both tests (IHC and ISH) from being reported as positive, negative or equivocal. Examples include inadequate specimen handling, artifacts (e.g., crushed or marked edge artifacts) that make interpretation difficult, analytical testing failure or controls that are not as expected. The test should be repeated if possible.

ISH reporting:

- *Positive*
  - Single-probe average HER2 copy number ≥6.0 signals/cell (Fig. 6.3).
  - Dual-probe HER2/CEP17 ratio ≥2.0 with an average HER2 copy number ≥4.0 signals per cell.
- *Negative*
  - Single-probe average HER2 copy number <4.0 signals/cell.
  - Dual-probe HER2/CEP17 ratio <2.0 with an average HER2 copy number <6.0 signals/cell.

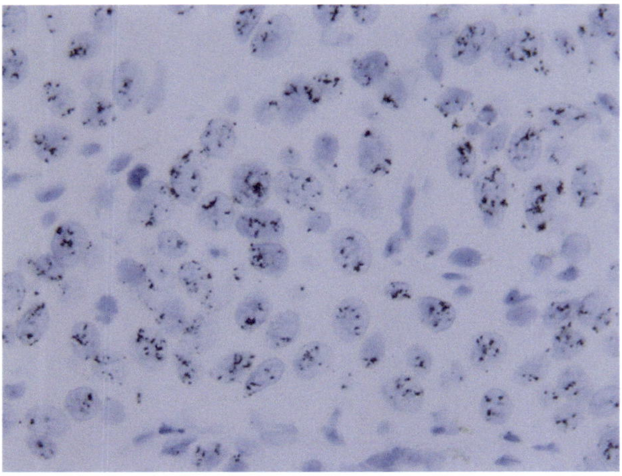

Fig. 6.3 Gene amplification of the same case with silver in situ hybridization (SISH). Numerous signals per nuclei forming many clusters

The 2018 update on recommendations for HER2 testing with ISH method cancelled an equivocal result. Instead, forced pathologists to make a judgement as positive or negative using combination of repeated IHC and dual-probe ISH method. According to final update, if the HER2/CEP 17 ratio ≥2.0 and average HER2 copy number is <4.0 the result should be negative after completion of a work-up. If the average HER2 copy number is ≥6.0 and the ratio is <2.0 the result should be positive after completion of a work-up [31].

Regarding preanalytical and analytical measures, these guidelines recommend a cold ischemic time as short as possible and less than 1 h. Only formalin-fixed, paraffin-embedded tumor tissue samples are considered appropriate for assay. Surgical specimens should be incised as soon as possible through the tumor to allow penetration of the fixative. The specimens are fixed in 10% neutral buffered formalin for 6–72 h, and routine processing and staining or probing are performed according to standardized analytically validated protocols [29].

Ki-67

Ki67 antigen is the most commonly used immunohistochemical marker of cell proliferation. It is expressed by proliferating cells in late G1, S and G2/M phases of the cell cycle. Several studies have shown that Ki67 expression correlates with other well-known markers of proliferation, such as the mitotic index, S-phase fraction, tyrosine kinase and bromodeoxyuridine incorporation.

The clinical utility of Ki67 has been reported in both the adjuvant setting as a prognostic and predictive marker and as an endpoint for neoadjuvant systemic therapy studies [32]. However, its routine clinical use is controversial due to problems of both preanalytical parameters and methodological differences in scoring.

The St Gallen breast cancer consensus panel endorses Ki67 as a means to differentiate Luminal A from Luminal B tumors. Acknowledging that the cut-point between Ki67 'high' versus 'low' tumors varies between laboratories, they accepted a level of <14% as having the best correlation with gene expression on the basis of the results of a single reference laboratory [33, 34]. However, the 14th St Gallen breast cancer panel declared that the minimum Ki-67 score for luminal B-like is 20–29% and that Ki-67 scores should be interpreted according to local laboratory values. For example, if a laboratory's median Ki-67 score is 20% in receptor-positive disease, scores of 30% and above are considered clearly high, whereas scores of 10% and below are considered low [35].

The International Ki67 in Breast Cancer Working Group is cautious in recommending the routine use of Ki67 [36]. Because of the lack of standardization of evaluation methods, Ki67 IHC is not recommended by CAP or ASCO [8].

Similar to other biomarkers, many variables (e.g., length of fixation, antigen retrieval method, choice of antibody clone) affect the results of Ki-67 scoring. Among several antibodies against Ki67, only the mouse monoclonal antibody MIB1 has been widely adopted for approximately two decades, but a recent rabbit monoclonal antibody, SP6, has shown similar performance to MIB1 for visual analysis and improved performance for image analysis [37].

Substantial variability in Ki67 scoring is observed among some of the world's most experienced laboratories, with moderate concordance at best [38] due to differences in scoring, such as tumor region selection, counting method (hot spot versus average), and subjective assessment of staining positivity.

Despite these difficulties, Ki67 can still provide useful information in pathology reports. When very low (a few percent), it can corroborate a Luminal A phenotype in the context of high ER and PR content; a very high Ki67 index can corroborate a Luminal B phenotype regardless of the percentage of ER/PR content; in high-grade triple-negative tumors, a Ki67 index of >50% is almost universal [32].

Gene Expression Tests

Several gene expression profiling assays have been developed in an attempt to predict the survival and response to therapies of breast cancer patients. These assays are based on the identification of prognostic gene signatures by using microarrays.

Perou [39] and his colleagues were the first to distinguish four molecular classes of breast cancer with their 'intrinsic' classification:

Luminal cancers are almost all ER positive, express cytokeratin 8 and 18 typical for the breast glands, and are divided into two categories:

Luminal A, which are mostly histologically low grade and express the highest levels of ER and ER-related genes and lowest levels of proliferation-related genes;

Luminal B, which tend to be of high grade with a worse prognosis, with an opposite pattern of gene expression compared with the Luminal A group.

HER2-enriched cancers show amplification and overexpression of the ERBB2 gene, do not express hormone receptors and have a poor prognosis.

A substantial proportion of breast cancers are HER2-positive but also express ER. They are classified as "luminal B" cancers.

Basal-like breast cancers overlay markedly with ER-, PgR-, and HER2-negative (triple negative) tumors, with poor prognosis and the expression of cytokeratins of the basal layer (for example, CK 5/6). They are characterized by the expression of genes that are usually found in the basal/myoepithelial layer of the normal breast, with high levels of proliferation-related genes.

Tumors that were initially classified as "normal breast-like" are now accepted as an artifactual group arising from the normal breast epithelium intermixed within the tumor.

More recently, additional subtypes have also been described [40]:

Molecular apocrine subtype features activation of androgen receptor signaling.

Interferon subtype is characterized by high expression of interferon regulated-genes, including STAT1.

Claudin-low comprises tumors that have transcriptomic features suggestive of a 'cancer stem cell-like' phenotype with high epithelial-mesenchymal transition (EMT) markers.

Studies have revealed that the most stable separation is between basal-like tumors and tumors classified as of another intrinsic subtype. Approximately 70–75% of cancers classified as basal-like by microarrays are triple negative by IHC, and only 70–75% of cases that are triple negative by IHC are basal-like by microarrays [41]. Furthermore, there is substantial discrepancy in HER2 status between IHC/FISH and microarray results [42].

Many groups have attempted to develop genomic tests based on genomic profiling with the expectation that this might better predict clinical outcome compared with standard pathological and clinical markers. The most common tests include the following:

MammaPrint This assay, which was developed by The Netherlands Cancer Institute in 2002, was the first prognostic signature described. Gene expression microarray analysis of breast cancer specimens from 78 node-negative patients less than 55 years of age was used to develop the 70-gene prognostic signature [43]. By comparing the expression profiles of tumors from patients who developed distant metastasis within 5 years and who did not, the researchers identified a prognostic signature. This signature was found to be a predictive parameter of outcome and predictive for chemotherapy response in patients with poor prognosis. It was also validated in several independent cohort studies and shown to add prognostic information beyond standard clinicopathological factors in both node-negative and positive patients [44–47].

Commercially available MammaPrint categorizes patient into two groups: (a) low risk (b) and high risk for breast cancer distant relapse within 10 years of the initial diagnosis. MammaPrint was developed originally for fresh frozen tissue but now has FDA clearance for the formalin-fixed paraffin-embedded (FFPE) version.

The international, prospective, phase III trial "microarray in node-negative and 1—3 positive lymph node disease may avoid chemotherapy" (MINDACT, NCT00433589) is designed to address whether chemotherapy can be safely avoided in patients who are predicted to be at low risk by the MammaPrint test but at high risk by clinical assessment with Adjuvant! Online [48]. MINDACT has shown that approximately 46% of patients who were at high clinical risk for recurrence defined using Adjuvant! Online might not require chemotherapy. These women had a low genomic risk for recurrence according to *MammaPrint*, a genomic signature that assists in predicting clinical outcomes in women with early-stage breast cancer [49].

Oncotype DX Test (Genomic Health, Redwood, CA, USA) This is a quantitative reverse transcriptase–polymerase chain reaction (RT–PCR) assay generated to measure gene expression in FFPE samples. It measures a panel of 21 genes, including 16 cancer-related (prognostic) genes plus five reference genes, and generates a recurrence score (RS) that classifies patients as at low (RS < 18), intermediate (RS 18–30), or high (RS ≥ 31) risk of recurrence [50]. The 10-year distant recurrence rates of each category are 6.8%, 14.3%, and 30.5%, respectively.

The test was originally designed to predict distant recurrence in 10 years in hormonal receptor-positive and node-negative breast cancers, and its role in lymph node-positive patients remains controversial [38].

Oncotype DX is included in the St Gallen, American Society of Clinical Oncology, and National Comprehensive Cancer Network (NCCN) guidelines as a decision tool enabling the identification of patients who are most likely to benefit from adjuvant chemotherapy and is indicated for women with node-negative, ER-positive breast cancer to determine prognosis in patients who are recommended to proceed with at least a 5-year course of endocrine therapy.

The Trial Assigning IndividuaLized Options for Treatment (Rx) (TAILORx) study demonstrated that a group of TAILORx trial participants with low 21-gene recurrence score (Oncotype DX® Recurrence Score®) results of 10 or less who received hormonal therapy alone without chemotherapy had a less than 1% chance of distant recurrence at 5 years [51].

PAM50 (Prosigna) The PAM50 ROR (NanoString Technologies, Seattle, WA, USA) score is based on a 50-gene test that was developed to identify intrinsic breast cancer subtypes. The ROR is derived from the expression profile of the 50 genes and includes information on tumor size as well. The ROR score has been validated in women with node-negative or node-positive disease and has been shown to classify women into low- or high-risk groups and to add prognostic information beyond that of clinical or IHC4 factors [52–54].

In the transATAC trial, the PAM50 ROR score provided more prognostic information than did RS, with fewer patients categorized as intermediate risk and more as high risk. It also provided at least as much information as IHC4 and may provide more information in the node-negative/HER2-negative group [55]. The ROR score was also evaluated in the ABCSG-8 (Austrian Breast and Colorectal Cancer Study Group 8) trial, in which postmenopausal women with early breast cancer were randomly assigned to receive tamoxifen or anastrozole for 5 years. In this large study, the ROR score was found to add significant prognostic information beyond that of clinical parameters for distant recurrence in the overall population and all subgroups. The study also confirmed the better discrimination between low- and high-risk groups in all subgroups [56].

The Genomic Grade Index (GGI) (MapQuant Dx) (Ipsogen, Marseille, France) is a 97-gene microarray signature that assigns a molecular grade.

The Breast Cancer Index (BCI) (BioTheranostics, San Diego, CA, USA) is a centrally performed qRT–PCR-based assay for use on FFPE tumor blocks.

The EndoPredict test (Sividon Diagnostics GmbH, Koln, Germany), also a qRT–PCR-based multigene assay, measures the expression of eight cancer genes and three housekeeping control genes (plus one gene to measure the presence of contaminating genomic DNA), which are then combined with the classical prognostic factors of tumor size and node status (EPclin score) to stratify patients with ER-positive HER2-negative cancer into a low or high risk of recurrence if treated with adjuvant endocrine therapy alone.

A trial comparing multiparameter tests (MammaPrint, Oncotype DX, Prosigna, IHC4, and IHC4-AQUA) [57] concluded that according to the existing evidence, the different tests provide broadly equivalent risk information for the population of women with ER-positive breast cancers. However, for individual patients, the tests may provide differing risk categorization and subtype information. There was marked disagreement across all tests. Indeed, for all tests, the level of agreement was “moderate”.

The major disadvantages of these tests are as follows:

They are informative only in hormone receptor-positive, lymph node-negative cases. Long-term recurrence risk cannot be predicted, except that shown in a study of Prosigna [57]. The cost effectiveness of these tests is another concern. They are performed in central laboratories, except Prosigna, which can be performed in appropriate local laboratories [54].

In the 8th version of the American Joint Commission of Cancer (AJCC) for breast cancer, which will be available in 2018, prognostic gene signatures will be integrated into the staging scheme as prognostic staging [58]:

For patients with hormone receptor-positive, HER2-negative, and lymph node-negative tumors, prognostic gene signatures (Oncotype DX, MammaPrint, Endopredict, BCI) with a low risk score regardless of T size place the tumor in the same prognostic category as T1a-T1b N0M0, and the tumor is staged using the AJCC prognostic stage group table as stage I [58].

References

1. Schnitt SJ. Classification and prognosis of invasive breast cancer: from morphology to molecular taxonomy: Long Course Article. Mod Pathol. 2010;23:S60–4.
2. Edge SB, Byrd DR, Carducci MA, Compton CC, editors. AJCC cancer staging manual. 7th ed. New York: Springer; 2009.

3. Elston CW, Gresham GA, Rao GS, Zebro T, Haybittle JL, et al. The cancer research campaign (Kings/Cambridge) trial for early breast cancer-pathological aspects. Brit J Cancer. 1982;45:655–69.
4. Fisher ER, Sass R, Fisher B. Pathologic findings from the National Surgical Adjuvant Project for breast cancer (protocol no 4). Discrimination for tenth year treatment failure. Cancer. 1984;53:712–23.
5. Carter GL, Allen C, Henson DE. Relation of tumour size, lymph node status, and survival in 24,740 breast cancer cases. Cancer. 1989;63:181–7.
6. Neville AM, Bettelheim R, Gelber RD, Säve-Söderbergh J, Davis BW, Reed R, et al. Factors predicting treatment responsiveness and prognosis in node-negative breast cancer. J Clin Oncol. 1992;10:696–705.
7. Lakhani S, Ellis IO, Tan PH, van de Vijver MJ, editors. World Health Organization classification of tumors, WHO classification of tumors of the breast. 2nd ed. Lyon: IARC; 2012.
8. Lester SC, Bose S, Chen YY, Connolly JL, de Baca ME, Fitzgibbons PL, et al. Members of the Cancer committee, College of American Pathologists. Protocol for the examination of specimens from patients with invasive carcinoma of the breast. Arch Pathol Lab Med. 2009;133(10):1515–38.
9. Zurrida S, Morabito A, Galimberti V, Luini A, Greco M, Bartoli C, et al. Importance of the level of axillary involvement in relation to traditional variables in the prognosis of breast cancer. Int J Oncol. 1999;15(3):475–80.
10. Giuliano AE, Hunt KK, Ballman KV, Beitsch PD, Whitworth PW, Blumencranz PW, et al. Axillary dissection vs no axillary dissection in women with invasive breast cancer and sentinel node metastasis: a randomized clinical trial. JAMA. 2011;305(6):569–75.
11. Elston CW, Ellis IO. Pathological prognostic factors in breast cancer I. The value of histological grade in breast cancer: experience from a large study with long-term follow-up. Histopathology. 1991;19:403–10.
12. Rakha EA, El-Sayed ME, Lee AH, Elston CW, Grainge MJ, Hodi Z, et al. Prognostic significance of Nottingham histologic grade in invasive breast carcinoma. J Clin Oncol. 2008;26:3153–8.
13. Rakha EA, Reis-Filho JS, Baehner F, Dabbs DJ, Decker D, et al. Breast cancer prognostic classification in the molecular era: the role of histological grade. Breast Cancer Res. 2010;12(4):207.
14. Pathology reporting of breast disease: a joint document incorporating the third edition of the NHS Breast Screening Programmes guidelines for pathology reporting in breast cancer screening and the second edition of The Royal College of Pathologists' minimum dataset for breast cancer histopathology. Sheffield; NHS Cancer Screening Programmes and The Royal College of Pathologists; 2005.
15. Ellis IO, Galea M, Broughton N, Locker A, Blamey RW, Elston CW. Pathological prognostic factors in breast cancer. II, histological type. Relationship with survival in a large study with long-term follow-up. Histopathology. 1992;20:479–89.
16. Pinder S, Ellis IO, Galea M, O'Rouke S, Blamey RW, Elston CW. Pathological prognostic factors in breast cancer—vascular invasion: relationship with recurrence and survival in a large series with long-term followup. Histopathology. 1994;24(1):41–7.
17. Rakha EA, Martin S, Lee AH, Morgan D, Pharoah PD, Hodi Z, et al. The prognostic significance of lymphovascular invasion in invasive breast carcinoma. Cancer. 2012;118(15):3670–80.
18. Bardou VJ, Arpino G, Elledge RM, Osborne CK, Clark GM. Progesterone receptor status significantly improves outcome prediction over estrogen receptor status alone for adjuvant endocrine therapy in two large breast cancer databases. J Clin Oncol. 2003;21(10):1973–9.
19. Rakha E, Ellis IO. Modern classification of breast cancer: should we stick with morphology or convert to molecular profile characteristics. Adv Anat Pathol. 2011;18(4):255–67.
20. Hammond ME, Hayes DF, Dowsett M, Allred DC, Hagerty KL, Badve S, et al. American Society of Clinical Oncology/College of American Pathologists guideline recommendations for immunohistochemical testing of estrogen and progesterone receptors in breast cancer. J Clin Oncol. 2010;28(16):2784–95.

21. Goldstein NS, Ferkowicz M, Odish E, Mani A, Hastah F. Minimum formalin fixation time for consistent estrogen receptor immunohistochemical staining of invasive breast carcinoma. Am J Clin Pathol. 2003;120:86–92.
22. Seidman AD, Berry D, Cirrincione C, Harris L, Muss H, Marcom PK, et al. Randomized phase III trial of weekly compared with every-3-weeks paclitaxel for metastatic breast cancer, with trastuzumab for all HER-2 overexpressors and random assignment to trastuzumab or not in HER-2 nonoverexpressors: final results of Cancer and Leukemia Group B protocol 9840. J Clin Oncol. 2008;26:1642–9.
23. Perez EA, Suman VJ, Davidson NE, Martino S, Kaufman PA, Lingle WL, et al. HER2 testing by local, central, and reference laboratories in specimens from the North Central Cancer Treatment Group N9831 intergroup adjuvant trial. J Clin Oncol. 2006;24(19):3032–8.
24. Dowsett M, Hanna WM, Kockx M, Penault-Llorca F, Rüschoff J, Gutjahr T, et al. Standardization of HER2 testing: results of an international proficiency-testing ring study. Mod Pathol. 2007;20(5):584–91.
25. Tuzlali S, Yavuz E, Canda T, Güray M, Geçer MO, Süllü Y, et al. In situ hybridization analysis of invasive breast carcinomas with immunohistochemically negative Her-2 status (a national multicenter study). Turk J Pathol. 2014;30(2):87–93.
26. Wolff AC, Hammond ME, Schwartz JN, Hagerty KL, Allred DC, Cote RJ, et al. American Society of Clinical Oncology/College of American Pathologists guideline recommendations for human epidermal growth factor receptor 2 testing in breast cancer. J Clin Oncol. 2007;25:118–45.
27. Middleton LP, Price KM, Puig P, Heydon LJ, Tarco E, Sneige N, et al. Implementation of American Society of Clinical Oncology/College of American Pathologists HER2 Guideline Recommendations in a tertiary care facility increases HER2 immunohistochemistry and fluorescence in situ hybridization concordance and decreases the number of inconclusive cases. Arch Pathol Lab Med. 2009;133:775–80.
28. Liu YH, Xu FP, Rao JY, Zhuang HG, Luo XL, Li L, et al. Justification of the change from 10% to 30% for the immunohistochemical HER2 scoring criterion in breast cancer. Am J Clin Pathol. 2009;132:74–9.
29. Wolff AC, Hammond ME, Hicks DG, Dowsett M, McShane LM, Allison KH, et al. Recommendations for human epidermal growth factor receptor 2 testing in breast cancer: American Society of Clinical Oncology/College of American Pathologists clinical practice guideline update. J Clin Oncol. 2013;31:3997–4013.
30. Wolff AC, Hammond ME, Hicks DG. American Society of Clinical Oncology/College of American Pathologists clinical practice guideline upcoming modifications. Proof thet clinical practice guidelines are living documents. Arch Pathol Lab Med. 2015;139(8):970–1.
31. Wolff AC, Hammond MEH, Allison KH, Harvey BE, Mangu PB, Bartlett JMS, et al. Human epidermal growth factor receptor 2 testing in breast cancer: American Society of Clinical Oncology/College of American Pathologists clinical practice guideline focused update. J Clin Oncol. 2018;36(20):2105–22. https://doi.org/10.1200/JCO.2018.77.8738.
32. Kos Z, Dabbs DJ. Biomarker assessment and molecular testing for prognostication in breast cancer. Histopathology. 2016;68:70–85.
33. Goldhirsch A, Winer EP, Coates AS, Gelber RD, Piccart-Gebhart M, Thürlimann B, et al. Personalizing the treatment of women with early breast cancer: highlights of the St Gallen International Expert Consensus on the Primary Therapy of Early Breast Cancer 2013. Ann Oncol. 2013;24:2206–23.
34. Cheang MCU, Chia SK, Voduc D, Gao D, Leung S, Snider J, et al. Ki67 index, HER2 status, and prognosis of patients with luminal B breast cancer. J Natl Cancer Inst. 2009;101:736–50.
35. Coates AS, Winer EP, Goldhirsch A, Gelber RD, Gnant M, Piccart-Gebhart M, et al. Tailoring therapies--improving the management of early breast cancer: St Gallen International Expert Consensus on the Primary Therapy of Early Breast Cancer 2015. Ann Oncol. 2015;26:1533–46.
36. Dowsett M, Nielsen TO, A'Hern R, Bartlett J, Coombes RC, Cuzick J, et al. Assessment of Ki67 in breast cancer: recommendations from the International Ki67 in Breast Cancer working group. J Natl Cancer Inst. 2011;103(22):1656–64.

37. Zabaglo L, Salter J, Anderson H, Quinn E, Hills M, Detre S, et al. Comparative validation of the SP6 antibody to Ki67 in breast cancer. J Clin Pathol. 2010;63(9):800–4.
38. Polley MY, Leung SC, McShane LM, Gao D, Hugh JC, Mastropasqua MG, et al. International Ki67 in Breast Cancer Working Group of the Breast International Group and North American Breast Cancer Group. An international Ki67 reproducibility study. J Natl Cancer Inst. 2013;105(24):1897–906.
39. Perou CM, Sørlie T, Eisen MB, van de Rijn M, Jeffrey SS, Rees CA, et al. Molecular portraits of human breast tumours. Nature. 2000;406:747–52.
40. Weigelt B, Geyer FC, Jorge S, Reis-Filho JS. Histological types of breast cancer: how special are they? Mol Oncol. 2010;4:192–208.
41. Foulkes WD, Smith IE, Reis-Filho JS. Triple-negative breast cancer. N Engl J Med. 2010;363:1938–48.
42. Dabbs DJ, Klein ME, Mohsin SK, Tubbs RR, Shuai Y, Bhargava R. High false-negative rate of HER2 quantitative reverse transcription polymerase chain reaction of the oncotype DX test: an independent quality assurance study. J Clin Oncol. 2011;29:4279–85.
43. van't Veer LJ, Dai H, van de Vijver MJ, He YD, Hart AA, Mao M, et al. Gene expression profiling predicts clinical outcome of breast cancer. Nature. 2002;415:530–6.
44. Bueno-de-Mesquita JM, Linn SC, Keijzer R, Wesseling J, Nuyten DS, van Krimpen C, et al. Validation of 70-gene prognosis signature in node-negative breast cancer. Breast Cancer Res Treat. 2009;117:483–95.
45. Mook S, Schmidt MK, Weigelt B, Kreike B, Eekhout I, van de Vijver MJ, et al. The 70-gene prognosis signature predicts early metastasis in breast cancer patients between 55 and 70 years of age. Ann Oncol. 2010;21:717–22.
46. Mook S, Schmidt MK, Viale G, Pruneri G, Eekhout I, Floore A, et al. The 70-gene prognosis signature predicts disease outcome in breast cancer patients with 1–3 positive lymph nodes in an independent validation study. Breast Cancer Res Treat. 2009;116:295–302.
47. Drukker CA, Bueno-De-Mesquita JM, Retel VP, van Harten WH, van Tinteren H, Wesseling J, et al. A prospective evaluation of a breast cancer prognosis signature in the observational RASTER study. Int J Cancer. 2013;133:929–36.
48. Rutgers E, Piccart-Gebhart MJ, Bogaerts J, Delaloge S, Veer LV, Rubio IT, et al. The EORTC 10041/BIG 03-04 MINDACT trial is feasible: results of the pilot phase. Eur J Cancer. 2011;47:2742–9.
49. Viale G, de Snoo FA, Slaets L, Bogaerts J, van't Veer L, Rutgers EJ, et al. MINDACT investigators. Immunohistochemical versus molecular (BluePrint and MammaPrint) subtyping of breast carcinoma. Outcome results from the EORTC 10041/BIG 3-04 MINDACT trial. Breast Cancer Res Treat. 2018;167(1):123–31.
50. Paik S, Shak S, Tang G, Kim C, Baker J, Cronin M, et al. A multigene assay to predict recurrence of tamoxifen-treated, node-negative breast cancer. N Engl J Med. 2004;351(27):2817–26.
51. Sparano JA, Gray RJ, Makowe DF, Pritchard KI, Albain KS, Hayes DF, et al. Prospective validation of a 21-gene expression assay in breast cancer. N Engl J Med. 2015;373:2005–14.
52. Parker JS, Mullins M, Cheang MC, Leung S, Voduc D, Vickery T, et al. Supervised risk predictor of breast cancer based on intrinsic subtypes. J Clin Oncol. 2009;27:1160–7.
53. Nielsen TO, Parker JS, Leung S, Voduc D, Ebbert M, Vickery T, et al. A comparison of PAM50 intrinsic subtyping with immunohistochemistry and clinical prognostic factors in tamoxifen-treated estrogen receptor-positive breast cancer. Clin Cancer Res. 2010;16:5222–32.
54. Nielsen T, Wallden B, Schaper C, Ferree S, Liu S, Gao D, et al. Analytical validation of the PAM50-based Prosigna Breast Cancer Prognostic Gene Signature Assay and nCounter Analysis System using formalin-fixed paraffin-embedded breast tumor specimens. BMC Cancer. 2014;14:177.
55. Dowsett M, Sestak I, Lopez-Knowles E, Sidhu K, Dunbier AK, Cowens JW, et al. Comparison of PAM50 risk of recurrence score with Oncotype DX and IHC4 for predicting risk of distant recurrence after endocrine therapy. J Clin Oncol. 2013;31:2783–90.

56. Gnant M, Filipits M, Greil R, Stoeger H, Rudas M, Bago-Horvath Z, et al. Predicting distant recurrence in receptor-positive breast cancer patients with limited clinicopathological risk: using the PAM50 risk of recurrence score in 1478 postmenopausal patients of the ABCSG-8 trial treated with adjuvant endocrine therapy alone. Ann Oncol. 2014;25:339–45.
57. Bartlett JM, Bayani J, Marshall A, Dunn JA, Campbell A, Cunningham C, et al. OPTIMA TMG. Comparing breast cancer multiparameter tests in the OPTIMA Prelim Trial: no test is more equal than the others. J Natl Cancer Inst. 2016;108(9):djw050. https://doi.org/10.1093/jnci/djw050.
58. Giuliano AE, Connolly JL, Edge SB, Mittendorf EA, Rugo HS, Solin LJ, et al. Breast Cancer-major changes in the American Joint Committee on Cancer eighth edition cancer staging manual. CA Cancer J Clin. 2017;67(4):290–303.

Part III
Radiologic Imaging

Chapter 7
Breast Imaging

Ravza Yilmaz

Introduction

The practice of breast imaging has transitioned through a wide variety of technological advances from the early days of direct-exposure film mammography to the current era of full-field digital mammography and tomosynthesis. Mammography is the best-proven imaging method for reducing breast cancer mortality. Breast ultrasonography (US) and magnetic resonance imaging (MRI) are often used as an adjuncts to mammography to increase the ability of the radiologist to detect cancer and assess the degree of disease. A substantial part of breast imaging practice involves breast interventional procedures. There are also now many developing breast-imaging technologies to assist in the formulation and confirmation of the diagnosis. In this chapter, we aim to provide core knowledge and clinical guidelines for performing and interpreting breast imaging in everyday practice.

Mammography

Mammography is a specialized radiography of the breast that uses X-rays to generate images of the breast. The purposes of mammography are early detection of breast cancer before symptoms (screening mammography) and diagnosis in patients with symptoms (diagnostic mammography).

Mammography can be performed using a film screen, phosphor-plate computer radiography or a digital technique. Preference should be given to full-field digital mammography, which has a number of relevant advantages, including a lower X-ray dose, higher image quality, possibility of post-processing, digital archiving,

R. Yilmaz (✉)
Istanbul Medical Faculty, Department of Radiology, Istanbul University, Istanbul, Turkey

A. Aydiner et al. (eds.), *Breast Cancer*, https://doi.org/10.1007/978-3-319-96947-3_7

image transmission and no chemical pollution [1, 2]. Digital mammography has significantly better detection performance than film-screen mammography in population-based breast cancer screening. This gain is largely due to enhanced depiction of microcalcifications, resulting in improved detection of both ductal carcinoma in situ (DCIS) and invasive carcinoma [3]. Breast doses in digital mammography are 22% lower per view than those in film-screen mammography [4]. Two-view digital and film-screen mammograms have a mean average glandular dose of 3.7 and 4.7 mGy, respectively [5].

Screening Mammography

Mammography is the only breast imaging examination that has been demonstrated to reduce breast cancer mortality. It is relatively inexpensive and widely available. Early detection through mass screening with mammography has the potential to reduce mortality. The cancer detection rate of screening mammography is approximately 2–7 per 1000 screened women, depending on the patient population [6].

Mammography is performed every 1, 2 or 3 years from the age of 40–50 years until around age 70–75, depending on national/regional screening programs. The recent recommendations of the American Cancer Society are as follows: (1) regular screening mammography starting at 45 years of age (strong recommendation); (2) annual screening mammography from 45 to 54 years of age (qualified recommendation); (3) from 55 years of age, transition to biennial or continuing annually (qualified recommendation); (4) opportunity to begin annual screening from 40 to 44 years (qualified recommendation); and (5) continued screening mammography as long as the woman's overall health is good and she has a life expectancy of ≥10 years (qualified recommendation) [7]. European guidelines suggest a 2-year interval for the general female population from 50 to 70 years of age [8].

With respect to screening, women should be aware that approximately 28% of cancers can be missed, especially in pre-menopausal women and in those with dense breasts [9]. Increased breast density strongly impacts the sensitivity of screening mammography, declining from 86 to 89% for almost entirely fatty breasts to only 62–68% for extremely dense breasts [10]. Nevertheless, mammography is the best-proven method for screening average-risk women.

Screening mammography is a standardized procedure composed of four views, two for each breast: the cranio-caudal (CC) projection and the medio-lateral oblique (MLO) projection (Fig. 7.1). Screening mammography is performed by a single specially trained technologist; the acquired images are usually read by two radiologists independently. If the examination is judged to not reveal any abnormality suspicious for malignancy, the woman receives a report explaining this result. If something suspicious is found, the woman is recalled for a customized assessment that can be variably composed of additional mammographic views, tomosynthesis, contrast enhanced mammography (CEM), US, MRI or needle biopsy.

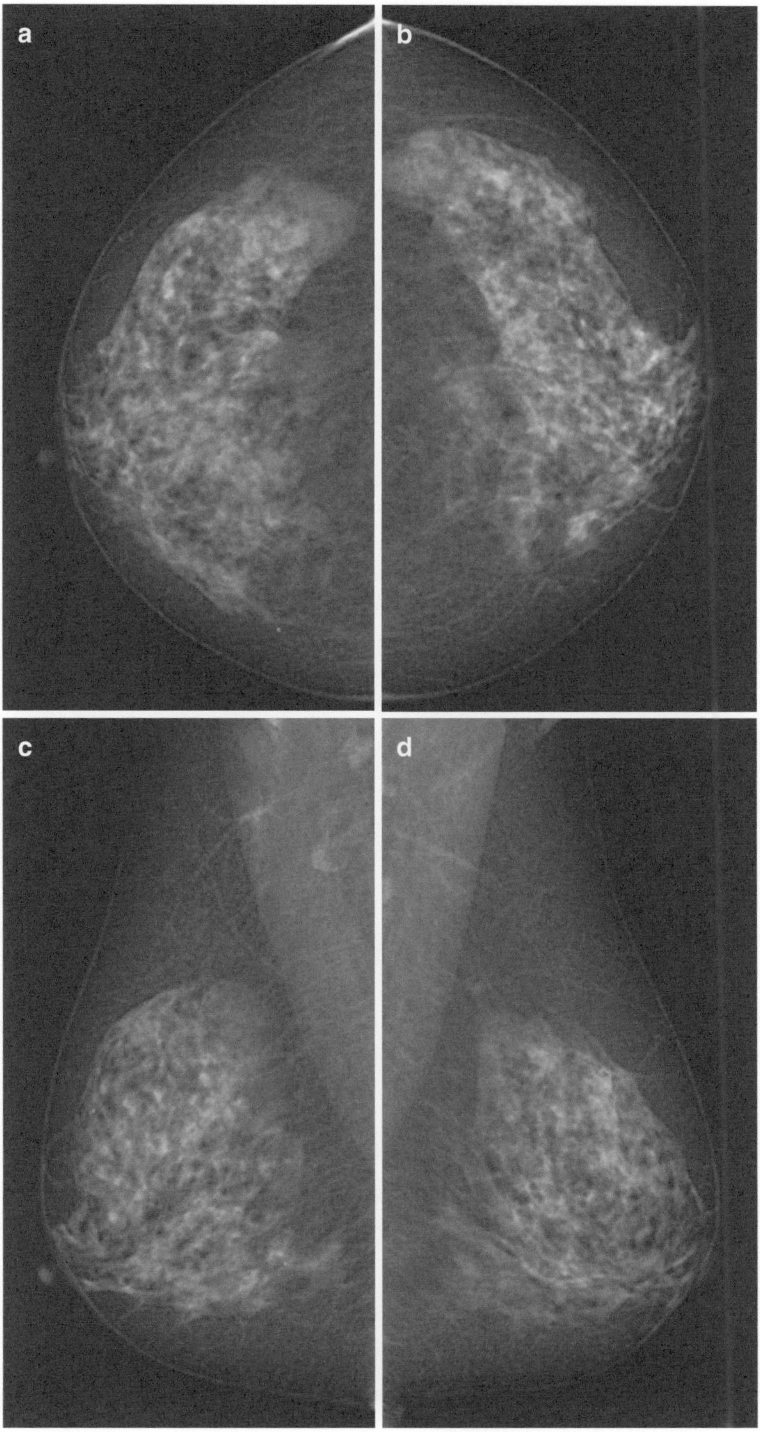

Fig. 7.1 Screening mammography in a 49-year-old asymptomatic woman. Bilateral digital cranio-caudal and mediolateral oblique views demonstrated heterogeneously dense breast tissue (**a–d**)

Diagnostic Mammography

A diagnostic mammography is performed in patients with clinical signs or symptoms of breast disease and in patients for whom further evaluation has been requested due to an abnormal screening mammogram or as a follow-up after prior imaging findings. When mammography is necessary in patients with symptoms, advantages always exceed disadvantages regardless of patient age. The patient waits in the department while the radiologist reviews the images; additional mammographic views and/or US may be obtained at that time to evaluate findings or symptoms. Comparison with previous mammography is very valuable and can allow the radiologist to detect a subtle developing malignancy. Spot compression and magnification are the mostly commonly used mammographic views to characterize a lesion or help image more of the breast tissue. Lateral, rolled CC, exaggerated CC, tangential, and cleavage views are used for the same purpose more rarely. Spot compression uses a smaller paddle to compress the breast focally, distinguish summation of normal tissue from a true mass, provide visibility of the lesion and evaluate the margins of a mass (Figs. 7.2 and 7.3). Magnification views are typically used to evaluate the morphology and distribution of microcalcifications; however, these mammographic views may also be helpful in characterizing the margins of a mass and architectural distortion (Fig. 7.4).

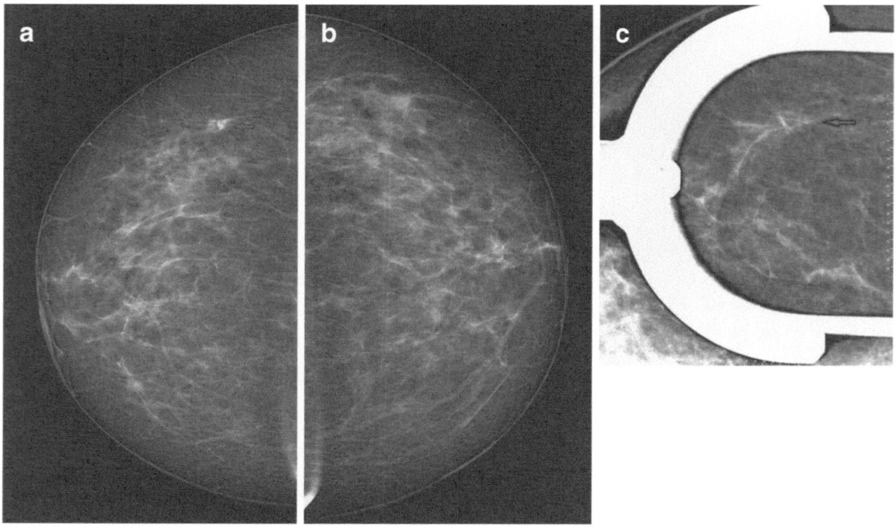

Fig. 7.2 First mammography in a 52-year-old asymptomatic woman. (**a**, **b**) Bilateral craniocaudal and mediolateral oblique views. In one view, an asymmetry was seen in the outer quadrant of the right breast. (**c**) Spot compression view showing decreased density and a lack of conspicuity of masses. Thus, the area was evaluated as a summation of normal tissue

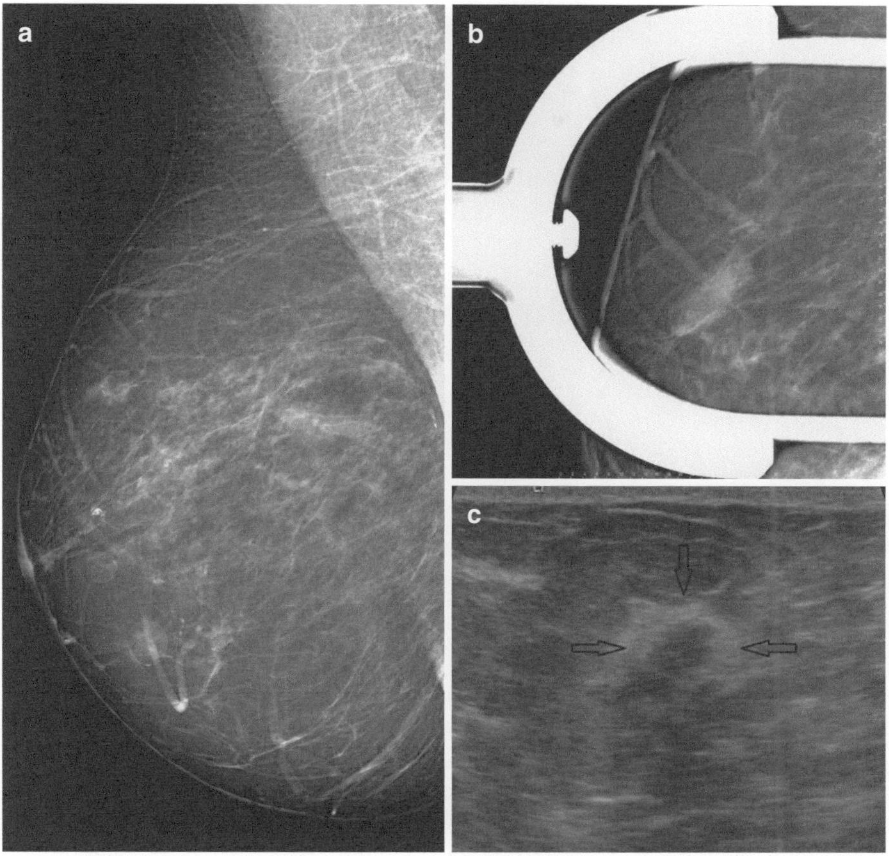

Fig. 7.3 Right MLO (**a**) and MLO spot compression (**b**) views showed a one-view asymmetry (*arrow*) in the upper anterior breast not seen on the CC view. Image from targeted US of the entire upper breast showed an oval hypoechoic mass with indistinct margins and an echogenic halo (*arrows*) (**c**). Subsequent ultrasound-guided biopsy revealed invasive ductal carcinoma

The mammographic lexicon includes category descriptions for breast composition or density, masses, calcifications, asymmetries, associated features, and location of the lesion. A mammographic report will begin by stating the breast density according to the allowed breast density lexicon as fatty, scattered, heterogeneously dense, and extremely dense. If a mass is seen, three descriptions are required: shape, margin, and density. The shape can be round, oval, or irregular. The margins can be circumscribed, obscured, microlobulated, indistinct, and spiculated. The density of the mass can be high density, equal density, low density, and fat containing. Of these descriptions, a mass that is an irregular shape with spiculated margins and high density is the most concerning for malignancy

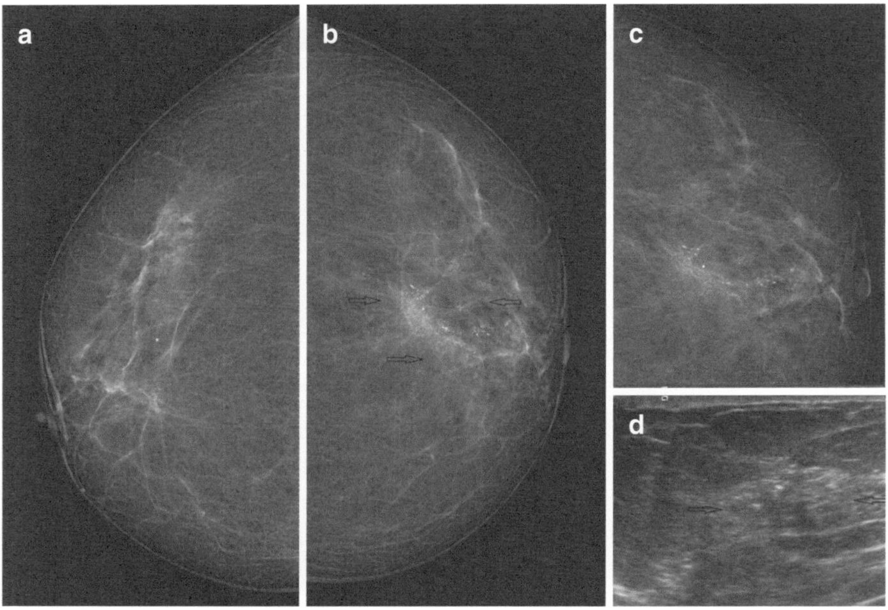

Fig. 7.4 A 48-year-old asymptomatic woman recalled from screening mammography (**a**, **b**). Spot magnification on craniocaudal mammogram demonstrated dense pleomorphic calcifications suspicious for malignancy (**c**). They are in a segmental distribution directed toward the nipple. An image from targeted US showed an irregular heterogenous mass with indistinct margins and echogenic calcifications (*arrows*) (**d**)

(Fig. 7.5). By contrast, a mass that is a round shape with circumscribed margins is more likely benign, especially if it is fat containing (Fig. 7.6). Malignant tumors rarely feature this appearance, but high density attracts attention (Fig. 7.7).

Architectural distortion refers to breast parenchymal architecture without a definable mass and can be due to malignant lesions, such as invasive cancer or DCIS, or to benign lesions, such as a radial scar or a complex sclerosing lesion (Fig. 7.8). The positive predictive value for malignancy is approximately 75% [11, 12]. Architectural distortion may be the earliest manifestation of breast cancer and is the most commonly missed abnormality on false-negative mammograms [13]. Distortion is best observed on magnified views or tomosynthesis images and is often subtle on US.

An asymmetry is seen on only one of the two standard mammographic views, either CC or MLO, lacks convex borders, may or may not contain interspersed fat, and occupies less than one quadrant of the breast. It is found on 3.3% of all screening mammograms [14]. Persistent asymmetries have been reported to be malignant in 10.3% of screening-detected cases [14]. A focal asymmetry has a similar appearance on both the CC and MLO views, lacks convex borders, and may contain interspersed fat. A developing asymmetry is a focal asymmetry that was not present on

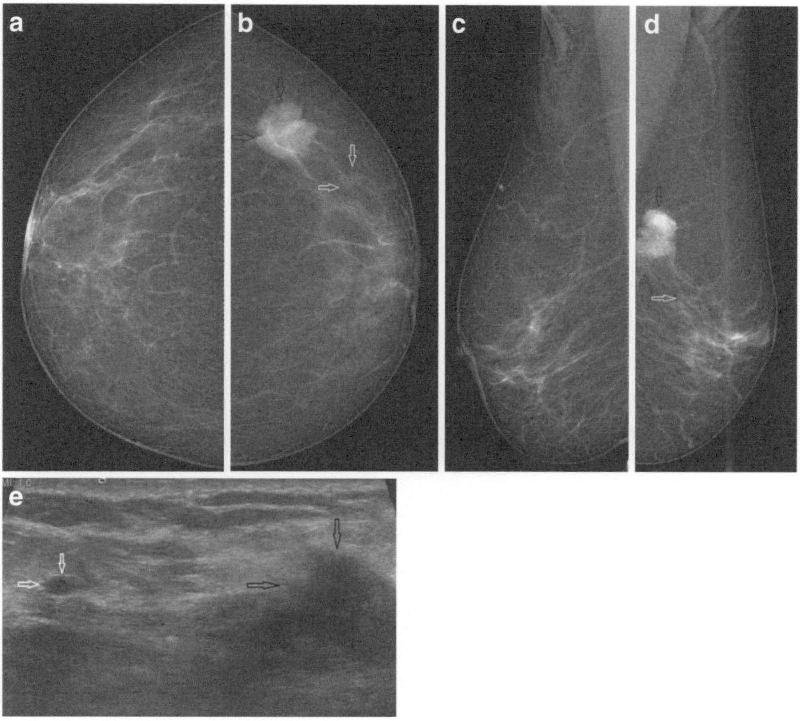

Fig. 7.5 A 61-year-old woman with a palpable lump in the left breast (**a**–**d**). CC and MLO mammograms of the left breast demonstrated a microlobulated dense mass in the upper outer quadrant corresponding to the palpable lump (*black arrow*). Lower-density opacity was observed in front of the identified mass on mammograms (*white arrows*) (**b**, **d**). US demonstrated an irregular hypoechoic mass with microlobulated and angulated margins (*black arrows*) and an ovoid hypoechoic mass with indistinct margins (*white arrows*), revealing multifocal invasive ductal carcinoma (**e**)

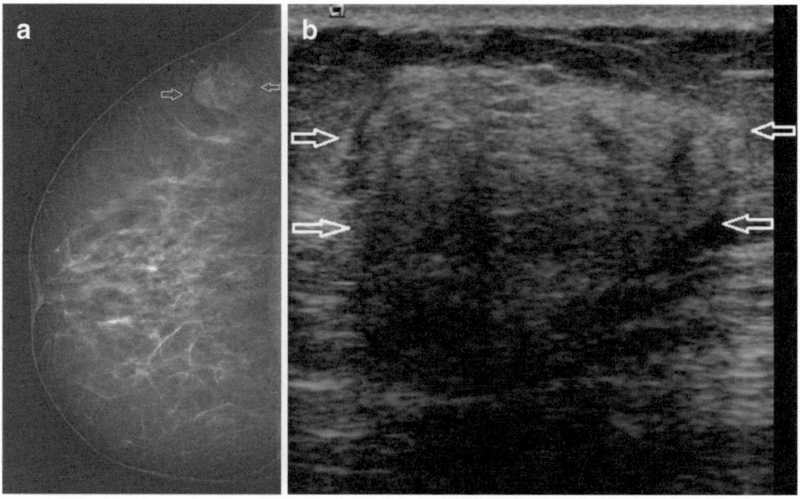

Fig. 7.6 Right CC views of a 36-mm circumscribed oval mass with a fat density typical of hamartoma (**a**). US showed a well-defined mass in the same area that was composed of hypoechoic and hyperechoic areas with posterior acoustic shadowing (**b**)

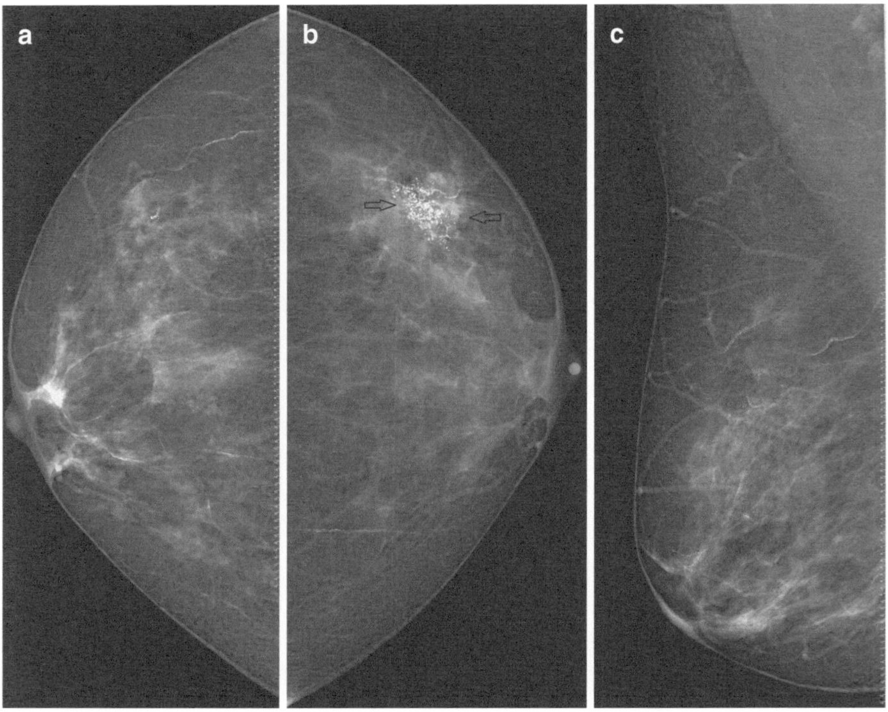

Fig. 7.7 A 40-year-old woman with a palpable lump in the left breast. Bilateral CC and MLO views demonstrated heterogeneously dense breast tissue and vascular calcifications (**a**–**d**). A spiculated dense mass within pleomorphic calcifications in the upper outer quadrant of the left breast and lymph nodes with a thick cortex (*stars*) were observed (**b**, **d**). Targeted US showed an irregular heterogenous mass with indistinct margins and echogenic calcifications (**e**) (*arrows*)

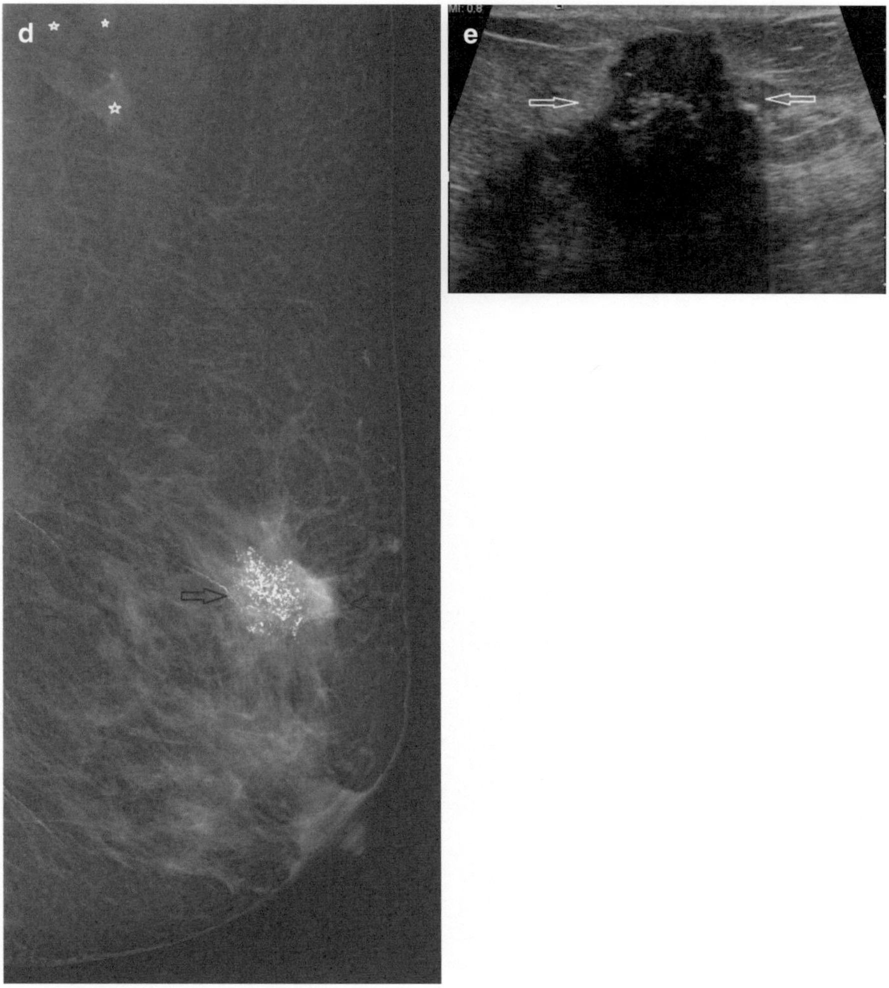

Fig. 7.7 (continued)

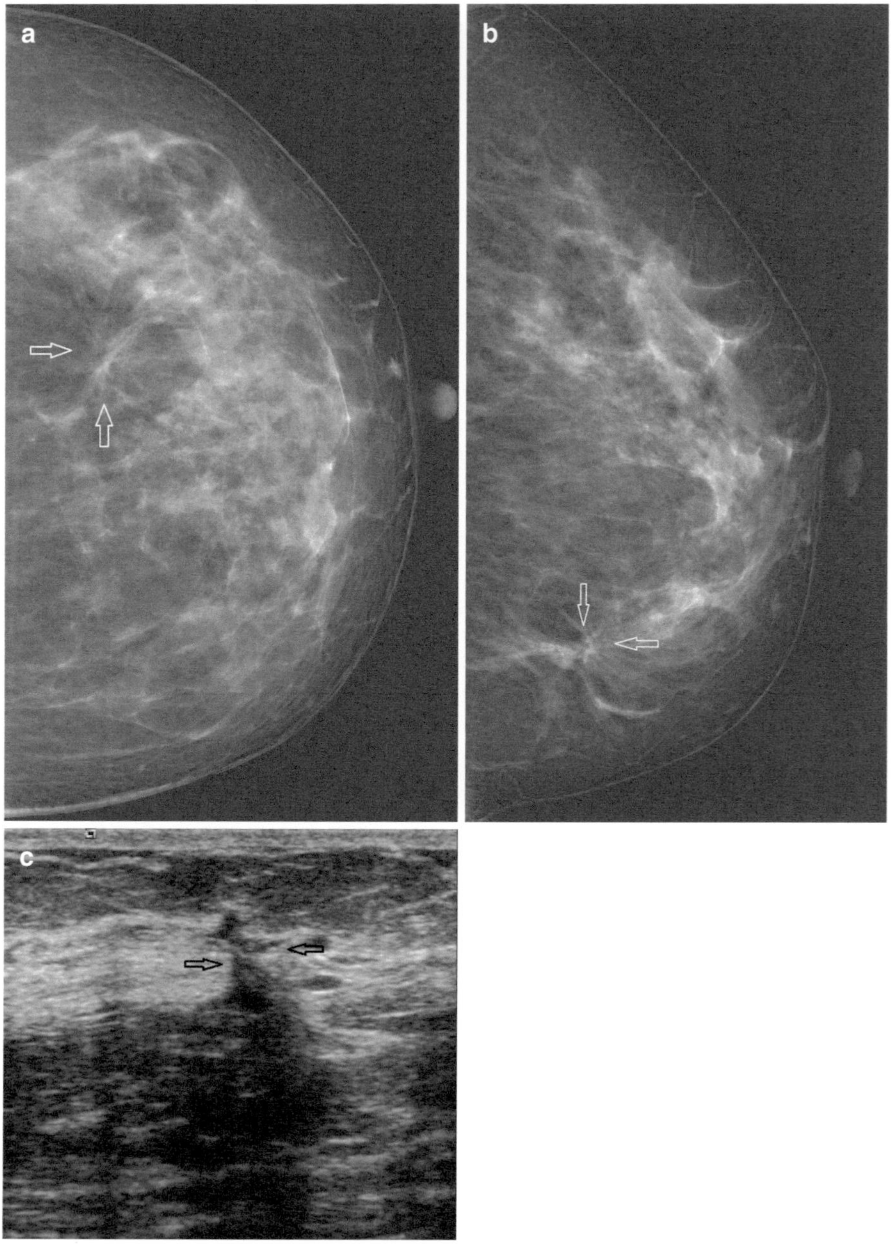

Fig. 7.8 A 57-year-old woman who presented for screening mammography. CC and ML mammograms showed architectural distortion (*arrows*) in the left breast (**a**, **b**). The US image showed an irregular hypoechoic 8-mm mass with posterior acoustic shadowing that corresponded to the mammographic finding (**c**). Core biopsy and surgical pathology revealed ductal carcinoma in situ

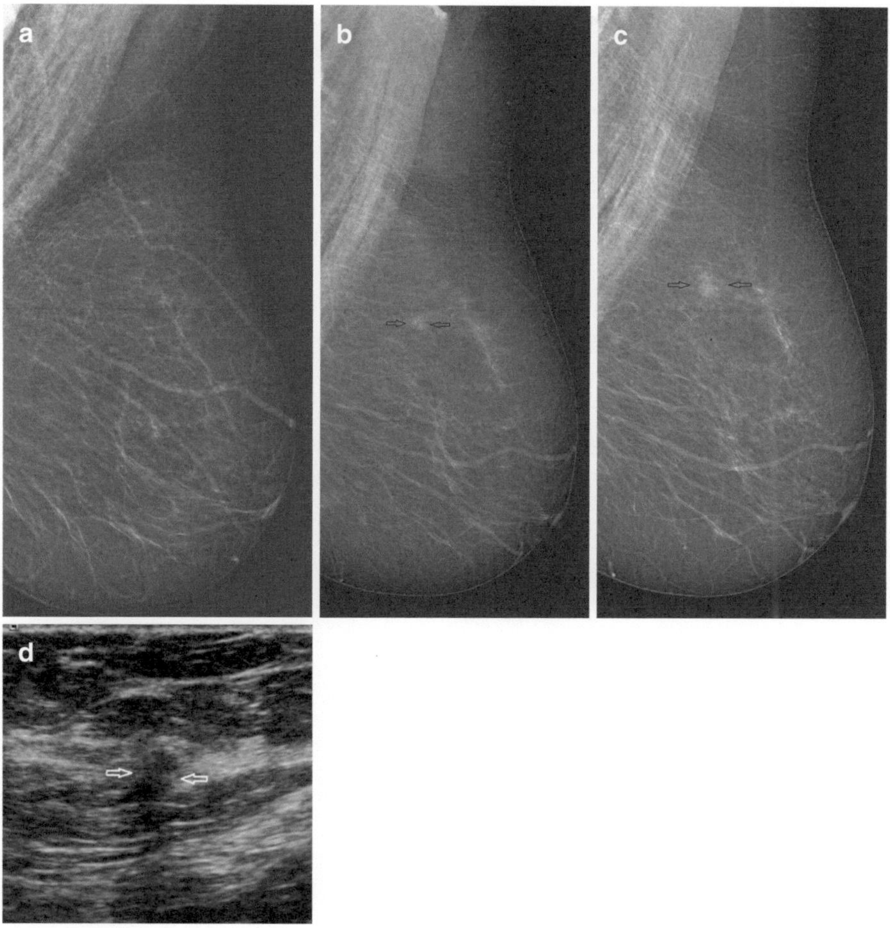

Fig. 7.9 A 63-year-old woman with developing asymmetry in the upper quadrant. The mediolateral oblique mammographic view from 2008 (**a**) showed no abnormal findings. The mammographic image from 2009 showed a focal asymmetry (**b**) that was enlarged in MLO from 2010 (**c**) (*arrows*). Targeted US showed an irregular hypoechoic 5-mm mass with indistinct margins (**d**)

the prior mammogram or has increased in size or conspicuity (Fig. 7.9). Developing asymmetries can have both benign and malignant causes. Some of the more common benign causes include cysts, fibrocystic changes, pseudoangiomatous stromal hyperplasia (PASH), scars, focal infections, weight loss or gain, trauma, fat necrosis, and hormone replacement therapy [15]. Malignant developing asymmetries may represent invasive ductal carcinoma (IDC), invasive lobular carcinoma (ILC), mixed IDC and ILC, invasive mucinous carcinoma, and ductal carcinoma in situ [15]. A developing asymmetry has a moderate likelihood of malignancy and is seen on 12.8% of screening and 26.7% of diagnostic mammograms [16].

Developing asymmetries identified at screening mammography can be further evaluated with diagnostic mammography, tomosynthesis, breast US, and MRI.

Calcifications were previously separated into three categories: typically benign, intermediate concern, and higher probability. They are now consolidated into two categories: typically benign and suspicious morphology. In the "typically benign" category, eggshell and lucent-centered calcifications have been combined into a new term, rim, whereas round and punctate calcifications are combined into the term round (Fig. 7.10). Amorphous, coarse heterogeneous, fine pleomorphic, and fine linear or fine linear branching calcifications are now placed in the "suspicious morphology" category (Fig. 7.11). Calcifications with suspicious morphology have an increased risk for malignancy, with a probability

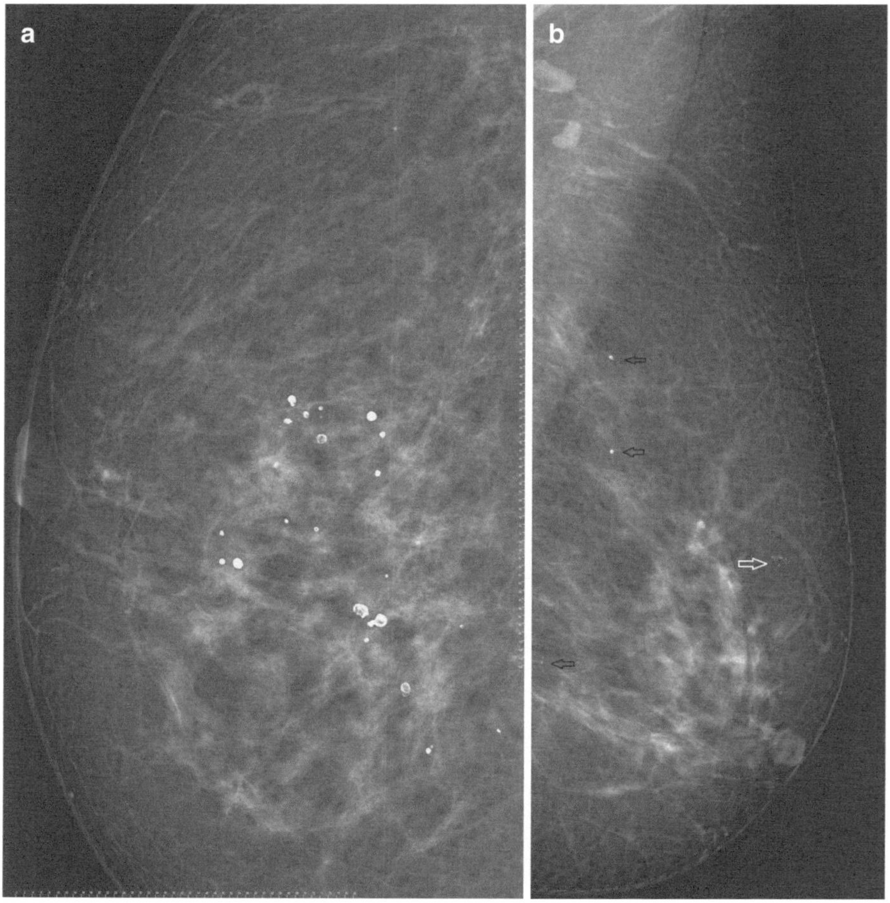

Fig. 7.10 First mammography in a 44-year-old asymptomatic woman. The right CC view showed typically benign round calcifications (**a**). Left MLO image of the same patient showed benign round calcifications (*black arrows*) and superficial lucent centered calcifications within the breast parenchyma (*white arrow*) (**b**). Left CC showed that these were skin calcifications (**c**)

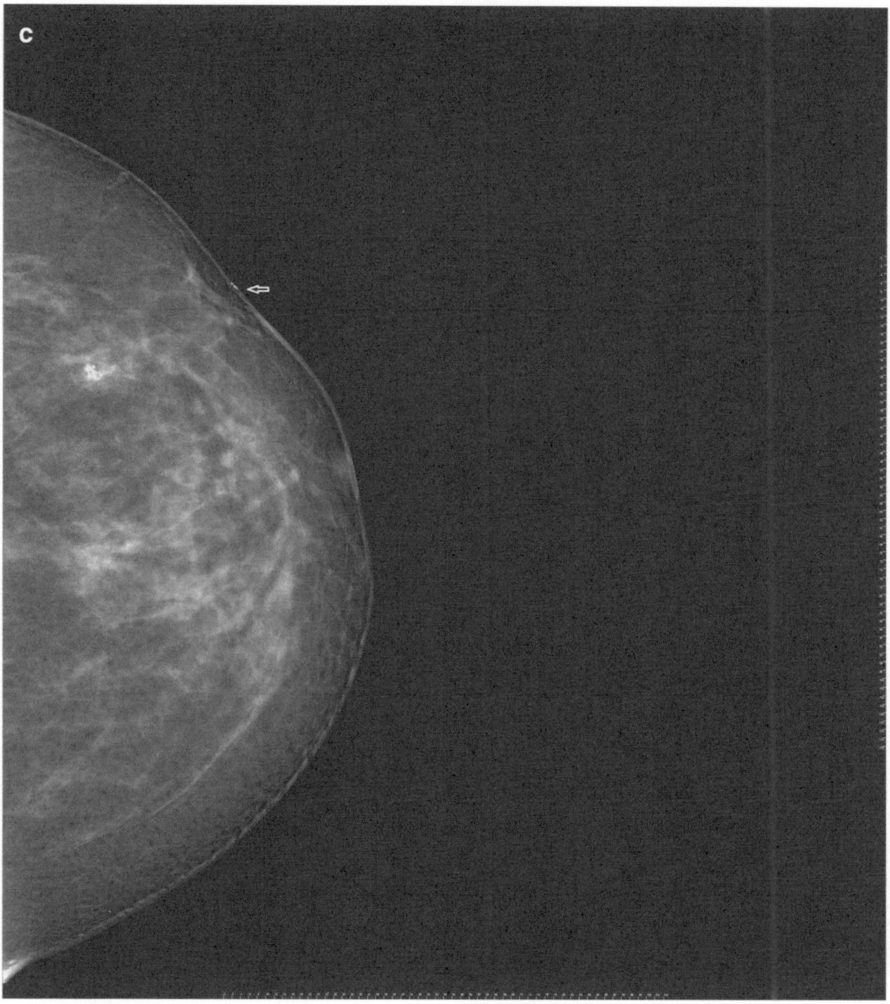

Fig. 7.10 (continued)

of 13% for coarse heterogeneous, 27% for amorphous, 50% for fine pleomorphic, and 78% for fine linear or fine linear branching calcifications [17]. The distribution of calcifications is also an important factor in characterizing calcifications as suspicious or benign. The distributions are diffuse, regional, grouped, linear, and segmental. Pleomorphic and linear calcifications in a segmental or ductal distribution are highly suspicious for DCIS. Calcifications that are believed to be probably benign, indicating a 2% or lower chance of malignancy, are usually recommended for follow-up mammography at 6-, 12-, and 24-month intervals. Calcifications that cannot be categorized definitively as benign or suspicious are reported as indeterminate and are usually also recommended for stereotactic biopsy.

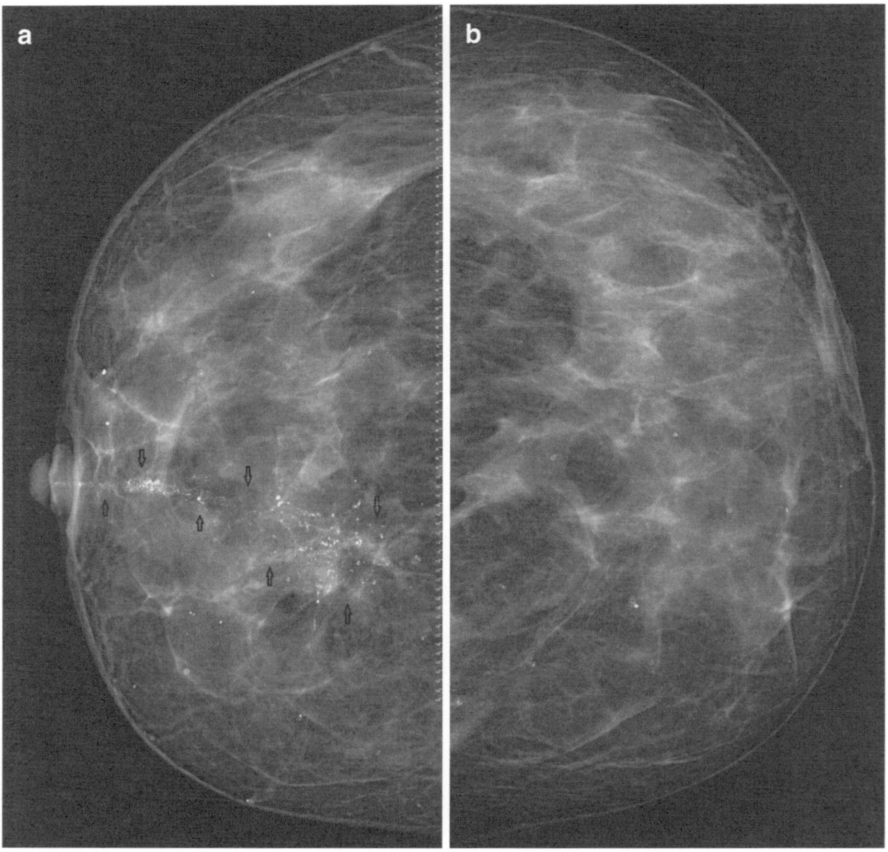

Fig. 7.11 A 40-year-old woman with a bloody nipple discharge in the right breast. Bilateral CC and MLO views demonstrated heterogeneously dense breast tissue and randomly distributed diffuse round calcifications (**a**–**d**). Malignant pleomorphic calcifications showing a segmental and linear distribution toward the nipple were observed on right CC and MLO mammograms (**a**, **c**)

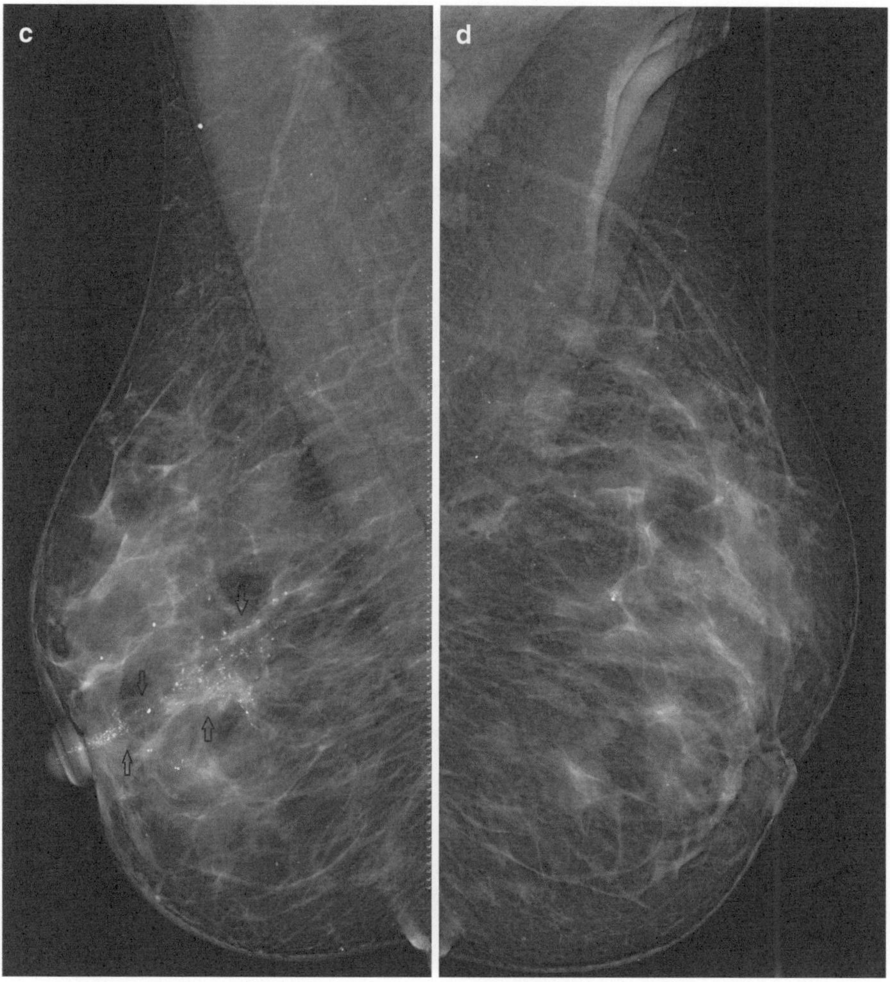

Fig. 7.11 (continued)

Ultrasonography

Ultrasonography uses high-frequency sound waves to produce images of internal organs and breast tissue. No X-rays are used. Among methods for imaging the breast, US is second to mammography because of its use for many years, its accessibility and relatively low cost, and the unique opportunity it affords for real-time guidance of needle biopsy and other interventional procedures.

Current indications for US examination of the breast include the following: (1) first examination (before mammography or MRI) for the evaluation of a palpable lump in women under age 30; (2) evaluation of a mass demonstrated on mammography; (3) evaluation of focal asymmetry or focal change in architecture on the mammogram compared with a previous study, performed after complete mammographic workup (additional views); (4) evaluation of suspicious finding requiring biopsy on MRI or a nuclear medicine study (in anticipation of US-guided biopsy); (5) guidance for intraoperative or percutaneous breast biopsy and aspiration; (6) evaluation of breast implants; (7) evaluation of lactating and pregnant women; (8) adjunctive examination to evaluate nipple discharge (after mammography); and (9) adjunctive examination to evaluate focal pain (after mammography). US can also be used to follow low-suspicion lesions and to evaluate the response to neoadjuvant chemotherapy.

US enables highly sensitive differentiation of benign breast lesions from malignant ones [18, 19]. Additional techniques, such as color Doppler and harmonic and compound imaging, can aid lesion analysis [20]. As technology continues to improve and the common practice of breast US increases, the diagnostic capabilities of breast US will expand.

Screening breast US is capable of detecting some cancers that are undetected by mammography and physical examination. For some states, US is recommended in mammography reports [21]. However, it has not been established that women will benefit from the incorporation of sonography into routine breast cancer screening programs.

US is useful in differentiating solid versus cystic breast lesions. A simple cyst should be anechoic with well-circumscribed margins upon acoustic enhancement due to greater sound transmission through the fluid than the surrounding breast tissue. A solid mass contains internal echoes. US features of benign lesions include well-defined margins, few gentle lobulations, a thin echogenic capsule and a horizontal axis parallel to the chest wall (Fig. 7.12). Cancers are generally hypoechoic relative to the brightly echogenic normal fibroglandular tissue. The following features suggest cancer: margins that are angulated, indistinct, microlobulated, or spiculated; acoustic shadowing; microcalcifications; ductal extension; an echogenic halo; and a taller than wide configuration (Fig. 7.13). Posterior acoustic shadowing is reported to occur in 60–97% of spiculated carcinomas. US is also the first modality used in patients with a suspected breast abscess because these patients often have too much pain to tolerate the compression required for mammography.

US is the primary nonsurgical method for evaluating axillary nodes [22]. The overall size of the node has very poor diagnostic accuracy for predicting metastasis, however, and in the absence of other associated findings, overall size should not be

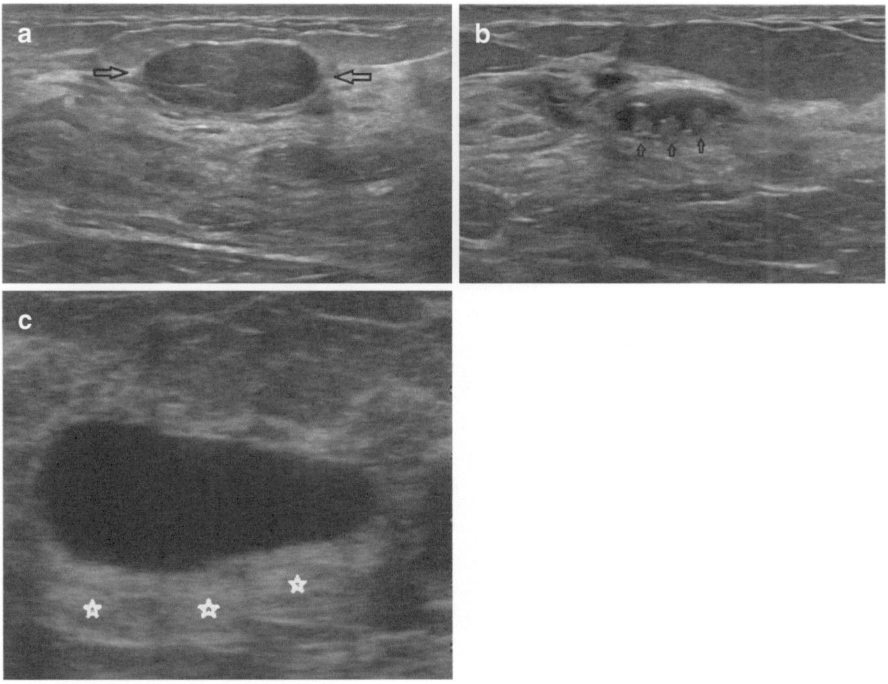

Fig. 7.12 A 49-year-old woman with a palpable lump in the right upper inner quadrant. A well-defined ovoid-shaped hypoechoic solid mass with a horizontal axis parallel to the chest was revealed as a fibroadenoma (**a**). A US image of the retroareolar region in the left breast showed multiple well-circumscribed hyperechoic millimetric masses within a dilated duct. Core biopsy revealed intraductal papillomatosis (**b**). In addition, US image of the upper outer left breast showed the characteristics of a simple cyst, that is, anechoic contents with an imperceptible wall and posterior acoustic enhancement (**c**)

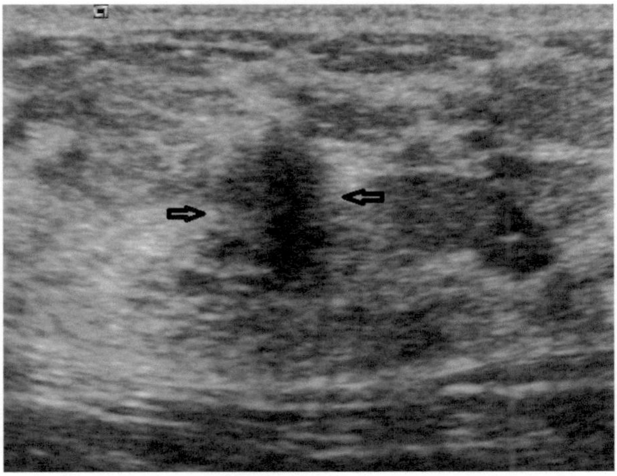

Fig. 7.13 Image from supplemental screening US of a 34-year-old patient with an intermediate risk for developing breast cancer showing an irregular hypoechoic mass with indistinct margins (*arrows*). The long axis of the mass was placed perpendicular to the skin. Ultrasound-guided biopsy revealed invasive ductal carcinoma

used as a criterion. The normal axillary lymph node should be oval and should have a smooth, well-defined margin. The cortex should be slightly hypoechoic and uniformly thin, measuring 3 mm or less (Fig. 7.14). Demonstrating arterial flow in the echogenic hilum is valuable for normal lymph nodes. Nodes that meet this description have a very high negative predictive value for excluding metastasis [22]. A focal cortical bulge or thickening, effacement of the fatty hilum or a rounded hypoechoic node, ill-defined contours and non-hilar blood flow are important findings for diagnosing abnormal nodes [23] (Fig. 7.15).

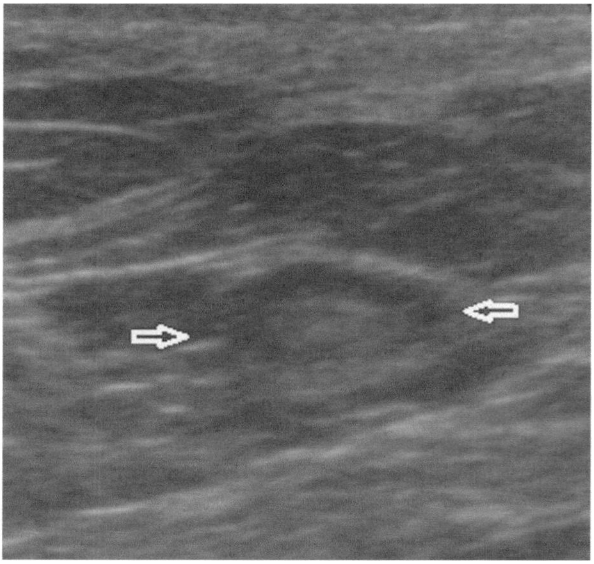

Fig. 7.14 Image from axilla US showing a normal-appearing ovoid-shaped lymph node with thin cortex and fatty hilum (*arrows*)

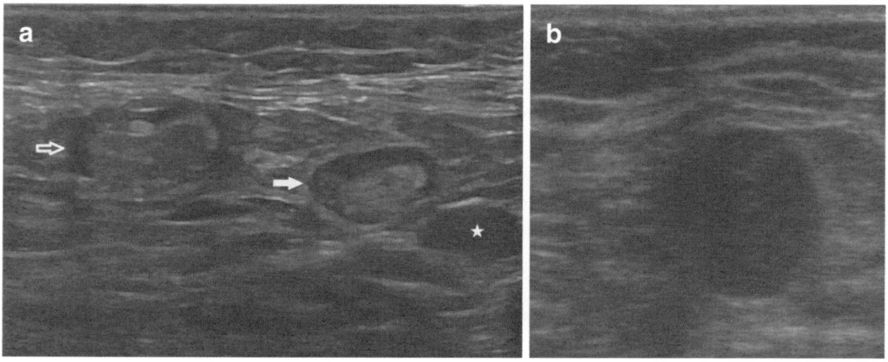

Fig. 7.15 A 56-year-old woman with a history of breast cancer presenting with axillary lymph nodes. US demonstrated a normal-appearing ovoid-shaped lymph node with a thin cortex (*open arrow*), a metastatic ovoid-shaped lymph node with an asymmetrical thick cortex (*closed arrow*) and a metastatic lymph node with a thick cortex (*star*) and absence of fatty hilum (**a**). An US image of the inferior axilla of the same patient showed a markedly enlarged spherical metastatic lymph node with a thick cortex and a lack of a visible hilum (**b**)

Magnetic Resonance Imaging

MRI is an established supplementary technique to mammography and US for the evaluation of suspicious breast lesions. As a diagnostic tool differing from mammography and US, MRI can show the tissue perfusion characteristics of masses on the breast parenchyma as well as morphological features. Although MRI has extremely high sensitivity in the diagnosis of breast cancer, reaching 89–100% for invasive cancers, specificity is only 72% and widely varies according to the criteria used in the differentiation of malignant from benign lesions [24–26]. Unfortunately, the moderate specificity of breast MRI, especially in the hands of inexperienced readers, can lead to more examinations rather than less. MRI is based on the use of (a) a strong magnetic field provided by a high-quality magnet; (b) low-energy radiofrequency waves radiated and received by special coils inside the magnet and positioned close to the investigated body part. The patient is placed in a prone position with the breasts hanging into a bilateral phased-array breast coil after placement of an intravenous catheter. However, to diagnose or exclude a cancer, intravenous administration of a gadolinium-based contrast material is required. When MRI is performed solely to evaluate silicone implant integrity, gadolinium is not necessary. Claustrophobia, implantable devices, allergic predisposition, and renal function should be checked.

Major clinical indications of MRI in breast diseases are suspicion of implant rupture, screening in high-risk women, solving difficult cases after standard imaging, local staging of breast cancer, suspicion of primary breast cancer in patients with metastatic axillary lymph nodes, differentiation of benign post-therapeutic changes, local recurrence in a treated breast, and monitoring neoadjuvant treatment efficacy (Fig. 7.16).

Normal fibroglandular tissue exhibits physiological enhancement, which can make detection of malignancy more difficult and increase the likelihood of false positives. The amount of background parenchymal enhancement is affected by hormonal status. To reduce this effect, elective or screening MR imaging must be scheduled between days 7 and 14 after the first day of the menstrual cycle. If MRI must be performed for another indication, speed may be more important than adequate scheduling.

Morphological analysis is performed by evaluating the shape, margin, and enhancement characteristics of the masses and the distribution and internal enhancement pattern of nonmass lesions. Kinetic analysis is performed by evaluating the initial enhancement rate and postinitial enhancement of the lesions. Although certain lesion characteristics, such as irregular or spiculated margins, rim enhancement, ductal or segmental enhancement, and rapid initial enhancement with a wash-out course, are highly suggestive of malignancy, certain lesion characteristics, such as smooth margins, less enhancement compared to the surrounding breast parenchyma, and nonenhancing internal septations are highly suggestive of benign disease (Figs. 7.17 and 7.18) [26]. A lack of enhancement is strongly suggestive of benignity but does not necessarily exclude malignancy.

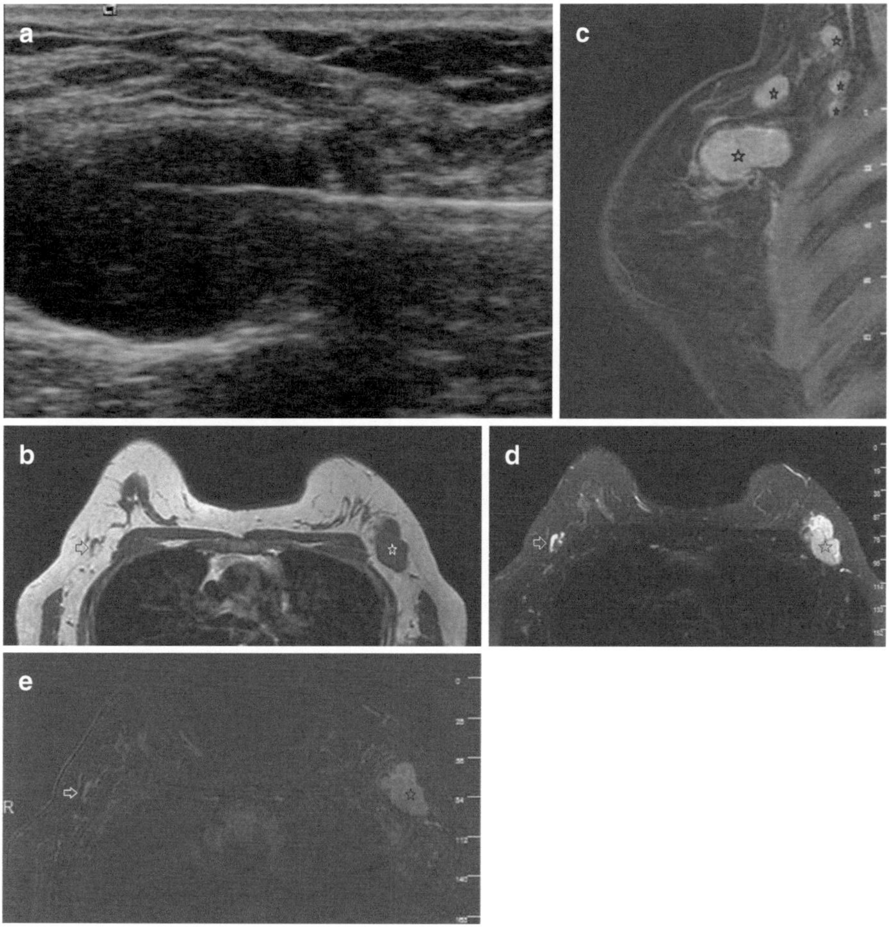

Fig. 7.16 Ultrasound-guided core biopsy of an axillary lymph node (**a**). Magnetic resonance imaging was performed to search for primary breast cancer in a patient with left metastatic axillary lymph nodes (*stars*) (**b–e**). Also a normal-appearing ovoid-shaped lymph node (*arrow*) was observed in the right axilla on MR images (**b**, **d**, **e**)

MRI is commonly used to assess the extent of disease preoperatively in patients newly diagnosed with breast cancer to aid surgical planning. MRI detects unsuspected cancer in the contralateral breast in 3% of these patients [27]. MRI detects additional disease in 27–34% of patients, resulting in wider surgical excision or mastectomy [28–30].

Diffusion-weighted imaging (DWI) was recently integrated into the standard breast MRI examination to increase the specificity of breast MRI. It is a noninvasive technique that measures the random motion of free water protons and characterizes the tissues with a mechanism that differs from T1 and T2 relaxation. For the quantification of this motion, apparent diffusion characteristic values are used.

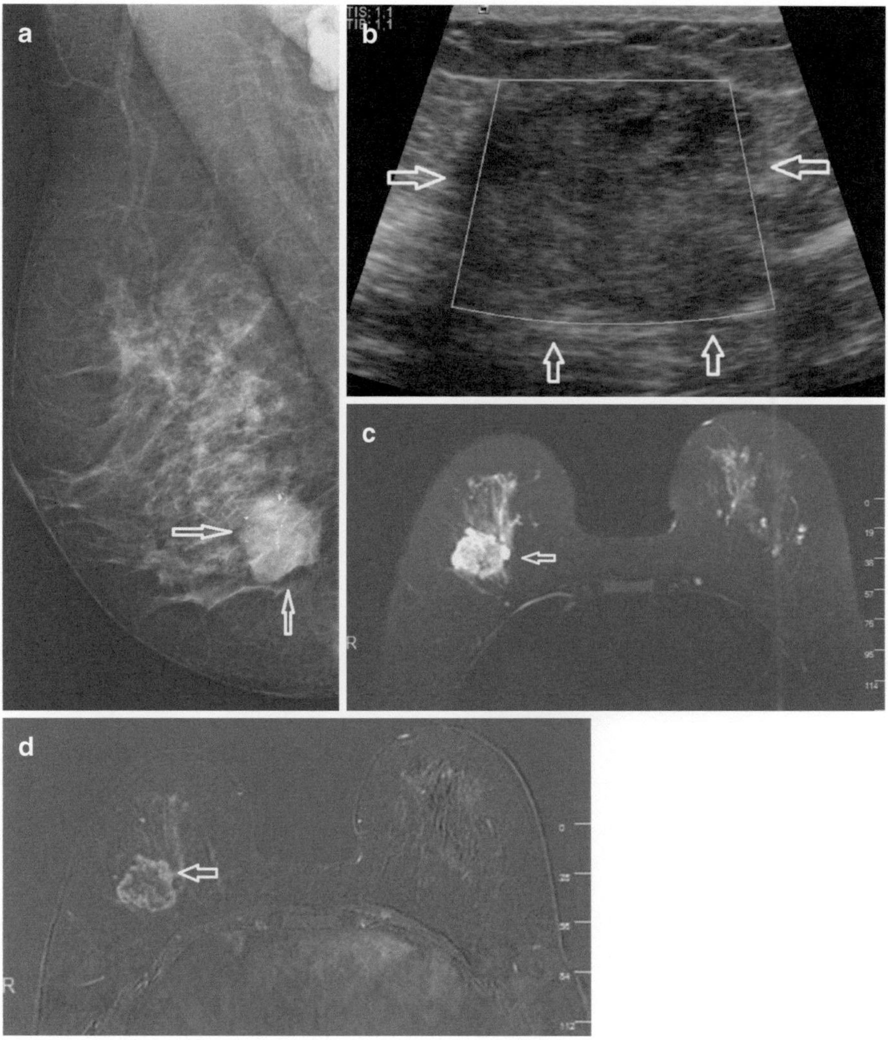

Fig. 7.17 A 51-year-old woman with a palpable lump in the right breast. Medio-lateral oblique mammogram demonstrated a microlobulated irregular dense mass in the inferior quadrant (**a**). Image from targeted US showed an irregular heterogenous mass with indistinct margins. The color Doppler US image revealed no flow within the mass (**b**). T2-weighted with fat saturation axial MR image showed a 2.5-cm hyperintense mass with irregular margins in the posterior location (**c**). T1-weighted gadolinium-enhanced early subtraction axial image showed the mass with rim enhancement (**d**). Surgical pathology revealed a mucinous breast cancer

Some recent studies have revealed the effectiveness of DWI for differentiating malignant from benign breast tumors [26, 31–33]. Kul et al. reported that a combined MRI protocol consisting of DCE-MRI and DWI provided 95.7% sensitivity and 89.2% specificity for the diagnosis of breast cancer [26].

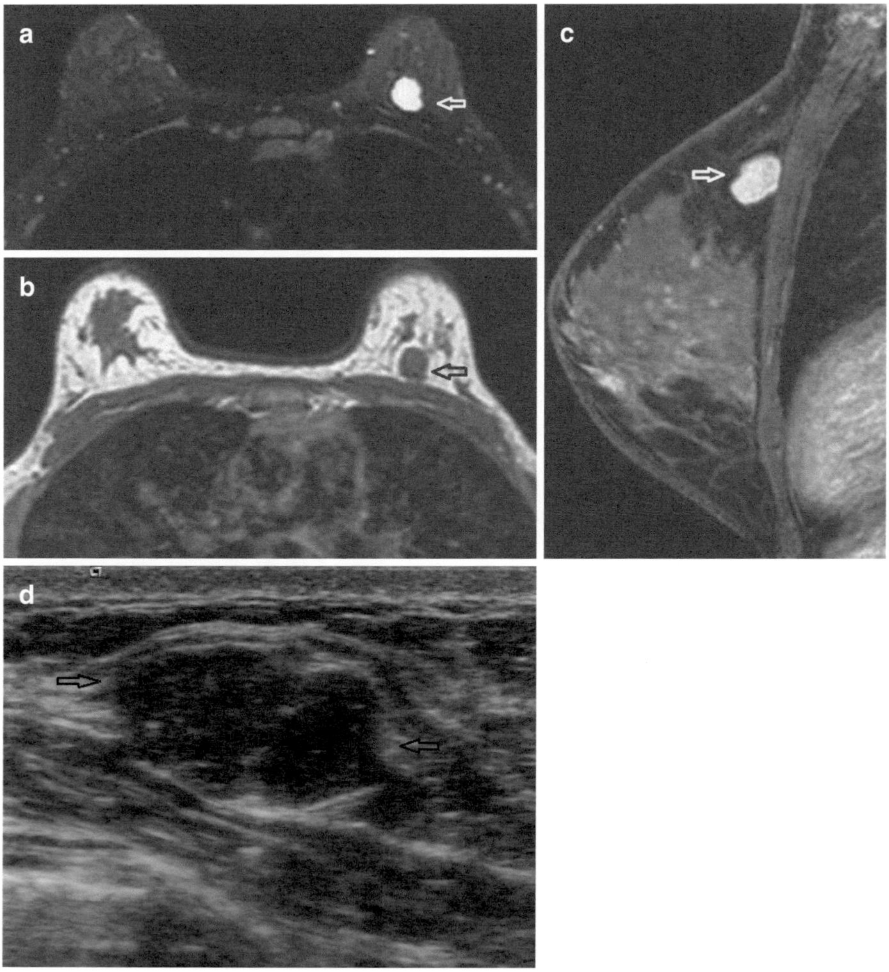

Fig. 7.18 A 43-year-old woman with fibroadenoma of the left breast. The T2-weighted with fat saturation axial MR image indicated a 2-cm hyperintense mass with circumscribed margins in the prepectoral location (**a**). The mass was observed as hypointense on precontrast T1-weighted image (**b**). Postcontrast T1-weighted sagittal MR image demonstrated the mass with homogeneous enhancement (**c**). The hypoechoic mass showed lobulation on US image (**d**)

New Imaging Methods

Tomosynthesis

Digital breast tomosynthesis (DBT) is an X-ray mammography technique that permits the three-dimensional reconstruction of the breast tissue and can be viewed as sequential sections through the breast. Tomosynthesis has been shown to increase the conspicuity of many lesions while reducing false-positive findings from summation of overlapping tissues [34]. Several studies of reductions in breast cancer screening recall rates have reported improved sensitivity and specificity with the use of DBT [35–38]. Specifically, in a study by Dang et al. 16% of invasive breast cancers were occult on conventional mammography versus 3% on DBT [39]. In another study, radiologists indicated that the availability of DBT would have eliminated use of US as part of the diagnostic process in 12% of cases [40]. There is concern about the increased radiation dose to the patient with the use of DBT. In a paper reporting results from the Oslo Trial (similar population and acquisition protocol, same system manufacturer), mean glandular doses per view of 1.58 mGy for digital mammography and 1.95 mGy for DBT were reported, representing a dose increase of 23% for tomosynthesis [41]. The use of synthetic 2D images with DBT is now FDA approved and would reduce the radiation dose to that of a standard mammogram while allowing the acquisition of both 2D and 3D images.

Contrast Enhanced Mammography

Contrast enhanced mammography is an FDA-approved technology that, similar to MRI, is based on the principle of imaging neovascularity. CEM requires approximately 8–10 min to perform and provides four low-energy views analogous to those obtained with 2D full-field digital mammography as well as four contrast-enhanced recombined images obtained after intravenous iodinated contrast. Similar to conventional mammography images, CEM images are acquired in cranio-caudal and mediolateral oblique views. Early studies have even demonstrated that the performance of CEM is superior to that of mammography alone in the diagnostic setting and comparable to the performance of MRI in women with known cancers [42–44]. For CEM, the mean glandular dose estimates vary according to breast density and are estimated to be 20–80% higher than those associated with standard 2D digital mammography alone but lower than those associated with DBT [45]. The additional dose should be kept in mind when deciding to use this examination, especially in patients who may be particularly sensitive to radiation [46].

Elastography

Breast elastography is emerging as an efficient tool to detect malignant solid lesions by measuring the tissue strain produced by compression. It is easily performed in clinical practice and adds only a short amount of time to breast ultrasonography. In breast ultrasonography, two elastographic techniques are popular and differ in the

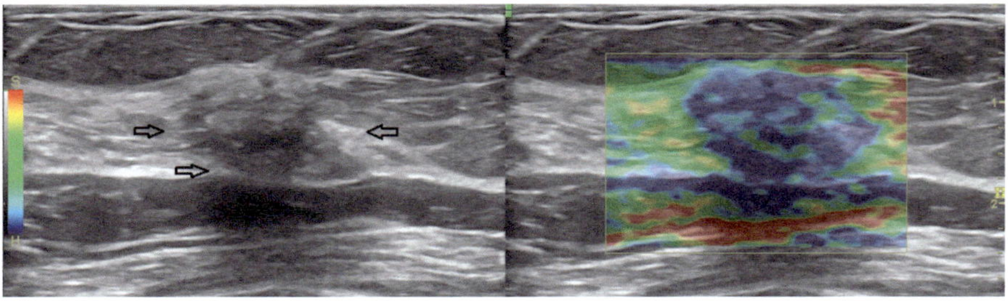

Fig. 7.19 Invasive carcinoma in a 35-year-old woman with pain in the left breast. Strain elastogram imaging revealed an irregular heterogeneous hyperechoic mass showing a predominantly blue lesion with some green portions (high hardness)

type of stress applied: strain and shear-wave elastography (SWE). Strain elastography produces an image based on the relative displacement of the tissue from an external (manual compression of the transducer) or patient source (Fig. 7.19). SWE using the acoustic radiation force induced by the US push pulse generated by the transducer provides quantitative elasticity parameters. SWE has been shown to be useful for differentiating benign breast lesions from malignant breast lesions and for characterizing breast masses categorized as BI-RADS categories 3 and 4A to attempt to reduce unnecessary breast biopsies [47]. SWE exhibits 86.5% sensitivity, 89.8% specificity and 88.3% accuracy in discriminating benign and malignant breast lesions [48]. It has been suggested that SWE enhances the diagnostic performance of ultrasonography, potentially improving the specificity of conventional ultrasonography.

Breast Imaging Reporting and Data System (BI-RADS)

The Breast Imaging Reporting and Data System (BI-RADS) is a classification system proposed by the American College of Radiology (ACR) in 1986; the original report was released in 1993. BI-RADS serves to standardize breast imaging reports, improve communication with referring physicians, and provide a quality assurance tool. The latest edition is BI-RADS 5, which was updated in 2013 [17]. The BI-RADS lexicon is a dictionary of descriptive terms used to describe a mammographic, US, or MRI finding. The ACR used scientific analysis and literature review to create a lexicon of descriptors shown to correlate with high predictive values associated with either benign or malignant disease. The other important aspect of the BI-RADS system is the category classification for the overall assessment of the imaging findings. This categorization provides an approximate risk of malignancy of a lesion from essentially zero to greater than 95%. The categorization and final assessment decrease ambiguity in recommendations. These assessment categories and recommendations are presented in Table 7.1.

Table 7.1 Assessment categories and recommendations of BI-RADS

Assessment	Management	Likelihood of cancer
Category 0: Incomplete—need additional evaluation and/or prior mammograms for comparison	Recall for additional imaging and/or comparison with prior examination(s)	N/A
Category 1: Negative	Routine mammography screening	Essentially 0% likelihood of malignancy
Category 2: Benign	Routine mammography screening	Essentially 0% likelihood of malignancy
Category 3: Probably benign	Short-interval (6-month) follow-up or continued surveillance mammography	>0% but ≤2% likelihood of malignancy
Category 4: Suspicious	Tissue diagnosis	>2% but <95% likelihood of malignancy
Category 4A: Low suspicion for malignancy		>2% but ≤10% likelihood of malignancy
Category 4B: Moderate suspicion for malignancy		>10 to ≤50% likelihood of malignancy
Category 4C: High suspicion for malignancy		>50 to <95% likelihood of malignancy
Category 5: Highly suggestive of malignancy	Tissue diagnosis	≥95% likelihood of malignancy
Category 6: Known biopsy-proven malignancy	Surgical excision when clinically appropriate	N/A

Image-Guided Biopsy

The decision to perform an image-guided biopsy includes the selection of the imaging modality to guide the biopsy and the type of biopsy device. Stereotactic, ultrasonography, and magnetic resonance imaging are most frequently used for biopsy guidance. Other imaging modalities that use nuclear metabolic agents such as fluorodeoxyglucose and sestamibi are infrequently used. In general, the modality used for imaging guidance should be the one that best demonstrates the lesion. If the pathology results are not concordant with the imaging finding, surgical excision or additional tissue sampling is recommended.

Ultrasonography-Guided Biopsy

Among imaging techniques used to evaluate breast abnormalities and guide interventions for tissue sampling or surgical excision, US is the most common method and the only one performed in real time. Patients and physicians prefer US guidance for its rapidity, comfort (the patient is supine or supine-oblique rather than prone as she would be for stereotactic or MRI-guided biopsies), reliability, and accuracy. US is the choice for biopsy of solid masses with automated biopsy devices using 12- or 14-gauge needles or with vacuum-assisted devices that yield larger specimens obtained with needles ranging from 8 to 12 gauge, as well as biopsy devices using other mechanisms (Fig. 7.20). US-guided 14-gauge core needle biopsy had a false-negative rate of 1.6% (11 of 671 malignancies) in non-palpable lesions [49]. A minimum of four specimens, preferably those that are nonfragmented and that sink, should be obtained by 14-gauge US-guided breast biopsy [50].

Suspicious calcifications usually undergo biopsy with stereotactic guidance. However, calcifications can be identified on US scans obtained with high-frequency transducers, particularly when associated with a mass. In these cases, US-guided biopsy may be performed instead of stereotactic biopsy, and specimen radiography should be performed to document calcifications in the tissue cores. Second-look US is commonly performed to locate a mass that correlates with an enhancing lesion seen on MRI. Biopsy can then be guided with US and accomplished more rapidly, in real time, and more comfortably for the patient than an MRI-guided biopsy.

US is also an excellent imaging guide for presurgical localization and for the aspiration of cysts and drainage of abscesses. Simple cysts do not require treatment; however, some patients desire US-guided aspiration for symptomatic relief. If a mass cannot be identified as a complicated cyst or a solid mass, aspiration may be performed initially. If the fluid is bloody, it should be sent for cytology. If no fluid can be aspirated, it can be assumed that the mass is solid, and a core biopsy may be performed. If the cyst contains a solid nodule, the nodule should undergo core biopsy prior to aspiration of the fluid.

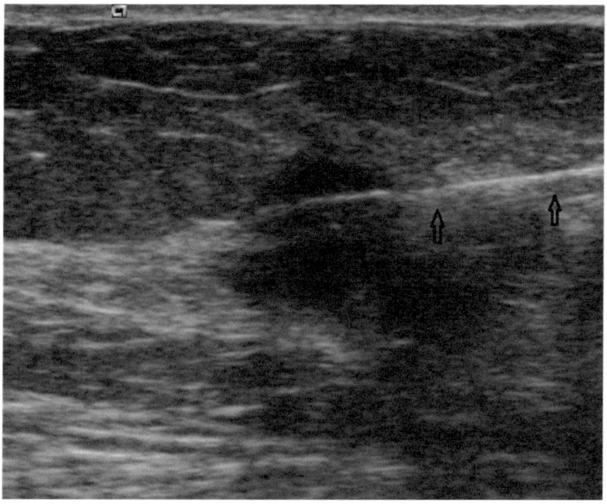

Fig. 7.20 Ultrasonography-guided core biopsy of the mass revealed an invasive ductal carcinoma. The hyperechoic line traversing the lesion is the biopsy needle (*arrows*)

Stereotactic-Guided Biopsy

Stereotactic breast biopsy is an X-ray-guided method that uses 3-dimensional images to localize and sample breast lesions discovered on mammography. The biopsy is performed primarily for microcalcifications but also includes masses, asymmetries, and architectural distortions that cannot be identified at US.

The patient is positioned either prone or seated, and the breast is compressed between the image receptor and the compression plate. Two 15-degree angled X-ray images of the lesion allow targeting by the radiologist to produce computer-generated coordinates that are transferred to the stereotactic biopsy device. An 8- to 11-gauge vacuum-assisted biopsy device is now the standard choice. The vacuum-assisted biopsy device retrieves a larger volume of tissue compared with core biopsy, minimizing the rate of histologic upgrades. At the end of the biopsy, a tissue marker ("biopsy clip") is placed to indicate the biopsy site and to localize the lumpectomy or excision. When the targeted lesion contains calcifications, a specimen radiograph is obtained to document the presence of calcifications within the tissue cores.

MRI-Guided Biopsy

Breast MR imaging can detect some suspicious lesions that are occult on mammography and US. Using the three-dimensional location information from MR imaging, some lesions can be identified with targeted US and sampled by using US guidance. However, this requires a good working knowledge of both modalities, the ability to translate the expected lesion position and appearance from one modality to another, and a meticulous radiologic-pathologic correlation when the results are returned to ensure that the US finding truly represents the lesion identified at MR imaging. If the lesion is only visualized with MR imaging, then MRI-guided biopsy is performed.

MRI-guided biopsy is difficult and troublesome for patients and radiologists because the patient is prone and requires intravenous administration of gadolinium for lesion visualization, breast compression for lesion targeting, and several MRI sequences to confirm accuracy. The usual practice after a benign MR biopsy result is to perform short-term follow-up MRI, 6 months after the procedure, due to a 1% rate of missed carcinoma [51, 52].

Preoperative Localization of Non-Palpable Breast Lesions

Approximately 25–30% of breast cancers are non-palpable at diagnosis and will require a localization technique to assist surgery [53, 54]. Wire-guided localization is the most frequently used method and entails the insertion of a wire via US, mammographic or MRI guidance on the day of operation to assist the surgeon in localizing the tumor intra-operatively (Fig. 7.21). An alternative is marking by a radioactive agent (radio-guided occult lesion localization; ROLL). In this technique, a titanium seed of iodine-125 is inserted into the tumor under mammographic or US guidance. A gamma probe is used intraoperatively by the surgeon to localize the non-palpable tumor and guide surgical excision. ROLL adds flexibility to clinical schedules as well as to the planning of the localization approach and surgical incision site. The seeds are placed internally, with no external wires extruding from the skin surface; patient satisfaction is markedly enhanced, and there is also no risk of wire dislodgement, migration, or transection with resultant loss of localization [55]. Localization tends to be more accurate and faster, the excision procedure is more elegant and simple to perform, and the cosmetic result seems to be better.

The major disadvantage of ROLL compared with wire localization is patient and environmental radiation exposure. However, there is no need for extra radiation-protection procedures because the dose exposure is far below the annual limit [56]. Another potential disadvantage of ROLL compared with wire localization is that seeds that are not initially placed in a satisfactory position generally cannot be removed preoperatively. A second seed (or wire) must then be placed to accurately localize the lesion, and both seeds are subsequently retrieved at surgery [55]. Disease recurrence rates and positive margin rates are similar for wire-guided localization and ROLL [57]. There was no difference in specimen size or re-excision rate for malignant lesions between the two methods [58]. Application of ROLL under MRI guidance can be performed for the preoperative localization of breast lesions detected only by MRI [59]. A specimen radiograph should be obtained at the time of surgery to confirm that the localized lesion has been removed, along with biopsy clips, wires, or radioactive seeds when the procedure is performed using mammographic guidance. Surgically placed markers, orthogonal sample views, and careful monitoring of the lesion and its relationship to the localizing markers permit an assessment of which margin is close.

High-Risk Screening

Breast cancer screening recommendations are based on risk factors. Women are considered at high risk of developing breast cancer if their estimated lifetime risk is 20% or greater based on family history, if they have a known or suspected BRCA or other high-risk genetic mutation, or if they had mantle radiation therapy to the chest prior to age 30. Lifetime risk is assessed using the Gail, Tyrer-Cuzick, BRCAPRO, and Claus models [60–62].

The Society of Breast Imaging and American College of Radiology recommend that women with a BRCA1 or BRCA2 gene mutation or those who have not been tested but have a first-degree relative with a known BRCA mutation have annual mammograms starting by age 30 but not before age 25. The recommendation for women with a greater than or equal to 20% lifetime risk for breast cancer based on

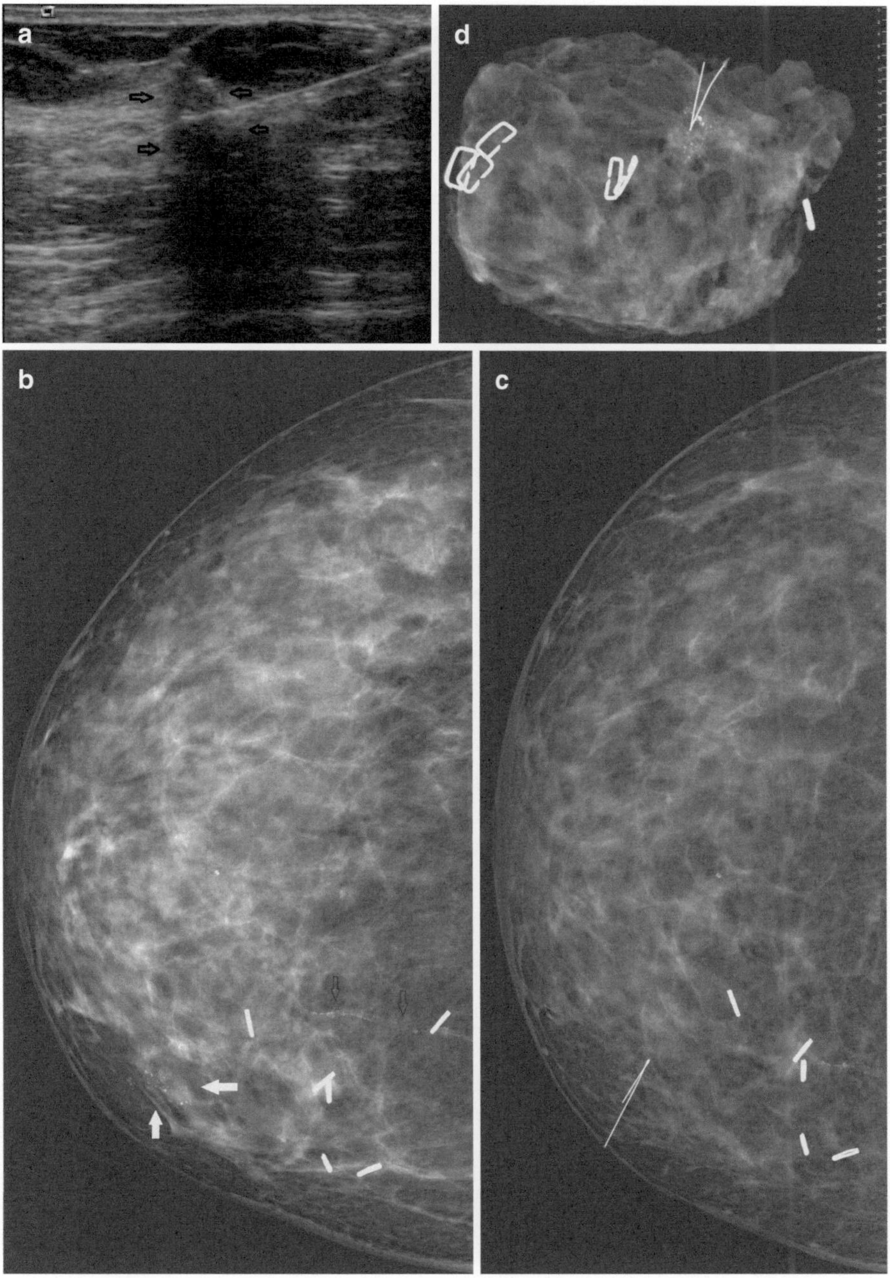

Fig. 7.21 Follow-up imaging of a 42-year-old woman 5 years after surgery for breast cancer. This image shows wire localization under US guidance of an irregular hypoechoic 5-mm non-palpable mass with posterior acoustic shadowing that including calcifications on mammograms (**a**). CC mammography shows malign calcifications (*arrows*) and clips from previous surgery in the inner of the right breast (**b**). This image shows the control mammography view after wire localization under US guidance (**c**). A specimen radiograph showing the excised mass within pleomorphic calcifications at the tip of the wire and operation clips (**d**). Postoperative ultimate pathology was high-grade in situ cancer compatible with core biopsy

family history is to have annual mammography starting by age 30 (but not before age 25) or 10 years earlier than the age of diagnosis of the youngest affected relative, whichever is later. For women who are at a high risk due to prior mantle radiation between the ages of 10–30, mammography is recommended starting 8 years after radiation therapy but not before age 25. Those women who have had a biopsy showing lobular carcinoma in situ, atypical lobular hyperplasia, atypical ductal hyperplasia, or DCIS should have annual mammograms from the time of diagnosis, regardless of age [63].

Supplemental screening with breast MRI is recommended for these patients at high risk for breast cancer. When data from 11 prospective studies were combined in a meta-analysis, the sensitivity was 77% for MR imaging alone, 94% for a combination of MR imaging and mammography, and 39% for mammography alone [64]. The highest sensitivity was achieved by using a combination of mammography and MR imaging. A modeling study reported that the most efficacious screening strategy for carriers of *BRCA* mutations was to start screening with MR imaging annually at age 25 and to add annual mammography at age 30; due to the high tumor growth rate and shorter lead time of BRCA-related breast cancers, alternating MR imaging and mammographic screening examinations at 6-month intervals may also be a clinically effective approach [65, 66]. Women with a history of chest irradiation are recommended to have a screening MRI annually starting 8 years after radiation therapy [48]. In the American College of Radiology Imaging Network 6666 trial, women cited their inability to tolerate the long acquisition time because of claustrophobia (25.4%) and time constraints (18.2%) as the primary reasons they refused MRI screening [67]. Short-protocol breast MRI can replace rutin-protocol MRI to screen patients at high breast cancer risk [68, 69].

US can be considered in high-risk women for whom MRI screening may be appropriate but who cannot have MRI for any reason or in women with dense breast tissue as an adjunct to mammography. A recent large multicenter trial concluded that in high-risk women, the use of screening US as a supplement to mammography in addition to screening mammography increases the detection of cancer by 3–4 per 1000 compared to mammography alone [21]. This increased detection rate does come at the cost of increased false positives. An average of 4.4% of women underwent biopsy due to screening US findings, with a positive predictive value (PPV) of 9.4% [21].

For intermediate-risk women (lifetime risk of 15–20%), US or MRI may be indicated as an adjunct to mammography depending upon specific risk factors [63]. However, CEM may also be an ideal alternative for women with an intermediate risk of breast cancer who may not be eligible for supplemental screening MRI [45].

Conclusion

Breast imaging is indispensable and the most important component of breast cancer diagnosis. Mammography is the standard imaging procedure for breast cancer detection and diagnosis. Breast US and MRI are frequently used adjuncts to mammography, and these techniques enhance the radiologist's ability to detect cancer and assess disease extent. Many developing technologies can assist the formulation and confirmation of a diagnosis, such as DBT, CEM, and elastography US.

Advances and ongoing improvements in imaging technologies have improved the sensitivity of breast cancer detection and diagnosis, but there is no single imaging modality that is capable of identifying and characterizing all breast abnormalities. Each modality is most beneficial when utilized according to individual traits such as age, risk, and breast density.

References

1. Sardanelli F, Aase H, Álvarez M, Azavedo E, Baarslag HJ, Balleyguier C, et al. Position paper on screening for breast cancer by the European Society of Breast Imaging and 30 national breast radiology bodies from Austria, Belgium, Bosnia and Herzegovina, Bulgaria, Croatia, Czech Republic, Denmark, Estonia, Finland, France, Germany, Greece, Hungary, Iceland, Ireland, Israel, Italy, Lithuania, Moldova, The Netherlands, Norway, Poland, Portugal, Romania, Serbia, Slovakia, Spain, Sweden, Switzerland, and Turkey. Eur Radiol. 2017;27:2737–43.
2. Prummel MV, Muradali D, Shumak R, Majpruz V, Brown P, Jiang H, et al. Digital compared with screen-film mammography: measures of diagnostic accuracy among women screened in the Ontario breast screening program. Radiology. 2016;278:365–73.
3. Bluekens AM, Holland R, Karssemeijer N, Broeders MJ, den Heeten GJ. Comparison of digital screening mammography and screen-film mammography in the early detection of clinically relevant cancers: a multicenter study. Radiology. 2012;265:707–14.
4. Hendrick RE, Pisano ED, Averbukh A, Moran C, Berns EA, Yaffe MJ, et al. Comparison of acquisition parameters and breast dose in digital mammography and screen-film mammography in the American College of Radiology Imaging Network digital mammographic imaging screening trial. AJR Am J Roentgenol. 2010;194:362–9.
5. Hendrick RE. Radiation doses and cancer risks from breast imaging studies. Radiology. 2010;257:246–53.
6. Rosenberg RD, Yankaskas BC, Abraham LA, Sickles DA, Lehman CD, Geller BM, et al. Performance benchmarks for screening mammography. Radiology. 2006;241:55–66.
7. American Cancer Society. What are the key statistics about breast cancer? 2017. http://www.cancer.org/cancer/breastcancer/detailedguide/breast-cancer-key-statistics. Accessed 22 Sept 2017.
8. Perry N, Broeders M, de Wolf C, Törnberg S, Holland R, von Karsa L. European guidelines for quality assurance in breast cancer screening and diagnosis. Fourth edition. Ann Oncol. 2008;19:614–22.
9. Sardanelli F, Fallenberg EM, Clauser P, Trimboli RM, Camps-Herrero J, Helbich TH, European Society of Breast Imaging (EUSOBI), with language review by Europa Donna–The European Breast Cancer Coalition, et al. Mammography: an update of the EUSOBI recommendations on information for women. Insights Imaging. 2017;8:11–8.
10. Freer PE. Mammographic breast density: impact on breast cancer risk and implications for screening. RadioGraphics. 2015;35:302–15.
11. Bahl M, Baker JA, Kinsey EN, Ghate SV. Architectural distortion on mammography: correlation with pathologic outcomes and predictors of malignancy. AJR Am J Roentgenol. 2015;205:1339–45.
12. Shaheen R, Schimmelpenninck CA, Stoddart L, Raymond H, Slanetz PJ. Spectrum of diseases presenting as architectural distortion on mammography: multimodality radiologic imaging with pathologic correlation. Semin Ultrasound CT MR. 2011;32:351–62.

13. Dibble EH, Lourenco AP, Baird GL, Ward RC, Maynard AS, Mainiero MB. Comparison of digital mammography and digital breast tomosynthesis in the detection of architectural distortion. Eur Radiol. 2018;28:3–10.
14. Sickles EA. Findings at mammographic screening on only one standard projection: outcomes analysis. Radiology. 1998;208:471–5.
15. Chesebro AL, Winkler NS, Birdwell RL, Giess CS. Developing asymmetries at mammography: a multimodality approach to assessment and management. RadioGraphics. 2016;36:322–34.
16. Leung JW, Sickles EA. Developing asymmetry identified on mammography: correlation with imaging outcome and pathologic findings. AJR Am J Roentgenol. 2007;188:667–75.
17. Rao AA, Feneis J, Lalonde C, Ojeda-Fournier H. A pictorial review of changes in the BI-RADS fifth edition. RadioGraphics. 2016;36:623–39.
18. Stavros AT, Thickman D, Rapp CL, Dennis MA, Parker SH, Sisney GA. Solid breast nodules: use of sonography to distinguish between benign and malignant lesions. Radiology. 1995;196:123–34.
19. Zonderland HM, Coerkamp EG, Hermans J, van de Vijver MJ, van Voorthuisen AE. Diagnosis of breast cancer: contribution of US as an adjunct to mammography. Radiology. 1999;213:413–22.
20. Mesurolle B, Helou T, El-Khoury M, Edwardes M, Sutton EJ, Kao E. Tissue harmonic imaging, frequency compound imaging, and conventional imaging: use and benefit in breast sonography. J Ultrasound Med. 2007;26:1041–51.
21. Hooley RJ, Greenberg KL, Stackhouse RM, Geisel JL, Butler RS, Philpotts LE. Screening US in patients with mammographically dense breasts: initial experience with Connecticut Public Act 09–41. Radiology. 2012;265:59–69.
22. Bedi DG, Krishnamurthy R, Krishnamurthy S, Edeiken BS, Le-Petross H, Fornage BD, et al. Cortical morphologic features of axillary lymph nodes as a predictor of metastasis in breast cancer: in vitro sonographic study. AJR Am J Roentgenol. 2008;191:646–52.
23. Ecanow JS, Abe H, Newstead GM, Ecanow DB, Jeske JM. Axillary staging of breast cancer: what the radiologist should know. RadioGraphics. 2013;33:1589–612.
24. Warren RML, Pointon L, Thompson D, Hoff R, Gilbert FJ, Padhani A, Easton D, et al. Reading protocol for dynamic contrast-enhanced MR images of the breast: sensitivity and specificity analysis. Radiology. 2005;236:779–88.
25. Peters NH, Borel Rinkes IH, Zuithoff NP, Mali WP, Moons KG, Peeters PH. Meta-analysis of MR imaging in the diagnosis of breast lesions. Radiology. 2008;246:116–24.
26. Kul S, Cansu A, Alhan E, Dinc H, Gunes G, Reis A. Contribution of diffusion-weighted imaging to dynamic contrast-enhanced MRI in the characterization of breast tumors. AJR Am J Roentgenol. 2011;196:210–7.
27. Lehman CD, Gastonis C, Kuhl CK, Hendrick RE, Pisano ED, Hanna L, et al. MRI evaluation of the contralateral breast in women with recently diagnosed breast cancer. N Engl J Med. 2007;356:1295–303.
28. Orel SG, Schnall MD, Powell CM, Hochman MG, Solin LJ, Fowble BL, et al. Staging of suspected breast cancer: effect of MR imaging and MR-guided biopsy. Radiology. 1995;196:115–22.
29. Liberman L, Morris EA, Dershaw DD, Abramson AF, Tan LK. MR imaging of the ipsilateral breast in women with percutaneously proven breast cancer. Am J Roentgenol. 2003;180:901–10.
30. Berg WA, Gutierrez L, NessAiver MS, Carter WB, Bhargavan M, Lewis RS, et al. Diagnostic accuracy of mammography, clinical examination, US and MR imaging in preoperative assessment of breast cancer. Radiology. 2004;233:830–49.
31. Tozaki M, Fukuma E. 1H MR spectroscopy and diffusion-weighted imaging of the breast: are they useful tools for characterizing breast lesions before biopsy? AJR Am J Roentgenol. 2009;193:840–9.
32. Partridge SC, Demartini WB, Kurland BF, Eby PR, White SW, Lehman CD. Differential diagnosis of mammographically and clinically occult breast lesions on diffusion-weighted MRI. J Magn Reson Imaging. 2010;31:562–70.

33. Yabuuchi H, Matsuo Y, Okafuji T, Kamitani T, Soeda H, Setoguchi T, et al. Enhanced mass on contrast-enhanced breast MR imaging: lesion characterization using combination of dynamic contrast-enhanced and diffusion-weighted MR images. J Magn Reson Imaging. 2008;28:1157–65.
34. Niklason LT, Christian BT, Niklason LE, Kopans DB, Castleberry DE, Opsahl-Ong BH, et al. Digital tomosynthesis in breast imaging. Radiology. 1997;205:399–406.
35. Caumo F, Bernardi D, Ciatto S, Macaskill P, Pellegrini M, Brunelli S, et al. Incremental effect from integrating 3D mammography (tomosynthesis) with 2D-mammography: increased breast cancer detection evident for screening centres in a population-based trial. Breast. 2014;23:76–80.
36. Haas BM, Kalra V, Geisel J, Raghu M, Durand M, Philpotts LE. Comparison of tomosynthesis plus digital mammography and digital mammography alone for breast cancer screening. Radiology. 2013;269:694–700.
37. Rose SL, Tidwell AL, Bujnoch LJ, Kushwaha AC, Nordmann AS, Sexton R Jr. Implementation of breast tomosynthesis in a routine screening practice: an observational study. AJR Am J Roentgenol. 2013;200:1401–8.
38. Rafferty EA, Park JM, Philpotts LE, Poplack SP, Sumkin JH, Halpern EF, et al. Assessing radiologist performance using combined digital mammography and breast tomosynthesis compared with digital mammography alone: results of a multicenter, multireader trial. Radiology. 2013;266:104–13.
39. Dang PA, Freer PE, Humphrey KL, Halpern EF, Rafferty EA. Addition of tomosynthesis to conventional digital mammography: effect on image interpretation time of screening examinations. Radiology. 2014;270:49–56.
40. Peppard HR, Nicholson BE, Rochman CM, Merchant JK, Mayo RC 3rd, Harvey JA. Digital breast tomosynthesis in the diagnostic setting: indications and clinical applications. RadioGraphics. 2015;35:975–90.
41. Skaane P, Bandos AI, Gullien R, Eben EB, Ekseth U, Haakenaasen U, et al. Comparison of digital mammography alone and digital mammography plus tomosynthesis in a population-based screening program. Radiology. 2013;267:47–56.
42. Lobbes MB, Lalji U, Houwers J, Nijssen EC, Nelemans PJ, van Roozendaal L, et al. Contrast-enhanced spectral mammography in patients referred from the best cancer screening programme. Eur Radiol. 2014;24:1668–76.
43. Dromain C, Balleyguier C, Adler G, Garbay JR, Delaloge S. Contrast-enhanced digital mammography. Eur J Radiol. 2009;69:34–42.
44. Jochelson MS, Dershaw DD, Sung JS, Heerdt AS, Thornton C, Moskowitz CS, et al. Bilateral contrast-enhanced dual-energy digital mammography: feasibility and comparison with conventional digital mammography and MR imaging in women with known breast carcinoma. Radiology. 2013;266:743–51.
45. Covington MF, Pizzitola VJ, Lorans R, Pockaj BA, Northfelt DW, Appleton CM, et al. The future of contrast-enhanced mammography. AJR Am J Roentgenol. 2018;210:292–300.
46. Jochelson MS, Pinker K, Dershaw DD, Hughes M, Gibbons GF, Rahbar K, et al. Comparison of screening CEDM and MRI for women at increased risk for breast cancer: a pilot study. Eur J Radiol. 2017;97:37–43.
47. Youk JH, Gweon HM, Son EJ. Shear-wave elastography in breast ultrasonography: the state of the art. Ultrasonography. 2017;36:300–9.
48. Itoh A, Ueno E, Tohno E, Kamma H, Takahashi H, Shiina T, et al. Breast disease: clinical application of US elastography for diagnosis. Radiology. 2006;239:341–50.
49. Schueller G, Jaromi S, Ponhold L, Fuchsjaeger M, Memarsadeghi M, Rudas M, et al. US-guided 14-gauge core-needle breast biopsy: results of a validation study in 1352 cases. Radiology. 2008;248:406–13.
50. Fishman JE, Milikowski C, Ramsinghani R, Velasquez MV, Aviram G. US-guided core-needle biopsy of the breast: how many specimens are necessary? Radiology. 2003;226:779–82.
51. Sung JS, Lee CH, Morris EA, Comstock CE, Dershaw DD. Patient follow-up after concordant histologically benign imaging-guided biopsy of MRI-detected lesions. AJR Am J Roentgenol. 2012;198:1464–9.

52. Li J, Dershaw DD, Lee CH, Kaplan J, Morris EA. MRI follow-up after concordant, histologically benign diagnosis of breast lesions sampled by MRI-guided biopsy. AJR Am J Roentgenol. 2009;193:850–5.
53. Skinner KA, Silberman H, Sposto R, Silverstein MJ. Palpable breast cancers are inherently different from nonpalpable breast cancers. Ann Surg Oncol. 2001;8:705–10.
54. Lovrics PJ, Cornacchi SD, Farrokhyar F, Garnett A, Chen V, Franic S, et al. The relationship between surgical factors and margin status after breast-conservation surgery for early stage breast cancer. Am J Surg. 2009;197:740–6.
55. Goudreau SH, Joseph JP, Seiler SJ. Preoperative radioactive seed localization for nonpalpable breast lesions: technique, pitfalls, and solutions. RadioGraphics. 2015;35:1319–34.
56. Rampaul RS, Dudley NJ, Thompson JZ, Burrell H, Evans AJ, Wilson AR, et al. Radioisotope for occult lesion localisation (ROLL) of the breast does not require extra radiation protection procedures. Breast. 2003;12:150–2.
57. Fung F, Cornacchi SD, Reedijk M, Hodgson N, Goldsmith CH, McCready D, et al. Breast cancer recurrence following radioguided seed localization and standard wire localization of nonpalpable invasive and in situ breast cancers: 5-year follow-up from a randomized controlled trial. Am J Surg. 2017;213:798–804.
58. Stelle L, Schoenheit T, Brubaker A, Tang X, Qu P, Cradock K, et al. Radioactive seed localization versus wire localization for nonpalpable breast lesions: a two-year initial experience at a large community hospital. Ann Surg Oncol. 2018;25:131–6.
59. Yilmaz MH, Kilic F, Icten GE, Aydogan F, Ozben V, Halac M, et al. Radio-guided occult lesion localisation for breast lesions under computer-aided MRI guidance: the first experience and initial results. Br J Radiol. 2012;85:395–402.
60. Gail MH, Brinton LA, Byar DP, Corle DK, Green SB, Schairer C, et al. Projecting individualized probabilities of developing breast cancer for white females who are being examined annually. J Natl Cancer Inst. 1989;81:1879–86.
61. Tyrer J, Duffy SW, Cuzick J. A breast cancer prediction model incorporating familial and personal risk factors. Stat Med. 2004;23:1111–30.
62. Gradishar WJ, Anderson BO, Balassanian R, Blair SL, Burstein HJ, Cyr A, et al. Breast cancer version 2.2015. J Natl Compr Cancer Netw. 2015;13:448–75.
63. Lee CH, Dershaw DD, Kopans D, Evans P, Monsees B, Monticciolo D, et al. Breast cancer screening with imaging: recommendations from the Society of Breast Imaging and the ACR on the use of mammography, breast MRI, breast ultrasound, and other technologies for the detection of clinically occult breast cancer. J Am Coll Radiol. 2010;7:18–27.
64. Warner E, Messersmith H, Causer P, Eisen A, Shumak R, Plewes D. Systematic review: using magnetic resonance imaging to screen women at high risk for breast cancer. Ann Intern Med. 2008;148:671–9.
65. Lowry KP, Lee JM, Kong CY, McMahon PM, Gilmore ME, Cott Chubiz JE, et al. Annual screening strategies in BRCA1 and BRCA2 gene mutation carriers: a comparative effectiveness analysis. Cancer. 2012;118:2021–30.
66. Lee MV, Katabathina VS, Bowerson ML, Mityul MI, Shetty AS, Elsayes KM, et al. BRCA-associated cancers: role of imaging in screening, diagnosis, and management. RadioGraphics. 2017;37:1005–23.
67. Berg WA, Blume J, Adams AM, Jong RA, Barr RG, Lehrer DE, et al. Reasons women at elevated risk of breast cancer refuse breast MR imaging screening: ACRIN 6666. Radiology. 2010;254:79–87.
68. Kuhl CK, Schrading S, Strobel K, Schild HH, Hilgers RD, Bieling HB. Abbreviated breast magnetic resonance imaging (MRI): first postcontrast subtracted images and maximum-intensity projection—a novel approach to breast cancer screening with MRI. J Clin Oncol. 2014;32:2304–10.
69. Dogan BE, Scoggins ME, Son JB, Wei W, Candelaria R, Yang WT, et al. American College of radiology-compliant short protocol breast MRI for high-risk breast cancer screening: a prospective feasibility study. AJR Am J Roentgenol. 2018;210:214–21.

Chapter 8
Nuclear Medicine Imaging in Breast Cancer

Cuneyt Turkmen

Introduction

Nuclear medicine is a medical specialty that targets molecules with radioactive substances (radiopharmaceuticals) for the diagnosis and treatment of disease. Nuclear medicine imaging, which includes single-photon emission computerized tomography (SPECT) and positron emission tomography (PET), can measure the cellular, molecular, and biochemical properties of neoplasms and normal tissues in vivo. Hybrid imaging systems such as PET/CT, PET/MR and SPECT/CT devices, which combine functional and anatomical information, can localize processes within the body to an anatomically identifiable or, in some instances, as yet unidentifiable structural alteration. While molecular imaging with PET is a rapidly emerging approach in breast cancer, conventional single-photon nuclear medicine imaging, including bone scintigraphy and sentinel lymph node scintigraphy, still has an important role in the management of breast cancer. Nuclear medicine imaging systems are designed primarily for whole-body imaging, which is one of the strengths of this modality. SPECT imaging uses nuclides such as 99mTc, which decay while emitting single γ-ray photons with different energies. In contrast to SPECT agents, PET agents use pharmaceuticals labeled with positron-emitting radionuclides, which are produced mainly by cyclotrons.

PET/CT is a molecular imaging exam that is commonly used to target cancer cells and is an essential component of staging and monitoring treatment for numerous types of cancer. Technological advancements in PET equipment via the development of new detectors and equipment designed specifically for breast imaging and the development of more specific radiopharmaceuticals for studying

---

C. Turkmen (✉)
Istanbul Medical Faculty, Department of Nuclear Medicine, Istanbul University, Istanbul, Turkey

A. Aydiner et al. (eds.), *Breast Cancer*, https://doi.org/10.1007/978-3-319-96947-3_8

the different biological processes of breast cancer will allow progress not only in diagnosing disease at an early stage but also in enabling personalized therapy for patients with breast cancer.

Scintimammography

Scintimammography is a functional imaging methodology that provides a noninvasive in vivo differentiation of malignant from benign processes and is helpful in clinical scenarios where mainstay anatomic modalities such as mammography, ultrasound and MRI are limited [1]. Scintimammography employs a wide range of instrumentation applications. In recent years, conventional planar scintimammography has been enhanced by SPECT and hybrid SPECT/CT and dedicated small field of view (FOV) breast-specific gamma imaging (BSGI) devices. Technetium-99m (Tc-99m) MIBI is the radiopharmaceutical of choice for SPECT studies in breast imaging [2]. Tc-99m MIBI is localized to the dense mitochondria characteristic of malignant cells, with its uptake dependent on regional blood flow, tumor angiogenesis, and increased metabolism and driven by plasma membrane potentials and mitochondrial membrane potentials [3, 4]. A number of studies have consistently shown that early tracer uptake reflects mitochondrial status, which is affected by both apoptosis and proliferation, whereas tracer clearance reflects the activity of drug transporters such as P-glycoprotein [5, 6]. Many clinical studies have highlighted that both proliferative activity and the apoptotic index correlate directly with Tc-99m MIBI uptake [7, 8].

The results of a recent meta-analysis that systematically evaluated the diagnostic value of BSGI and MRI in the same cohort of patients with breast cancer showed that compared with MRI, BSGI had comparable sensitivity (84% vs. 89%) but higher specificity (82% vs. 39%) and diagnostic efficacy (AUC 0.93 vs. 0.72), indicating excellent diagnostic performance [9]. Given the high specificity of scintimammography, a positive scintigraphic finding would support a recommendation of an invasive evaluation. Many well-known factors, including tumor type (poorly differentiated DCIS, lobular and tubulolobular carcinomas), size (<1 cm), cellularity, blood supply and cell viability, can cause a false negative result on scintimammography [10, 11]. Scintimammography also has limitations in detecting axillary lymph nodes and delineating adjacent lesions. However, the combined functional and morphological information provided by SPECT-CT significantly increases the diagnostic value of noninvasive detection of axillary lymph node invasion by breast cancer; the sensitivity of SPECT-CT 1.4 times higher (from 55% to 75%) than that of CT, with excellent specificity (97% and 89%) and comparable overall accuracy (82% and 84%) [12]. Breast benign hyperplasia lesions such as fibrocystic change and fibroadenoma can also cause false positive results in scintimammography. An effective radiation dose was estimated to be 5.9–9.4 mSv compared to 0.44 mSv for digital mammography [13].

Another potential clinical application of Tc-99m MIBI scintimammography is to predict the response to neoadjuvant chemotherapy in patients with breast cancer. Tc-99m MIBI scintimammography has also been used for decades to monitor the treatment response to neoadjuvant chemotherapy. In a recent meta-analysis, for all 14 studies included, pooled sensitivity was 0.86 (95% CI: 0.78–0.92), and pooled specificity was 0.69 (95% CI: 0.64–0.74) for the accuracy of Tc-99m MIBI scintimammography in the prediction of neoadjuvant chemotherapy response in breast cancer [14]. These results indicate that Tc-99m MIBI scintimammography could yield high sensitivity but low specificity, which must be considered cautiously in clinical practice. This analysis suggests that a negative scintimammography result does not fully exclude the presence of a residual tumor, especially remaining ductal carcinoma in situ or residual tumor less than 1 cm in size. Subgroup analysis also showed that performing early mid-treatment Tc-99m MIBI scintimammography (using the reduction rate of one or two cycles or within the first half-courses of chemotherapy compared with baseline) was superior to later (after three courses or more) or post-treatment scintimammography for predicting neoadjuvant chemotherapy response. Lee et al. reported that MRI had added value to scintimammography in the detection of residual tumor after neoadjuvant chemotherapy and that scintimammography could help locate tumors after therapy that were false negative on MRI. However, a direct comparison between MRI and scintimammography was statistically insignificant. Thus, it is suggested that a combination of scintimammography and MRI in the prediction of treatment response would be more accurate [15].

Sentinel Lymph Node Scintigraphy

Axillary lymph node status, a major prognostic factor in early-stage breast cancer, provides important information for individualized surgical treatment. Therefore, sentinel lymph node biopsy is the standard surgical procedure for staging clinically tumor-free regional nodes in patients with early-stage breast cancer. Axillary lymph node dissection is no longer recommended in these patients as it only adds to arm morbidity without conferring any prognostic or staging benefit [16]. Sentinel lymph node biopsy has become the standard of care for the primary treatment of early breast cancer and has replaced axillary lymph node dissection to stage clinically node-negative patients, thus reducing axillary lymph node dissection-associated morbidity.

Sentinel lymph node biopsy is based on the notion that tumors drain in an orderly manner through the lymphatic system. Therefore, the sentinel lymph node is the first to be affected by metastasis if the tumor has spread, and a tumor-free sentinel lymph node suggests that it is highly unlikely that other nodes will be affected. Sentinel lymph node scintigraphy using radiolabeled colloids provides surgeons with a visual map to guide accurate localization of sentinel nodes and atypical drainage patterns. Although lymphoscintigraphy and sentinel lymph node biopsy have been used to stage many solid cancers, these procedures are most commonly performed in patients with breast cancer and melanoma. In the sentinel lymph node biopsy procedure, general recommendations require lymphoscintigraphy for quality control because it can improve accuracy (especially in extra-axillary lymph nodes) and reduce surgical morbidity [17]. Lymphatic mapping reveals lymphatic ducts and nodes and helps locate sentinel lymph nodes. SPECT/CT considerably improves the topographic localization of sentinel lymph nodes by providing more accurate staging of breast cancer patients. Intraoperative detection of sentinel lymph nodes is usually radio guided by a γ-probe. Recently, several portable γ-cameras have been developed to provide an overview of radioactive "hot spots" in all surgical fields to verify the completeness of sentinel lymph node excision. Recent developments include combining conventional γ-probes with position and orientation tracking systems such as so-called free-hand SPECT, which permits virtual reconstruction in a 3-dimensional environment.

Identification of the sentinel node is crucial to the success of sentinel lymph node biopsy, and with a detection rate between 94% and 100%, preoperative sentinel node imaging is ideally suited for this purpose [18–21]. Recent multi-institutional studies have revealed sentinel lymph node biopsy false-negative rates ranging from 5.5% to 16.7%, higher than the target set by the 2005 ASCO guidelines (<5%) [22, 23]. Unfortunately, sentinel lymph node biopsy remains an unstandardized procedure surrounded by many unresolved controversies concerning the technique itself. The radiopharmaceuticals commonly used for sentinel lymph node biopsy are 99mTc-sulfur colloid (particle size, 15–5000 nm), 99mTc-nanocolloid (5–100 nm), and 99mTc-antimony trisulfide (3–30 nm). There is general agreement that a radiocolloid measuring 100–200 nm should be considered the best compromise between fast lymphatic drainage and optimal retention in sentinel lymph nodes [24]. The literature supports the use of small volumes (0.3–0.4 mL) with high specific activity to improve sentinel lymph node detection. Currently, the criterion standard for sentinel lymph node detection is based on use of radiotracer alone or in combination with blue dye, especially when the sentinel lymph node is suspected to be diffusely metastatic [25]. Currently, no clinical consensus exists on the optimal site of injection of the radioactive tracer or blue dye. Superficial (periareolar, subareolar, intradermal, subdermal) and deep (peritumoral, intratumoral) injections within the breast have been reported widely for radioactive tracer administration [22, 26]. A recent meta-analysis comparing superficial and deep injections of radioactive tracer demonstrated no significant difference between the two injection sites in the sentinel lymph node identification rate on lymphoscintigraphy and during intraoperative sentinel lymph node biopsy [27]. The rate of extra-axillary sentinel lymph node identification was significantly greater when deep rather than superficial injection was used (OR 3.00, 1.92–4.67).

Several contraindications for sentinel lymph node biopsy include grossly palpable nodes and inflammatory breast cancer. For some patients, sentinel lymph node biopsy may not be helpful because accurate sentinel lymph node removal may be challenging after prior surgery or radiation. Studies of inflammatory breast cancer report sentinel lymph node identification rates of only 80%–85% with a relatively high false negative rate (6.18%) [28]. Since the publication of the updated ASCO guidelines in 2017, no new data are available that support the benefit of sentinel lymph node biopsy in women with large or locally advanced invasive breast cancers (T3/T4) and inflammatory breast cancer [29]. Sentinel lymph node biopsy is not recommended for women who have DCIS when surgery is planned. Sentinel lymph node biopsy is instead recommended for smaller tumors (T1 and T2), multiple tumors, DCIS when mastectomy is planned, for older or obese patients, in male patients with breast cancer, and in patients with prior breast or axillary surgery. Sentinel lymph node biopsy may be offered before or after neoadjuvant systemic therapy, but the procedure appears to be less accurate after neoadjuvant systemic therapy.

Today, the prognostic relevance of isolated tumor cells and micrometastases is negligible. Two multi-institutional randomized studies demonstrated an identification rate of sentinel lymph node biopsy of 98% in cN0 stage I/II breast cancer patients [30, 31]. Thus, sentinel lymph node biopsy could prevent axillary lymph node dissection for sentinel lymph node-negative women. In the ACOSOG Z0010 trial, occult metastases were detected in 9% of cases, but no differences were observed in disease-free survival and overall survival [32]. The 10-year follow-up data of the NSABP B-32 trial, which demonstrated a prevalence of occult metastases of 15.9%, revealed small differences in disease-free survival and overall survival that were statistically significant but not clinically significant. Therefore, complete axillary lymph node dissection in cases of sentinel lymph node micrometastases is no longer recommended [33].

Bone Scintigraphy

The skeleton is the most common site for metastases from breast cancer. The skeleton is affected in approximately 50%–70% of patients with relapse and is the only metastatic site of disease in 28%–44% of patients [34]. It is important to detect bone metastases at an early stage to minimize skeleton-related events and to allow the determination of a response as early as possible to limit toxicity and accelerate the therapeutic transition in nonresponding patients. Imaging has always played a key role in the diagnosis of bone metastases in breast cancer, and planar 99mTc-diphosphonate bone scanning remains widely used. Its lack of specificity has been improved with the addition of SPECT and SPECT/CT. Despite improved accuracy in staging of the skeleton, evidence of efficacy and consensus regarding effective monitoring of a treatment response are lacking. Although radiographs have been used historically to determine a response by lesion resolution or sclerosis, this method has been recognized as insensitive and may take at least 6 months to yield a confident assessment of a response. Abnormal accumulation of 99mTc-labeled diphosphonates is related to changes in local blood flow and osteoblastic activity, events that are secondary in most bone metastases that are seeded in the bone marrow. The mechanism of accumulation means that the uptake of 99mTc-labeled diphosphonates is not specific for metastatic disease and may make the differentiation of increased reparative osteoblastic activity after successful treatment (flare) from unresponsive progressive disease impossible for several months. The problem of the flare phenomenon, which makes the differentiation of progression from a temporary healing osteoblastic response to successful therapy difficult for 3–6 months, has also been recognized for many years and has been described after chemotherapy and endocrine therapy in breast cancer [35]. Limitations with bone scintigraphy are reported when measuring treatment response in breast cancer, with only 52% of responders showing scintigraphic improvement, and 62% of nonresponders showing scintigraphic deterioration at 6–8 months [36].

Positron Emission Tomography/Computed Tomography

Positron emission tomography combined with computed tomography (PET/CT) has received increasing attention in recent years for the diagnosis, staging and follow-up of various malignancies. Positron emission tomography-computed tomography with 2-[fluorine-18]-fluoro-2-deoxy-D-glucose (FDG) has been established as an effective modality for evaluation of cancer.

Currently, PET is not used in breast cancer screening or in diagnosing primary breast cancer, mainly due to the high prevalence of false negative results, particularly for tumors with a diameter smaller than 1 cm and tumors with low metabolic activity. Inferior sensitivity of PET in primary breast cancer detection has been reported compared to ultrasonography, magnetic resonance imaging (MRI) and mammography [37]. The metabolic activity of breast tumors is variable. For example, invasive lobular breast cancer has a considerably lower ^{18}F-FDG uptake than invasive ductal cancer does. The relatively high physiological glucose uptake in surrounding mammary tissue is another difficulty for the detection of tumors with low metabolic activity. The highest glucose uptake is observed for high-grade tumors, triple-negative tumors (ER−, PgR−, HER2−) and inflammatory breast cancer [38, 39].

In early-stage breast cancer with clinically negative axilla, ^{18}F-FDG PET/CT is not recommended because its role is limited in the initial staging and treatment planning in most patients. In regional staging, ^{18}F-FDG PET/CT is less sensitive than sentinel lymph node biopsy in assessing axillary lymph node involvement. The low prevalence of distant metastases and the risk of false-positive findings detract from the usefulness of ^{18}F-FDG PET/CT for distant staging in these patients [40]. In contrast, in patients with positive axilla, especially those with locally advanced breast cancer, ^{18}F-FDG PET/CT can be useful prior to surgery or neoadjuvant chemotherapy, based on the high rate of detection of distant metastases, ranging from 6% to 26% [41]. The percentage of patients with extra-axillary lymph node involvement detected by PET/CT in locally advanced breast cancer ranges from 10% to 29% [42, 43]. The superiority of ^{18}F-FDG PET/CT with respect to conventional

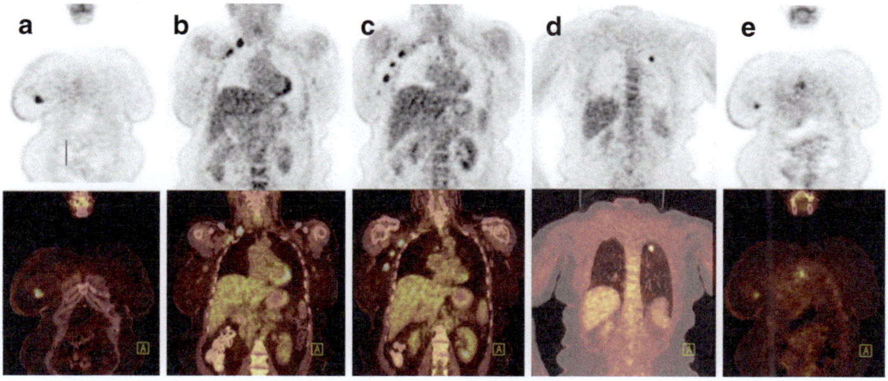

Fig. 8.1 A 54-year-old woman with ER−, PR−, and HER2-positive right breast invasive ductal carcinoma. PET coronal images demonstrate a corresponding FDG-avid mass consistent with the known carcinoma (**a**), metastatic lymph nodes in the right supraclavicular and axillary region (**b**, **c**), a metastatic nodule in the apicoposterior segment of the left lung (**d**) and bone metastasis in the sternum (**e**)

imaging for detecting extra-axillary lymph nodes and metastatic disease is more relevant in locally advanced breast cancer (Fig. 8.1). ^{18}F-FDG PET/CT changes the initial treatment in 1%–8% of patients with early-stage breast cancer, in 7%–13% of those with locally advanced breast cancer and in up to 52% of those with more aggressive tumors, such as inflammatory breast cancer [44, 45].

In addition to staging, the level of ^{18}F-FDG uptake by a primary tumor has prognostic value in many types of cancer. With respect to the semiquantitative information from ^{18}F-FDG PET/CT, the prognostic impact of the glycolytic activity (SUVmax) of the primary breast tumor is controversial. Whereas some authors found no association between tumor ^{18}F-FDG uptake and prognosis [46, 47], others reported that patients with high tumor uptake had worse outcomes [48, 49]. Furthermore, a single and reproducible SUVmax has not been established; cutoff values range from 3 to 6. The evidence for the prognostic value of SUVmax in axillary lymph nodes is also limited, although higher values have been associated with higher recurrence rates [50, 51].

Changes in tumor metabolic activity have been shown to be an early indicator of treatment effectiveness for breast cancer, mainly in the neoadjuvant setting. A decrease in tumor metabolic activity offers both assessment of the treatment response after the completion of therapy and early prediction of therapeutic effectiveness after the first or second cycle of chemotherapy. Identifying nonresponding patients on the basis of changes in tumor metabolic activity early during treatment could facilitate a change from an ineffective to a more effective treatment approach. Rousseau et al. studied 64 stage II and III breast cancer patients at multiple cycles during neoadjuvant chemotherapy and found a marked decrease in ^{18}F-FDG uptake in nearly all patients who achieved a greater than 50% therapeutic effect [52]. Performing ^{18}F-FDG PET after the second cycle of treatment potentially provides a more accurate prediction of treatment response. Using a 40% decrease in the SUV,

Rousseau et al. identified a negative predictive value of 68% for identifying nonresponders after the first cycle; this value increased to 85% after the second cycle. Schwarz-Dose et al. confirmed in 104 patients that the greater the reduction in tumor metabolic activity early during neoadjuvant treatment, the more likely the patients would achieve a pathologic response [53]. After the first cycle of chemotherapy, tumor metabolic activity decreased by 50% ± 18% in pathologic responders; in comparison, the decrease in pathologic nonresponders was 36% ± 20%. Of note, all breast carcinomas (23%) with a baseline SUV less than 3.0 did not respond to chemotherapy. A recent meta-analysis including 19 studies with more than 900 patients found that the best cutoff for a response was a decrease in ^{18}F-FDG uptake ranging from 55% to 65% [54]. Although the sensitivity and specificity for identifying patients responding to treatment were limited (84% and 66%, respectively), the negative predictive value for identifying nonresponders was high (91%).

Changes in the sizes of bone metastases are particularly difficult to evaluate with conventional imaging as sclerotic lesions do not disappear and lytic lesions can show sclerotic changes as an indicator of a treatment response (Fig. 8.2). Two studies demonstrated a high sensitivity of ^{18}F-FDG PET/CT for the detection of osseous metastases in patients with newly diagnosed metastatic breast cancer, and the metabolic activity of osseous breast cancer metastases provided prognostic information [55, 56]. In a retrospective analysis, bone metastases in 102 patients

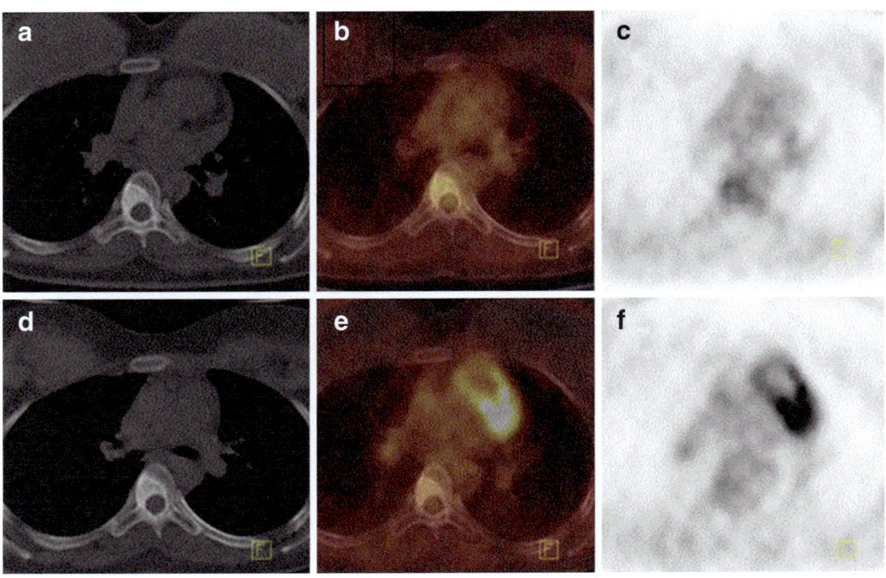

Fig. 8.2 A 64-year-old woman with a history of left invasive ductal cancer, status postmastectomy, imaged for surveillance. ^{18}F-FDG PET-CT images showed sclerotic bone metastasis in the thoracic vertebrae (**a**), which demonstrated mild FDG uptake on the fused (**b**) and PET images (**c**). After chemotherapy, while there was no chance of a sclerotic component of lesion on CT images (**d**), fused (**e**) and PET/CT (**f**) images showed decreased metabolic activity corresponding to therapeutic response at the same location

were assessed with ^{18}F-FDG PET/CT before and after treatment, and a decrease in ^{18}F-FDG uptake was a significant predictor of response duration in univariate and multivariate analyses [57].

The early detection and accurate restaging of recurrent breast cancer are of significant importance for applying optimal therapeutic strategies to achieve better prognosis and lower mortality. For breast cancer with suspicious recurrence, however, there is no standard follow-up protocol to date, and further examination of radiologic imaging, such as CT, bone scintigraphy, MRI, and PET, may be needed. ^{18}F-FDG-PET or PET/CT is a valuable technique for acquiring functional information for early detection of whole-body multifocal malignant lesions and enables the diagnosis of missed or incorrect recurrence offered by conventional imaging modalities. Because it allows better discrimination between posttreatment scar or fibrosis and viable tumor tissue, PET/CT is efficient for detecting locoregional recurrence, especially in the chest wall, axilla, and extraaxillary lymph nodes basins, with better performance than CT or MRI. A recent meta-analysis systematically summarized the overall diagnostic value of ^{18}F-FDG PET or PET/CT for the diagnosis of recurrence in suspicious breast cancer. The pooled sensitivity was 0.90 (95% CI: 0.88–0.92), indicating a higher capacity for PET analysis in the early detection of recurrent breast cancer [58]. In addition, the pooled specificity was 0.81 (95% CI: 0.78–0.84), demonstrating a relatively higher ability to exclude recurrence in suspicious breast cancer compared with other imaging modalities, such as CT or MRI. In other words, a negative PET result can indicate the absence of recurrent breast cancer with 81% probability.

^{18}F-NaF is a positron emitter that is used for bone imaging. The mechanism of uptake is quite similar to those of ^{99m}Tc-MDP and ^{18}F-NaF. Chemisorption of ^{18}F-NaF to hydroxyapatite results in conversion to fluoroapatite and a hydroxyl group. Studies comparing the utility of ^{18}F-NaF PET/CT with ^{99m}Tc-MDP whole-body bone scintigraphy have shown that ^{18}F-NaF PET/CT generally has higher sensitivity and specificity than bone scan. The higher uptake of ^{18}F-NaF compared to ^{99m}Tc-MDP in the skeleton and faster blood clearance yield a better target/background ratio in a shorter time period. Factors contributing to the success of ^{18}F-NaF PET/CT include the following: ^{18}F-NaF uptake in both lytic and blastic metastasis, sectional imaging advantages for the whole body and easy detection of small lesions due to the improved resolution of PET technology, and better visualization of bone marrow lesions [59]. In addition to ^{18}F-FDG and ^{18}F-NaF, other radiopharmaceuticals have been used in both pre-clinical and clinical settings in breast cancer. Radiolabeled hypoxia-avid compounds such as ^{18}F-labeled fluoromisonidazole or ^{18}F-FMISO can be used to evaluate oxygenation status in experimental or human tumors. This PET radiotracer has affinity for hypoxic cells with functional nitroreductase enzymes; therefore, it accumulates in activated cells but not in necrotic cells. ^{18}F-labeled fluorothymidine, or ^{18}F-FLT, has been proposed as an early molecular imaging biomarker able to evaluate treatment response with taxanes [60]. The uptake of FLT is also correlated with the Ki-67 labeling index, another proliferation parameter, in breast cancer. Some studies have presented a strong correlation of FLT uptake with cell proliferation in untreated patients with breast cancer, enabling detection of response as early as 1 week after chemotherapy. Pio et al. compared ^{18}F-FDG and ^{18}F-FLT imaging in 14 patients with newly diagnosed primary or metastatic breast cancer for monitoring and predicting tumor response to chemotherapy [61]. The group concluded that ^{18}F-FLT may be more accurate than ^{18}F-FDG 2 weeks after the end of the first course of chemotherapy for predicting longer-term efficacy of chemotherapy for women with breast cancer. ^{18}F-labeled fluoroestradiol or ^{18}F-FES is a novel radiopharmaceutical that non-invasively measures ER expression in tumors and has emerged as a valuable method for predicting response to hormone therapy in recurrent or metastatic breast cancer patients [62, 63]. The level of ^{18}F-FES uptake predicts the likelihood of a response to tamoxifen and aromatase inhibitor treatment, as supported by some studies, and could be of use in assessing the treatment response in groups with recurrent or metastatic breast cancer [64].

Positron Emission Tomography/Magnetic Resonance Imaging

PET/MR imaging is particularly interesting as a possible improvement over PET/CT oncologic whole-body imaging because MR imaging provides improved lesion detection in the brain, breast, liver, kidneys, and bones compared with CT. In focused breast and whole-body settings, PET/MR imaging can bring metabolic, anatomic, spectroscopic, and diffusion- and perfusion-based data together in a single examination. In whole-body imaging for breast cancer, PET/MR imaging has been shown to provide improved sensitivity over PET/CT, particularly for breast cancers, liver metastases, and bone metastases [65, 66]. In local staging, PET and MR imaging appear to be complimentary, with MR imaging providing greater accuracy for satellite lesions and PET providing greater sensitivity for axillary nodes. PET/MR imaging has been shown to be more likely than PET/CT to determine the correct maximum diameter of the tumor (T stage), which may be useful in surgical and oncologic planning [67]. In imaging metastatic disease, PET and MR imaging are again complimentary, with MR imaging providing high sensitivity and PET tempering the relatively low specificity of diffusion-weighted imaging (DWI). PET/MR imaging has also been shown to detect brain metastases.

When separated out by sequence, dynamic contrast-enhanced (DCE) MR imaging has been shown to be most useful for breast and brain lesions, DWI has been shown to be most useful for liver and bone metastases, and PET has been shown to be most useful for lymph node metastases [66]. These variable strengths highlight the advantage of multimodality imaging. In particular, combining PET and DWI may be important because PET has been shown to greatly improve the specificity of DWI in whole-body imaging [68]. In addition, omitting whole-body CT from the PET examination can decrease the radiation dose by half [66]. These data suggest a wider role for PET/MR imaging in breast cancer staging and surveillance, particularly in young patients and in patients undergoing serial examinations.

Conclusion

The general advantage of nuclear medicine imaging is that tumor-seeking radiopharmaceuticals accumulate in cancer lesions, which makes scintimammography and PET fundamentally different from radiological techniques that image the tumor mainly on the basis of morphological alterations. Scintimammography is indicated for the study of breast lesions in patients in whom mammography or MRI is nondiagnostic or difficult to interpret; it may also be useful for assessing and even predicting the response to chemotherapy. Although whole-body FDG PET imaging does not have sufficient utility in the detection of primary disease and is not optimized to replace the sentinel lymph node procedure for initial axillary staging, FDG PET scanning has efficacy superior to that of conventional imaging for the detection of locoregional and metastatic spread in the appropriate patient population and has better diagnostic performance for the detection of skeletal metastasis compared with routine bone scanning. The major roles for PET/CT in breast cancer are detection and localization of metastasis, monitoring the response to treatment and early detection of recurrence. On the basis of the abovementioned evidence, nuclear medicine techniques, integrated with radiological techniques, offer an interesting opportunity to improve the diagnostic imaging yield in breast cancer, which will eventually lead to better patient management.

References

1. Brem R, Rechtman L. Nuclear medicine imaging of the breast: a novel, physiological approach to breast cancer detection and diagnosis. Radiol Clin N Am. 2010;48:1055–74.
2. de Cesare A, Giuseppe DV, Stefano G, Crescentini G, Fiori E, Bonomi M, et al. Single photon emission computed tomography (SPECT) with technetium-99m sestamibi in the diagnosis of small breast cancer and axillary lymph node involvement. World J Surg. 2011;35:2668–72.
3. Jacobsson H. Single-photon-emission computed tomography (SPECT) with 99mTechnetium sestamibi in the diagnosis of small breast cancer and axillary node involvement. World J Surg. 2011;35:2673–4.
4. Lee J, Rosen E, Mankoff D. The role of radiotracer imaging in the diagnosis and management of patients with breast cancer: part 1 – overview, detection and staging. J Nucl Med. 2009;50:569–81.
5. Delmon-Moingeon LI, Piwnica-Worms D, Van den Abbeele AD, Holman BL, Davison A, Jones AG. Uptake of the cation hexakis(2-methoxyisobutylisonitrile)-technetium-99m by human carcinoma cell lines in vitro. Cancer Res. 1990;50:2198–202.
6. Carvalho PA, Chiu ML, Kronauge JF, Kawamura M, Jones AG, Holman BL, et al. Subcellular distribution and analysis of technetium-99m-MIBI in isolated perfused rat hearts. J Nucl Med. 1992;33:1516–22.
7. Archer CD, Parton M, Smith IE, Ellis PA, Salter J, Ashley S, et al. Early changes in apoptosis and proliferation following primary chemotherapy for breast cancer. Br J Cancer. 2003;89:1035–41.
8. Cutrone JA, Yospur LS, Khalkhali I, Tolmos J, Devito A, Diggles L, et al. Immunohistologic assessment of technetium-99m-MIBI uptake in benign and malignant breast lesions. J Nucl Med. 1998;39:449–53.

9. Zhang A, Li P, Liu Q, Song S. Breast-specific gamma camera imaging with 99mTc-MIBI has better diagnostic performance than magnetic resonance imaging in breast cancer patients: a meta-analysis. Hell J Nucl Med. 2017;20(1):26–35.
10. Brem RF, Petrovitch I, Rapelyea JA, Young H, Teal C, Kelly T. Breast-specific gamma imaging with 99mTc-Sestamibi and magnetic resonance imaging in the diagnosis of breast cancer-a comparative study. Breast J. 2007;13(5):465–9.
11. Meissnitzer T, Seymer A, Keinrath P, Holzmannhofer J, Pirich C, Hergan K, et al. Added value of semi-quantitative breast-specific gamma imaging in the work-up of suspicious breast lesions compared to mammography, ultrasound and 3-T MRI. Br J Radiol. 2015;88(1051):20150147.
12. Novikov SN, Krzhivitskii PI, Kanaev SV, Krivorotko PV, Ilin ND, Jukova LA, et al. Axillary lymph node staging in breast cancer: clinical value of single photon emission computed tomography-computed tomography (SPECT-CT) with 99mTc methoxyisobutylisonitrile. Ann Nucl Med. 2015;29(2):177–83.
13. Hendrick RE. Radiation doses and cancer risks from breast imaging studies. Radiology. 2010;257:246–53.
14. Guo C, Zhang C, Liu J, Tong L, Huang G. Is Tc-99m sestamibi scintimammography useful in the prediction of neoadjuvant chemotherapy responses in breast cancer? A systematic review and meta-analysis. Nucl Med Commun. 2016;37(7):675–88.
15. Lee HS, Ko BS, Ahn SH, Son BH, Lee JW, Kim HJ, et al. Diagnostic performance of breast-specific gamma imaging in the assessment of residual tumor after neoadjuvant chemotherapy in breast cancer patients. Breast Cancer Res Treat. 2014;145:91–100.
16. Bromham N, Schmidt-Hansen M, Astin M, Hasler E, Reed MW. Axillary treatment for operable primary breast cancer. Cochrane Database Syst Rev. 2017;4(1):CD004561.
17. Johnson MT, Guidroz JA, Smith BJ, Graham MM, Scott-Conner CE, Sugg SL, et al. A single institutional experience of factors affecting successful identification of sentinel lymph node in breast cancer patients. Surgery. 2009;146:671–6.
18. Caruso G, Cipolla C, Costa R, Morabito A, Latteri S, Fricano S, et al. Lymphoscintigraphy with peritumoral injection versus lymphoscintigraphy with subdermal periareolar injection of technetium-labeled human albumin to identify sentinel lymph nodes in breast cancer patients. Acta Radiol. 2014;55:39–44.
19. Somasundaram SK, Chicken DW, Waddington WA, Bomanji J, Ell PJ, Keshtgar MRS. Sentinel node imaging in breast cancer using superficial injections: technical details and observations. Eur J Surg Oncol. 2009;35:1250–6.
20. Aliakbarian M, Memar B, Jangjoo A, Zakavi SR, Reza Dabbagh Kakhki V, Aryana K, et al. Factors influencing the time of sentinel node visualization in breast cancer patients using intradermal injection of the radiotracer. Am J Surg. 2011;202:199–202.
21. Mudun A, Sanli Y, Ozmen V, Turkmen C, Ozel S, Eroglu A, et al. Comparison of different injection sites of radionuclide for sentinel lymph node detection in breast cancer: single institution experience. Clin Nucl Med. 2008;33:262–7.
22. Hindie E, Groheux D, Brenot-Rossi I, Rubello D, Moretti JL, Espié M. The sentinel node procedure in breast cancer: nuclear medicine as the starting point. J Nucl Med. 2001;52:405–14.
23. Lyman GH, Giuliano AE, Somerfield MR, Benson AB 3rd, Bodurka DC, Burstein HJ, et al. American Society of Clinical Oncology guideline recommendations for sentinel lymph node biopsy in early-stage breast cancer. J Clin Oncol. 2005;23:7703–20.
24. G M, Rubello D, Tardelli E, Giammarile F, Mazzarri S, Boni G, et al. Sentinel lymph node biopsy in breast cancer: indications, contraindications, and controversies. Clin Nucl Med. 2016;41(2):126–33.
25. Giammarile F, Alazraki N, Aarsvold JN, Audisio RA, Glass E, Grant SF, et al. The EANM and SNMMI practice guideline for lymphoscintigraphy and sentinel node localization in breast cancer. Eur J Nucl Med Mol Imaging. 2013;40:1932–47.
26. Sun X, Liu JJ, Wang YS, et al. Roles of preoperative lymphoscintigraphy for sentinel lymph node biopsy in breast cancer patients. Jpn J Clin Oncol. 2010;40:722–5.
27. Ahmed M, Purushotham AD, Horgan K, Klaase JM, Douek M. Meta-analysis of superficial versus deep injection of radioactive tracer and blue dye for lymphatic mapping and detection of sentinel lymph nodes in breast cancer. Br J Surg. 2015;102(3):169–81.

28. Hidar S, Bibi M, Gharbi O, Tebra S, Trabelsi A, Korbi S, et al. Sentinel lymph node biopsy after neoadjuvant chemotherapy in inflammatory breast cancer. Int J Surg. 2009;7:272–5.
29. Lyman GH, Somerfield MR, Bosserman LD, Perkins CL, Weaver DL, Giuliano AE. Sentinel lymph node biopsy for patients with early-stage breast cancer: American Society of Clinical Oncology clinical practice guideline update. J Clin Oncol. 2017;35(5):561–4.
30. Veronesi U, Paganelli G, Viale G, Luini A, Zurrida S, Galimberti V, et al. Sentinel-lymph-node biopsy as a staging procedure in breast cancer: update of a randomised controlled study. Lancet Oncol. 2006;7:983–90.
31. Krag DN, Anderson SJ, Julian TB, Brown AM, Harlow SP, Ashikaga T, et al. Technical outcomes of sentinel lymph-node resection and conventional axillary-lymph-node dissection in patients with clinically node-negative breast cancer: results from the NSABP B-32 randomised phase III trial. Lancet Oncol. 2007;8:881–8.
32. Hunt KK, Ballman KV, McCall LM, Boughey JC, Mittendorf EA, Cox CE, et al. Factors associated with localregional recurrence after a negative sentinel node dissection: results of the ACOSOG Z0010 trial. Ann Surg. 2012;256:428–36.
33. Goldhirsch A, Wood WC, Coates AS, Gelber RD, Thürlimann B, Senn HJ, et al. Strategies for subtypes dealing with the diversity of breast cancer: highlights of the St. Gallen International Expert Consensus on the Primary Therapy of Early Breast Cancer 2011. Ann Oncol. 2011;22:1736–47.
34. Jung SY, Rosenzweig M, Sereika S, Linkov F, Brufsky A, Weissfeld JL. Factors associated with mortality after breast cancer metastasis. Cancer Causes Control. 2012;23:103–12.
35. Schneider JA, Divgi CR, Scott AM, Macapinlac HA, Seidman AD, Goldsmith SJ, et al. Flare on bone scintigraphy following Taxol chemotherapy for metastatic breast cancer. J Nucl Med. 1994;35:1748–52.
36. Coombes RC, Dady P, Parsons C, Rose C, Tubiana-Hulin M, Bastit P, et al. Assessment of response of bone metastases to systemic treatment in patients with breast cancer. Cancer. 1983;52:610–4.
37. Choi YJ, Shin YD, Kang YH, Lee MS, Lee MK, Cho BS, et al. The effects of preoperative ^{18}F-FDG PET/CT in breast cancer patients in comparison to the conventional imaging study. J Breast Cancer. 2012;15:441–8.
38. Groheux D, Giacchetti S, Moretti JL, Porcher R, Espié M, Lehmann-Che J, et al. Correlation of high ^{18}F-FDG uptake to clinical, pathological and biological prognostic factors in breast cancer. Eur J Nucl Med Mol Imaging. 2011;38:426–35.
39. Tchou J, Sonnad SS, Bergey MR, Basu S, Tomaszewski J, Alavi A, et al. Degree of tumor FDG uptake correlates with proliferation index in triple negative breast cancer. Mol Imaging Biol. 2010;12:657–62.
40. Jeong YJ, Kang DY, Yoon HJ, Son HJ. Additional value of F-18 FDG PET/CT for initial staging in breast cancer with clinically negative axillary nodes. Breast Cancer Res Treat. 2014;145:137–42.
41. Manohar K, Mittal BR, Bhoil A, Bhattacharya A, Singh G. Role of ^{18}F-FDG PET/CT in identifying distant metastatic disease missed by conventional imaging in patients with locally advanced breast cancer. Nucl Med Commun. 2013;34:557–61.
42. Seo MJ, Lee JJ, Kim HO, Chae SY, Park SH, Ryu JS, et al. Detection of internal mammary lymph node metastasis with (18)F-fluorodeoxyglucose positron emission tomography/computed tomography in patients with stage III breast cancer. Eur J Nucl Med Mol Imaging. 2014;41:438–45.
43. Fuster D, Duch J, Paredes P, Velasco M, Muñoz M, Santamaría G, et al. Preoperative staging of large primary breast cancer with [^{18}F]fluorodeoxyglucose positron emission tomography/computed tomography compared with conventional imaging procedures. J Clin. 2008;26:4746–51.
44. Groheux D, Giacchetti S, Espié M, Vercellino L, Hamy AS, Delord M, et al. The yield of ^{18}F-FDG PET/CT in patients with clinical stage IIA, IIB, or IIIA breast cancer: a prospective study. J Nucl Med. 2011;52:1526–34.
45. Segaert I, Mottaghy F, Ceyssens S, De Wever W, Stroobants S, Van Ongeval C, et al. Additional value of PET-CT in staging of clinical stage IIB and III breast cancer. Breast J. 2010;16:617–24.

46. Champion L, Lerebours F, Cherel P, Edeline V, Giraudet AL, Wartski M, et al. ^{18}F-FDG PET/CT imaging versus dynamic contrast-enhanced CT for staging and prognosis of inflammatory breast cancer. Eur J Nucl Med Mol Imaging. 2013;40:1206–13.
47. Joo Hyun O, Choi WH, Han EJ, Choi EK, Chae BJ, Park YG, et al. The prognostic value of (18)F-FDG PET/CT for early recurrence in operable breast cancer: comparison with TNM stage. Nucl Med Mol Imaging. 2013;47:263–7.
48. Aogi K, Kadoya T, Sugawara Y, Kiyoto S, Shigematsu H, Masumoto N, et al. Utility of (18)F FDG-PET/CT for predicting prognosis of luminal-type breast cancer. Breast Cancer Res Treat. 2015;150:209–17.
49. Kadoya T, Aogi K, Kiyoto S, Masumoto N, Sugawara Y, Okada M, et al. Role of maximum standardized uptake value in fluorodeoxyglucose positron emission tomography/computed tomography predicts malignancy grade and prognosis of operable breast cancer: a multi-institute study. Breast Cancer Res Treat. 2013;141:269–75.
50. García Vicente AM, Soriano Castrejón A, López-Fidalgo JF, Amo-Salas M, Muñoz Sanchez Mdel M, Álvarez Cabellos R, et al. Basal ^{18}F-FDG PET/CT as a prognostic biomarker in patients with locally advanced breast cancer. Eur J Nucl Med Mol Imaging. 2015;42:1804–13.
51. Song BI, Lee SW, Jeong SY, Chae YS, Lee WK, Ahn BC, et al. ^{18}F-FDG uptake by metastatic axillary lymph nodes on pretreatment PET/CT as a prognostic factor for recurrence in patients with invasive ductal breast cancer. J Nucl Med. 2012;53:1337–44.
52. Rousseau C, Devillers A, Sagan C, Ferrer L, Bridji B, Campion L, et al. Monitoring of early response to neoadjuvant chemotherapy in stage II and III breast cancer by [^{18}F]fluorodeoxyglucose positron emission tomography. J Clin Oncol. 2006;24:5366–72.
53. Schwarz-Dose J, Untch M, Tiling R, Sassen S, Mahner S, Kahlert S, et al. Monitoring primary systemic therapy of large and locally advanced breast cancer by using sequential positron emission tomography imaging with [^{18}F]fluorodeoxyglucose. J Clin Oncol. 2009;27:535–41.
54. Wang Y, Zhang C, Liu J, Huang G. Is ^{18}F-FDG PET accurate to predict neoadjuvant therapy response in breast cancer? A meta-analysis. Breast Cancer Res Treat. 2012;131:357–69.
55. Morris PG, Lynch C, Feeney JN, Patil S, Howard J, Larson SM, et al. Integrated positron emission tomography/computed tomography may render bone scintigraphy unnecessary to investigate suspected metastatic breast cancer. J Clin Oncol. 2010;28:3154–9.
56. Morris PG, Ulaner GA, Eaton A, Fazio M, Jhaveri K, Patil S, et al. Standardized uptake value by positron emission tomography/computed tomography as a prognostic variable in metastatic breast cancer. Cancer. 2012;118:5454–62.
57. Tateishi U, Gamez C, Dawood S, Yeung HW, Cristofanilli M, Macapinlac HA. Bone metastases in patients with metastatic breast cancer: morphologic and metabolic monitoring of response to systemic therapy with integrated PET/CT. Radiology. 2008;247:189–96.
58. Xiao Y, Wang L, Jiang X, She W, He L, Hu G. Diagnostic efficacy of ^{18}F-FDG-PET or PET/CT in breast cancer with suspected recurrence: a systematic review and meta-analysis. Nucl Med Commun. 2016;37(11):1180–8.
59. Schirrmeister H, Guhlmann A, Kotzerke J, Santjohanser C, Kühn T, Kreienberg R. Early detection and accurate description of extent of metastatic bone disease in breast cancer with fluoride ion and positron emission tomography. J Clin Oncol. 1999;17:2381–9.
60. Dittmann H, Jusufoska A, Dohmen BM, Smyczek-Gargya B, Fersis N, Pritzkow M, et al. 3′-deoxy-3′-[^{18}F]fluorothymidine (FLT) uptake in breast cancer cells as a measure of proliferation after doxorubicin and docetaxel treatment. Nucl Med Biol. 2009;36:163–9.
61. Pio BS, Park CK, Pietras R, Hsueh WA, Satyamurthy N, Pegram MD, et al. Usefulness of 3′-[F-18]fluoro-3′-deoxythymidine with positron emission tomography in predicting breast cancer response to therapy. Mol Imaging Biol. 2006;8:36–42.
62. Peterson LM, Mankoff DA, Lawton T, Yagle K, Schubert EK, Stekhova S, et al. Quantitative imaging of estrogen receptor expression in breast cancer with pet and ^{18}F-fluoroestradiol. J Nucl Med. 2008;49:367–74.
63. Kenny LM, Al-Nahhas A, Aboagye EO. Novel PET biomarkers for breast cancer imaging. Nucl Med Commun. 2011;32:333–5.

64. Linden HM, Stekhova SA, Link JM, Gralow JR, Livingston RB, Ellis GK, et al. Quantitative fluoroestradiol positron emission tomography imaging predicts response to endocrine treatment in breast cancer. J Clin Oncol. 2006;24:2793–9.
65. Melsaether AN, Raad RA, Pujara AC, Ponzo FD, Pysarenko KM, Jhaveri K, et al. Comparison of whole-body (18)F FDG PET/MR imaging and whole-body (18)F FDG PET/CT in terms of lesion detection and radiation dose in patients with breast cancer. Radiology. 2016;281(1):193–202.
66. Catalano OA, Nicolai E, Rosen BR, Luongo A, Catalano M, Iannace C, et al. Comparison of CE-FDG-PET/CT with CE-FDG-PET/MR in the evaluation of osseous metastases in breast cancer patients. Br J Cancer. 2015;112:1452–60.
67. Grueneisen J, Nagarajah J, Buchbender C, Hoffmann O, Schaarschmidt BM, Poeppel T, et al. Positron emission tomography/magnetic resonance imaging for local tumor staging in patients with primary breast cancer: a comparison with positron emission tomography/computed tomography and magnetic resonance imaging. Investig Radiol. 2015;50:505–13.
68. Heusner TA, Kuemmel S, Koeninger A, Hamami ME, Hahn S, Quinsten A, et al. Diagnostic value of diffusion-weighted magnetic resonance imaging (DWI) compared to FDG PET/CT for whole-body breast cancer staging. Eur J Nucl Med Mol Imaging. 2010;37:1077–86.

Part IV
Preoperative Systemic Therapy for Breast Cancer

Chapter 9
Preoperative Systemic Therapy for Operable Breast Cancer

Yesim Eralp

Introduction

A number of large-scale trials have established the role of neoadjuvant chemotherapy in operable and locally advanced breast cancer [1–4]. The common denominator in these studies is the significant association of complete pathologic response with not only breast conservation but also a prominent improvement in odds of survival ranging between 50% and 67% [5–8]. Consequently, the ultimate goal of induction treatment has been to improve pathologic complete response (pCR) rates with different combinations administered at variable schedules. The incorporation of taxanes has resulted in higher pCR rates ranging between 18% and 34%, with the range dependent on the biology of the tumor. Nevertheless, we have unfortunately reached a plateau in response rates, despite utilization of further strategies such as dose-dense regimens or the incorporation of newer agents such as capecitabine, vinorelbine or gemcitabine in combinations, even when used as part of a response-adopted approach [7–9]. Data from these trials and others have suggested that an early clinical response to treatment may also be used to predict a higher probability of pCR at surgery. The main objective of predefining a pCR is to select the best chemotherapy regimen for a given patient. This would also enable treating physicians to switch to better regimens early in the course of treatment and prevent unnecessary toxicity from an ineffective combination. In other words, by using a "patient-tailored" approach, it would be hypothetically possible to improve the chance of pCR, which may ultimately lead to an improvement in survival. Some clinicopathological variables, such as a lack of hormone receptors and a high grade, have already been shown to be associated with

Y. Eralp (✉)
Internal Medicine, Medical Oncology, Istanbul University, Institute of Oncology, Istanbul Medical Faculty, Department of Medical Oncology, Istanbul, Turkey

A. Aydiner et al. (eds.), *Breast Cancer*, https://doi.org/10.1007/978-3-319-96947-3_9

an improved response to neoadjuvant chemotherapy. Energetic efforts to identify molecular determinants or groups of genetic variables in specific patterns, namely, the "genetic signatures" of response, are in their early stages of development, and as of yet there is no reliable predictor of pCR.

The main advantage of preoperative systemic treatment is the incorporation of genomic analyses in the clinical setting, thereby enabling studies of the molecular predictors of response to a given treatment and providing insight into the biology of the tumor. In fact, to carry this approach one step further, recent neoadjuvant trials have focused on investigating the role of various biological agents in treating distinct biological subgroups before confirmation by larger-scale adjuvant trials.

Basic Considerations

Pathologic Complete Response

Randomized trials have provided substantial and consistent evidence of a positive correlation with pCR and outcome, as summarized in Table 9.1. Therefore, pCR has been universally accepted as the primary endpoint in nearly all neoadjuvant trials. However, the definition of pCR remains somewhat controversial, and there appears to be substantial heterogeneity in this definition across different trials, leading to difficulty in comparing outcomes. As summarized in Table 9.2, definitions range from no invasive disease in the breast only to no invasive or non-invasive tumor deposits in the breast and lymph nodes (ypT0N0). Most of these definitions have shown a significant association with disease-free survival (DFS) or overall survival (OS). In a meta-analysis of seven neoadjuvant German trials including data from 3332 patients, no invasive or non-invasive residuals in both the breast and lymph nodes was the most sensitive definition of pCR predicting a better outcome in terms of OS and DFS [21]. These data conflict with the most recent meta-analysis reporting individual patient data from 12 large randomized trials,

Table 9.1 Pathologic complete response classification systems and correlations with outcome

Author/group	pCR definition	Outcome correlation
Fisher/NSABP [8]	Breast: no invasive tumor	OS; DFS
Kuerer/MD Anderson CC [7]	Breast and lymph nodes: no invasive tumor	OS; DFS
Pierga/Institut Curie [10]	Breast and lymph nodes: no invasive tumor	OS; DFS
Van der Hage/EORTC [2]	Breast and lymph nodes: no malignant cells	OS
Ogston/Aberdeen [11]	Breast: no invasive tumor	OS; DFS
Von Minckwitz/GBCSG [12]	Breast and lymph nodes: no invasive or non-invasive tumor	OS; DFS

pCR pathologic complete response, *OS* overall survival, *DFS* disease-free survival

Table 9.2 Survival outcomes of neoadjuvant chemotherapy and pathologic complete response rates

Author	Regimen	pCR (%)	pCR site	P	DFS, EFS (%)	p	OS (%)	p
Aberdeen [13]	CVAP	16	B		77		84	
	CVAP-D	34		0.034	90 (3-yr DFS)	0.03	97 (3-yr OS)	0.05
AGO [6]	EP	10	BL		50		77	
	E-P	18		0.008	70 (5-yr DFS)	0.011	83 (5-yr OS)	0.04
SICOG [14]	EP q3 wk	6	BL		55		69	
	EPCis q wk	16		0.02	73 (5-yr DMFS)	0.04	82 (5-yr OS)	0.07
NOAH [15]	AP-P-CMF	19	BL		56		79	
	AP-P-CMF + Trastz	38		0.001	71 (3-yr EFS)	0.013	87 (3-yr OS)	NS
NSABP B-27 [5]	AC-surgery	13	BL		59		74	
	AC-surgery-D	14.5			62		75	
	AC-D-surgery	26		<0.001	62 (8-yr DFS)	NS	75 (8-yr OS)	NS
ACCOG [16]	AC	16	BL		NA		NA	
	AD	12		NS		NS		NS
MDA [17]	CAF	8	BL		89		NA	
	P	17		NS	94 (2-yr DFS)	NS		NS
Baldni [18]	CED	2.6	BL		48		52	
	dd CEF	4.1		NS	60 (5-yr DFS)	NS	54 (5-yr OS)	NS
TOPIC [19]	AC	25	BL		63		74	
	ECisF	24		NS	62 (5-yr RFS)	NS	82 (5-yr OS)	NS
TOPIC 2 [20]	AC	12	BL					
	VE	12		NS	HR: 1.18 (2-yr DFS)	NS	HR: 1.41 (2-yr OS)	NS

pCR pathologic response rate, *dd* dose-dense, *Cis* cisplatin, *AC* adriamycin-cyclophosphamide, *D* docetaxel, *EC* epirubicin-cyclophosphamide, *CEF* fluorouracil-epirubicin-cyclophosphamide, *ED* epirubicin-docetaxel, *CED* cyclophosphamide-epirubicin-docetaxel, *AP* adriamycin-paclitaxel, *D* docetaxel, *CVAP* cyclophosphamide-vincristine-adriamycin-prednisolone, *VE* vincristine-epirubicin, *wk* week, *B* breast, *BL* breast and lymph nodes, *yr* year, *OS* overall survival, *DFS* disease-free survival, *RFS* relapse-free survival, *DMFS* distant metastasis-free survival
$p < 0.05$ denotes statistically significant difference, *NS* not significant

which showed that the presence of in situ carcinoma in the breast does not influence the favorable effect of pCR on OS [hazard ratio (HR) ypT0ypN0 vs ypT0/isypN0 vs ypT0/is: 0.36, 0.36 vs 0.51, respectively]. According to this meta-analysis, the definition of pCR should be no invasive tumor in the breast and lymph nodes (ypT0/isypN0) [22].

Predictive Biomarkers

With the evolution of molecular and genetic testing in modern oncology, numerous multi-gene signatures with potential predictive and prognostic roles have been identified. However, correlative validation studies have shown that these classifiers not only are associated with substantially different outcomes but also display a wide variation in response to standard chemotherapy regimens. Nevertheless, trials evaluating the role of biomarkers have consistently concluded that tumors with a high proliferative capacity as assessed by a high Ki-67 level or grade, hormone receptor negativity or HER-2 positivity display a high probability of response and a higher chance of survival in those with a pCR. Although, molecular tests specifically developed to predict pCR have not demonstrated any predictive superiority over the combination of standard clinicopathological parameters (ER status, grade, and age), there are emerging data that some tests that have been compared with a survival endpoint may have a role in identifying patients who may or may not benefit from chemotherapy. A retrospective evaluation of gene expression profiling data from eight studies including 996 patients revealed that the addition of an immunogenic genomic module to clinical characteristics significantly increased the accuracy in predicting pCR in the HER-2 subgroup [12]. In the remaining intrinsic subgroups as assessed by the PAM50 assay, there were no specific genomic signatures that would identify patients who would benefit from standard neoadjuvant chemotherapy. I-SPY, a multi-center trial reported recently, prospectively evaluated the role of multigene classifiers as well as standard pathological biomarkers in 237 patients treated with neoadjuvant anthracycline and taxane-based chemotherapy [23]. This trial confirmed the general consensus that highly proliferative tumors respond better to chemotherapy as pCR rates were approximately 5–9% for luminal A tumors or those with a low Ki-67 level, as well as those with low-risk genomic profiles (ROR-S, wound healing signature, PAM-50, 70-gene classifier). By contrast, high-risk and HER-2-positive tumors showed pCR rates of 35% and 54%, respectively [23, 24]. In terms of outcome, patients with luminal or low-risk tumors had longer survival rates but lower pCR rates, as also reported in a meta-analysis of individual patient data across 12 large randomized neoadjuvant trials and the recently reported GEPARTRIO trial [22, 25]. As expected, for higher-risk patients, pCR improved the chances for a better outcome. In multivariate analysis, most molecular signatures and clinical stages improved the ability to predict RFS, suggesting that molecular classifiers can identify patients with a favorable prognostic profile among the non-pCR hormone receptor-positive subtypes. The wound-healing signature was the most accurate classifier in identifying lower-risk patients, consistent with previous studies suggesting that the tumor microenvironment and inflammatory response may have relevant roles in the pathogenesis of breast cancer.

Response-Guided Treatment

Accurate early-response assessment during chemotherapy is an important part of the neoadjuvant treatment strategy to identify patients who are unlikely to benefit from the given regimen. There are substantial data from randomized trials showing a strong correlation between achieving pCR and favorable long-term survival, as summarized previously in this chapter. As expected, a poor or minimal response usually suggests a poorer outcome. Numerous neoadjuvant trials have evaluated the role of early response to standard chemotherapy regimens in selecting subsequent non-cross-resistant agents. An earlier study by the MD Anderson group randomized patients with a larger than 1 cm^2 residual tumor burden following five cycles of anthracycline-based combination to either five more cycles of the same regimen or to 5 cycles of a different combination including vinblastine, methotrexate and fluorouracil [26]. Despite the limited sample size, there was a trend for survival advantage for patients treated with the alternative regimen ($p = 0.08$). Contradicting this data, the TAX 301 Aberdeen Trial showed no advantage in switching to docetaxel in patients who were unresponsive to four cycles of an anthracycline-based combination [13]. Nevertheless, there was a significant increase in the pCR rate (31% vs 15%) when responding patients received four more cycles of docetaxel, which translated into a survival advantage in these pathologically complete responding patients. The recently reported GEPARTRIO trial, which included 2090 patients who initially received two cycles of the docetaxel/doxorubicin/cyclophosphamide (TAC) regimen, randomized non-responding patients to six more cycles of the same regimen or to two cycles of TAC, followed by four cycles of the vinorelbine and capecitabine combination [27]. Although an earlier report failed to show an advantage in terms of pCR in the experimental group, an updated analysis suggested a significant survival advantage favoring response-guided treatment that was limited to patients in the luminal A and luminal B subgroups [25, 27]. The results of this study highlight the fact that in patients with hormone receptor-positive tumors, pCR may not be a good surrogate endpoint for survival because these patients receive the most effective regimen in the adjuvant setting. Despite accumulating data suggesting that neoadjuvant chemotherapy may be tailored according to the response early during the course of treatment, some questions remain to be resolved before adoption as a standard approach.

Chemotherapy Regimens

The significant survival advantage achieved by adjuvant chemotherapy demonstrated in earlier studies led to trials investigating the role of neoadjuvant chemotherapy toward the end of the last century. The potential benefit of systemic

Table 9.3 Earlier neoadjuvant studies comparing neoadjuvant versus adjuvant anthracycline-based regimens

Trial	n	Disease status	Regimen	pCR	Local recurrence	p	DFS	P	OS	p
NSABP B-18 [1]	1523	T1-3N0-1	4 AC-surgery	13%[a]	13%		58%		72%	
			Surgery-4 AC	NA	10%	NS	55%[b]	NS	72%[b]	NS
EORTC [2]	689	T1c-T4b N0-1	4 FEC-surgery	4%	10%		65%		82%	
			Surgery-4 FEC	NA	9%	NS	70%[c]	NS	84%[c]	NS
ECTO [4]	1355	T2-3N0-1	4 AT-4CMF-surgery	23%	4.6%		72%		84%	
			Surgery-4 AT-4CMF	NA	4.1%	NS	76%		85%	
			Surgery-4 A-4CMF	NA			69%[d]	NS	82%[d]	NS

pCR pathologic complete response, *DFS* disease-free survival, *OS* overall survival, *NA* not applicable, *NS* not significant, *AC* adriamycin-cyclophosphamide, *FEC* fluorouracil-epirubicin-cyclophosphamide, *AT* adriamycin-docetaxel, *CMF* cyclophosphamide-methotrexate-fluorouracil
[a]Ratio of patients with pathologically node-positive disease was significantly lower in the neoadjuvant group (59% vs 43%, $p < 0.001$)
[b]At 8 years
[c]At 4 years
[d]At 7 years

chemotherapy given as primary treatment had been initially reported by De Lena et al. [28], who showed a significant improvement in overall survival with neoadjuvant doxorubicin and vincristine combination administered before irradiation compared to radiation alone in locally advanced breast cancer. Pivotal trials investigating the role of PSC basically compared four to eight cycles of anthracycline-based regimens given as neoadjuvant versus adjuvant treatment in patients with operable clinical T1-3N0-1 disease [1, 2, 4]. None of these trials were able to show a difference in outcomes between these approaches, as summarized in Table 9.3.

One Step Higher to Improved Response Rates: Integration of Newer-Generation Agents

Taxanes

Encouraged by the favorable results achieved in the adjuvant setting, taxanes were swiftly incorporated in anthracycline-based combinations in the hope of improving response rates in the neoadjuvant setting. As anticipated, taxanes resulted in higher pathologic complete response rates compared to non-taxane regimens. The largest of these trials was NSABP B-27, which randomized 2411 patients with operable breast cancer to four cycles of AC alone, four cycles of AC followed by four cycles of docetaxel before surgery, or four cycles of neoadjuvant AC followed by surgery and four cycles of adjuvant docetaxel [3]. The significantly increased pCR rate (14% vs 26%, $p > 0.001$) compared to the standard referent regimen and manageable toxicity profile set AC followed by docetaxel as the state-of-the-art approach in the neoadjuvant setting. Nevertheless, despite a nearly twofold increase in the pCR rate, the B-27 trial failed to show a significant difference in overall survival, possibly related to the inadequate sample size, which lacked sufficient power to detect a small expected improvement of 3–5%, as seen in adjuvant taxane trials [5].

The favorable impact of taxanes on response rates is summarized in Table 9.4. Overall, these trials have shown that six to eight cycles of anthracycline and taxane-based combinations, either in sequence or given concomitantly, yield higher pathologic complete response rates compared to non-taxane-based regimens. In trials that have evaluated the role of dose-dense chemotherapy, the response rate was not demonstrated to be substantially higher compared to standard dose regimens. In fact, the PREPARE trial, which investigated the role of a dose-dense regimen incorporating anthracyclines, taxanes and alkylating agents, showed that despite the higher pCR rate (21% vs 14%), outcomes in terms of DFS (3 year 75.8 vs 78.8%) and OS (3 year 88.4 vs 91.8%) were not different [35]. Although there appears to be an incremental pCR benefit in the hormone

Table 9.4 Benefit of taxanes with respect to clinical and pathologic response rates

Trial	Regimen	cRR (%)	pCR (%)
Therasse [29]	ddEC × 6	27	14
	CEF × 6	31	10
Romieu [30]	AP × 4	20	17
	AP × 6	32	32[a]
Dieras [31]	AP × 4	89	16
	AC × 4	70	10
Steger [32]	ED × 3	–	7.7
	ED × 6	–	18.6[a]
Han [33]	ED × 6	82	24[a]
	ED × 4	72	11
Evans [16]	AD × 6	70	16
	AC × 6	61	12
Von Minckwitz [34]	ddAD × 4	75	7
	AC × 4-D × 4	85	14.3[a]
Bear [3]	AC × 4	85	13
	AC × 4-D × 4	91	26[a]
Smith [13]	CVAP × 8	64	15
	CVAP × 4-D × 4	85	31[a]
Von Minckwitz [27]	TAC × 6	48.2	21.0
	TAC × 8	52.9	23.5

cRR clinical response rate, *pCR* pathologic response rate, *dd* dose-dense, *AC* adriamycin-cyclophosphamide, *EC* epirubicin-cyclophosphamide, *CEF* fluorouracil-epirubicin-cyclophosphamide, *ED* epirubicin-docetaxel, *AP* adriamycin-paclitaxel, *D* docetaxel, *CVAP* cyclophosphamide-vincristine-adriamycin-prednisolone, *TAC* docetaxel-adriamycin-cyclophosphamide

[a]$p < 0.05$

receptor-negative subtype, considering the added toxicity, dose-dense or –intense regimens incorporating a standard weekly dose of paclitaxel or 3-weekly docetaxel should not be used outside of a clinical trial setting.

Capecitabine

The favorable response rates attained by capecitabine in the metastatic setting have led to studies evaluating the role of capecitabine in the neoadjuvant setting. The GEPARQUATTRO trial, which is the largest in sample size, randomized 1495 patients with T1-4N0-3M0 patients to single-agent docetaxel, sequential docetaxel and capecitabine or concomitant docetaxel and capecitabine following four cycles of epirubicin/cyclophosphamide (EC) [36]. The study failed to show a significant improvement in pCR rates, and there was a higher rate of serious non-hematological toxicity with the combination. Similarly, a phase III trial by the Austrian Breast and Colorectal Study Group (ABCSG-24) revealed no difference between a triplet combination of epirubicin, docetaxel and capecitabine and the doublet [37]. Furthermore, in the NSABP B-40 trial, investigators reported a 29.7% pCR rate for the combination of docetaxel and capecitabine, which was somewhat lower than that for single-agent docetaxel (32.7%) [38].

Despite discouraging data from single studies and a recent meta-analysis of pooled data [39], a meta-analysis including individual patient data of 966 patients from German neoadjuvant trials suggested a significantly increased rate of pCR with a hazard ratio of 1.62 by multivariate analysis ($p = 0.02$) [21].

Until further data from ongoing trials including triple-negative patients are reported, there appears to be no role for incorporating capecitabine in standard anthracycline- and taxane-based neoadjuvant chemotherapy regimens.

Gemcitabine

Gemcitabine has established activity when combined with paclitaxel in patients with advanced breast cancer. Preliminary data from the first randomized trial testing the role of this combination in the neoadjuvant setting failed to detect an advantage in terms of pCR compared to single-agent paclitaxel following four cycles of the EC regimen [40]. Similarly, the addition of gemcitabine to docetaxel yielded a lower pCR rate (31.8%) compared to docetaxel (32.7%) in the NSABP B-40 trial [38]. In conclusion, there exists no evidence supporting a role for adding gemcitabine in the neoadjuvant setting.

Vinorelbine

There are limited data on the role of vinorelbine in the neoadjuvant setting. In a considerably resistant patient population, a vinorelbine and capecitabine combination yielded a pCR rate of 6%, which was not different than that observed for the standard TAC combination [27]. In another phase III trial, the epirubicin-vinorelbine combination resulted in similar pCR (12%) and mastectomy rates as found for AC [20]. Based on these data, there seems to be no role for vinorelbine in the neoadjuvant setting.

Nano-Albumin-Bound Paclitaxel (nab-Pac)

Following approval of this agent for first-line treatment for those progressing within 6 months of adjuvant chemotherapy or second-line treatment of metastatic breast cancer, numerous phase II studies investigated the role of nab-Pac for earlier disease. However, almost all of these studies used this agent in combination with carboplatin and bevacizumab, which yielded encouraging response rates, especially in the triple-negative subgroup, of 53–59% [41–43].

A phase III study that evaluated the role of nab-Pac in the neoadjuvant setting was recently reported [44]. In the GEPARSEPTO trial, 1204 patients were randomized to two arms: standard paclitaxel weekly at 80 mg/m^2 for 12 weeks or nab-Pac weekly at 150 mg/m^2 for 12 weeks followed by four cycles of EC. Patients with Her-2-positive disease received pertuzumab and trastuzumab throughout the treatment period (n:400). Use of nab-paclitaxel resulted in a significant benefit in the whole patient group, with an absolute 9% incremental improvement in the pCR rate (pCR: 38% vs 29%, $p < 0.001$). A planned subgroup analysis showed a significantly improved pCR rate of 48.2% in the triple-negative subgroup (n:275 patients), with a hazard ratio of 2.69 ($p < 0.001$) and a trend for an improved 4-year DFS rate (78% vs 68%; HR:0.66; 95% CI: 0.42–1.04) [45]. Nevertheless, the 25.7% pCR rate of the standard arm in the triple-negative group is considerably lower than previously reported pCR rates for similar combinations, including 34.5% in the GEPARSIXTO trial and 41% in the CALGB 40603 trials [46, 47]. However, as a subgroup analysis, this result should be regarded with caution; based on the favorable outcome in the advanced setting, it would seem feasible to use this agent in the absence of effective targeted regimens. Nevertheless, it should be noted that further confirmatory data are required to establish the role of nab-Paclitaxel for triple-negative breast cancer.

Carboplatin

The role of carboplatin as neoadjuvant treatment was evaluated in the context of triple-negative and Her-2 positive breast cancer. In triple-negative disease, a small phase II trial [48] failed to show a benefit with carboplatin added to docetaxel compared to single-agent docetaxel following four cycles of a standard anthracycline-based combination, whereas two larger randomized trials [46, 47] yielded significantly higher pCR rates, with increments of 13–16% (Table 9.5). Notably, both of these trials also incorporated bevacizumab as part of the combination regimens. Furthermore, a subgroup analysis in the GEPARSIXTO trial revealed that the addition of carboplatin provided benefit, regardless of the germline BRCA mutation

Table 9.5 Platin-based neoadjuvant chemotherapy and pathologic complete response rates

Author	Regimen	n	pCR (%)	p	DFS (%)	p
Alba [48]	EC-D	46	30		NA	
	EC-DC	48	30	NS	NA	NA
Von Minckwitz [46]	LdP-Bev	157	37		76.1%	
	LdPC-Bev	158	53	0.005	85.8% (3-yr DFS)	0.03
Sikov [47, 49]	P-ddAC (±Bev)	218	41		71%	
	PC-ddAC (±Bev)	225	54	0.0029	76% (3-yr DFS)	NS

pCR pathologic response rate, *dd* dose-dense, *AC* adriamycin-cyclophosphamide, *EC* epirubicin-cyclophosphamide, *D* docetaxel, *C* carboplatin, *Ld* liposomal doxorubicin, *P* paclitaxel, *Bev* bevacizumab, *yr* year, *DFS* disease-free survival, *NS* not significant, *NA* not applicable. The difference with $p < 0.05$ is significant.

status [Odds Ratio (OR): 2.09 for wild-type patients; $p = 0.005$ vs OR: 1.6 for germline carriers; $p = 0.41$] [50]. In the triple-negative subgroup of the recently reported German Adapt trial, which incorporates a risk-adapted neoadjuvant strategy, 4 cycles of a nab-pac and carboplatin combination yielded a significantly improved pCR rate compared to four cycles of nab-pac and gemcitabine (45.9% vs 28.7%, $p < 0.001$) [51]. Although germline BRCA status has not been consistently linked with response to platin-based chemotherapy, there is clinical evidence suggesting that somatic mutations in the BRCA gene or the homologous repair pathway (HRD) may be potentially associated with platin responsiveness. A validation study from a pooled analysis of three neoadjuvant studies including triple-negative patients demonstrated that tumors with a high HRD score were more likely to achieve pCR (53% vs 18%) with a hazard ratio of 4.64 ($p < 0.0001$) irrespective of BRCA status [52]. In light of the data showing significantly improved response rates, it would be reasonable to use platin-based regimens in triple-negative patients, who otherwise lack effective treatment options. The future of triple-negative disease holds promise as results from trials incorporating biomarker-driven strategies, including PARP inhibitors and PD-1 inhibitor-based combinations, are awaited with enthusiasm.

In Her-2-positive disease, the role of carboplatin as part of a non-anthracycline-based regimen combined with dual blockade (TCH-Lapatinib and TCH-Pertuzumab) was investigated in two phase II trials, which each yielded pCR rates of 52% [53, 54]. Following encouraging response rates, especially in hormone receptor-negative patients, the TCHP regimen was further evaluated in two phase III trials. In the TRAIN-II trial, 27 weeks of this combination was compared to a standard anthracycline- and taxane-based combination with a similar total duration. Overall, the pCR rates were similar in both arms (68% vs 67%, NS), including in hormone receptor (HR)-positive patients (55 vs 51%; NS). Nevertheless, the numerically higher pCR rate in HR-negative patients (84% vs 89%; NS) led to concerns regarding omission of anthracyclines in this subset [55]. Furthermore, in the phase III KRISTINE trial, the standard TCHP arm yielded a 56% pCR rate, in concordance with previous results utilizing the same regimen and confirming the efficacy of this combination [56]. When we put these data in context, non-anthracycline-based combinations incorporating carboplatin with taxanes, in addition to pertuzumab-based dual Her-2 blockade, have shown favorable pCR rates and should be considered in all patients who are eligible for neoadjuvant treatment, especially in those with cardiac comorbidities. In

HR-negative patients, who are considered to harbor high-risk disease, omission of anthracyclines remains a matter of debate, and the decision should be individualized. The role of dual Her-2 blockade within the context of neoadjuvant treatment is further discussed in detail below.

Biological Agents

Her-2-Targeting Agents

Trastuzumab

Trastuzumab-based combinations have opened a new era for the treatment of early- and advanced-stage Her-2-positive breast cancer. One of the earlier studies in the neoadjuvant setting was a small randomized pilot trial in operable patients that showed a pCR of 65.2% [57]. This unprecedented pCR rate has been confirmed by subsequent larger randomized trials that evaluated the role of trastuzumab as part of standard anthracycline- and taxane-based regimens. One of these, the NOAH trial, had a unique design that allowed the concomitant use of anthracycline and trastuzumab. In that trial, the combination regimen yielded a pCR rate of 38% and a 5-year EFS of 71% in the HER-2-positive patient subset, significantly higher than pCR rate of 19% ($p = 0.001$) and EFS rate of 56% ($p = 0.013$) in the control arm. The updated data after a median follow-up period of 5.4 years showed a significant advantage in terms of overall survival, with a hazard ratio of 0.66 ($p = 0.05$) [15]. In terms of cardiac toxicity, there were no differences with respect to grade 3 and 4 cardiac events; only 2 patients (2%) developed a transient grade 3 left ventricular dysfunction in the trastuzumab arm. In the GEPARQUATTRO trial, which was originally designed to test the efficacy of capecitabine in the neoadjuvant setting, trastuzumab was allowed as part of treatment in the HER-2-positive subgroup. The pCR rate, including residual ductal carcinoma in situ (DCIS), was reported as 48.9% among 340 HER-2-positive patients. In patients who were unresponsive to four cycles of EC, the pCR rate in HER2-positive group was five times that in the HER2-negative cohort (16.7% vs 3.3%), again confirming the role of trastuzumab even in patients with anthracycline-resistant disease [58].

Second-Generation Anti-Her-2 Agents and Dual Blockade

Lapatinib

Lapatinib, a dual EGFR tyrosine kinase inhibitor, has already been established as an active agent in the metastatic setting. In the GEPARQUINTO trial, lapatinib (L) was tested head-to-head with trastuzumab (H) as part of a standard regimen consisting of four cycles of EC followed by 4 cycles of docetaxel (T). Of 620 eligible patients, 30.3% in the ECH-TH group achieved pCR, a significant increase compared to the

ECL-TL arm (22.7%) (p = 0.04) [59]. The Neo-Altto trial evaluated the role of lapatinib either as a single agent or in combination with trastuzumab compared to trastuzumab for 6 weeks followed by 12 weeks of weekly paclitaxel added to the three randomized arms before surgery. Despite an amendment for dose reduction in the lapatinib arms due to increased grade 3 and 4 diarrhea and hepatic toxicity, there was a higher pCR rate with dual blockade (51.3%) compared to-single agent trastuzumab (29.5%) or lapatinib (24.7%) (p = 0.0001) [60]. Nevertheless, a subsequent study by the CALGB with a similar design that was reported recently showed no advantage of dual targeted therapy in terms of pCR (56% vs 46%) [61]. The NSABP B41 trial, which differed slightly from the others in design, was a phase III trial that investigated the role of dual blockade following four cycles of an anthracycline-based combination followed by surgery. In this trial, the pCR rate in the combination arm was 60%, which was marginally significant compared to the unexpectedly high pCR rate for the trastuzumab and chemotherapy combination (52.5%; p = 0.056) [62]. Although the pCR rate in hormone receptor-negative patients was numerically higher than that in endocrine-responsive patients, the difference was not significant. The high rate of non-cardiac adverse effects favored trastuzumab as the single agent of choice. Given these data, there is as yet no evidence supporting the role of lapatinib as a single agent or in the context of dual Her-2 blockade.

Pertuzumab

Pertuzumab is a monoclonal antibody that inhibits ligand-dependent signaling between HER-2 and HER-3 receptors and thus has a complementary effect with trastuzumab. With encouraging data in metastatic patients as both a first-line and subsequent treatment option, pertuzumab was also evaluated in the neoadjuvant setting. Initially, feasibility and potential cardiotoxicity were evaluated in the phase II TRYPHENA trial, which incorporated dual blockade with pertuzumab and trastuzumab in combination with a standard anthracycline-based and taxane-based regimen, as well as a non-anthracycline-based TCH combination and FEC followed by docetaxel, trastuzumab and pertuzumab. This trial confirmed the cardiac safety of dual blockade. In addition, the high pCR rate reaching 66% supported the efficacy of non-anthracycline combinations in Her-2-positive disease [54].

In the NEO-SPHERE trial, women with operable or locally advanced or inflammatory breast cancer were randomized to receive four cycles every 3 weeks of docetaxel, trastuzumab; or docetaxel, trastuzumab and pertuzumab; the doublet of the two monoclonal antibodies; or docetaxel and pertuzumab [63]. Following surgery, patients in the docetaxel-containing arms received adjuvant FEC for three cycles and trastuzumab every 3 weeks for 1 year. The remaining patients received four cycles of docetaxel followed by three cycles of FEC with trastuzumab in the adjuvant setting. The in-breast pCR rate for pertuzumab added to the conventional trastuzumab and docetaxel combination was 46.8%, which was significantly higher than the pCR rates of 24% for the pertuzumab and docetaxel doublet and 29% for the trastuzumab and docetaxel combination. Furthermore, there was a small subset of patients (16.8%) that achieved pCR with the double-antibody regimen, raising a hypothetical question of whether there is really a group of patients who do not require any chemotherapy at all [63]. There was some concern regarding toxicity because the triplet combination resulted in more neutropenia and febrile neutropenia, and there was one treatment-related death with fulminant hepatitis. Based on the significantly higher pCR rate for the combination, pertuzumab received FDA approval in 2013 for the neoadjuvant treatment of Her-2-amplified breast cancer. An updated survival analysis showed numerically higher 5-year progression-free survival in the dual-blockade group compared with the standard arm of trastuzumab and docetaxel (86 vs 81%). Although the confidence intervals are large and overlapping, these results suggest a higher efficacy of the pertuzumab, trastuzumab and chemotherapy combination [64]. In light of accumulating data, further studies are needed to identify predictive markers that would help accurately define patients who would benefit from combined treatment strategies. Despite a lack of profound survival benefit with dual blockade, it seems feasible to utilize pertuzumab and trastuzumab combination in the neoadjuvant setting, based on evidence showing improved outcomes with increased pCR rates.

TDM-1

Trastuzumab emtansine is a new-generation conjugated monoclonal antibody bound with a tubulin inhibitor (maytansine). Based on successful results in trastuzumab-resistant disease as a second-line treatment in the advanced setting, TDM-1 was steadily incorporated in neoadjuvant trials. In the I-SPY trial, which followed an adapted strategy, patients harboring one of the three predictive signatures were more likely to achieve pCR with the TDM-1 and pertuzumab combination than in the standard trastuzumab paclitaxel arm [65]. The KRISTINE trial was a phase III trial comparing 6 cycles of the TCHP regimen to a non-chemotherapy doublet of the TDM-1 and pertuzumab combination. This trial yielded a lower pCR rate with the investigational regimen compared to the platin-based combination (44 vs 56%) [56], in line with the recently reported Marianne trial, which showed a lack of benefit of the TDM-1 and pertuzumab regimen in the first-line advanced setting [66].

The data on dual blockade in Her-2-positive disease are summarized in Table 9.6.

Anti-Angiogenic Agents

Bevacizumab

Bevacizumab, a monoclonal antibody targeting VEGF, has unfortunately been withdrawn by the FDA for indication as a treatment option for metastatic breast cancer patients in light of recent data that failed to show a significant overall survival advantage despite favorable DFS rates. In the neoadjuvant setting, two trials

Table 9.6 Dual Her-2 blockade as neoadjuvant chemotherapy and pathologic complete response rates with respect to hormone receptor status

Trial	Phase	n	Regimen	pCR (whole population)	pCR (HR positive)	pCR (HR negative)
Lapatinib						
NeoAltto [60]	III	455	TL (6 wk)-TL/Pac (12 wk)	47%[a]	42%[a]	61%[a]
			T (6 wk)-T/Pac (12 wk)	27%	22%	37%
			L (6 wk-L/Pac (12 wk)	20%	16%	34%
CALGB 40601 [61]	III	305	TL/Pac (16 wk)	56%	41%	79%[a]
			T/Pac	46%	41%	54%
			L/Pac	32%	29%	37%
NSABP B-41 [62]	III	529	ACx4-TL/Pac (16 wk)	60%	55%	70%
			ACx4-T/Pac (16 wk)	49%	46%	58%
			ACx4-L/Pac (16 wk)	47%	42%	55%
TRIO-US B07 [53]	II	128	LT (3 wk)-DCTL (18 wk)	52%	40%	67%
CHERLOB [67]	II	121	TL/Pac (12 wk)-FEC × 4	47%[a]	29%	41%
			T/Pac (12 wk)-FEC × 4	25%	–	–
			L/Pac (12 wk)-FEC × 4	26%	–	–
Pertuzumab						
NEOSPHERE [63]	II	417	DTP (12 wk)	39%[a]	26%	63%
			DT	23%	20%	37%
			DP	18%	17%	30%
			TP	11%	6%	29%
TRYPHENA [54]	II	225	FEC/TP (9 wk)-DTP (9 wk)	52%	–	–
			FEC (9 wk)-DTP (9 wk)	45%	–	–
			DCTP (18 wk)	52%	–	–
KRISTINE [56]	III	432	DCTP (18 wk)	56%[a]	45%	73%
			TDM-1/P (18 wk)	44%	38%	54%
NSABP B-7 [68]	II	126	Neratinib/PT (16 wk)-AC × 4	50%	30%	74%

Table 9.6 (continued)

Trial	Phase	n	Regimen	pCR (whole population)	pCR (HR positive)	pCR (HR negative)
ISPY 2 [65]	II	46/52	TP/Pac (12 wk)-AC × 4	54%	44%	74%
			TDM-1/P (12 wk)-AC × 4	52%	46%	64%
TRAIN-II [55]	III	438	FEC/TP (9 wk)-TP/Pac (18 wk)	67%	51%	89%
			TP/Pac (27 wk)	68%	55%	84%

pCR pathologic response rate, *HR* hormone receptor, *AC* adriamycin-cyclophosphamide, *FEC* fluorouracil-epirubicin-cyclophosphamide, *Pac* paclitaxel, *D* docetaxel, *C* carboplatin, *L* lapatinib, *P* pertuzumab, *T* trastuzumab, *wk* week
[a]$p < 0.05$ (vs standard arm)

evaluated the role of this antibody in combination with various cytotoxic regimens. In a subset of the GEPARQUINTO trial, HER-2-negative patients were randomized to four cycles of EC with bevacizumab and continued to four cycles of docetaxel plus bevacizumab if responsive to EC and to chemotherapy-only arms. This trial failed to show a benefit in terms of pCR of the addition of bevacizumab in the general population (17.5% vs 15%), with a subgroup benefit in the receptor-negative subset [69]. To evaluate the role of capecitabine and gemcitabine, a subsequent study by the NSABP Group (NSABP B-40) randomized 1206 patients to docetaxel followed by four cycles of AC and a second randomization with or without bevacizumab. In this trial, the addition of bevacizumab significantly increased the pCR rate, which was the primary endpoint, from 28.2% to 34.5% ($p = 0.02$), with greater benefit observed in the hormone receptor-positive subset [38]. Recently, an overall survival advantage was also reported that was most evident in this subgroup [70]. Nevertheless, it is not clear if the benefit observed in this trial is due to a compensatory effect in the context of a lower dose of docetaxel in the two thirds of patients who received the antibodies. In the CALGB 40603 trial, which included triple-negative patients, addition of bevacizumab resulted in an 8% incremental benefit over the 44% pCR rate achieved with the platin-based combination ($p = 0.057$). However, bevacizumab was associated with an increased incidence of grade 3 hypertension, febrile neutropenia, bleeding and thromboembolic complications [47]. In the updated survival analysis, use of bevacizumab failed to result in a significant improvement in EFS or OS [49]. In conclusion, considering the conflicting evidence regarding the efficacy of bevacizumab within distinct molecular subgroups and the lack of a valid predictive marker, bevacizumab cannot be considered standard in the neoadjuvant setting at this time.

M-TOR Inhibitors

Everolimus

Mammalian target of rapamycin (m-TOR) is a valid target that is frequently disrupted in breast cancer pathogenesis. The accumulation of favorable data in combination with hormonal and cytotoxic agents led to the randomized GEPARQUINTO trial, which evaluated the role of everolimus in combination with paclitaxel as a second randomization in patients who were resistant to neoadjuvant EC with or without bevacizumab. The trial was stopped prematurely after 395 patients were randomized due to completion of the main trial. In terms of pCR, there was no difference between study arms (3.6% vs 5.6%). Almost half of the patient group had to stop treatment due to side effects in the combination arm, and there were concerns about whether everolimus attenuated the cytotoxic effects of paclitaxel with inhibition of cell cycle progression. In addition, there was no indication of any subgroup that might benefit from the addition of everolimus to paclitaxel in this resistant group of patients [71].

Conclusion

Neoadjuvant chemotherapy offers an ideal setting to identify regimens or agents that could be prioritized for adjuvant confirmatory trials and to identify biomarkers or genomic signatures that would predict response or resistance to a given regimen. Numerous trials performed over the last three or four decades have provided valuable information on the biology of breast cancer, as well as efficacy data that helped to improve treatment strategies in earlier stages. There exists substantial evidence from meta-analyses suggesting that pCR is an important surrogate endpoint for outcome in most subgroups, and it is now argued that costly, time-consuming large trials may be spared for agents showing a high pCR rate with survival advantage in the neoadjuvant setting. With the advent of molecular diagnostic techniques and translational medicine, the last decade has proved to be an exciting era for oncology research. Nevertheless, the more we examine the basic mechanisms of oncogenesis, the deeper in the abyss of the cancer enigma we find ourselves. There appears to be much more to be accomplished than ever to develop better treatment options for patients with breast cancer.

In conclusion, preoperative systemic chemotherapy is a valuable research tool for identifying predictive molecular biomarkers and a valid treatment option for patients with early-stage breast cancer. However, the decision to treat a patient with neoadjuvant chemotherapy requires careful clinical judgment and multidisciplinary evaluation by an experienced team.

References

1. Wolmark N, Wang J, Mamounas E, Bryant J, Fisher B. Preoperative chemotherapy in patients with operable breast cancer: nine-year results from National Surgical Adjuvant Breast and Bowel Project B-18. J Natl Cancer Inst Monogr. 2001;30:96–102.
2. van der Hage JA, van de Velde CJ, Julien JP, Tubiana-Hulin M, Vandervelden C, Duchateau L, et al. Preoperative chemotherapy in primary operable breast cancer: results from the European Organization for Research and Treatment of Cancer trial 10902. J Clin Oncol. 2001;19:4224–37.
3. Bear HD, Anderson S, Smith RE, Geyer CE Jr, Mamounas EP, Fisher B, et al. Sequential preoperative or postoperative docetaxel added to preoperative doxorubicin plus cyclophosphamide for operable breast cancer National Surgical Adjuvant Breast and Bowel Project Protocol B-27. J Clin Oncol. 2006;24:2019–27.
4. Gianni L, Baselga J, Eiermann W, Porta VG, Semiglazov V, Lluch A, et al. Phase III trial evaluating the addition of paclitaxel to doxorubicin followed by cyclophosphamide, methotrexate, and fluorouracil, as adjuvant or primary systemic therapy: European Cooperative Trial in Operable Breast Cancer. J Clin Oncol. 2009;27:2474–81.
5. Rastogi P, Anderson SJ, Bear HD, Geyer CE, Kahlenberg MS, Robidoux A, et al. Preoperative chemotherapy: updates of National Surgical Adjuvant Breast and Bowel Project Protocols B-18 and B-27. J Clin Oncol. 2008;26:778–85.
6. Untch M, Mobus V, Kuhn W, Muck BR, Thomssen C, Bauerfeind I, et al. Intensive dose-dense compared with conventionally scheduled preoperative chemotherapy for high-risk primary breast cancer. J Clin Oncol. 2009;27:2938–45.
7. Kuerer HM, Newman LA, Smith TL, Ames FC, Hunt KK, Dhingra K, et al. Clinical course of breast cancer patients with complete pathologic primary tumor and axillary lymph node response to doxorubicin-based neoadjuvant chemotherapy. J Clin Oncol. 1999;17:460–9.
8. Fisher B, Bryant J, Wolmark N, Mamounas E, Brown A, Fisher ER, et al. Effect of preoperative chemotherapy on the outcome of women with operable breast cancer. J Clin Oncol. 1998;16:2672–85.
9. Ring AE, Smith IE, Ashley S, Fulford LG, Lakhani SR. Oestrogen receptor status, pathological complete response and prognosis in patients receiving neoadjuvant chemotherapy for early breast cancer. Br J Cancer. 2004;91(12):2012–7.
10. Pierga JY, Mouret E, Diéras V, Laurence V, Beuzeboc P, Dorval T, et al. Prognostic value of persistent node involvement after neoadjuvant chemotherapy in patients with operable breast cancer. Br J Cancer. 2000;83(11):1480–7.
11. Ogston KN, Miller ID, Payne S, Hutcheon AW, Sarkar TK, Smith I, et al. A new histological grading system to assess response of breast cancers to primary chemotherapy: prognostic significance and survival. Breast. 2003;12(5):320–7.
12. von Minckwitz G, Untch M, Blohmer JU, Costa SD, Eidtmann H, Fasching PA, et al. Definition and impact of pathologic complete response on prognosis after neoadjuvant chemotherapy in various intrinsic breast cancer subtypes. J Clin Oncol. 2012;30(15):1796–804.
13. Smith IC, Heys SD, Hutcheon AW, Miller ID, Payne S, Gilbert FJ, et al. Neoadjuvant chemotherapy in breast cancer: significantly enhanced response with docetaxel. J Clin Oncol. 2002;20(6):1456–66.
14. Frasci G, D'Aiuto G, Comella P, D'Aiuto M, Di Bonito M, Ruffolo P, et al. Preoperative weekly cisplatin, epirubicin, and paclitaxel (PET) improves prognosis in locally advanced breast cancer patients: an update of the southern Italy Cooperative Oncology Group (SICOG) randomised trial 9908. Ann Oncol. 2010;21:707–16.
15. Gianni L, Eiermann W, Semiglazov V, Lluch A, Tjulandin S, Zambetti M, et al. Neoadjuvant chemotherapy with trastuzumab followed by adjuvant trastuzumab versus neoadjuvant chemotherapy alone, in patients with HER2-positive locally advanced breast cancer (the NOAH

trial): follow-up of a randomised controlled superiority trial with a parallel HER2-negative cohort. Lancet Oncol. 2014;15:640–7.
16. Evans TR, Yellowlees A, Foster E, Earl H, Cameron DA, Hutcheon AW, et al. Phase III randomized trial of doxorubicin and docetaxel versus doxorubicin and cyclophosphamide as primary medical therapy in women with breast cancer: an anglo-celtic cooperative oncology group study. J Clin Oncol. 2005;23(13):2988–95.
17. Buzdar AU, Singletary SE, Theriault RL, Booser DJ, Valero V, Ibrahim N, et al. Prospective evaluation of paclitaxel versus combination chemotherapy with fluorouracil, doxorubicin, and cyclophosphamide as neoadjuvant therapy in patients with operable breast cancer. J Clin Oncol. 1999;17:3412–7.
18. Baldini E, Gardin G, Giannessi PG, Evangelista G, Roncella M, Prochilo T, et al. Accelerated versus standard cyclophosphamide, epirubicin and 5-fluorouracil or cyclophosphamide, methotrexate and 5-fluorouracil: a randomized phase III trial in locally advanced breast cancer. Ann Oncol. 2003;14:227–32.
19. Smith IE, A'Hern RP, Coombes GA, Howell A, Ebbs SR, Hickish TF, TOPIC Trial Group, et al. A novel continuous infusional 5-fluorouracil-based chemotherapy regimen compared with conventional chemotherapy in the neoadjuvant treatment of early breast cancer: 5 year results of the TOPIC trial. Ann Oncol. 2004;15:751–8.
20. Chua S, Smith IE, A'Hern RP, Coombes GA, Hickish TF, Robinson AC, TOPIC Trial Group, et al. Neoadjuvant vinorelbine/epirubicin (VE) versus standard adriamycin/cyclophosphamide (AC) in operable breast cancer: analysis of response and tolerability in a randomised phase III trial (TOPIC 2). Ann Oncol. 2005;16:1435–41.
21. von Minckwitz G, Untch M, Nüesch E, Loibl S, Kaufmann M, Kümmel S, et al. Impact of treatment characteristics on response of different breast cancer phenotypes: pooled analysis of the German neo-adjuvant chemotherapy trials. Breast Cancer Res Treat. 2011;125(1):145–56.
22. Cortazar P, Zhang L, Untch M, Mehta K, Costantino JP, Wolmark N, et al. P athological complete response and long-term clinical benefit in breast cancer: the CTNeoBC pooled analysis. Lancet. 2014;384(9938):164–72.
23. Esserman LJ, Berry DA, Cheang MC, I-SPY 1 TRIAL Investigators, et al. Chemotherapy response and recurrence-free survival in neoadjuvant breast cancer depends on biomarker profiles: results from the I-SPY 1 TRIAL (CALGB 150007/150012; ACRIN 6657). Breast Cancer Res Treat. 2012;132(3):1049–62.
24. Esserman LJ, Berry DA, DeMichele A, Yau C, Perou CM, Carey L, et al. Pathologic complete response predicts recurrence-free survival more effectively by cancer subset: results from the I-SPY 1 TRIAL-CALGB 150007/150012, ACRIN 6657. J Clin Oncol. 2012;30(26):3242–9.
25. von Minckwitz G, Blohmer JU, Costa S, Denkert C, Eidtmann H, Eiermann W, et al. Response guided neoadjuvant chemotherapy for breast cancer—results of the GeparTrio trial. J Clin Oncol. 2013;31:3623–30.
26. Thomas E, Holmes FA, Smith TL, Buzdar AU, Frye DK, Fraschini G, et al. The use of alternate, non-cross-resistant adjuvant chemotherapy on the basis of pathologic response to a neoadjuvant doxorubicin-based regimen in women with operable breast cancer: long-term results from a prospective randomized trial. J Clin Oncol. 2004;22(12):2294–302.
27. von Minckwitz G, Kümmel S, Vogel P, Hanusch C, Eidtmann H, Hilfrich J, German Breast Group, et al. Neoadjuvant vinorelbine-capecitabine versus docetaxel-doxorubicin-cyclophosphamide in early nonresponsive breast cancer: phase III randomized GeparTrio trial. J Natl Cancer Inst. 2008;100(8):542–51.
28. De Lena M, Zucali R, Viganotti G, Valagussa P, Bonadonna G. Combined chemotherapy-radiotherapy approach in locally advanced (T3b–T4) breast cancer. Cancer Chemother Pharmacol. 1978;1:53–9.
29. Therasse P, Mauriac L, Welnicka-Jaskiewicz M, Bruning P, Cufer T, Bonnefoi H, EORTC, et al. Final results of a randomized phase III trial comparing cyclophosphamide, epirubicin, and fluorouracil with a dose-intensified epirubicin and cyclophosphamide + filgrastim as neoadjuvant treatment in locally advanced breast cancer: an EORTC-NCIC-SAKK multicenter study. J Clin Oncol. 2003;21(5):843–50.

30. Romieu G, Tubiana-Hulin M, Fumoleau P, Namer M, Delva R, et al. A multicenter randomized phase II study of 4 or6 cycles of adriamycin/Taxol (paclitaxel) (AT) as neoadjuvant treatment of breast cancer (BC). Ann Oncol. 2002;13(Suppl 5):33–9.
31. Diéras V, Fumoleau P, Romieu G, Tubiana-Hulin M, Namer M, Mauriac L, et al. Randomized parallel study of doxorubicin plus paclitaxel and doxorubicin plus cyclophosphamide as neoadjuvant treatment of patients with breast cancer. J Clin Oncol. 2004;22(24):4958–65.
32. Steger GG, Kubista E, Hausmaninger H, Gnant M, Tausch C, Lang A, et al. 6 vs. 3 cycles of epirubicin/docetaxel + G-CSF in operable breast cancer: results of ABCSG-14. J Clin Oncol. 2004;22(Suppl 14S):A553.
33. Han S, Kim J, Lee J, Chang E, Gwak G, Cho H, et al. Comparison of 6 cycles versus 4 cycles of neoadjuvant epirubicin plus docetaxel chemotherapy in stages II and III breast cancer. Eur J Surg Oncol. 2009;35(6):583–7.
34. von Minckwitz G, Raab G, Caputo A, Schütte M, Hilfrich J, Blohmer JU, et al. Doxorubicin with cyclophosphamide followed by docetaxel every 21 days compared with doxorubicin and docetaxel every 14 days as preoperative treatment in operable breast cancer: the GEPARDUO study of the German Breast Group. J Clin Oncol. 2005;23:2676–85.
35. Untch M, von Minckwitz G, Konecny GE, Conrad U, Fett W, Kurzeder C, Arbeitsgemeinschaft Gynäkologische Onkologie PREPARE Investigators, et al. PREPARE trial: a randomized phase III trial comparing preoperative, dose-dense, dose-intensified chemotherapy with epirubicin, paclitaxel, and CMF versus a standard-dosed epirubicin-cyclophosphamide followed by paclitaxel with or without darbepoetin alfa in primary breast cancer--outcome on prognosis. Ann Oncol. 2011;22(9):1999–2006.
36. von Minckwitz G, Rezai M, Loibl S, Fasching PA, Huober J, Tesch H, et al. Capecitabine in addition to anthracycline- and taxane-based neoadjuvant treatment in patients with primary breast cancer: phase III GeparQuattro study. J Clin Oncol. 2010;28(12):2015–23.
37. Steger GG, Greil R, Jakesz R, Lang A, Mineritsch B, Melbinger-Zeinitzer E, et al. Final results of ABCSG-24, a randomized phase III study comparing epirubicin, docetaxel, and capecitabine (EDC) to epirubicin and docetaxel (ED) as neoadjuvant treatment for early breast cancer and comparing ED/EDC + trastuzumab (T) to ED/EDC as neoadjuvant treatment for early HER-2 positive breast cancer. Cancer Res. 2009;69(24 Suppl):564s. abstract 1081.
38. Bear HD, Tang G, Rastogi P, Geyer CE Jr, Robidoux A, Atkins JN, et al. Bevacizumab added to neoadjuvant chemotherapy for breast cancer. N Engl J Med. 2012;366(4):310–20.
39. Li Q, Jiang Y, Wei W, Yang H, Liu J. Clinical efficacy of including Capecitabine in Neoadjuvant chemotherapy for breast cancer: a systematic review and meta-analysis of randomized controlled trials. PLoS One. 2013;8(1):e53403.
40. Earl HM, Vallier A, Hiller L, Fenwick N, Young J, Iddawela M, et al. Effects of the addition of gemcitabine and paclitaxel-first sequencing in neoadjuvant sequential epirubicin, cyclophosphamide and paclitaxel for women with high-risk early breast cancer (Neo-tAnGo): an open-label 2 × 2 factorial randomized phase III trial. Lancet. 2014;15(2):201–12.
41. Snider JN, Schwartzberg L, Young RR, Yunus F, Allen JW, Verrier C, et al. Pathologic complete response with weekly nanoparticle albumin bound paclitaxel plus carboplatin followed by doxorubicin plus cyclophosphamide with concurrent bevacizumab for triple negative breast cancer. J Clin Oncol. 2013;31:1068.
42. Mrozek E, Lustber MB, Knopp MV, Spigos DG, Yang X, Houton LA, et al. Phase II trial of neoadjuvant chemotherapy with weekly nanoparticle albumin bound paclitaxel, carboplatin and bevacizumab in women with clinical stages II-III breast cancer: pathologic response prediction by changes in angiogenic volüme by dynamic contrast enhanced magnetic resonance imaging. J Clin Oncol. 2010;28:604.
43. Sinclair NF, Abu-Khalaf MM, Rizack T, Rosati K, Chung G, Legare RD, et al. Neoadjuvant weekly nanoparticle albumin bound paclitaxel, carboplatin plus bevacizumab with or without dose-dense doxorubicin-cyclophosphamide plus B in ER+/Her-2 negative and triple negative breast cancer: a BrUOG study. J Clin Oncol. 2012;30:1045.
44. Untch M, Jackisch C, Schneeweiß A, Conrad B, Aktas B, Denkert C, et al. Nanoparticle-based paclitaxel versus solvent-based paclitaxel in neoadjuvant chemotherapy with weekly

for h early breast cancer (GeparSepto-GBG 69): a randomized phase III trial. Lancet Oncol. 2016;17(3):345–56.
45. Schneeweiss A, Jackisch C, Schmatloch S, Aktas B, Denkert C, Schem C, et al. Survival analysis of the prospectively randomized phase III GeparSepto trial comparing neoadjuvant chemotherapy with weekly nab-paclitaxel with solvent-based paclitaxel followed by anthracycline-cyclosphosphamide for patients with early breast cancer—GBG69. 40th SABCS; 2017 Dec 3–9; GS3-05.
46. von Minckwitz G, Schneeweiss A, Loibl S, Salat C, Denkert C, Rezai M, et al. Neoadjuvant carboplatin in patients with triple-negative and HER2-positive early breast cancer (GeparSixto; GBG 66): a randomised phase 2 trial. Lancet Oncol. 2014;15(7):747–56.
47. Sikov WM, Berry DA, Perou CM, Singh B, Cirrincione CT, Tolaney SM, et al. Impact of the addition of carboplatin and/or bevacizumab to neoadjuvant once-per-week paclitaxel followed by dose-dense doxorubicin and cyclophosphamide on pathologic complete response rates in stage II to III triple-negative breast cancer: CALGB 40603 (Alliance). J Clin Oncol. 2015;33(1):13–21.
48. Alba E, Chacon JI, Lluch A, Anton A, Estevez L, Cirauqui B, et al. A randomized phase II trial of platinum salts in basal-like breast cancer patients in the neoadjuvant setting. Results from the GEICAM/2006-03, multicenter study. Breast Cancer Res Treat. 2012;136(2):487–93.
49. Sikov WM, Berry DA, Perou CM, Singh, B., Cirrincione, C., Tolaney, S, et al. Event-free and overall survival following neoadjuvant weekly paclitaxel and dose -dense AC +/− carboplatin and/or bevacizumab in triple-negative breast cancer: Outcomes from CALGB 40603 (Alliance) 38th Annual SABCS; 2015 Dec 8–12; Abstract S2-05.
50. von Minckwitz G, Schneeweiss A, Loibl S, Salat CT, Rezai M, Zahm DM, et al. Early survival analysis of the randomized phase II trial investigating the addition of carboplatin to neoadjuvant therapy for triple-negative and HER2-positive early breast cancer (GeparSixto). SABCS; 2015 Dec 8–12; abstr S2-04.
51. Gluz O, Nitz U, Liedtke C, Christgen M, Grischke EM, Forstbauer H, et al. Comparison of neoadjuvant nab-paclitaxel + carboplatin vs nab paclitaxel+gemcitabine in triple-negative breast cancer: randomized WSG-ADAPT-TN trial results. J Natl Cancer Inst. 2017;109(12):628–37. https://doi.org/10.1093/jnci/djx258.
52. Telli ML, Timms KM, Reid J, Hennessy B, Mills GB, Jensen KC, et al. Homologous recombination deficiency (HRD) score predicts response to platinum-containing neoadjuvant chemotherapy in patients with triple-negative breast cancer. Clin Cancer Res. 2016;22(15):3764–73.
53. Hurvitz SA, Miller JM, Dichman R, Perez AT, Patel R, Zehngebot LM, et al. Final analysis of a phase II 3-arm randomized trial of neoadjuvant trastuzumab or lapatinib or the combination of trastuzumab and lapatinib, followed by six cycles of docetaxel and carboplatin with trastuzumab and/or lapatinib in patients with HER2 breast cancer (TRIO-US B07) [SABCS abstract S1–S2]. Cancer Res. 2013;73(Suppl):24.
54. Schneeweiss A, Chia S, Hickish T, Harvey V, Eniu A, Hegg R, et al. Pertuzumab plus trastuzumab in combination with standard neoadjuvant anthracycline-containing and anthracycline-free chemotherapy regimens in patients with HER2-positive early breast cancer: a randomized phase II cardiac safety study (TRYPHAENA). Ann Oncol. 2013;24(9):2278–84.
55. Van Ramshorst MS, van Werkhoven E, Mandjes IA, Kemper I, Dezentje VO, Oving IM, et al. A phase III trial of neoadjuvant chemotherapy with or without anthracyclines in the presence of dual HER2-blockade for HER2+ breast cancer: the TRAIN-2 study (BOOG 2012-03). ASCO 2017 Annual Meeting; 2017 June 2–6; Chicago, IL. J Clin Oncol. 2017;35(Suppl 15):507.
56. Hurvitz SA, Martin M, Symmans WF, Jung KH, Huang CS, Thompson AM, et al. Neoadjuvant trastuzumab, pertuzumab, and chemotherapy versus trastuzumab emtansine plus pertuzumab in patients with HER2-positive breast cancer (KRISTINE): a randomised, open-label, multicentre, phase 3 trial. Lancet Oncol. 2018;19(1):115–26.
57. Buzdar AU, Ibrahim NK, Francis D, Booser DJ, Thomas ES, Theriault RL, et al. Significantly higher pathologic complete remission rate after neoadjuvant therapy with trastuzumab, paclitaxel, and epirubicin chemotherapy: results of a randomized trial in human epidermal growth factor receptor 2-positive operable breast cancer. J Clin Oncol. 2005;23:3676–85.

58. Untch M, Rezai M, Loibl S, Fasching PA, Huober J, Tesch H, et al. Neoadjuvant treatment with trastuzumab in HER2-positive breast cancer: results from the GeparQuattro study. J Clin Oncol. 2010;28(12):2024–31.
59. Untch M, Loibl S, Bischoff J, Eidtmann H, Kaufmann M, Blohmer JU, Arbeitsgemeinschaft Gynäkologische Onkologie-Breast (AGO-B) Study Group, et al. Lapatinib versus trastuzumab in combination with neoadjuvant anthracycline-taxane-based chemotherapy (GeparQuinto, GBG 44): a randomised phase 3 trial. Lancet Oncol. 2012;13(2):135–44.
60. Baselga J, Bradbury I, Eidtmann H, Di Cosimo S, de Azambuja E, Aura C, NeoALTTO Study Team, et al. Lapatinib with trastuzumab for HER2-positive early breast cancer (NeoALTTO): a randomised, open-label, multicentre, phase 3 trial. Lancet. 2012;379(9816):633–40.
61. Carey LA, Berry DA, Cirrincione CT, Barry WT, Pitcher BN, Harris LN, et al. Molecular heterogeneity and response to neoadjuvant human epidermal growth factor receptor 2 targeting in CALGB 40601, a randomized phase III trial of paclitaxel plus trastuzumab with or without Lapatinib. J Clin Oncol. 2016;34(6):542–9.
62. Robidoux A, Tang G, Rastogi P, Geyer CE Jr, Azar CA, Atkins JN, et al. Lapatinib as a component of neoadjuvant therapy for HER2-positive operable breast cancer (NSABP protocol B-41): an open-label, randomised phase 3 trial. Lancet Oncol. 2013;14(12):1183–92.
63. Gianni L, Pienkowski T, Im YH, Roman L, Tseng LM, Liu MC, et al. Efficacy and safety of neoadjuvant pertuzumab and trastuzumab in women with locally advanced, inflammatory, or early HER2-positive breast cancer (NeoSphere): a randomised multicentre, open-label, phase 2 trial. Lancet Oncol. 2012;13(1):25–32.
64. Gianni L, Pienkowski T, Im YH, Tseng LM, Liu MC, Lluch A, et al. 5-year analysis of neoadjuvant pertuzumab and trastuzumab in patients with locally advanced, inflammatory, or early-stage HER2-positive breast cancer (NeoSphere): a multicentre, open-label, phase 2 randomised trial. Lancet Oncol. 2016;17(6):791–800.
65. DeMichele AM, Moulder S, Meredith B, Yee D, Wallace A, Chien J, et al. Efficacy of T-DM1 + pertuzumab over standard therapy for HER2+ breast cancer: results from the neoadjuvant I-SPY 2 TRIAL. AACR Annual Meeting; 2016 April 16–20; CT042.
66. Perez EA, Barrios C, Eiermann W, Toi M, Im YH, Conte P, et al. Trastuzumab emtansine with or without pertuzumab versus trastuzumab plus taxane for human epidermal growth factor receptor 2-positive, advanced breast cancer: primary results from the phase III MARIANNE study. J Clin Oncol. 2017;35(2):141–8.
67. Guarneri V, Frassoldati A, Bottini A, Cagossi K, Bisagni G, Sarti S, et al. Preoperative chemotherapy plus trastuzumab, lapatinib, or both in human epidermal growth factor receptor 2-positive operable breast cancer: results of the randomized phase II CHER-LOB study. J Clin Oncol. 2012;30(16):1989–95.
68. Jacobs SA, Robidoux A, Garcia JMP, Abraham J, La Verde N, Orcutt JM, et al. NSABP FB-7: A phase II randomized trial evaluating neoadjuvant therapy with weekly paclitaxel (P) plus neratinib (N) or trastuzumab (T) or neratinib and trastuzumab (N+T) followed by doxorubicin and cyclophosphamide (AC) with postoperative T in women with locally advanced HER2-positive breast cancer. Thirty-Eighth Annual CTRC-AACR San Antonio Breast Cancer Symposium; 2015 Dec 8–12; San Antonio, TX; PD5-04.
69. von Minckwitz G, Eidtmann H, Rezai M, Fasching PA, Tesch H, Eggemann H, German Breast Group; Arbeitsgemeinschaft Gynäkologische Onkologie–Breast Study Groups, et al. Neoadjuvant chemotherapy and bevacizumab for HER2-negative breast cancer. N Engl J Med. 2012;366(4):299–309.
70. Bear HD, Tang G, Rastogi P, Geyer CE Jr, Liu Q, Robidoux A, et al. Neoadjuvant plus adjuvant bevacizumab in early breast cancer (NSABP B-40 [NRG oncology]): secondary outcomes of a phase 3, randomised controlled trial. Lancet Oncol. 2015;16(9):1037–48.
71. Huober J, Fasching PA, Hanusch C, Rezai M, Eidtmann H, Kittel K, et al. Neoadjuvant chemotherapy with paclitaxel and everolimus in breast cancer patients with non-responsive tumours to epirubicin/cyclophosphamide (EC) ± bevacizumab- results of the randomised GeparQuinto study (GBG 44). Eur J Cancer. 2013;49(10):2284–93.

Chapter 10
Preoperative Systemic Therapy for Non-Inflammatory Locally Advanced Breast Cancer

Serkan Keskin and Adnan Aydiner

Introduction

Neoadjuvant therapy refers to the systemic treatment of breast cancer prior to definitive surgical therapy (i.e., preoperative therapy). Neoadjuvant therapy should be considered for women with large clinical stage IIA, stage IIB, and T3N1M0 tumors who meet the criteria for breast-conserving therapy except tumor size and wish to undergo breast-conserving therapy and for patients with locally advanced breast cancer (LABC). LABC has always included a heterogeneous group of presentations. According to the American Joint Committee on Cancer (AJCC) staging system, LABC technically can include a patient with a clinically apparent internal mammary or paraclavicular node as well as the more commonly accepted presentations, which include a primary breast cancer larger than 5 cm, disease fixed to the chest wall or involving the skin, or bulky palpable disease in the axilla. Inflammatory breast cancer can also be called LABC.

The primary objective of neoadjuvant therapy is to improve the surgical outcomes in patients for whom a primary surgical approach is technically not feasible and in patients with operable breast cancer who desire breast conservation but for whom either a mastectomy is required or a partial mastectomy would result in a poor cosmetic outcome [1–3] (Figs. 10.1, 10.2, 10.3, 10.4, and 10.5). Although it was hypothesized that overall survival would improve with earlier initiation of systemic therapy in patients at risk of distant recurrence, clinical studies have not yet demonstrated a mortality benefit for pre-versus postoperative delivery of systemic

S. Keskin
Internal Medicine, Department of Medical Oncology, Memorial Hospital, Istanbul, Turkey
e-mail: serkan.keskin@memorial.com.tr

A. Aydiner (✉)
Internal Medicine, Medical Oncology, Istanbul Medical Faculty, Department of Medical Oncology, Institute of Oncology, Istanbul University, Istanbul, Turkey

A. Aydiner et al. (eds.), *Breast Cancer*, https://doi.org/10.1007/978-3-319-96947-3_10

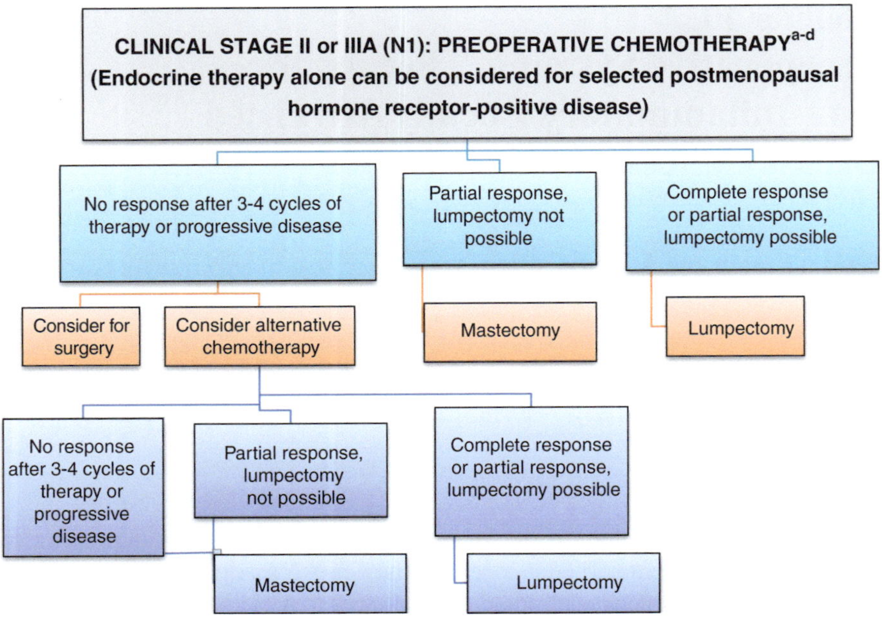

Fig. 10.1 Management of patients receiving neoadjuvant therapy for breast conserving surgery (stage II or IIIA with N1). [a]HER2-targeted therapy: According to the version 1.0 2018 NCCN Guidelines, patients with HER2- positive disease should receive "pertuzumab + trastuzumab + chemotherapy" in the neoadjuvant setting. The St Gallen 2017 Consensus Panel supported dual anti-HER2 therapy as an acceptable regimen with neoadjuvant taxane, trastuzumab and pertuzumab in such patients and considered anthracycline-taxane and anti-HER2 treatments as the best options. [b]Stage II–III triple-negative disease: If provided to patients with triple-negative tumors, the preferred regimen should include an anthracycline and a taxane. Although the available data are insufficient, a platinum-based regimen may be considered only in patients with a known BRCA mutation. Anthracyclines followed by taxanes is an acceptable regimen for BRCA-mutant TNBC. Dose-dense chemotherapy requiring growth factor support may also be an option. [c]Neoadjuvant cytotoxic therapy should be discussed as an option and provided frequently to patients with "Luminal A-like" tumors, only if conservative surgery would not otherwise be feasible. Neoadjuvant chemotherapy should be administered to T2 and T3 tumors (N0-N1) meeting BCS criteria except tumor diameter, or to triple negative and HER-2-positive patients. [d]Neoadjuvant endocrine therapy without cytotoxics represents a reasonable option for some selected postmenopausal patients with endocrine-responsive disease. The duration of treatment must be at least 4–6 months, and treatment can be provided until a maximal response is reached

therapy. However, achieving a pathologic complete response (pCR) to neoadjuvant therapy is associated with favorable disease-free and OS in early-stage breast cancer. The correlation between pathologic response and long-term outcomes in patients with early-stage breast cancer is strongest for patients with triple-negative breast cancer, less so for HER2-positive disease, and lowest for hormone-positive disease. Neoadjuvant therapy is most appropriate for patients likely to have a good locoregional response, regardless of tumor size at presentation, including those with HER2-positive *or* triple-negative breast cancers (TNBC) [4–7]. By contrast, patients with HER2-negative, ER-positive (luminal A) breast cancers are *less likely* to have

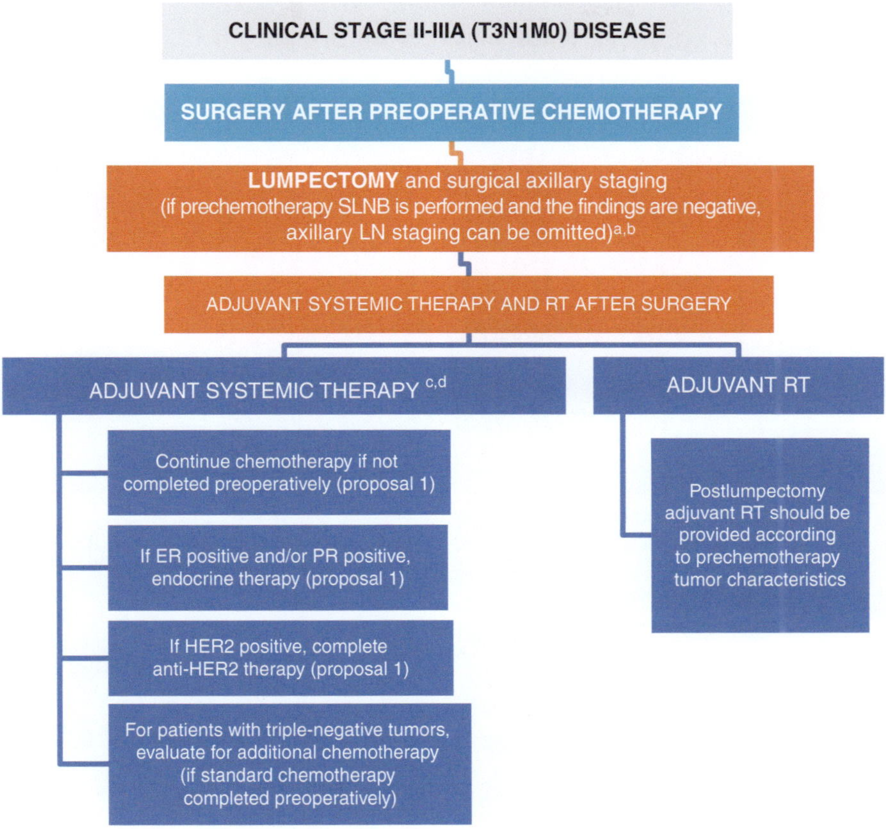

Fig. 10.2 Locoregional and adjuvant systemic treatment after neoadjuvant therapy: Lumpectomy. [a]In a patient who is clinically node positive at presentation and is downstaged after chemotherapy, sentinel lymph node (SLN) biopsy is appropriate. If SLN is positive, axillary lymph node dissection must be performed. After downstaging, resection of the entire area of the original primary tumor is not necessary (if there is shrinkage in the tumor). MR imaging is recommended in patients who will undergo BCS after neoadjuvant therapy. Clinical examination and radiological imaging modalities (USG, MMG, MR imaging) are used to evaluate the tissue to be excised (shrinking or patching). However, if the tumor response is patchy, the original tumor area should be removed with clean surgical margins. If diffuse live tumor cells are observed in the excised lumpectomy specimen after neoadjuvant chemotherapy, re-excision should be performed, even if there is no surgical margin involvement. [b]Consider adjuvant bisphosphonate therapy in postmenopausal (natural or induced) patients receiving adjuvant therapy. [c]Additional adjuvant systemic chemotherapy may be given to patients who are considered to have an inadequate response according to postoperative pathology (adjuvant chemotherapy may be given if the pathological response to neoadjuvant taxane-anthracycline is inadequate in triple-negative tumors). In a randomized clinical trial, adjuvant capecitabine has been shown to be beneficial in triple-negative patients. However, there is no other study confirming this suggestion. [d]HER2-targeted therapy: When indicated, trastuzumab can be administered with RT and together with endocrine therapy. According to the version 1.0 2018 NCCN Guidelines, "pertuzumab + trastuzumab" should be used as anti-HER2 treatment in neoadjuvant treatment, and pertuzumab can be continued in adjuvant treatment in ≥T2 and ≥N1 HER2-positive patients. Pertuzumab use in adjuvant therapy can be considered in node-positive, patients with locally advanced tumors according to APHINITY study results. According to a randomized controlled trial, 1-year neratinib use after 1-year administration of trastuzumab reduced the recurrence rate. This benefit was obvious especially in ER-positive, HER-2-positive disease. However, diarrhea is an important side effect

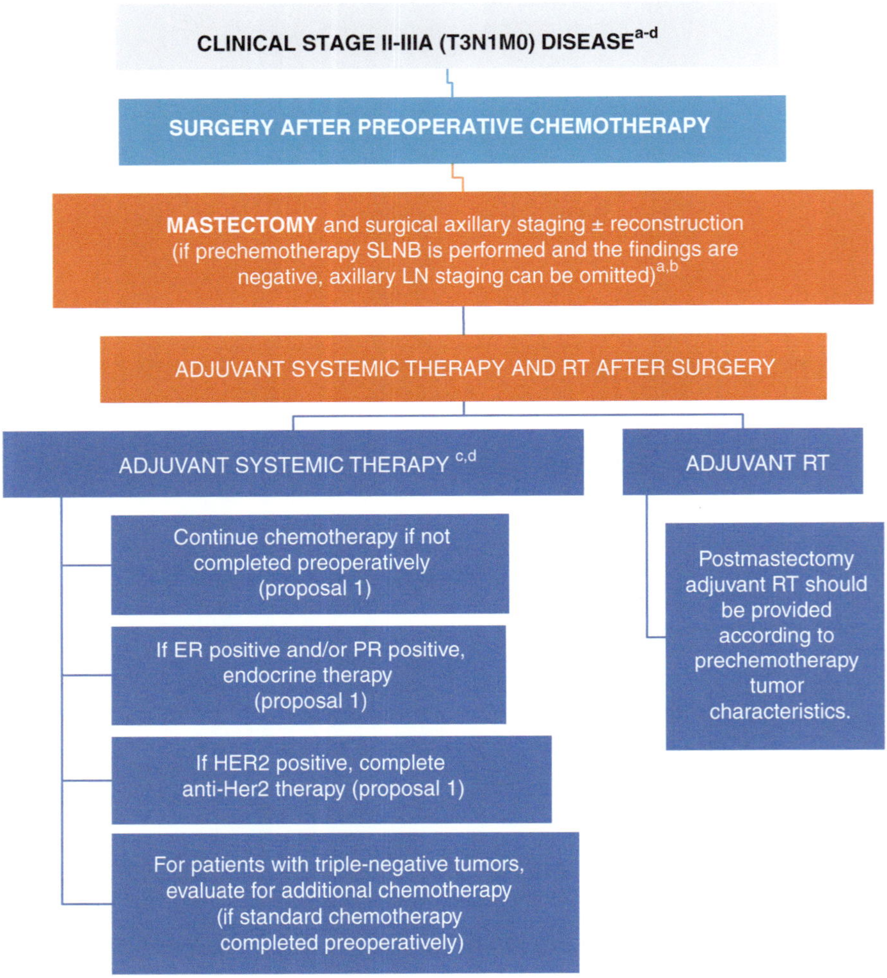

Fig. 10.3 Locoregional and adjuvant systemic treatment after neoadjuvant therapy: Mastectomy. [a]In a patient who is clinically node positive at presentation and is downstaged after chemotherapy, sentinel lymph node (SLN) biopsy is appropriate. If SLN is positive, axillar lymph node dissection must be performed. [b]Consider adjuvant bisphosphonate therapy in postmenopausal (natural or induced) patients receiving adjuvant therapy. [c]Additional adjuvant systemic chemotherapy is controversial in triple-negative tumor patients, who are considered to have an inadequate response in postoperative pathology, and 31% of the panelists did not recommend additional treatment in the 2017 St. Gallen consensus meeting. Furthermore, 49% of the panelists recommended capecitabine, 7% recommended platinum, 9% recommended (in BRCA-positive patients) platinum, and 4% recommended metronomic treatment. Additional adjuvant systemic chemotherapy may be given to patients who are considered to have an inadequate response according to postoperative pathology (adjuvant chemotherapy may be given if the pathological response to neoadjuvant taxane-anthracycline is inadequate in triple-negative tumors). In a randomized clinical trial, adjuvant capecitabine was shown to be beneficial in triple-negative patients. However, there is no other study confirming this suggestion. [d]HER2-targeted therapy: When indicated, trastuzumab can be administered with RT and together with endocrine therapy. "Pertuzumab + trastuzumab" should be used as anti-HER2 treatment in neoadjuvant treatment, and pertuzumab can be continued in adjuvant treatment. According to the results of a randomized study, 1-year administration of trastuzumab after neratinib use for 1 year reduced the recurrence rate. This benefit was obvious, especially in ER-positive, HER-2-positive disease. However, diarrhea is an important side effect

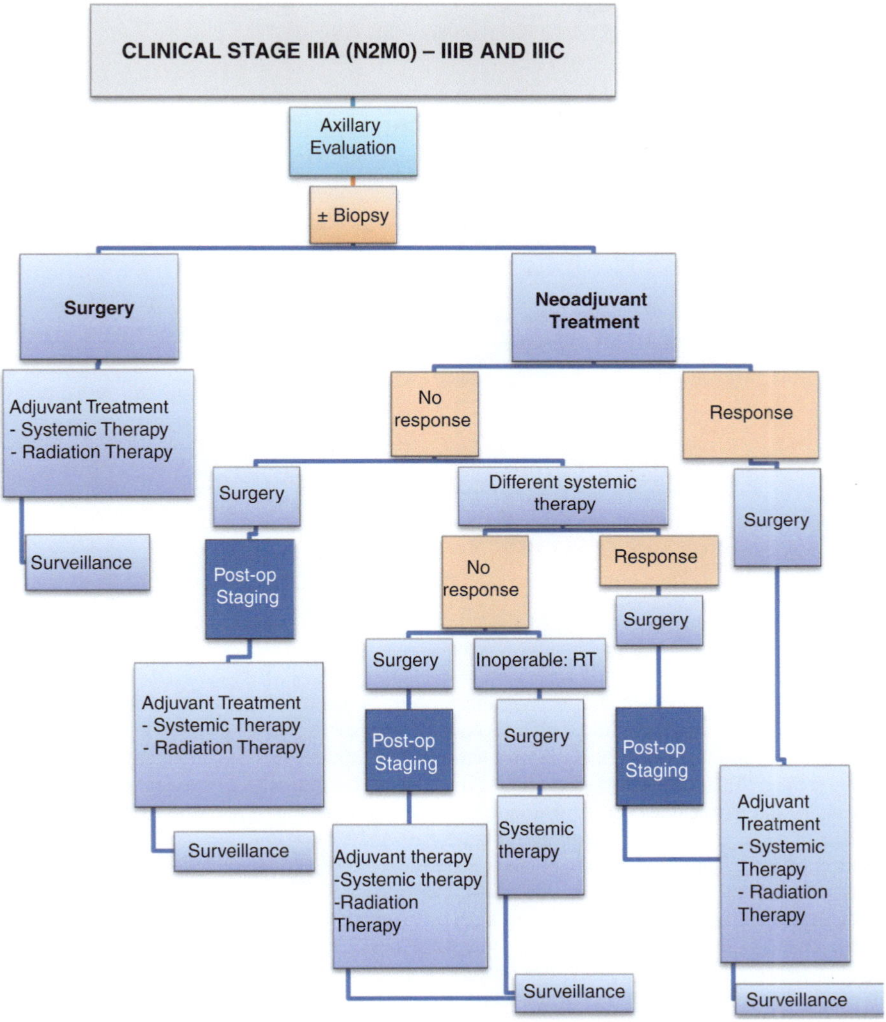

Fig. 10.4 Locoregional and adjuvant systemic treatment for clinical stage IIIA (N2M0)—IIIB and IIIC disease (non-inflammatory)

a clinical or pathological complete response (pCR) to neoadjuvant therapy [4, 6]. The rates of pCR to neoadjuvant therapy among TNBC patients range from 30% to 50%, whereas the pCR rate for HER2-negative, hormone receptor-positive patients is generally less than 10%. However, while TNBC patients who achieve pCR appear to have a prognosis similar to that of patients with other breast cancer subtypes, TNBC patients with more than minimal residual disease at surgery have a higher risk of early distant disease recurrence [7].

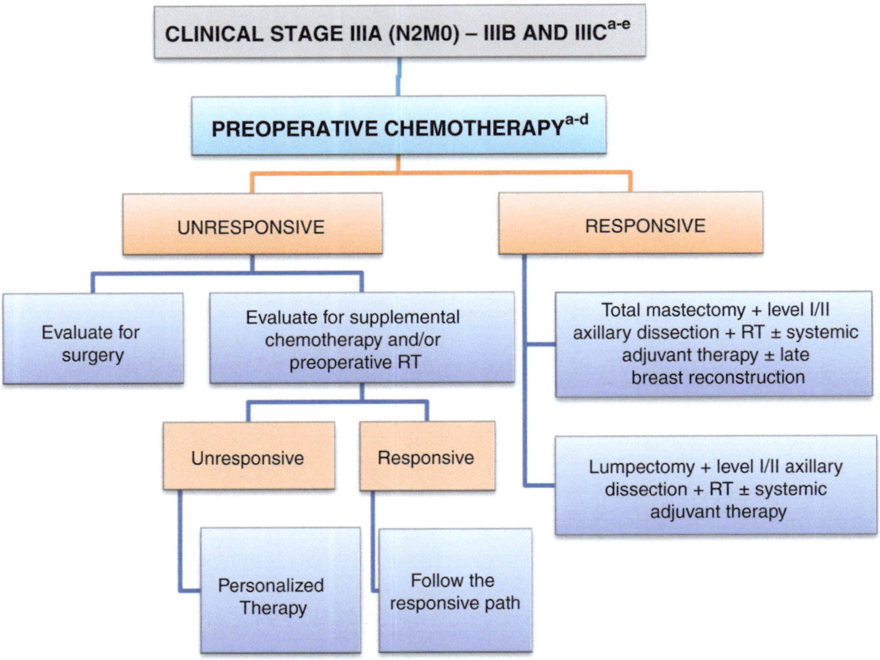

Fig. 10.5 Surgical approach after neoadjuvant systemic treatment for patients with clinical stage IIIA (N2M0)—IIIB and IIIC breast cancer (non-inflammatory). [a]HER2-targeted therapy: Patients with HER2- positive disease should receive anti-HER2 treatment plus chemotherapy in the neoadjuvant setting. "Pertuzumab + trastuzumab" should be used as anti-HER2 treatment in neoadjuvant treatment, and pertuzumab can be continued in adjuvant treatment. According to the results of a randomized study, 1-year administration of trastuzumab after neratinib use for 1 year reduced the recurrence rate. This benefit was obvious especially in ER-positive, HER-2-positive disease. However, diarrhea is an important side effect. The rate of pCR is lower when neoadjuvant ado-trastuzumab emtansine (TDM-1) is given with pertuzumab than for chemotherapy-trastuzumab-pertuzumab (TCHP) treatment. [b]For triple-negative breast cancer (TNBC), the regimen should contain anthracyclines and taxanes. The addition of carboplatin to the treatment increases the rate of pathologic complete response (pCR), which prolongs disease-free survival. Although the available data are insufficient, a platinum-based regimen may be considered only in patients with a known BRCA mutation. Anthracyclines followed by taxanes is an acceptable regimen for BRCA-mutant TNBC. In an adaptive study, the addition of veliparib and carboplatin to the treatment increased the rate of pCR. Dose-dense chemotherapy requiring growth factor support may also be an option. [c]Data regarding the use of nab-paclitaxel instead of paclitaxel in neoadjuvant chemotherapy are inconsistent.[d]Neoadjuvant endocrine therapy shows a high response rates in patients with low genomic scores. [e]Consider adjuvant bisphosphonate therapy in postmenopausal (natural or induced) patients receiving adjuvant therapy

Treatment Options

The options for neoadjuvant treatment include chemotherapy, endocrine therapy, and the incorporation of biological therapy in appropriate patients. Much of the information regarding neoadjuvant therapy comes from trials utilizing chemotherapy, with recent studies assessing the role of biologics.

For women with HER2-negative, estrogen-receptor (ER)- and/or progesterone-receptor (PR)-positive breast cancers who are not candidates for initial resection, we suggest neoadjuvant chemotherapy rather than endocrine therapy [8, 9]. While few of these patients will achieve a clinical or pathologic complete response, tumor shrinkage may enable surgery for some unresectable patients and breast conservation for some borderline patients. Neoadjuvant therapy is typically indicated in women with larger tumors and/or locally advanced breast cancer. In such situations, most premenopausal women should receive chemotherapy rather than endocrine therapy. If a premenopausal woman refuses (or is not a good candidate for) neoadjuvant chemotherapy, we suggest proceeding to surgical treatment, if possible, rather than attempting neoadjuvant endocrine therapy.

Most postmenopausal women for whom neoadjuvant treatment is indicated receive chemotherapy, although endocrine therapy may be offered as an alternative for some women. While historically neoadjuvant endocrine therapy (NET) has been reserved for patients with substantial comorbid health problems who would not tolerate chemotherapy, it is increasingly seen as a viable alternative for other patients, especially those with human epidermal growth factor receptor 2 (HER2)-negative, HR-positive tumors that are strongly ER positive. In such patients, NET may enable improved surgical outcomes and cosmesis.

The response to endocrine therapy has been shown to correlate with levels of ER expression, as quantified by the Allred score. In a study of 324 postmenopausal women with HR-positive breast cancer randomly assigned to 4 months of tamoxifen or letrozole, response rates among those with Allred scores of 7–8 were >60% for letrozole and approximately 30–45% for tamoxifen, whereas the response rate for patients with Allred scores of 0–2 was 0% [10].

Several trials have also investigated the role of endocrine therapy in combination with other targeted therapies. These include combinations of endocrine therapy with everolimus, celecoxib, zoledronic acid, gefitinib, lapatinib, and palbociclib. Although general combination therapy is associated with a higher response rate, given the lack of survival data and concern about added toxicity, combination therapy cannot be recommended for routine clinical practice. Several ongoing trials are investigating the role of combination therapy, including the combination of aromatase inhibitors with cyclin-dependent kinase (CDK) 4/6 inhibitors (NeoMONARCH), PI3K inhibitors (LORELEI), and dual endocrine therapy (ALTERNATE).

For patients with HER2-positive breast cancer who are not candidates for surgery or who have larger tumors (T2-T3) and desire breast-conserving surgery, we recommend the addition of anti-HER2 therapy to neoadjuvant therapy over chemotherapy alone.

Several chemotherapy regimens have been studied as preoperative systemic therapy. The regimens recommended in the adjuvant setting are appropriate for consideration in the preoperative systemic therapy setting [11, 12]. The outcomes of neoadjuvant therapy were demonstrated in a 2007 meta-analysis that included data for 5500 women participating in 1 of 14 trials reported between 1991 and 2001 [13]. Compared to adjuvant chemotherapy, neoadjuvant therapy resulted in equivalent overall survival (hazard ratio [HR] 0.98, 95% CI 0.87–1.09) and disease-free survival (HR 0.97, 95% CI 0.89–1.07) and a reduction in the likelihood of modified radical mastectomy (HR 0.71, 95% CI 0.67–0.75).

The choice of specific chemotherapy drugs and regimens should be based on tumor biology and intrinsic subsets (i.e., triple negative, estrogen receptor positive, HER2 positive) [12–14]. There is no reason to assume that regimens administered in the adjuvant setting would be less active when used prior to surgery. Because a reduction in tumor size to permit surgery is the primary objective of neoadjuvant therapy, all planned treatment should be administered *prior* to definitive surgery, provided there is no evidence of disease progression during treatment.

Multiple studies have demonstrated that anthracycline-based regimens incorporating a taxane (either concurrently or in sequence with anthracycline-based regimens) are associated with increased response rates in the neoadjuvant setting compared to the use of non-taxane-containing regimens [15]. Ongoing clinical research is examining whether the addition of non-cross-resistant agents with demonstrated activity in metastatic breast cancer might improve the clinical and pathologic response rates observed with the use of an anthracycline and/or a taxane. However, there is no evidence that this approach improves survival outcomes or response rates. Thus, we suggest not administering additional agents with standard anthracycline- and taxane-based neoadjuvant therapy (Table 10.1).

Table 10.1 Neoadjuvant therapy in HER2-negative breast cancer

Study	Experimental regimen	Control regimen	No. of patients	pCR definition applied to breast (B) or breast and lymph nodes (B/LN)	pCR, %	p
Anthracycline and taxane-based vs *anthracycline-based regimens*						
Diéras et al. [16]	AP	AC	200	B/LN	8 vs 6	NS
Rastogi et al. [17]	AC-T	AC	1609	B	26 vs 13	<0.0001
Evans et al. [18]	AT	AC	363	B/LN	16 vs 12	0.43
Intensified/dose-dense vs *standard-dose regimens*						
Baldini et al. [19]	ddFEC	FEC	150	B/LN	4.1 vs 2.6	0.95
Walker et al. [20]	AC-wT	AC-3wT	89	B	8 vs 11	0.9
Arun el al [21]	ddFAC	FAC	199	B/LN	13 vs 9	NS

AC doxorubicin, cyclophosphamide, *AT* doxorubicin, docetaxel, *Edd-Pdd* dose-dense epirubicin, dose-dense paclitaxel, *EP* epirubicin, paclitaxel, *ET* epirubicin, docetaxel, *FAC* fluorouracil, doxorubicin, cyclophosphamide, *FEC* fluorouracil, epirubicin, cyclophosphamide, *P* paclitaxel, *pCR* pathologic complete response, *T* Docetaxel, *NS* non-significant

There is a small body of evidence suggesting that the use of endocrine therapy may be equivalent to chemotherapy in postmenopausal women. However, until more data are available, we recommend chemotherapy for most patients in the neoadjuvant setting.

HER2-Directed Therapy

The benefit of adding trastuzumab to chemotherapy was demonstrated in a pooled analysis of two randomized studies that evaluated neoadjuvant therapy with or without trastuzumab [22]. The addition of trastuzumab to chemotherapy resulted in an improvement in the rate of pCR (43% versus 20%; relative risk for achieving pCR [RR] 2.07, 95% CI 1.41–3.03); a reduction in the relapse rate (26% versus 39%; RR for relapse 0.67, 95% CI 0.48–0.94); and a trend toward a lower mortality rate (13% versus 20%; RR for mortality 0.67, 95% CI 0.39–1.15) that did not reach statistical significance.

Pertuzumab is a recombinant humanized monoclonal antibody that inhibits the ligand-dependent dimerization of HER2 and its downstream signaling. Pertuzumab and trastuzumab bind to different epitopes of the HER2 receptor and have complementary mechanisms of action. When administered together in HER2-positive tumor models and in humans, pertuzumab and trastuzumab provide a greater overall anti-tumor effect than either alone. Because the combination of pertuzumab and trastuzumab exhibited a significant overall survival benefit in a metastatic setting, it has also been examined in the neoadjuvant setting [23]. The combination of trastuzumab plus pertuzumab was evaluated in the neoadjuvant setting with responses noted even without the use of chemotherapy. These results are fascinating not only because of the higher pCR rate associated with chemotherapy plus trastuzumab and pertuzumab but also because of the frequency of pCR associated with dual HER2-targeted therapy alone, particularly in patients with ER-negative disease [23–29] (Table 10.2).

Treatment Evaluation

Patients receiving neoadjuvant systemic therapy should be followed by clinical exam at regular intervals during treatment to ensure that the disease is not progressing. At the end of treatment, an assessment of tumor response is important to help guide the surgical approach.

There are no formal guidelines regarding the ideal assessment strategy during neoadjuvant treatment. Our approach is as follows:

- For patients on neoadjuvant therapy, we perform a clinical examination every 2–4 weeks (i.e., prior to each cycle of treatment). This should include evaluation of the affected breast and ipsilateral axilla.

Table 10.2 Neoadjuvant therapy in HER2-positive breast cancer

	No. of patients	Treatment arms	pCR (breast and nodes)	p	3-yr DFS
GeparQuinto [24]	309	ECH → TH	31.3%	<0.05	84.8%
	311	ECL → TL	21.7%		83.7%
NeoALTTO [25]	149	H → HP	27.6%		76% (3-yr EFS)
	154	L → LP	20.0%	0.13	78%
	152	HL → HLP	46.9%	0.001	84%
CHER-LOB [26]	36	HP → FECH	25%		N/A
	39	LP → FECL	26.3%		N/A
	46	HLP → FECHL	46.7%		N/A
NSABP B-41 [27]	177	AC → HP	52.5% (breast)		N/A
	171	AC → LP	53.2% (breast)	0.9852	N/A
	171	AC → HLP	62.0% (breast)	0.095	N/A
CALGB 40601 [28]	120	HP	40% (breast)		N/A
	67	LP	32% (breast)		N/A
	118	HLP	51% (breast)	0.11	N/A
NeoSphere [29]	107	TH	29% (breast)		81% (5-yr PFS)
	107	PerHT	45.8% (breast)	0.01412	86%
	107	PerH	24% (breast)		73%
	96	PerH	16.8% (breast)		73%
TPYPHENA [23]	73	PerHFEC → PerTH	61.6% (breast)		87%
	77	FEC → PerTH	57.3% (breast)		88%
	77	TcarboHPer	66.2% (breast)		90%

pCR pathologic complete response, *EFS* event-free survival, *E* epirubicin, *C* cyclophosphamide, *H* trastuzumab, *T* Docetaxel, *L* lapatinib, *P* paclitaxel, *F* 5-fluorouracil, *NSABP* National Surgical Adjuvant Breast and Bowel Project, *A* doxorubicin, *CALGB* Cancer and Leukemia Group B, *Per* pertuzumab, *carbo* carboplatin, *yr* year, *PFS* progression-free survival, *DFS* disease-free survival

- For patients undergoing neoadjuvant endocrine therapy, we perform clinical evaluations every 4–8 weeks. The response to treatment is expected to take a longer time to become evident.
- Imaging studies (ultrasound [US] or magnetic resonance imaging [MRI]) should only be performed if disease progression is suspected based on clinical exam.

Prognosis

The prognosis of patients with breast cancer who undergo neoadjuvant therapy correlates with the pathological response observed at the time of surgery, but it is also influenced by presenting clinical stage and tumor characteristics (particularly hormone receptor and HER2 status). Clinical response is not an accurate predictor of pathological response, and achieving a pCR in the breast and axilla is a better predictor of survival than a clinical complete response is.

The prognostic significance of pCR for survival endpoints has been evaluated in several meta-analyses [30, 31]. The largest of these was conducted by the Collaborative

Trials in Neoadjuvant Breast Cancer (CTNeoBC) working group and included 12 randomized trials and nearly 12,000 patients [30]. Their major findings were as follows. Patients who achieved pCR had significant improvements in event-free survival (hazard ratio [HR] 0.48, $p < 0.001$) and overall survival ([OS] HR 0.36, $p < 0.001$) compared to patients who did not achieve pCR. The inclusion of patients with residual ductal carcinoma in situ (DCIS) only (ypT0/is, ypN0) did not diminish the benefit of achieving pCR for event-free survival and overall survival. However, the inclusion of patients with residual axillary nodal involvement in the definition of pCR reduced its prognostic value for both event-free survival and overall survival. pCR rates and improvement in event-free survival for patients who achieved pCR varied by breast cancer subtype:

- Hormone receptor (HR)-positive, HER2-negative, grade 1 to 2: 8% (HR for event-free survival 0.63, $p = 0.07$)
- HR-positive, HER2-negative, grade 3: 16% (HR 0.27, $p < 0.001$)
- HR-positive, HER2-positive (treated with a trastuzumab-containing regimen): 31% (HR 0.58, $p = 0.001$)
- HR-negative, HER2-negative (triple-negative): 34% (HR 0.24, $p < 0.001$)
- HR-negative, HER2-positive (treated with a trastuzumab-containing regimen): 50% (HR 0.25, $p < 0.001$)

Despite these results, the threshold of benefit (defined by an increase in the pCR rate) associated with an improvement in event-free survival and/or overall survival is not clear. The investigators hypothesized that the lack of an association may have been due to the heterogeneous patient populations in many of the studies, the relatively low pCR rates (even in the "superior" treatment arm), and/or the lack of effective targeted agents for many of the patient populations studied.

Conclusion

In conclusion, preoperative systemic chemotherapy is a valuable research tool to identify predictive molecular biomarkers and a valid treatment option for patients with early-stage or locally advanced breast cancer. However, the decision regarding neoadjuvant treatment should be made after discussion of the patient's clinical, histological, and imaging characteristics by a multidisciplinary oncology board.

References

1. van der Hage JA, van de Velde CJ, Julien JP, Tubiana-Hulin M, Vandervelden C, Duchateau L. Preoperative chemotherapy in primary operable breast cancer: results from the European Organization for Research and Treatment of Cancer trial 10902. J Clin Oncol. 2001;19(22):4224–37.
2. Gralow JR, Burstein HJ, Wood W, Hortobagyi GN, Gianni L, von Minckwitz G, et al. Preoperative therapy in invasive breast cancer: pathologic assessment and systemic therapy issues in operable disease. J Clin Oncol. 2008;26(5):814–9.

3. Davidson NE, Morrow M. Sometimes a great notion—an assessment of neoadjuvant systemic therapy for breast cancer. J Natl Cancer Inst. 2005;97(3):159–61.
4. Shannon C, Smith I. Is there still a role for neoadjuvant therapy in breast cancer? Crit Rev Oncol Hematol. 2003;45(1):77–90.
5. Coates AS, Colleoni M, Goldhirsch A. Is adjuvant chemotherapy useful for women with luminal a breast cancer? J Clin Oncol. 2012;30(12):1260–3.
6. Untch M, Fasching PA, Konecny GE, Hasmuller S, Lebeau A, Kreienberg R, et al. Pathologic complete response after neoadjuvant chemotherapy plus trastuzumab predicts favorable survival in human epidermal growth factor receptor 2-overexpressing breast cancer: results from the TECHNO trial of the AGO and GBG study groups. J Clin Oncol. 2011;29(25):3351–7.
7. Carey LA, Dees EC, Sawyer L, Gatti L, Moore DT, Collichio F, et al. The triple negative paradox: primary tumor chemosensitivity of breast cancer subtypes. Clin Cancer Res. 2007;13(8):2329–34.
8. Berry DA, Cirrincione C, Henderson IC, Citron ML, Budman DR, Goldstein LJ, et al. Estrogen-receptor status and outcomes of modern chemotherapy for patients with node-positive breast cancer. JAMA. 2006;295(14):1658–67.
9. Barroso-Sousa R, Silva DD, Alessi JV, Mano MS. Neoadjuvant endocrine therapy in breast cancer: current role and future perspectives. Ecancermedicalscience. 2016;10:609.
10. Ellis MJ, Coop A, Singh B, Mauriac L, Llombert-Cussac A, Janicke F, et al. Letrozole is more effective neoadjuvant endocrine therapy than tamoxifen for ErbB-1- and/or ErbB-2-positive, estrogen receptor-positive primary breast cancer: evidence from a phase III randomized trial. J Clin Oncol. 2001;19(18):3808–16.
11. Schott AF, Hayes DF. Defining the benefits of neoadjuvant chemotherapy for breast cancer. J Clin Oncol. 2012;30(15):1747–9.
12. Gianni L, Mansutti M, Anton A, Calvo L, Bisagni G, Bermejo B, et al. Comparing neoadjuvant nab-paclitaxel vs paclitaxel both followed by anthracycline regimens in women with ERBB2/HER2-negative breast cancer—the Evaluating Treatment with Neoadjuvant Abraxane (ETNA) Trial: a randomized phase 3 clinical trial. JAMA Oncol. 2018;4(3):302–8.
13. Mieog JS, van der Hage JA, van de Velde CJ. Neoadjuvant chemotherapy for operable breast cancer. Br J Surg. 2007;94(10):1189–200.
14. von Minckwitz G, Kummel S, Vogel P, Hanusch C, Eidtmann H, Hilfrich J, et al. Neoadjuvant vinorelbine-capecitabine versus docetaxel-doxorubicin-cyclophosphamide in early nonresponsive breast cancer: phase III randomized GeparTrio trial. J Natl Cancer Inst. 2008;100(8):542–51.
15. von Minckwitz G, Rezai M, Loibl S, Fasching PA, Huober J, Tesch H, et al. Capecitabine in addition to anthracycline- and taxane-based neoadjuvant treatment in patients with primary breast cancer: phase III GeparQuattro study. J Clin Oncol. 2010;28(12):2015–23.
16. Dieras V, Fumoleau P, Romieu G, Tubiana-Hulin M, Namer M, Mauriac L, et al. Randomized parallel study of doxorubicin plus paclitaxel and doxorubicin plus cyclophosphamide as neoadjuvant treatment of patients with breast cancer. J Clin Oncol. 2004;22(24):4958–65.
17. Rastogi P, Anderson SJ, Bear HD, Geyer CE, Kahlenberg MS, Robidoux A, et al. Preoperative chemotherapy: updates of National Surgical Adjuvant Breast and Bowel Project Protocols B-18 and B-27. J Clin Oncol. 2008;26(5):778–85.
18. Evans TR, Yellowlees A, Foster E, Earl H, Cameron DA, Hutcheon AW, et al. Phase III randomized trial of doxorubicin and docetaxel versus doxorubicin and cyclophosphamide as primary medical therapy in women with breast cancer: an anglo-celtic cooperative oncology group study. J Clin Oncol. 2005;23(13):2988–95.
19. Baldini E, Gardin G, Giannessi PG, Evangelista G, Roncella M, Prochilo T, et al. Accelerated versus standard cyclophosphamide, epirubicin and 5-fluorouracil or cyclophosphamide, methotrexate and 5-fluorouracil: a randomized phase III trial in locally advanced breast cancer. Ann Oncol. 2003;14(2):227–32.
20. Walker LG, Eremin JM, Aloysius MM, Vassanasiri W, Walker MB, El-Sheemy M, et al. Effects on quality of life, anti-cancer responses, breast conserving surgery and survival with neoadjuvant docetaxel: a randomised study of sequential weekly versus three-weekly

docetaxel following neoadjuvant doxorubicin and cyclophosphamide in women with primary breast cancer. BMC Cancer. 2011;11:179.
21. Arun BK, Dhinghra K, Valero V, Kau SW, Broglio K, Booser D, et al. Phase III randomized trial of dose intensive neoadjuvant chemotherapy with or without G-CSF in locally advanced breast cancer: long-term results. Oncologist. 2011;16(11):1527–34.
22. Petrelli F, Borgonovo K, Cabiddu M, Ghilardi M, Barni S. Neoadjuvant chemotherapy and concomitant trastuzumab in breast cancer: a pooled analysis of two randomized trials. Anti-Cancer Drugs. 2011;22(2):128–35.
23. Schneeweiss A, Chia S, Hickish T, Harvey V, Eniu A, Waldron-Lynch M, et al. Long-term efficacy analysis of the randomised, phase II TRYPHAENA cardiac safety study: Evaluating pertuzumab and trastuzumab plus standard neoadjuvant anthracycline-containing and anthracycline-free chemotherapy regimens in patients with HER2-positive early breast cancer. Eur J Cancer. 2018;89:27–35.
24. Untch M, von Minckwitz G, Gerber B, Schem C, Rezai M, Fasching PA, et al. Survival analysis after neoadjuvant chemotherapy with trastuzumab or lapatinib in patients with human epidermal growth factor receptor 2-positive breast cancer in the GeparQuinto (G5) Study (GBG 44). J Clin Oncol. 2018;36(13):1308–16.
25. de Azambuja E, Holmes AP, Piccart-Gebhart M, Holmes E, Di Cosimo S, Swaby RF, et al. Lapatinib with trastuzumab for HER2-positive early breast cancer (NeoALTTO): survival outcomes of a randomised, open-label, multicentre, phase 3 trial and their association with pathological complete response. Lancet Oncol. 2014;15:1137–46.
26. Guarneri V, Frassoldati A, Bottini A, Cagossi K, Bisagni G, Sarti S, et al. Preoperative chemotherapy plus trastuzumab, lapatinib, or both in human epidermal growth factor receptor 2-positive operable breast cancer: results of the randomized phase II CHER-LOB study. J Clin Oncol. 2012;30(16):1989–95.
27. Robidoux A, Tang G, Rastogi P, Geyer CE Jr, Azar CA, Atkins JN, et al. Lapatinib as a component of neoadjuvant therapy for HER2-positive operable breast cancer (NSABP protocol B-41): an open-label, randomised phase 3 trial. Lancet Oncol. 2013;14(12):1183–92.
28. Carey LA, Berry DA, Cirrincione CT, Barry WT, Pitcher BN, Harris LN, et al. Molecular heterogeneity and response to Neoadjuvant human epidermal growth factor receptor 2 targeting in CALGB 40601, a randomized phase III trial of paclitaxel plus Trastuzumab with or without Lapatinib. J Clin Oncol. 2016;34(6):542–9.
29. Gianni L, Pienkowski T, Im YH, Tseng LM, Liu MC, Lluch A, et al. 5-year analysis of neoadjuvant pertuzumab and trastuzumab in patients with locally advanced, inflammatory, or early-stage HER2-positive breast cancer (NeoSphere): a multicentre, open-label, phase 2 randomized trial. Lancet Oncol. 2016;17(6):791–800.
30. Cortazar P, Zhang L, Untch M, Mehta K, Costantino JP, Wolmark N, et al. Pathological complete response and long-term clinical benefit in breast cancer: the CTNeoBC pooled analysis. Lancet. 2014;384(9938):164–72.
31. Kong X, Moran MS, Zhang N, Haffty B, Yang Q. Meta-analysis confirms achieving pathological complete response after neoadjuvant chemotherapy predicts favourable prognosis for breast cancer patients. Eur J Cancer. 2011;47(14):2084–90.

Chapter 11
Inflammatory Breast Cancer

Nilufer Guler

Introduction

Inflammatory breast carcinoma (IBC) is a rare and aggressive subtype of breast carcinoma that is diagnosed clinically [1–5]. IBC is characterized by skin changes that are suggestive of infection and inflammation, usually with fairly abrupt onset and rapid progression. The duration of symptoms before diagnosis is usually less than 3 months [1–5]. The most common symptoms are a feeling of warmth and heaviness, itching, nipple retraction, and pain in the affected breast. IBC is frequently misdiagnosed as cellulitis or acute mastitis. Acute-phase radiation dermatitis, sarcoma or lymphoma of the breast, inflammatory metastatic melanoma, and Paget's disease of the nipple can also mimic IBC.

The minimum diagnostic criteria for the diagnosis of IBC are the following [6–8]:

- Rapid onset of breast erythema (with a palpable border), edema and/or dermal edema (peau d'orange), and/or warm breast, with or without an underlying palpable mass;
- A duration of symptom history of no more than 6 months;
- Erythema occupying at least one third of the breast;
- Pathological confirmation of invasive carcinoma.

Primary IBC is classified as T4d according to the American Joint Commission for Cancer (AJCC) staging system and is staged as IIIB, IIIC, or IV according to nodal involvement and distant metastases [7, 8]. IBC is not an entity of locally advanced breast carcinoma (LABC) but is completely separate according to epidemiological and molecular evidence. The outcomes of these two diseases are quite

N. Guler (✉)
Hacettepe University Cancer Institute, Department of Medical Oncology, Ankara, Turkey
e-mail: nguler@hacettepe.edu.tr

A. Aydiner et al. (eds.), *Breast Cancer*, https://doi.org/10.1007/978-3-319-96947-3_11

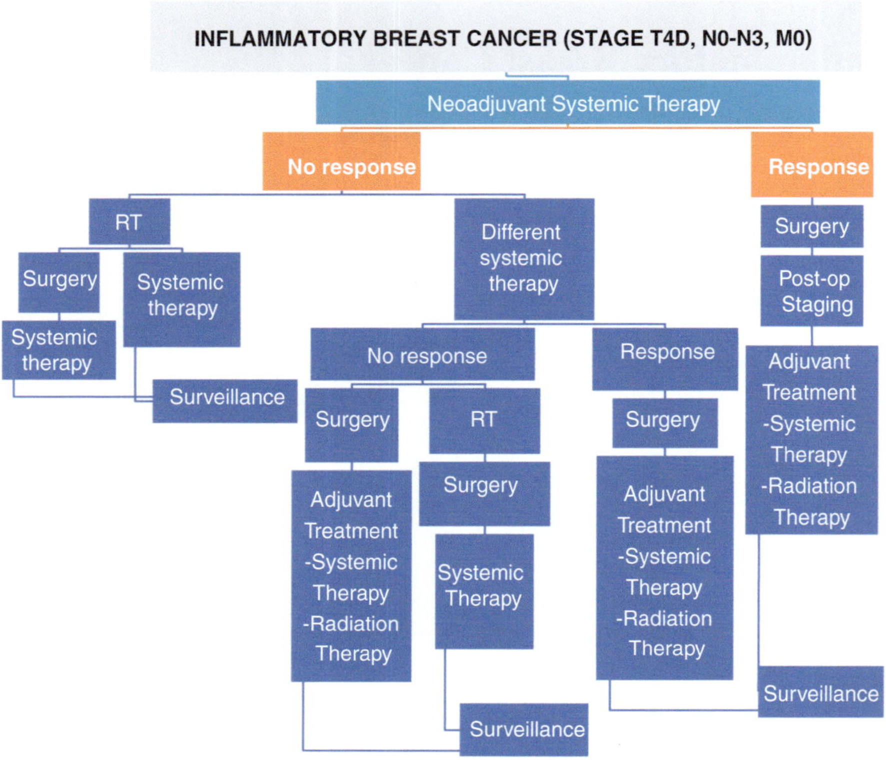

Fig. 11.1 Management of inflammatory breast cancer

different: younger age at diagnosis, higher tumor grade, and the absence of the estrogen receptor (*ER*) in the tumor are more suggestive of primary IBC than LABC [1, 2, 4]. In addition, a distinction must be made between primary and secondary IBC [2]. In primary IBC, skin alterations and carcinoma develop concurrently from the previously healthy breast, whereas in secondary IBC, inflammatory skin alterations appear subsequent to malignancy development [1, 2, 4, 5] (Fig. 11.1).

Epidemiology, Etiology, and Risk Factors

The reported incidence of IBC varies due to a lack of consensus regarding the case definition for the disease [9]. In the United States, the incidence of IBC ranges from 1% to 6% [10–12]. Data from the SEER program have demonstrated that the age-adjusted incidence rates for IBC increased significantly between 1988–1990 and 1997–1999 (from 2.0 to 2.5 cases/100,000 woman-years; $P < 0.001$) [13]. The incidence of IBC is significantly higher in African-American women than in Caucasian women (3.1/100,000 woman-years vs. 2.2/100,000 woman-years, respectively)

[13]. The incidence is lowest among Asian Pacific Islander women (0.7 cases/100,000 woman-years) [14]. In Morocco, Egypt, Algeria, and Tunisia, the reported incidence rates are very high, and nearly 10–15% of all breast cancers are stated to present as IBC [15–18].

IBC generally has an early onset. The maximal peak age at diagnosis is approximately 50 years. According to the SEER database, the median age at diagnosis is lower in patients with IBC (58.8 years) than in patients with non-T4 breast cancer (61.7 years, $P < 0.0001$) and LABC (66.2 years, $P < 0.0001$) [13]. In addition, race seems to be an important risk factor, as African-American women are at a higher risk of developing the disease. The age of onset also varies according to race and ethnicity [14]. Compared to Caucasians, African-Americans present at a younger age of onset (median age 55.2 versus 58.1 years) with an inferior prognosis. However, Hispanic women present with the youngest average age (median 50.5 years) at the initial diagnosis of IBC.

Possible risk factors for IBC are young age at first birth (<20 years), pregnancy (21–26% of IBC cases develop during or after pregnancy), lactation (longer cumulative duration of breastfeeding history), increased BMI (>26.65; the odds ratio for IBC vs. other types of BC is 2.45), blood group A, and rural residency [1–4, 12, 19–22]. However, it should be recognized that these risk factors are currently based on smaller studies and have not been well-established.

Immunological factors have been examined in Tunisian studies. Immunodeficiency was not observed, but the results suggested that a hyperimmune response may be the cause of this rapidly progressing breast cancer [23, 24].

Because of the rapid onset and clinical characteristics of IBC, the involvement of viral infection was suggested by Pogo et al. [25]. They detected *human mammary tumor virus (HMTV),* a provirus structure with 96% homology with *mouse mammary tumor virus (MMTV),* in 71% of IBC cases compared to 40% of non-IBC cases in American patients [25]. *HMTV*-positive IBC was significantly higher in breast cancer patients in Tunisia (74%) compared with those in the United States (36%), Italy (38%), Argentina (31%), and Vietnam (0.8%) [26]. Another study from Egypt demonstrated that *human cytomegalovirus* (*HCMV*) infection enhances the expression and activation of transcription factor *NF*-kB (*nuclear factor*-kB/*p65′*, which controls different cytokines) signaling in IBC patients [27]. *HCMV* infection may be associated with the etiology and progression of IBC versus non-IBC. The relationship between viral etiology and IBC is under investigation in the United States [2].

Although the median age of IBC is younger than that of non-IBC, *BRCA1, BRCA2,* and *PTEN* do not play a strong role in IBC. *BRCA* testing is not routinely recommended, except in cases with a strong family history [8]. In one retrospective study, there was no statistically significant difference ($P = 0.169$) in the rate of *BRCA1* and *BRCA2* mutations between IBC (35.9%; total 39 patients) and non-IBC (26.1%; total 992 patients) [28]. In another study, the percentage of patients with a positive family history was 13% in IBC cases and 8% in non-IBC [19]. This difference was not statistically significant. Family history was significantly more common in IBC cases than in non-IBC cases (20% versus 5%, respectively) in one Pakistani study [29].

Imaging Studies

Mammography is the least sensitive and least effective method for the diagnosis of IBC and detects only 43% of breast parenchymal lesions [30]. Therefore, IBC is usually not detected by mammographic scanning. The most common signs of IBC by mammography are skin thickening and trabecular distortion; a mass is often visible by ultrasonography (USG) [5, 6, 31]. Both the mammary tissue and local lymph nodes should be evaluated by USG. Axillary lymph node metastases are detected in 90% of all patients. Parenchymal lesions in the breasts can be identified in nearly 95% of IBC patients by USG, which is also a useful method for obtaining biopsies from lesions. Recently, magnetic resonance imaging (MRI) has become a popular method for visualizing the breast. The reported success rates of MRI, USG, and mammography in detecting parenchymal lesions in patients with proven IBC are 100%, 95% and 80%, respectively [31]. Although MRI appears to be the best method, it is not recommended for routine diagnostic imaging and is advised only under two conditions [6]: when parenchymal lesions cannot be detected with mammography or USG and when patients are recruited for research studies that evaluate the use of MRI of the breast in the diagnosis of IBC.

Local-regional disease is present in all patients diagnosed with IBC; however, approximately 30% of patients have metastatic disease at the time of diagnosis. Therefore, a systemic staging workup [e.g., computed tomography, bone scintigraphy, ^{8}F FDG PET/CT (fluorodeoxyglucose positron emission tomography/computed tomography)] should be performed in every patient [1–5, 6, 8]. In addition, cross-sectional imaging of the neck and an evaluation of infra- and supraclavicular lymph nodes during radiological imaging and planning of radiotherapy are equally important [6].

Tissue Sampling and Pathology

Preoperative systemic chemotherapy (PSC) is the standard therapy for IBC treatment [1–5]. Sufficient tissue sampling from the parenchymal lesion in the affected breast during the pretreatment period is essential for both future treatment planning and subsequent research studies [1–4, 6]. The presence of an invasive cancer, the identification of the histological type and grade of the tumor, and the expression of the *ER*, progesterone receptor (*PR*), and *HER2* should be clarified with utmost care. If there is doubt about metastasis in the axillary and/or supraclavicular lymph nodes, image-guided core biopsies and analysis of prognostic and predictive markers are suggested [6]. For patients who meet the diagnostic criteria for IBC, obtaining at least two skin punch biopsies to determine dermal lymphatic invasion (DLI) is recommended. Apart from their significance in indicating the presence of DLI, these biopsies are also important for the diagnosis of invasive cancer in patients with no detectable intraparenchymal breast lesions or regional metastases. The best site for sampling is believed to be the region with the most significant color alteration on the breast skin

[6]. A 2- to 8-mm biopsy specimen taken from that region is sufficient to demonstrate the presence of DLI. However, although DLI is responsible for the clinically observed inflammatory alterations in IBC, it is not necessary for diagnosis [6, 8, 32].

All pathological subtypes of invasive adenocarcinoma can be associated with IBC [4, 32, 33]. IBC is also rarely seen in male patients [34]. IBC is often in the form of ductal carcinoma. It is a highly angiogenic and invasive type of cancer that is characterized by a high histological grade and *HER2* positivity with a high rate of *ER* negativity. *p53* mutations are common (70% in IBC and 48% in non-IBC, $P = 0.0238$) [29].

There are three subtypes of IBC: clinicopathologically apparent IBC, clinically apparent IBC, and pathological (occult) IBC [2]. Two population-based studies used this classification for IBC to demonstrate that patients with occult IBC have better disease-free survival (DFS) (5-year DFS 51.6% vs. 25.6%, respectively) and OS than patients with clinically apparent IBC (5-year OS 40% vs. 28.6%, respectively) [35, 36].

The molecular subtypes of IBC are the same as those of non-IBC (luminal, triple negative, and *HER2* positive). Twenty to forty percent of all IBC cases are triple negative (TN), whereas 15–20% of non-IBC cases display this molecular subtype [37].

Preoperative Systemic Therapy

Historically, radical mastectomy was the primary modality for treating IBC. Surgery alone resulted in a very poor prognosis and a 5-year survival of less than 5%, with a median survival of 12–32 months [38, 39]. Over the past 30 years, the treatment of IBC has significantly evolved. Because of the systemic nature of the disease, adding radiotherapy (RT) after surgery increased only locoregional control without increasing OS [40–42]. The addition of preoperative systemic chemotherapy (PSC) (also referred to as neoadjuvant, preoperative, or induction) before surgery and RT has been associated with significantly increased survival rates of 30–50% for 5-year survival and 24% for 15-year survival [43–48].

Breast-conserving surgery is not suggested for IBC because it is a disease that often has a diffuse character [1–4]. Mastectomy and axillary lymph node dissection are the optimal surgical procedure. A clinical response evaluation by physical examination and imaging techniques may underestimate the extent of residual disease [1–5, 8, 46, 47]. The removal of all gross disease is important because skin lymphatic involvement may extend beyond the area of visible skin changes. After mastectomy, postmastectomy RT to the chest wall and axillary, infraclavicular, and supraclavicular, and internal mammary lymph nodes (if involved; consider internal mammary nodes if not clinically involved) is part of standard multimodality treatment [1–4, 8, 48].

Historically, primary systemic treatment included only chemotherapy (CT). However, in recent years, some targeted therapies have been used together with CT based on tumor characteristics. Survival was analyzed in IBC cases who were treated before and after October 2006 at MD Anderson Cancer Center (MDACC) [49]. The date October 2006 was chosen because this date was the beginning of anti-*HER2* usage in standard neoadjuvant chemotherapies (NACT) and the opening of a multidisciplinary IBC clinic. Before this date, 3-year OS was 63%; after this date, the rate increased to 82% ($P = 0.02$). Multivariate analysis demonstrated that anti-*HER2* therapies (HR = 0.38; 95% CI 0.17–0.84; $P = 0.02$) and *ER* positivity (HR = 0.032; CI 0.14–0.74, $P = 0.01$) are important factors for survival.

Randomized clinical trials assessing therapy have not been performed because of the rare occurrence of the disease. Many of the cases are evaluated in protocols in the same way as the LABC study. Data are gathered from one-armed studies and retrospective case series [43–48].

Treatment should begin with NACT. There is no standard primary CT regimen or combination. However, anthracyclines and taxanes are constant members of current primary chemotherapy regimens. The optimal sequence, dose, duration, and intensity of the CT regimen remain to be defined, and the optimal sequence and type of locoregional therapy have not yet been resolved.

Preoperative Systemic Chemotherapy

In pre-1970 clinical trials, IBC cases were excluded because of their rarity and poor overall prognosis. Most IBC cases were treated with the same regimens used for the treatment of non-IBC cases. In recent years, CT trials specifically designed for patients with IBC have increased. The response to PSC has prognostic significance. Patients with pCR (complete clearance of the tumor in the breast and axilla) have a significantly increased DFS rate. Here, I would like to discuss PSC chronologically.

MDACC is the most experienced center for IBC. Since 1974, MDACC has been planning prospective studies on only IBC patients. As of 2010, 242 IBC patients had been enrolled in clinical trials. These studies demonstrated that PSC is necessary for this group of patients. The response to NACT is a surrogate marker for long-term survival. The survival of patients without a response to NACT is shorter than those with a response. In one study, NACT was applied to 175 IBC patients [50]. After NACT and surgery, 61 of the 175 patients had residual disease in the breast and axillary lymph nodes. The 5-year relapse-free survival (RFS) was 82.5% and the OS was 78.6% in patients with pCR after NACT, but in the group with residual disease after NACT, RFS was 37.1%, and OS was 25.4%.

First CMF (cyclophosphamide, methotrexate, 5-fluorouracil) and similar regimens, then anthracycline-containing CT regimens, and finally taxanes have been used for NACT in IBC (Fig. 11.2).

Anthracyclines

Active chemotherapy applications for IBC began in 1970. Anthracycline-containing NACT studies involving 15–192 patients have reported improvements in response rates from 20% to 93% and in complete response (CR) rates from 4% to 55% [41]. pCR ratios improved from 3% to 16% [45].

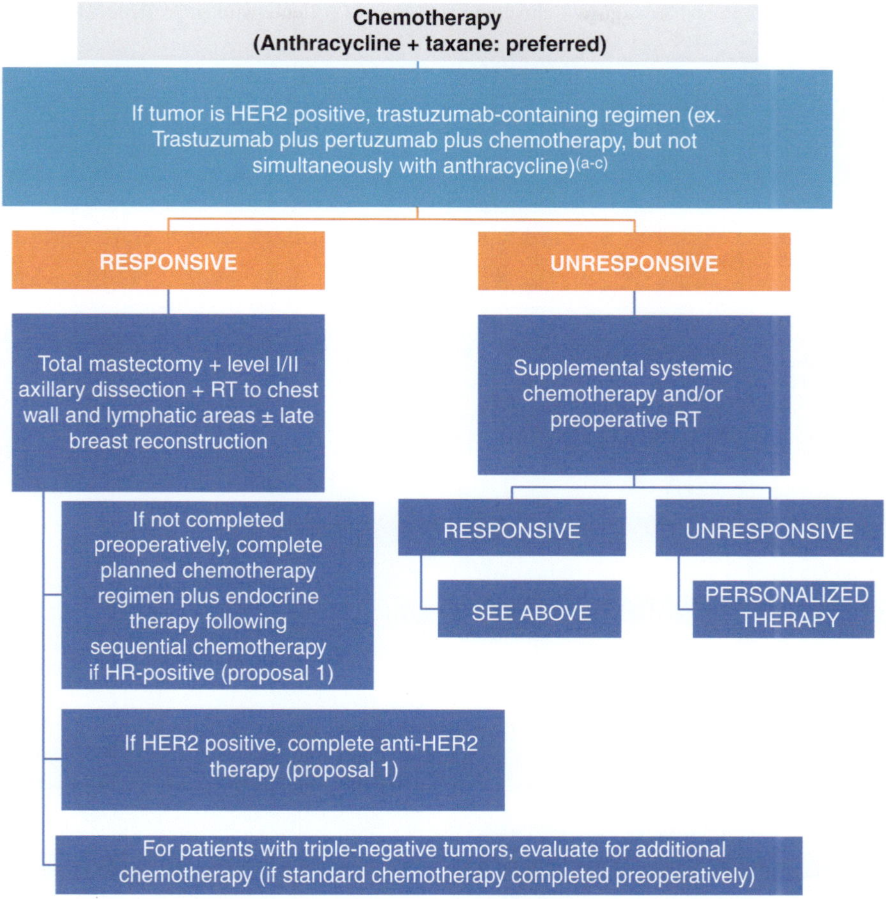

Fig. 11.2 Locoregional and systemic treatment of inflammatory breast cancer. [a]HER2-targeted therapy: Trastuzumab + pertuzumab + chemotherapy should be administered to HER2-positive patients in neoadjuvant therapy. Pertuzumab can be added to adjuvant treatment. [b]If an inadequate response to chemotherapy is considered on postoperative pathological examination, additional adjuvant chemotherapy can be given (e.g., treatment including capecitabine or platinum in TNBC), despite the completion of preoperative chemotherapy. [c]Consider adjuvant bisphosphonate therapy in postmenopausal (natural or induced) patients receiving adjuvant therapy

The use of CMF ± VP (vincristine-prednisone) and FAC (fluorouracil-doxorubicin-cyclophosphamide) combinations for NACT in 38 IBC cases was reviewed retrospectively [51] (Table 11.1). The overall response rate (ORR) was 57% in the CMF ± VP group and 100% in the FAC group; the median OS was 18 months in the CMF ± VP group and 30 months in the FAC group. Harris et al. evaluated the long-term follow-up of combined modality therapy in 54 IBC patients [46] (Table 11.1). CMF or CAF (cyclophosphamide-doxorubicin-fluorouracil) was applied as PSC. The clinical CR rate was 52% in patients treated with PSC with or without preoperative radiotherapy. pCR was achieved in 37% (13 patients) of the PSC and RT group and 12% (2 patients) of the PSC-only group. The 10-year overall

Table 11.1 Important neoadjuvant chemotherapy trials in patients with stage III inflammatory breast cancer [43, 46, 47, 51–56]

Study group	Chemotherapy protocol	*n*	ORR% (complete + partial)	Median survival (months)	DFS %	OS %
MDACC	FAC-RT-FAC	40	80	38	–	–
Protocol A	FAC-RT-CMF					
MDACC	FAC-surgery	23	57	38	–	–
Protocol B	FAC-RT					
MDACC	FACVP-surgery	43	76	64	–	–
Protocol C	FACVP-CMF-RT					
MDACC protocol D	FACVP-surgery-FACVP or FACVP ± MV or MV according to the response to induction CT	72	77	34+		
MDACC-Ueno-whole group [53]	FAC ± VP	178	72	37	32 (5-year) 28 (10-year) 28 (15-year)	40 (5-year) 35 (10-year)
Bauer et al. [51]	CMF ± VP	38	57	18	–	–
	FAC		100	30		
Harris et al. [46]	CMF or CAF	54	54		–	56 (5-year)
Low et al. [47]	CAFM	46	46	–	–	27 (10-year) 20 (15-year)
Cristofanilli et al. [54]	FAC-3 weekly P-surgery-FAC-weekly P-RT	44	77	46		74 (2-year OS)
Cristofanilli et al. [55]	FAC	178	72	–	39 (3-yearPFS)	53 (3-year)
	FAC-P (weekly or 3-weekly)	62	79		46 (3-yearPFS)	71 (3-year)

survival was 46% in patients who achieved pCR and 31% in patients with residual disease in the breast and axilla ($P = 0.09$).

A total of 107 stage III breast cancer patients were included in one prospective, randomized NCI study [47] (Table 11.1). Forty-six of the patients had IBC. CAF and methotrexate were applied as NACT until the maximal response was achieved. The median follow-up time was 16.8 years. ORR was 57% within IBC patients.

Two hundred forty-two IBC patients who were enrolled between 1974 and 2001 were examined in five study protocols by MDACC [43, 52–56]. A total of 178 patients received neoadjuvant therapy with four different chemotherapy regimens containing anthracycline [52, 53, 56] (Table 11.1).

- Protocol A (First Protocol): Patients received FAC neoadjuvant therapy first and then received radiotherapy, followed by FAC or CMF therapies.

- Protocol B (Second Protocol): Patients received FAC neoadjuvant therapy first and then surgery, followed by adjuvant FAC and radiotherapy.
- Protocol C (Third Protocol): Patients received FACVP (fluorouracil-doxorubicin-cyclophosphamide-vincristine prednisone) as induction therapy first and then surgery, followed by FACVP and CMF radiotherapy.
- Protocol D (Fourth Protocol): Patients received FACVP as induction therapy and then surgery. After surgery, patients with complete responses received adjuvant FACVP.

Patients with partial responses (tumors that decreased in diameter by more than half) received FACVP with MV (methotrexate-vincristine). Patients received MV therapy only when tumors decreased in diameter by approximately 25–50%.

The response rate for all studies was 72%, and the clinical CR rate was 12% [44, 53, 56] (Table 11.1). There were no differences within the four studies in terms of DFS and OS. The median survival was 37 months. The DFS for 5, 10, and 15 years was 32%, 28% and 28%, respectively. The 15-year DFS for patients with complete or partial responses who received induction chemotherapy was 44% and 31%, respectively, and the 15-year OS was 51% and 31%, respectively. The 15-year DFS and OS of patients whose responses were less than partial with induction chemotherapy decreased to 7%. These results indicate the importance of the response to induction chemotherapy for prognosis.

VP or MV therapy combinations in the third and fourth study protocols had no effect on DFS and OS. Surgery after a poor response to NACT did not alter local relapse risk. Surgery and RT application instead of RT-only as a local therapy did not affect DFS and OS. At the 20-year follow-up, the local relapse rate was 20% [53]. Distant metastasis was observed in 39% of patients, and central nervous system (CNS) metastasis was observed in 9% of patients.

Taxanes

The effect of taxane use in NACT for IBC cases was investigated in 1994 and included 44 patients in an MDACC study (Protocol E) [54] (Table 11.1). FAC chemotherapy was used as NACT and adjuvant therapy in all patients. Paclitaxel (P) was added to the therapy regimen of patients with stable disease or who had a minor response to NACT during the preoperative period, and P was added as an adjuvant therapy in all patients. NACT and then surgery, followed by adjuvant chemotherapy and then radiotherapy, were applied. The objective/clinical response rate was 77% (vs. 72% in regimens containing only anthracycline), and the median survival time was 46 months (vs. 37 months in regimens containing only anthracycline). The results were not statistically significant.

In another study, anthracycline-based and taxane-based NACT protocols were compared in patients with IBC. Group 1 included 178 patients who received anthracycline-containing induction chemotherapy, and group 2 included 62 patients

Table 11.2 MDACC comparison of neoadjuvant-only anthracycline and anthracycline-taxane-containing chemotherapy protocols in patients with inflammatory breast cancer [53, 55]

Parameter	Group 1	Group 2
n	178 patients	62 patients
Follow-up years	1973–1993	1994–2000
Median follow-up (months)	148 (85–283)	45 (21–99)
Chemotherapy protocol	FAC-based regimens	FAC followed by 3 weekly P or weekly high-dose P
ORR	72%	79%
3-year PFS	39%	46% $p = 0.19$
3-year OS	53%	71% $p = 0.12$
pCR rate	10%	25%
ER-negative tumors	33%	65%
Median PFS (*ER*-negative group)	18 months	27 months $p = 0.042$
Median OS (*ER*-negative group)	32 months	54 months $p = 0.035$
3-year PFS (*ER*-negative group)	31%	39%
3-year OS (*ER*-negative group)	43%	71%

who received taxane-containing chemotherapy (Tables 11.1 and 11.2) [54, 55]. The median follow-up period was 148 months (range: 85–283 months) for group 1 and 45 months (range: 21–99 months) for group 2. The 3-year OS was 71% in group 2 and 53% in group 1. In conclusion, P is an important agent in IBC therapy. The 3-year OS for patients with *ER*-negative tumors in groups 1 and 2 was 43% and 71%, respectively (32 months and 54 months, respectively ($P = 0.03$)); progression-free survival (PFS) was 31% and 39%, respectively (18 and 27 months, respectively; $P = 0.04$). Taxanes are clearly more effective, particularly in *ER*-negative tumors. The pCR ratio was 10% in the FAC-only group and 25% in the anthracycline-P group; this difference was statistically significant ($P = 0.012$).

A retrospective analysis substantiated these findings using data from 308 IBC patients who were observed between 1980 and 2000 in a study performed in England [57]. In the 1990s, taxane-containing chemotherapy regimens (AP, cisplatin, P) were superior to anthracycline-containing chemotherapy regimens in terms of the 10-year BCSS (43.7% and 23.6%, respectively, $P = 0.03$).

In the GeparTrio trial, an anthracycline and taxane combination (docetaxel/doxorubicin/cyclophosphamide (TAC)) was used as NACT [58]. Participants were stratified by stage (93 IBC, 194 LABC, and 1777 operable breast cancers) and randomized to arms with six or eight cycles of TAC or two cycles of TAC followed by four cycles of vinorelbine/capecitabine chemotherapy. pCR rates and ORRs were not significantly different between IBC and LABC patients (8.6% vs. 11.3% for pCR, respectively; 71% vs. 69.6% for ORR, respectively) but were significantly lower compared with operable breast cancer (17.7% and 83.4%, respectively; $P = 0.002$ and $P < 0.001$, respectively). In IBC patients, there was a nonsignificant trend toward higher pCR rates with a response at midcourse in patients who received eight cycles of TAC compared with those patients who received only six cycles (17.2% vs. 3.3%; $P = 0.103$).

These studies demonstrate that anthracyclines and taxanes are important and necessary as primary chemotherapies for IBC. pCR rates are higher with the use of weekly paclitaxel regimens [59, 60]. The optimal dosage and sequence of anthracycline-taxane remain under investigation (taxane first followed by anthracycline, anthracycline first followed by taxane, or an anthracycline-taxane combination).

Other Chemotherapies

Dose-dense chemotherapy and high-dose chemotherapy with stem cell support may be effective for some selected patient groups. Survival advantages were observed in small, phase II studies (3–4 year DFS of 45–65% and OS of 52–89%), but because there have been no prospective, randomized studies of these protocols, they are not standard and are not suggested except in clinical research trials [1, 2, 45, 61–67].

An international expert panel on IBC recommended a minimum of six cycles of PSC be administered over a course of 4–6 months before surgery [6]. If the response is insufficient, different CT regimens or RT can be applied [6, 8]. RT is applied after surgery, and if the CT program is not completed before surgery, it should be completed during the postoperative period.

Targeted Therapies

Anti-HER2 Therapies

The *HER2* positivity ratio in IBC is very high and varies between 42% and 57% [1–4, 37, 38]. *HER2* positivity is important for the prognosis of non-IBC, but its importance for IBC is not known. A retrospective study that included 179 stage III IBC patients determined that *HER2* positivity or negativity is not related to relapse-free survival (RFS) [68]. Another study of more than 2000 patients conducted in California demonstrated improved breast cancer-specific survival (BCSS) in *HER2*-positive patients compared to *HER2*-negative patients (HR, 0.82; 95% CI 0.68–0.99) [69].

Although the prognostic importance of *HER2* for IBC is not known, *HER2* positivity is important for predicting the response to anti-*HER2* therapies in HER2-positive patients. Trastuzumab (Tr) is a monoclonal antibody against HER2 and the first of the anti-HER2 agents. The addition of Tr to anthracycline- and taxane-containing PSC regimens yielded a significantly increased response and improved survival compared to non-Tr PSC regimens [5, 67, 69–74]. The increase in the pCR rate from 17% to 62.5% was also statistically significant. Unfortunately, the studies included many LABC cases and fewer IBC cases. Studies including only IBC cases are very rare.

Dawood et al. reported that the pCR rate was 62.5% in *HER2*+ IBC cases receiving NACT combined with Tr therapy, and the 2-year PFS was 59.4% [74]. In that study, 3 of the 16 IBC patients had metastatic disease at the beginning of treatment. Forty-eight *HER2*+ LABC (IBC-containing) patients were enrolled in a study by Hurley et al. [75]. Docetaxel-cisplatin-Tr was applied as induction therapy. After chemotherapy, surgery, adjuvant chemotherapy and radiotherapy were performed consecutively. OS was 100% in patients with pCR. In patients with residual disease after NACT, the OS rate ranged from 76% to 83%.

In another study including 9 IBC and 22 LABC patients, docetaxel and Tr were applied as the primary chemotherapy, and the CR rate was 40% [76].

The NOAH (neoadjuvant Herceptin) trial was a prospective, open-label, phase 3, multicenter, randomized study [77]. *HER2*-positive, locally advanced ($n = 174$) or IBC ($n = 61$) cases were enrolled in the study. The patients received anthracycline-based and taxane-based NACT alone or with 1 year of Tr (concurrently with NACT and continued after surgery). A parallel group with *HER2*-negative disease was included and received NACT alone. The relapse, progression, and mortality risks were statistically significantly decreased in the Tr group compared with the CT-only group. The pCR ratio was twofold higher in the Tr group than in the CT-only group (38% and 19%, respectively). After a median follow-up of 5.4 years, the event-free survival (EFS) benefit of the addition of Tr was maintained in patients with *HER2*-positive disease [78]. The 5-year EFS was 58% in the Tr group and 43% in the CT group (HR, 0.64; 95% CI 0.44–0.93; $P = 0.016$). Similarly, during that time period, EFS was strongly associated with pCR in patients who received Tr. In that study, 27% of *HER2*(+) patients had IBC. The 3-year EFS was 70.1% in the Tr group and 53.3% in the CT-only group ($P = 0.0007$). The pCR (complete disappearance of the tumors from both the breast and lymph nodes) rate was 48% in the Tr group and only 13% in the CT-only group ($P = 0.002$) [79].

Tr should be started in the induction chemotherapy period for the treatment of *HER2*-positive LABC or IBC patients. Although there has been no prospective randomized study, Tr therapy should be extended to 1 year. An anthracycline-Tr combination is not suggested because of enhanced cardiotoxicity [5, 6, 8].

Lapatinib is another anti-*HER2*-targeted drug (reversible dual inhibitor of both *HER1* and *HER2*), and studies with lapatinib or lapatinib with paclitaxel are ongoing [80–82]. The clinical RR was 80% for 21 IBC patients who received a lapatinib-paclitaxel combination [81]. In one multicenter, open-label, phase II study with 49 IBC patients, a lapatinib-paclitaxel combination was used as NACT [82]. Patients were divided into two groups: cohort A was positive for *HER2* 2+ or 3+ by immunohistochemical (IHC) methods or FISH (fluorescence in situ hybridization) ± epidermal growth factor receptor (*EGFR*) expression; cohort B was *HER2* negative/ EGFR positive. *HER2* 3+ or FISH-positive patients were analyzed separately. First, patients received lapatinib for only 14 days, followed by 12 weeks of lapatinib and paclitaxel weekly. Cohort B was stopped because of slow enrollment and a lack of efficacy in IBC patients with *HER2*-negative/*EGFR*-positive tumors enrolled in a parallel study, EGF103009. Thirty-five patients completed the study and underwent surgery. The pCR rate of cohort A was 18.2%, and the clinical RR was 78.6% for all groups and 78.1% in the *HER2* 3+ group. The clinical RR was 31% in the *HER2*-positive group receiving only lapatinib, and the pCR rate was 17.6% in all patients who underwent surgery after therapy. The most common side effects of lapatinib were diarrhea and skin eruptions. Lapatinib is currently suggested only for clinical research studies and not for routine clinical applications, and it should only be administered to patients who have *HER2*-positive BC.

In one German randomized, phase III trial (GeparQuinto, GBG 44 trial), lapatinib versus trastuzumab in combination with neoadjuvant anthracycline-taxane-based chemotherapy were compared in the neoadjuvant setting [83]. IBC cases were also included in the study (83 patients had T4d disease). A total of 620 patients were randomly assigned in a 1/1 ratio to receive neoadjuvant therapy with four cycles of EC (epirubicin + cyclophosphamide) every 3 weeks and four cycles of docetaxel (D) with either Tr (every 3 weeks for eight cycles) or lapatinib (L: 1000–1250 mg/day throughout all cycles) before surgery. Of the 620 patients, 309 received ECTr-DTr, and 311 received ECL-DL. The pCR rate was 30.3% in the ECTr-DTr group and 22.7% in the ECL-DL group. The difference was statistically significant ($P = 0.04$). This study demonstrated that the pCR rate was significantly lower in the lapatinib + CT group compared to the Tr + CT group. The investigators concluded that unless long-term outcome data showed different results, lapatinib should not be used outside of clinical trials as a single anti-*HER2* treatment in combination with NACT.

In one prospective randomized study, a lapatinib plus Tr combination was compared to Tr and lapatinib (NeoALTTO trial) [84]. Only early breast cancer patients were enrolled in this study. The NeoALTTO trial demonstrated that dual anti-HER2 inhibition with Tr + lapatinib combined with weekly P significantly increased the proportion of patients achieving pCR (51.3%; 95% CI 43.1–59.5) in the combination group compared with Tr alone (29.5%; 95% CI 22.437.5) and lapatinib alone (24.7%; 95% CI 18.132.3). The difference was statistically significant ($P = 0.0001$). EFS and OS did not differ between treatment groups. However, the 3-year EFS and 3-year OS were significantly improved in women who achieved pCR (HR 0.38, $P = 0.0003$, and HR 0.35, $P = 0.005$, respectively) [85]. The findings from this study confirmed that pCR after neoadjuvant anti-HER2 therapy is an important prognostic factor for survival.

The NeoSphere study was a multicenter, open-label, phase II randomized trial. IBC cases (29 of 417 patients) were also enrolled in this study. Tr and another anti-*HER2* targeted agent, pertuzumab, were used during the preoperative CT period [86]. The pCR ratio was higher in the pertuzumab + Tr + docetaxel combination arm then in the Tr + docetaxel combination arm (39.3% vs. 21.5%; $p = 0.0063$). The TRYPHANEA study, a phase II cardiac safety study, was a randomized, three-arm study [87]. Overall, 225 *HER2*-positive LABC, IBC and operable breast cancer patients were enrolled in the study. In the first arm, 5-fluorouracil, epirubicin, cyclophosphamide [FEC] + trastuzumab (H) + pertuzumab (P) was followed by docetaxel + H + P. In the second arm, FEC only was followed by docetaxel + H + P. In the third arm, a docetaxel + carboplatin + H + P combination was administered. The pCR ratio was similar in all treatment groups but was the highest in the third arm (66.2%). After these two studies, the Food and Drug Administration (FDA) approved

Table 11.3 Pathological complete response and survival rates according to neoadjuvant chemotherapy protocol in inflammatory breast cancer

	Type of study			
Trial	NACT protocol	*n*	pCR rate	Survival
Ueno et al. [53]	Retrospective	178	10%	15-year DFS 28%
	Anthracycline-containing regimens			10-year OS 35%
Cristofanili et al. [55]	Retrospective	62	25%	3-year PFS 46%
	Anthracycline + paclitaxel			3-year OS 71%
Dawood et al. [74]	Retrospective	16 (3 patients	62.5%	2-year PFS
	Anthracycline + paclitaxel + trastuzumab in HER2-positive patients	With stage 4 disease)		59.4%
Baselga et al. [79]	Prospective randomized study	61		3-year EFS
	(NOAH trial)		48% (+Tr) vs. 13% (−Tr)	70.1% (+Tr) vs. 53.3% (−Tr)
	Anthracycline + taxane ± trastuzumab in HER2-positive patients			

the use of the H + P + docetaxel combination as NACT for *HER2*-positive LABC, IBC, and early breast cancer (>2 cm tumor or axillary lymph node positive) [88].

The pCR rates and survival after anthracycline, anthracycline + taxane, and CT + trastuzumab-containing NACT regimens were used to treat IBC are outlined in Table 11.3.

In another study, a new anti-*HER2* agent, afatinib (an oral tyrosine kinase inhibitor and irreversible binder of *HER1, HER2,* and *HER4*), was compared to Tr and lapatinib in the neoadjuvant setting for patients with *HER2*-positive stage IIIA, B, C, and IBC [89]. A total of 29 patients were randomized to afatinib (n = 10), lapatinib (n = 8), or trastuzumab (n = 11). These drugs were administered for a duration of 6 weeks until the patients underwent surgery. The ORR was determined for eight afatinib-, six lapatinib-, and four trastuzumab-treated patients. Drug-related adverse events were recorded in all afatinib-treated patients and commonly included diarrhea, acneiform dermatitis, and paronychia. Diarrhea and rash were documented in six of eight lapatinib-treated patients. The authors concluded that afatinib demonstrated more favorable clinical activity than lapatinib and trastuzumab did for neoadjuvant treatment of HER2-positive LABC and IBC.

Antiangiogenic Therapies

Vascular endothelial growth factor (*VEGF*) expression is increased in IBC. Therefore, anti-angiogenic drugs have been suggested as therapy targets. The anti-angiogenic drug bevacizumab has been used together with chemotherapy in induction therapy but did not meet expectations [1–4, 48, 71, 90, 91]. NCI-0173 was a small, phase II study that included 21 patients and assessed the efficacy of doxorubicin and docetaxel combined with bevacizumab in the preoperative treatment of LABC/IBC cases [92]. The clinical RR was 67%, and the pCR rate was 5%. The BEVERLY-2 study was a multicenter, one-armed, open-label, phase II study performed in France with *HER2*-positive non-metastatic IBC patients [93]. First, four cycles of a FEC-bevacizumab combination were applied, followed by four cycles of a docetaxel-bevacizumab-Tr combination every 21 days. Forty-two (8%) of 52 patients completed eight cycles of therapy, and 49 patients (94%) underwent surgery. The pCR rate was 63.5%. The 3-year DFS rate was 68%, and the OS rate was 90%; the 3-year DFS rate for patients who achieved pCR was 80%. Astheny and vomiting were reported as the most common side effects. In the other part of this study, the numbers of circulating tumor cells (CTCs) and circulating endothelial cells (CECs) were counted before the study began, at the fifth cycle, before surgery, during the postoperative period, and during the first year [94]. The 3-year DFS was 95% in patients with pCR, and these patients were CTC-free after treatment. For baseline (before treatment) patient CTC numbers of <1 and >1, 3-year survival was 81% and 43%, respectively; this difference was statistically significant ($P = 0.01$). Prognostic importance was not detected for CEC. This study is important in terms of demonstrating the prognostic effect of CTC. In another study, CTCs were determined to be a strong predictor of worse prognosis in patients with newly diagnosed IBC [95].

Semaxanib (*SU5416*) is an organic small receptor tyrosine kinase inhibitor that inhibits *VEGF*-mediated signaling through *VEGFR2*. The effectiveness of a doxorubicin and semaxanib combination was investigated in 18 stage IIIB and IBC patients in a phase IB study [96]. Median survival has not yet been provided. After treatment, the density of microvessels and blood flow through the tumor decreased. Neutropenia was reported as a factor in dose-limiting toxicity. Congestive heart failure was monitored in four patients (22%).

Antiangiogenic drug studies continue with pazopanib, a new multi-targeted tyrosine kinase inhibitor.

New Targets

There are many ongoing targeted therapy drug studies (*p53* gene therapy, *p53* stabilizer agents, proteasome inhibitors, *Tie-2* kinase inhibitors, *E-cadherin* inhibitors, phosphatidyl-inositol-3-kinase inhibitors, farnesyltransferase inhibitors, etc.) [1–4, 44, 48, 71, 90, 91]. *p53* mutations are associated with decreased responses to CT and decreased survival outcomes.

EGFR overexpression occurs in 30% of IBC cases. Mortality risk is increased with increased expression of *EGFR* and chemokine receptors (*CXCR4* and *CCR7*) in IBC [97]. The 5-year OS was 24.8% in an IHC analysis of CXCR4-positive patients and 42.3% in the negative group. The 5-year OS was 20% in an IHC analysis of

CCR7-positive patients and 41.9% in the negative group. These genes have been announced as new targets for therapy. The effectiveness of the human-*EGFR* antibody panitumumab and chemotherapy (nanoparticle paclitaxel and carboplatin) combination will be investigated in *HER2*-negative IBC cases during the preoperative period.

A deficiency in the Ras signaling pathway member low-affinity insulin-like growth binding protein (*LIBC/WINT1*) and overexpression of Ras homolog gene family member C (*RhoC*) guanosine triphosphatase (*GTPase*) have been established in IBC [98]. In situ hybridization analysis of paraffin blocks demonstrated that LIBC deficiency was 80% in IBC cases and 21% in non-IBC cases ($P = 0.0013$). The *RhoC GTPase* overexpression rate was 90% in IBC cases and 38% in non-IBC cases ($P = 0.0095$). These genes may be a target for the treatment of IBC. Farnesyltransferase inhibitors (*FTIs*) inhibit RhoC and angiogenesis. *FTIs* have been investigated for IBC. The FTI tipifarnib (T) enhances the antitumor effects of chemotherapy in vitro, has activity in metastatic breast cancer, and enhances the pCR rate of neoadjuvant AC chemotherapy. In one phase I-II trial, T plus weekly P and 2-week AC CT were tested as a neoadjuvant treatment for HER2-negative *ER* and/or PR-positive LABC (stratum A: 33 patients) and IBC (stratum B: 22 patients) irrespective of *ER/PR* expression [99]. The breast pCR rate was 18% in stratum A and 4% in stratum B. These results are insufficient to indicate the use of FTIs for the neoadjuvant treatment of IBC.

Anaplastic lymphoma kinase (*ALK*) gene amplification or overexpression may occur in IBC [100, 101]. IBC patients are currently being evaluated for the presence of *ALK* genetic abnormalities and, when eligible, enrolled into clinical trials evaluating *ALK*-targeted therapies (the small-molecule dual tyrosine kinase *cMET/ALK* inhibitor crizotinib).

Endocrine Therapies

ER and *PgR* negativity are higher in IBC than in other types of breast cancer [1–4, 32, 33]. Some studies have reported that up to 83% of IBC tumors are *ER* negative [102, 103]. HR negativity is associated with a more aggressive clinical course, shorter survival, and poor prognosis. The median survival for HR-positive IBC is superior to that of HR-negative IBC according to the SEER data (4 vs. 2 years; $P = 0.0001$) [13].

There are no studies of neoadjuvant hormonal therapy in primary IBC. Antiestrogen therapy should be applied after induction therapy and adjuvant chemotherapy are completed for HR-positive patients [6, 8]. Antiestrogen therapy should include either tamoxifen (±ovarian suppression) or an aromatase inhibitor depending on the patient's menopausal status. The minimum period for use is 5–7 years.

The anti-inflammatory and cholesterol-lowering effects of statins suggest they may have antitumor effects as well. The effect of statins on IBC was determined in a cohort study conducted by MDACC [104]. PFS was improved in patients who received hydrophobic statins (atorvastatin, pravastatin, rosuvastatin) (HR, 0.49; 95% CI 0.28–0.84; $P < 0.01$). No significant response was observed in patients who received lipophilic statins (fluvastatin, lovastatin, simvastatin). The mechanism of this effect is not known. Double-blind, prospective randomized studies are needed to explain this effect.

Monitoring the Response to Treatment

The international IBC consensus panel recommends that monitoring of the response to PSC entails a combination of physical examination and imaging techniques [6]. Physical examination of the breast and regional lymph nodes for response may be conducted every 6–9 weeks [105]. The breasts are usually photographed during the examination because the response to treatment can be monitored by the reduction in erythema and edema [106]. After completing therapy, radiological evaluation should be performed and compared with the initial examination data. If necessary, radiological evaluation can be performed in the middle of the treatment course to confirm or refute the clinical findings.

Mammography and USG are recommended for radiological evaluation. MRI may be a better option to evaluate the response to therapy if it is available and affordable [5, 6]. In one trial, FDG-PET/CT was used to evaluate the response to NACT [107]. Thirty-two patients were included in the study. In patients with CR according to PET/CT imaging, only 26% had pCR. In conclusion, more research is needed on the use of PET/CT to evaluate the response to therapy.

Follow-Up After Therapy

After the completion of treatment, regular history, physical examination, and mammography are recommended for follow-up by the American Society of Clinical Oncology (ASCO) and the European Society of Medical Oncology (ESMO) [108, 109]. Physical examinations should be performed at 3- to 6-month intervals for the first 3 years, every 6–12 months for years 4 and 5, and annually thereafter. Yearly mammography of the other breast is suggested by ASCO [108]. The examination of local lymph nodes with yearly USG has been suggested, although the data are insufficient [6]. Genetic consultations are particularly important for patients with a family history of breast and ovarian cancer [8]. Prophylactic contralateral mastectomy should not be performed unless there are risk factors that make this obligatory. Routine performance of other radiological examinations, blood tests, and tumor markers are not suggested in asymptomatic patients. Distant metastases are common during the follow-up period of the disease. Metastasis was observed in 203 of 478 stage III IBC patients at a median observation time of 29 months [110].

The most common metastasis locations were the bone (28%), lung (21%), liver (21%), and CNS (21%). CNS metastasis was most frequent in *HER2*-positive and triple-negative subtypes, as with non-IBC subtypes ($P = 0.001$).

Conclusion

Multimodal therapy (PST, surgery, and radiotherapy) is the main treatment method for IBC [1–6, 8, 111] (Fig. 11.1). Currently, anthracycline- and taxane-containing chemotherapy protocols as PSC are preferred (with the addition of trastuzumab in *HER2+* patients). Following PSC, surgical assessment is suggested. A modified radical mastectomy can be performed in patients with recovered skin eruption. Next, adjuvant RT is applied. In patients with no response to PSC, additional systemic CT and/or preoperative RT is planned. Trastuzumab therapy should be started during the NACT period with taxanes and extended to 1 year for *HER2*-positive patients. Antiestrogen therapy is suggested for at least 5 years for HR-positive patients. New combined CT regimens and new targeted therapies are being investigated to increase the pCR ratio and survival times.

In recent years, an international congress devoted to IBC has been planned [112]. Opening specific IBC clinics similar to that established by MDACC will improve outcomes and promote well-designed research trials.

CAF cyclophosphamide-doxorubicin-fluorouracil, *CMF* cyclophosphamide-methotrexate-fluorouracil, *CMF ± VP* CMF plus/minus vincristine-prednisone, *DFS* disease-free survival, *FAC* fluorouracil-doxorubicin-cyclophosphamide, *FACVP* FAC plus vincristine-prednisone, *FACVP-MV* FACVP plus methotrexate and vinblastine, *MDACC* MD Anderson Cancer Center, *ORR* overall response rate, *OS* overall survival, *P* paclitaxel, *PFS* progression-free survival, *RT* radiotherapy

ER estrogen receptor, *FAC* fluorouracil-doxorubicin-cyclophosphamide, *MDACC* MD Anderson Cancer Center, *ORR* overall response rate (complete + partial response), *OS* overall survival, *P* paclitaxel, *pCR* pathological complete response, *PFS* progression-free survival

DFS disease-free survival, *EFS* event-free survival, *NACT* neoadjuvant chemotherapy, *NOAH* neoadjuvant Herceptin trial, *pCR* pathological complete response, *PFS* progression-free survival, *OS* overall survival, *Tr* trastuzumab

References

1. Barsky SH, Mrozek E, Love R. Inflammatory breast cancer. In: Bland KI, Copeland III EM, editors. The breast comprehensive management of benign and malignant diseases. 4th ed. Philadelphia: Saunders; 2009. p. 1393–402.
2. Dean-Colomb WM, Cristofanilli M. Inflammatory breast cancer. In: Kantarjian HM, Wolff RA, Koller CA, editors. The MD Anderson manual of medical oncology. 2nd ed. Beijing: Mc Graw-Hill; 2011. p. 712–29.

3. Woodward WE, Cristofanilli M. Inflammatory breast cancer. Semin Radiat Oncol. 2009;19:256–65.
4. Overmoyer B, Pierce LJ. Inflammatory breast cancer. In: Harris JR, Morrow M, Osborne JK, editors. Disease of the breast. 5th ed. Philadelphia: Wolters Kluwer; 2015. p. 800–15.
5. Yamauchi H, Woodward WA, Valero V, Alvarez RH, Lucci A, Buchholz TA, et al. Inflammatory breast cancer: what we know and what we need to learn. Oncologist. 2012;17:891–9.
6. Dawood S, Merajver SD, Viens P, Vermeulen PB, Swain SM, Buchholz TA, et al. International expert panel on inflammatory breast cancer: consensus statement for standardized diagnosis and treatment. Ann Oncol. 2011;22:515–23.
7. Rabban J. Breast. In: Edge SB, Byrd DB, Compton CC, Fritz AG, Grene FI, Trotti A, editors. AJCC cancer staging manual. 7th ed. Chicago: Springer; 2010. p. 345–77.
8. National Comprehensive Cancer Network (NCCN). NCCN clinical practice guideline in oncology. Breast Cancer v. 1.2018. www.nccn.org.
9. Hirko KA, Soliman AS, Banerjee M, Ruterbusch J, Harford JB, Merajver SD, et al. A comparison of criteria to identify inflammatory breast cancer cases from medical records and the surveillance, epidemiology and end results data base, 2007–2009. Breast J. 2014;20:185–91.
10. Levine PH, Venerosa C. The epidemiology of inflammatory breast cancer. Semin Oncol. 2008;35:11–6.
11. Dawood S, Cristofanilli M. What progress have we made in managing inflammatory breast cancer? Oncology (Willingston Park). 2007;21:673–9.
12. Anderson WF, Schairer C, Chen BE, Hance KW, Levine PH. Epidemiology of inflammatory breast cancer (IBC). Breast Dis. 2005;22:9–23.
13. Hance KW, Anderson WF, Devesa SS, Young HA, Levine PH. Trends in inflammatory breast carcinoma incidence and survival: the surveillance, epidemiology, and end results program at the National Cancer Institute. J Natl Cancer Inst. 2005;97:966–75.
14. Wingo PA, Jamison PM, Young JL, Gargiullo P. Population-based statistics for women diagnosed with inflammatory breast cancer. Cancer Causes Control. 2004;15:321–8.
15. Corbex M, Bouzbid S, Boffetta P. Features of breast cancer in developing countries, examples from North-Africa. Eur J Cancer. 2014;50:1808–18.
16. Slaoui M, Razine R, Ibrahimi A, Attaleb M, Mzibri ME, Amrani M. Breast cancer in Morocco: a literature review. Asian Pac J Cancer Prev. 2014;15:1067–74.
17. Chiedozi LC. Rapidly progressing breast cancer in Nigeria. Eur J Surg Oncol. 1987;13:505–9.
18. Maalej M, Frikha H, Salem B, Daoud J, Bouaouina N, Ben Abdallah M, et al. Breast cancer in Tunisia: clinical and epidemiological study. Bull Cancer. 1999;86:302–6.
19. Chang S, Buzdar AU, Hursting SD. Inflammatory breast cancer and body-mass index. J Clin Oncol. 1998;16:3731–5.
20. Chang S, Alderfer JR, Asmar L, Buzdar AU. Inflammatory breast cancer survival: the role of obesity and menopausal status at diagnosis. Breast Cancer Res Treat. 2000;64:157–63.
21. Schairer C, Li Y, Frawley P, Graubard BI, Wellman RD, Buist DS, et al. Risk factors for inflammatory breast cancer and other invasive breast cancer. J Natl Cancer Inst. 2013;105:1373–84.
22. Mohamed MM, Al-Raawi D, Sabet SF, El-Shinawi M. Inflammatory breast cancer: new factors contribute to disease etiology: review. J Adv Res. 2013;6:526–35.
23. Levine PH, Mourali N, Tabbane F, Loon J, Terasaki P, Tsang P, et al. Studies on the role of cellular immunity and genetics in the etiology of rapidly progressing breast cancer in Tunisia. Int J Cancer. 1981;27:611–5.
24. Mourali N, Levine PH, Tabanne F, Belhassen S, Bahi J, Bennaceur M, et al. Rapidly progressing breast cancer (poussee evolutive) in Tunisia: studies on delayed hypersensitivity. Int J Cancer. 1978;22:1–3.
25. Pogo BG, Holland JF, Levine PH. Human mammary tumor virus in inflammatory breast cancer. Cancer. 2010;116(11 suppl):2741–4.
26. Levine PH, Pogo BG, Klouj A, Coronel S, Woodson K, Melana SM, et al. Increasing evidence for a human breast carcinoma virus with geographic differences. Cancer. 2004;101:721–6.
27. El-Shinawi M, Mohamed HT, El-Ghonaimy EA, Tantawy M, Younis A, Schneider RJ, et al. Human cytomegalovirus infection enhances NF/kB/p65 signaling in inflammatory breast cancer patients. PLoS One. 2013;8:1–10.

28. Gutierrez-Barrera AM, Turco DL, Alvarez RH, Litton JK, Valero V, Hortobagyi GN, et al. BRCA mutations in women with inflammatory breast cancer. J Clin Oncol. 2010;(ASCO breast cancer symposium abstracts) 28:Abstract 192.
29. Aziz SA, Pervez S, Khan S, Kayani N, Azam SI, Rahbar MH. Case control study of prognostic markers and disease outcome in inflammatory carcinoma breast: a unique clinical experience. Breast J. 2001;7:398–404.
30. Chow CK. Imaging in inflammatory breast carcinoma. Breast Dis. 2005;22:45–54.
31. Yang WT, Le-Petross HT, Macapinlac H, Carkaci S, Gonzalez-Angulo AM, Dawood S, et al. Inflammatory breast cancer: PET/CT, MRI, mammography and ultrasonography findings. Breast Cancer Res Treat. 2008;109:417–26.
32. Morgensztern D. Breast pathology. In: Silva OE, Zurrida S, editors. Breast cancer, a practical guide. 3rd ed. Edinburgh: Elsevier; 2005. p. 84–94.
33. Stamatakos MD. Invasive breast cancer. In: Jacops L, Finlayson CA, editors. Early diagnosis and treatment of cancer: breast cancer. Philadelphia: Saunders-Elsevier; 2011. p. 21–54.
34. Abner A, Kaufman M, Pories S, Gauvin G. Unusual presentations of malignancy. Case 1. Male inflammatory (?) breast cancer. J Clin Oncol. 2001;19:3288–9.
35. Amparo RS, Angel CD, Ana LH, Antonio LC, Vicente MS, Carlos FM, et al. Inflammatory breast carcinoma: pathological or clinical entity? Breast Cancer Res Treat. 2000;64:269–73.
36. Lucas FV, Perez-Mesa C. Inflammatory carcinoma of the breast. Cancer. 1978;41:1595–605.
37. Li J, Gonzalez-Angulo AM, Allen PK, Yu TK, Woodward WA, Ueno NT, et al. Triple-negative subtype predicts poor overall survival and high locore-gional relapse in inflammatory breast cancer. Oncologist. 2011;16:1675–83.
38. Taylor G, Meltzer A. Inflammatory carcinoma of the breast. Am J Cancer. 1938;33:33–49.
39. Kell MR, Morrow M. Surgical aspects of inflammatory breast cancer. Breast Dis. 2005;22:67–73.
40. Bruckman JE, Harris JR, Levene MB, Chaffey JT, Hellman S. Results of treating stage III carcinoma of the breast by primary radiation therapy. Cancer. 1979;43:985–93.
41. Perez CA, Fields JN. Role of radiation therapy for locally advanced and inflammatory carcinoma of the breast. Oncology. 1979;1:81–94.
42. Barker JL, Nelson AJ, Montague ED. Inlammatory carcinoma of the breast. Radiology. 1976;121:173–6.
43. Singletary SE, Ames FC, Buzdar AU. Management of inflammatory breast cancer. World J Surg. 1994;18:87–92.
44. Cristofanilli M, Buzdar AU, Hortobagyi GN. Update on the management of inlammatory breast cancer. Oncologist. 2003;8:141–8.
45. Giordano SH. Update on locally advanced breast cancer. Oncologist. 2003;8:521–30.
46. Harris EE, Schultz D, Bertsch H, Fox K, Glick J, Solin LJ. Ten-year outcome after combined modality therapy for inlammatory breast cancer. Int J Radiat Oncol Biol Phys. 2003;55:1200–8.
47. Low JA, Berman AW, Steinberg SM, Danforth DN, Lippman ME, Swain SM. Long-term follow-up for locally advanced and inlammatory breast cancer patients treated with multimodality therapy. J Clin Oncol. 2004;22:4067–74.
48. Sinclair S, Swain SM. Primary systemic chemotherapy for inlammatory breast cancer. Cancer. 2010;116(11 suppl):2821–8.
49. Tsai CJ, Li J, Gonzales-Angulo AM, Allen PK, Woodward WA, Ueno NT, et al. Outcomes after multidisciplinary treatment of inlammatory breast cancer in the era of neoadjuvant HER-2 directed therapy. Am J Clin Oncol. 2015;38(3):242–7.
50. Hennessy BT, Gonzales-Angulo AM, Hortobagyi GN, Cristofanilli M, Kau SW, Broglio K, et al. Disease-free and overall survival after pathologic complete disease remission of cytologically proven inlammatory breast carcinoma axillary lymph node metastases after primary systemic chemotherapy. Cancer. 2006;106:1000–6.
51. Bauer RL, Busch E, Levine F, Edge SB. Therapy for inflammatory breast cancer: impact of doxorubicin based therapy. Ann Surg Oncol. 1995;2:288–94.

52. Koh EH, Buzdar AU, Ames FC, Koh EH, Buzdar AU, Ames FC, et al. Inflammatory carcinoma of the breast: results of a combined modality approach-M.D. Anderson Cancer Center experience. Cancer Chemother Pharmacol. 1990;27:94–100.
53. Ueno NT, Buzdar AU, Singletary SE, Ames FC, McNeese MD, Holmes FA, et al. Combined modality treatment of inflammatory breast cancer. Twenty years experience at M.D. Anderson Cancer Center. Cancer Chemother Pharmacol. 1997;40:321–9.
54. Cristofanilli M, Buzdar AU, Sneige N, Smith T, Wasaff B, Ibrahim N, et al. Paclitaxel in the multi-modality treatment for inlammatory breast carcinoma. Cancer. 2001;92:1775–82.
55. Cristofanilli M, Gonzalez-Angulo AM, Buzdar AU, Kau SW, Frye DK, Hortobagyi GN. Paclitaxel significantly improves the prognosis in ER negative inlammatory breast cancer. The M.D. Anderson Cancer Center experience (1974-2000). Breast Cancer Res Treat. 2002;76(suppl 1):S158a.
56. Buzdar AU, Singletary SE, Booser DJ, Frye DK, Wasaff B, Hortobagyi GN. Combined modality treatment of stage III and inlammatory breast cancer. M.D. Anderson Cancer Center experience. Surg Oncol Clin N Am. 1995;4:715–34.
57. Panades M, Olivotto IA, Speers CH, Shenkier T, Olivotto TA, Weir L, et al. Evolving treatment strategies for inlammatory breast cancer: a population based survival analysis. J Clin Oncol. 2005;23:1941–50.
58. Costa SD, Loibl S, Kaufmann M, Zahm DM, Hilfrich J, Huober J, et al. Neoadjuvant chemotherapy shows similar response in patients with inlammatory or locally advanced breast cancer when compared with operable breast cancer: a secondary analysis of the GeparTrio trial data. J Clin Oncol. 2010;28:83–91.
59. Cristofanilli M, Fratarcangeli T, Esteva F, Rosales M, Booser D, Ibrahim M, et al. Weekly high dose paclitaxel has significant antitumor activity in inlammatory breast cancer (IBC). Proceeding of the ECCO 11. Eur J Cancer. 2001;37:S173.
60. Green MC, Buzdar AU, Smith T, Ibrahim NK, Valero V, Rosales MF, et al. Weekly paclitaxel improves pathologic complete remission in operable breast cancer when compared with paclitaxel once every 3 weeks. J Clin Oncol. 2005;23(25):5983–92.
61. Chevallier B, Roche H, Olivier JP, Chollet P, Hurteloup P. Inlammatory breast cancer: pilot study of intensive induction chemotherapy (FEC-HD) results in a high histologic response rate. Am J Clin Oncol. 1993;16:223–8.
62. Cagnoni PJ, Nieto Y, Shpall EJ, Bearman SI, Baron AE, Ross M, et al. High-dose chemotherapy with autologous hematopoietic progenitor-cell support as part of combined modality therapy in patients with inflammatory breast cancer. J Clin Oncol. 1998;16:1661–8.
63. Dazzi C, Cariello A, Rosti G, Tienghi A, Molino A, Sabbatini R, et al. Neoadjuvant high dose chemotherapy plus peripheral blood progenitor cells in inflammatory breast cancer: a multicenter phase II pilot study. Haematologica. 2001;86:523–9.
64. Viens P, Palangie T, Janvier M, Fabbro M, Roché H, Delozier T. First-line high-dose sequential chemotherapy with r-GCSF and repeated blood stem cell transplantation in untreated inflammatory breast cancer: toxicity and response (PEGASE 02 trial). Br J Cancer. 1999;81:449–56.
65. Somlo G, Frankel P, Chow W, Leong L, Margolin K, Morgan R Jr. Prognostic indicators and survival in patients with stage IIIB inflammatory breast carcinoma after dose-intense chemotherapy. J Clin Oncol. 2004;10:1839–48.
66. Cheng YC, Rondon G, Yang Y, Smith TL, Gajewski JL, Donato ML. The use of high dose cyclophosphamide, carmustine, and thitepa plus autologous hematopoietic stem cell transplantation as consolidation therapy for high risk primary breast cancer after primary surgery or neoadjuvant chemotherapy. Biol Blood Marrow Transplant. 2004;10:794–804.
67. Viens P, Tarpin C, Roche H, Bertucci F. Systemic therapy of inflammatory breast cancer from high-dose chemotherapy to targeted therapies: the French experience. Cancer. 2010;116(11 suppl):2829–36.
68. Dawood S, Broglio K, Gong Y, Yang WT, Cristofanilli M, Kau SW. Prognostic significance of *HER2* status in women with inflammatory breast cancer. Cancer. 2008;112:97–103.

69. Zell JA, Tsang WY, Taylor TH, Mehta RS, Anton-Culver H. Prognostic impact of human epidermal growth factor like receptor 2 and hormone receptor status in inflammatory breast cancer (IBC): analysis of 2.014 IBC cases from the California Cancer Registry. Breast Cancer Res. 2009;11:R9.
70. Buzdar AU, Valero V, Ibrahim NK, Francis D, Broglio KR, Theriault RL, et al. Neoadjuvant therapy with paclitaxel followed by 5 fluorouracil, epirubicin and cyclophosphamide chemotherapy and concurrent trastuzumab in *HER2* positive operable breast cancer: an update of the initial randomized study population and data of additional patients treated with the same regimen. Clin Cancer Res. 2007;13:228–33.
71. Cristofanilli M. Novel targeted therapies in inflammatory breast cancer. Cancer. 2010;116(11 suppl):2837–9.
72. Dawood S, Gonzales Angulo AM, Peintinger F, Broglio K, Symmans WF, Kau SW, et al. Efficacy and safety of neoadjuvant trastuzumab combined with paclitaxel and epirubicin: a retrospective review of the MD Anderson experience. Cancer. 2007;110:1195–200.
73. Chang HR. Trastuzumab-based neoadjuvant therapy in patients with HER2-positive breast cancer. Cancer. 2010;116:2856–67.
74. Dawood S, Gong Y, Broglio K, Buchholz TA, Woodward W, Lucci A, et al. Trastuzumab in primary inflammatory breast cancer, high pathologic response rates and improved outcome. Breast J. 2010;16:529–32.
75. Hurley J, Doliny P, Reis I, Silva O, Gomez-Fernandez C, Velez P, et al. Docetaxel, cisplatin, and trastuzumab as primary systemic therapy for human epidermal growth factor receptor 2-positive locally advanced breast cancer. J Clin Oncol. 2006;24:1831–8.
76. Van Pelt AE, Mohsin S, Elledge RM, Hilsenbeck SG, Gutierrez MC, Lucci A Jr, et al. Neoadjuvant trastuzumab and docetaxel in breast cancer: preliminary results. Clin Breast Cancer. 2003;4:348–53.
77. Gianni L, Eiermann W, Semiglazov V, Manikhas A, Lluch A, Tjulandin S, et al. Neoadjuvant chemotherapy with trastuzumab followed by adjuvant trastu-zumab versus neoadjuvant chemotherapy alone, in patients with HER-2-positive locally advanced breast cancer (the NOAH trial): a randomised controlled superiority trial with a parallel *HER2*-negative cohort. Lancet. 2010;375:377–84.
78. Gianni L, Eiermann W, Semiglazov V, Lluch A, Tjulandin S, Zambetti M, et al. Neoadjuvant and adjuvant trastuzumab in patients with HER-2-positive locally advanced breast cancer (the NOAH trial): follow-up of a randomised controlled superiority trial with a parallel *HER2*-negative cohort. Lancet Oncol. 2014;15:640–7.
79. Baselga J, Semiglazov V, Manikhas GM. Efficacy of neoadjuvan trastuzumab in patients with inflammatory breast cancer: data from the NOAH (neoadjuvant herceptin) phase III trial (abstract 2030) (ECCO meeting 2007). Eur J Cancer. 2007;5:193.
80. Hall PS, Hanby A, Cameron DA. Lapatinib for inflammatory breast cancer. Lancet Oncol. 2009;10:538–9.
81. Cristofanelli M, Boussen J, Baselga J. Phase II combination study of lapatinib and paclitaxel as neo-adjuvant therapy in patients with newly diagnosed inflammatory breast cancer. Breast Cancer Res Treat. 2006;100:1A. Abstract.
82. Boussen H, Cristofanilli M, Zaks T, Desilvio M, Salazar V, Spector N. Phase II study to evaluate the efficacy and safety of neoadjuvant lapatinib plus paclitaxel in patients with inflammatory breast cancer. J Clin Oncol. 2010;28:3248–55.
83. Untch M, von Minckwitz G, Gerber B, Schem C, Rezai M, Fasching PA, et al. Survival analysis after neoadjuvant chemotherapy with trastuzumab or lapatinib in patients with human epidermal growth factor receptor 2-positive breast cancer in the GeparQuinto (G5) Study (GBG 44). J Clin Oncol. 2018;36(13):1308–16.
84. Baselga J, Bradbury I, Eidtmann H, Di Cosimo S, de Azambuja E, Aura C, et al. Lapatinib with trastu-zumab for *HER2* positive early breast cancer (NeoALTTO). A randomized, open label, multicen-tre phase III trial. Lancet. 2012;379:633–40.
85. Azambuja E, Holmes AP, Piccart M, Holmes E, Di Cosimo S, Swaby F, et al. Lapatinib with trastuzumab for *HER2* positive early breast cancer (NeoALTTO): survival outcomes of a

randomised, open-label, multicentre, phase 3 trial and their association with pathological complete response. Lancet Oncol. 2014;15:1137–46.
86. Gianni L, Pienkowski T, Im YH, Tseng LM, Liu MC, Lluch A, et al. 5-year analysis of neoadjuvant pertuzumab and trastuzumab in patients with locally advanced, inflammatory, or early-stage HER2-positive breast cancer (NeoSphere): a multicentre, open-label, phase 2 randomised trial. Lancet Oncol. 2016;17(6):791–800.
87. Schneeweiss A, Chia S, Hickish T, Harvey V, Eniu A, Waldron-Lynch M, et al. Long-term efficacy analysis of the randomised, phase II TRYPHAENA cardiac safety study: Evaluating pertuzumab and trastuzumab plus standard neoadjuvant anthracycline-containing and anthracycline-free chemotherapy regimens in patients with HER2-positive early breast cancer. Eur J Cancer. 2018;89:27–35.
88. Amiri-Kordestani L, Wedam S, Zhang L, Tang S, Tilley A, Ibrahim A, et al. First FDA approval of neoadjuvant therapy for breast cancer: pertuzumab for the treatment of patients with *HER2*-positive breast cancer. Clin Cancer Res. 2014;20:5359–64.
89. Riawi MF, Aleixo SB, Rozas AA, Nunes de Matos Neto J, Caleffi M, Figueira AC, et al. A neoadjuvant, randomized, open-label phase II trial of afatinib versus trastuzumab versus lapatinib in patients with locally advanced HER2-positive breast cancer. Clin Breast Cancer. 2015;15(2):101–9.
90. Yamauchi H, Cristofanilli M, Nakamura S, Hortobaghy GN, Ueno NT. Molecular targets for treatment of inflammatory breast cancer. Nat Rev Clin Oncol. 2009;6:387–94.
91. Monneur A, Bertucci F, Viens P, Gonçalves A. Systemic treatment of inflammatory breast cancer: an overview. Bull Cancer. 2014;101:1080–8.
92. Wedam SB, Low JA, Yang SX, Chow CK, Choyke P, Danforth D, et al. Antiangiogenic and antitumor effects of bevacizumab in patients with inflammatory and locally advanced breast cancer. J Clin Oncol. 2006;24:769–77.
93. Pierga JY, Petit T, Delozier T, Ferrero JM, Campone M, Gligorov J, et al. Neoadjuvant bevacizumab, trastuzumab, and chemotherapy for primary inflammatory *HER2* positive breast cancer (BEVERLY-2): an open-label, single-arm phase II study. Lancet Oncol. 2012;13:375–84.
94. Pierga JY, Petit T, Levy C, Ferrero JM, Campone M, Gligorov J, et al. Pathological response and circulating tumor cell count identifies treated *HER2+* inflammatory breast cancer patients with excellent prognosis: BEVERLY-2 survival data. Clin Cancer Res. 2015;21(6):1298–304.
95. Mego M, Giordano A, De Giorgi U, Masuda H, Hsu L, Giuliano M, et al. Circulating tumor cells in newly diagnosed inflammatory breast cancer. Breast Cancer Res. 2015;17:2.
96. Overmoyer B, Fu P, Hoppel C, Radivoyevitch T, Shenk R, Persons M, et al. Inflammatory breast cancer as a model disease to study tumor angiogenesis: results of a phase IB trial of combination *SU5416* and doxorubicin. Clin Cancer Res. 2007;13:5862–8.
97. Cabioglu N, Gong Y, Islam R, Broglio KR, Sneige N, Sahin A, et al. Expression of growth factor and chemokine receptors: new insights in the biology of inflammatory breast cancer. Ann Oncol. 2007;18:1021–9.
98. van Golen KL, Wu ZF, Qiao XT, Bao LW, Merajver SD. RhoC GTPase, a novel transforming oncogene for human mammary epithelial cells that partially recapitulates the inflammatory breast cancer pheno-type. Cancer Res. 2000;60:5832–8.
99. Andreopoulou E, Vigoda IS, Hershman DL, Hershman DL, Raptis G, Vahdat LT, et al. Phase I-II study of farnesyl transferase inhibitor tipifarnib plus sequential weekly paclitaxel and doxorubicin-cyclophosphamide in i/ER2/neu-negative inflammatory carcinoma and non-inflammatory estrogen-receptor positive breast carcinoma. Breast Cancer Res. 2013;141:429–35.
100. Krisnamurthy S, Woodward W, Yang W, Reuben JM, Tepperberg J, Ogura D, et al. Status of the anaplastic lymphoma kinase *(ALK)* gene in inflammatory breast carcinoma. Springerplus. 2013;2:409.
101. Robertson FM, Petricoin EF III, Van Laere SJ, Bertucci F, Chu K, Fernandez SV, et al. Presence of anaplastic lymphoma kinase in inflammatory breast cancer. Springerplus. 2013;2:497.
102. Harvey HA, Lipton A, Lawrence BV, White DS, Wells SA, Blumenschein G, et al. Estrogen receptor status in inflammatory breast carcinoma. J Surg Oncol. 1982;21:42–4.

103. Nguyen DM, Sam K, Tsimelzon A, Li X, Wong H, Mohsin S, et al. Molecular heterogeneity of inflammatory breast cancer: a hyperproliferative phenotype. Clin Cancer Res. 2006;12:5047–54.
104. Brewer TM, Masuda H, Liu DD, Shen Y, Liu P, Iwamoto T, et al. Statin use in primary inflammatory breast cancer: a cohort study. Br J Cancer. 2013;109:318–24.
105. Kaufmann M, von Minckwitz G, Bear HD, Buzdar A, McGale P, Bonnefoi H, et al. Recommendations from an international expert panel on the use of neoadjuvant (primary) systemic treatment of operable breast cancer: new perspectives 2006. Ann Oncol. 2007;18:1927–34.
106. Dushkin H, Cristofanilli M. Inflammatory breast cancer. J Natl Compr Cancer Netw. 2011;9(2):233–40. quiz 241
107. Woodward WA, Buchholz TA. Unpublished observations from Yamauchi H, Woodward WA, Valero V, et al. Inflammatory breast cancer: what we know and what we need to learn. Oncologist. 2012;17:891–9.
108. Khatcheressian JL, Hurley P, Bantug E, Esserman LJ, Grunfeld E, Halberg F, et al. Breast cancer follow-up and management after primary treatment: American Society of Clinical Oncology clinical practice guideline update. J Clin Oncol. 2013;3:961–5.
109. Senkus E, Kyriakides S, Penault-Llorca P, Poortmans P, Thompson A, Zackrisson S, et al. Primary breast cancer: ESMO clinical practice guidelines for diagnosis, treatment and follow-up. Ann Oncol. 2013;24(supplement 6):vi7–23.
110. Matro JM, Cristofanilli M, Hughes ME, Hughes ME, Ottesen RA, Weeks JC, et al. Inflammatory breast cancer management in the National Comprehensive Cancer Network: the disease, recurrence pattern, and outcome. Clin Breast Cancer. 2015;15:1–7.
111. Guler N, Karabulut B, Koçdor MA. Locally advanced breast cancer-2010 Istanbul Breast Cancer Consensus Meeting. J Breast Health. 2011;7:68–89.
112. van Golen KL, Cristofanilli M. The third international inflammatory breast cancer conference. Breast Cancer Res. 2013;15:318.

Part V
Surgical Approach for Breast Cancer

Part V
Surgical Approach for Breast Cancer

Chapter 12
In Situ Cancer Treatment

Hasan Karanlik and Abdullah Igci

Introduction

The most common types of breast carcinoma in situ are lobular carcinoma in situ (LCIS) and ductal carcinoma in situ (DCIS). The work-up for in situ carcinomas includes patient history, physical examination, bilateral mammography and careful review of pathology. Estrogen receptor (ER) positivity should be assessed in DCIS but is not recommended in LCIS patients. Breast MRI is not currently a routine work-up examination for in situ carcinomas but may be useful for selected patients.

Lobular Carcinoma In Situ

LCIS or lobular neoplasia cells resemble cancer cells growing in the lobules of breast tissue that do not spread beyond the walls of the lobules. LCIS develops only in the female breast. These cells contain a normal nuclear/cytoplasmic ratio. Mucoid globules in the cytoplasm are a characteristic feature. LCIS is usually an incidental finding on pathology specimens and is usually located near microcalcifications lying in the adjacent tissue. LCIS is observed nearly ten times more often in white women than African women. Women harboring LCIS can develop invasive breast cancer in 25–35% of cases, and 65% of subsequent invasive breast cancer is ductal in origin. Lobular neoplasia is considered a risk factor for invasive breast cancer in

H. Karanlik
Department of Surgical Oncology, Institute of Oncology, Istanbul University, Istanbul, Turkey

A. Igci (✉)
General Surgery, Istanbul Medical Faculty, Department of Surgery, Istanbul University, Istanbul, Turkey
e-mail: aigci@istanbul.edu.tr

A. Aydiner et al. (eds.), *Breast Cancer*, https://doi.org/10.1007/978-3-319-96947-3_12

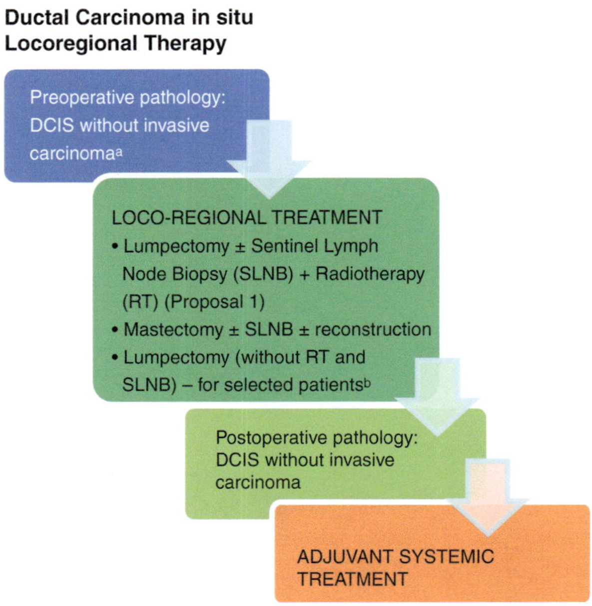

Fig. 12.1 Management of patient with ductal carcinoma in situ (DCIS). [a]Preoperative MR imaging is recommended in DCIS. The specimen should be evaluated with X-ray imaging. Radiation therapy after breast-conserving surgery is the standard treatment in DCIS. The disease-free surgical margin should be adequate. In cases undergoing BCS, a surgical margin of 2 mm or above is considered safe only in those with DCIS. If the invasive tumor is <1 mm in DCIS, the surgical border safety is evaluated according to DCIS. If the invasive focus is >1 mm in DCIS, the surgical margin width should be evaluated according to the invasive cancer. A sufficient surgical margin should be decided together with clinical, radiological and pathological findings. The decision regarding the "sufficient surgical margin" should be made according to findings such as additional radiological foci (multiple foci, microcalcification), invasive lobular carcinoma, presence of more than one surgical margin and persistence of surgical marginal proximity in re-excision. [b]ER-positive, postmenopausal case, advanced age, low-grade tumors

both breasts rather than a precursor lesion. Therefore, cancer can develop in either breast and not only the one harboring the lesion.

Disagreement exists about whether a surgical excision should be performed of the area of LCIS diagnosed by core needle biopsy. Most of the studies have shown that around 25% of patients with LCIS diagnosed by core needle biopsy will be upgraded to having invasive cancer or DCIS after excisional biopsy [1]. Determining of the subtypes of the LCIS based on core needle biopsy may be helpful to differentiate patients who can be spared a surgical excision. Pleomorphic LCIS and/or multifocal/multicentric LCIS may behave similarly to DCIS; thus, surgical excision with negative margins may be considered (Fig. 12.1) [2]. More than 4 foci of LCIS may also strengthen the possibility for upstaging on surgical excision. The usual type of LCIS found on core biopsy (affecting less than 4 terminal units in a single core), without imaging discordance, may be managed by radiological follow-up. All LCIS patients should be counseled on risk-reduction strategies [1].

Recommendations

Pleomorphic LCIS and/or multifocal/multicentric LCIS may behave similarly to DCIS; thus, surgical excision with negative margins may be considered.

In asymptomatic women with LCIS, the routine use of bone scanning, liver ultrasonography and chest radiography cannot be recommended for baseline staging.

Ductal Carcinoma In Situ

Ductal carcinoma in situ or intraductal carcinoma is considered non-invasive or pre-invasive breast cancer. The pathological appearance is the proliferation of cells lining the ducts, resulting in papillary growth within duct but without spreading beyond the walls of ducts to surrounding tissue. Early lesions do not harbor atypia or pleomorphism. The papillary growths (papillary growth pattern) then start to fill the lumen of the duct, and atypical cells have hyperchromasia and loss of polarity (cribriform growth pattern). Eventually, these pleomorphic cells with mitosis obliterate the ducts (solid growth pattern). Intensive growth causes necrosis at the center due to decreased blood supply (comedo growth pattern). These necrotic centers contain calcium deposits and appear on mammograms. No spread or invasion occurs theoretically because the cells cannot spread outside the breast tissue. DCIS is considered a pre-cancer of high risk, as some cases may progress to become invasive cancer. Paget's disease of the breast is characterized by eczema-form changes accompanied by erosion and ulceration of the nipple and areolar epidermis. This condition is primarily correlated with DCIS; additionally, it can be accompanied by invasive ductal carcinoma. The diagnosis is determined based on the microscopic observation of Paget cells in a skin biopsy. The width of the lesion is evaluated via mammography and MRI in patients for whom breast-conserving surgery is planned.

The standard treatment for DCIS is breast-conserving lumpectomy with negative surgical margins (without axillary intervention) and whole-breast radiation [3]. If negative margins cannot be attained by breast-conserving surgery or if disease is extensive (>4 cm of disease or disease in more than one quadrant), mastectomy must be performed [4]. For non-palpable disease, needle localization or other image-guided techniques are utilized to guide surgical resection. Specimen mammography is usually performed for margin assessment.

Patients should be evaluated for hereditary breast cancer risk, and genetic counseling should be provided to DCIS patients with high-risk features.

The role of axillary staging in patients with DCIS is limited. The probability of a positive SLN is 7–9%, and most metastases are found as micrometastases or isolated tumor cells [5, 6]. Nearly 20–40% of patients are diagnosed with a coincidence of invasive cancer at needle core biopsy for the primary tumor, and the risk increases with palpable mass, poorly differentiated DCIS, younger age and extensive disease [7, 8]. Sentinel node biopsy should be routinely performed in patients with high-grade ductal carcinoma in situ who will undergo mastectomy or for whom breast-conserving surgery will compromise the performance of a future SLN biopsy because of wide excision in an anatomic location (e.g., tail of the breast) [9].

Re-excision is not required for surgical margins of 2–5 mm in DCIS. Multifocality and an increasing number of close or involved margins have been identified as predictive of additional disease on re-excision. These factors may be surrogate markers of an increased extent of disease. If the surgical margin is less than 1 mm at the skin or chest wall, boost radiation at a higher dose to the involved site should be provided instead of re-excision [10]. Recent consensus guidelines issued jointly by the Society of Surgical Oncology and the American Society for Radiation Oncology, which recommend "no ink on tumor" as the standard for an adequate margin in invasive cancer, caution that these findings cannot be extrapolated to DCIS [11].

Recommendations

The routine use of bone scanning, liver ultrasonography and chest radiography cannot be recommended for baseline study in asymptomatic DCIS patients. Routine MRI utility for breast assessment of DCIS patients is not recommended.

MRI may be performed in case of the following:

- Divergence among clinical examination, mammography and ultrasound
- Need for treatment planning due to difficulty in interpretation of disease extent (both bilateral and multicentric disease).

In case of multicentricity, lumpectomy is not recommended (*Proposal 1*).

The standard treatment for DCIS is breast-conserving surgery with negative surgical margins (without axillary intervention) and whole-breast radiation (*Proposal 1*).

If negative margins cannot be attained by breast-conserving surgery for DCIS, mastectomy must be performed.

Patients with high-risk DCIS should be evaluated for hereditary breast cancer, and genetic counselling should be provided.

Sentinel node biopsy should be routinely performed in patients with high-grade DCIS

- who will undergo mastectomy and
- for whom BCS will not allow further SNB due to anatomic location (e.g., tail of the breast).

Surgical margins of at least 2 mm should be achieved.

Re-excision is not required for surgical margins of 2–5 mm.

Estrogen receptors and progesterone receptors should be tested in all DCIS patients (*Proposal 1*).

Immediate breast reconstruction should be offered to all patients with DCIS treated with mastectomy (*Proposal 1*).

Treatment

If total mastectomy is performed with negative margins, adjuvant irradiation is not required. When nipple-sparing mastectomy and reconstruction are performed, irradiation of the nipple-areola complex is not standard. Breast tissue inadvertently left under the skin flaps should not be an indication for postoperative radiotherapy.

In cases treated with BCS, adjuvant radiotherapy using partial-breast irradiation (PBI) techniques is under investigation in randomized trials; such an approach is to be considered "with caution" according to the American Society for Radiation Oncology and other groups [12–14]. Intraoperative radiation therapy and electronic brachytherapy should not be offered regardless of technique outside of clinical trial [12]. Lumpectomy without radiotherapy has been investigated in prospective and randomized trials in patients considered to be at low risk of local recurrence [15, 16]. In such low-risk DCIS patients, whole-breast radiotherapy should be considered in the decision-making process with the patient, accounting for age, comorbidities, radiation risks, patient preferences, and salvage options [17]. Radiotherapy following breast-conserving surgery is optional in DCIS patients with low-risk features (>60 years of age, ER positive, tumor diameter <1 cm, low grade, negative margins, no palpable mass) [18]. For a patient to be considered a low-risk DCIS case, the following criteria must be present: mammographic detection, no palpable mass, small tumor, ER positive, nuclear grade I or II, and clear surgical margins of at least 3 mm [17]. All other DCIS cases treated with lumpectomy are candidates for whole-breast irradiation [19–22].

The marked reduction in recurrence rates following tamoxifen for 5 years in women with ER-positive DCIS reported by the NSABP B-24 trial resulted in increased use of tamoxifen as an adjuvant therapy. Despite this reduction ratio, 5-year tamoxifen is not routinely prescribed worldwide. The benefit of tamoxifen in ER-negative DCIS patients to reduce the risk of breast cancer recurrence after breast-conserving surgery and radiotherapy is uncertain, and tamoxifen should not be routinely recommended to ER-negative DCIS patients. Tamoxifen may be given to reduce the contralateral breast cancer risk in ER-positive DCIS patients after mastectomy (Tables 12.1 and 12.2) [23, 24].

Table 12.1 Adjuvant systemic therapy of ductal carcinoma in situ

Risk reduction treatment for the ipsilateral breast after breast-conserving surgery
Tamoxifen for 5 years:
For ER- or PgR-positive patients who have undergone breast-conserving surgery (BCS) and RT
Benefit of tamoxifen is not definite for ER-negative patients
Patients treated with excision only
Aromatase inhibitor for 5 years[a]
For ER-positive or PgR-positive postmenopausal patients who have undergone BCS and RT
Risk-mitigating treatment for the contralateral breast
Counseling for risk reduction

[a]The primary endpoint of NSABP B-35, a phase III trial comparing anastrozole to tamoxifen, each given for 5 years, was breast cancer-free interval (BCFI), defined as the time from randomization to any breast cancer (BC) event including local, regional, or distant recurrence or contralateral disease, invasive or DCIS. In conclusion, anastrozole provided a significant improvement compared to tamoxifen for BCFI, which was seen later in the study, primarily in women <60 years old. In the IBIS-II DCIS trial, anastrozole was shown to reduce recurrence, similar to tamoxifen

Table 12.2 DCIS—monitoring and follow-up[a]

Medical history and physical examination
Every 6 months for 5 years
Once a year thereafter
Mammography
Once a year (if BCS is performed, at months 6–12 following RT)

[a]If treated with tamoxifen monitor according to breast cancer risk mitigation guidelines

Recommendations

Patients treated with BCS for DCIS with other than low-risk features are candidates for whole-breast irradiation (*Proposal 1*).

Radiotherapy is optional in patients treated with BCS for DCIS with low-risk features.

Boost radiation at a higher dose to surgical margins of less than 1 mm at the skin or chest wall should be provided instead of re-excision.

Adjuvant hormonotherapy is recommended for patients with ER-positive DCIS (*Proposal 1*).

Tamoxifen may be given to reduce contralateral breast cancer risk in ER-positive DCIS patients after mastectomy.

Conclusions

Classic LCIS does not require surgical treatment. There is evidence to support the existence of histologically aggressive variants of LCIS (e.g., "pleomorphic" LCIS), which may have a greater potential than classic LCIS to develop into invasive lobular carcinoma. Surgeons may consider complete excision with negative margins for pleomorphic LCIS.

Most DCIS patients with limited disease may be treated with wide local excision or with re-excision in which negative margins are achieved. Patients with widespread disease (i.e., disease in two or more quadrants) require total mastectomy with SLN biopsy. Complete ALND is not recommended in the absence of proven axillary metastatic disease in patients with apparent pure DCIS or mammographically detected DCIS with microcalcifications. However, a small proportion of women with pure DCIS on initial biopsy will have invasive breast cancer at the time of the definitive surgical procedure and thus will ultimately require ALN staging. In patients with seemingly pure DCIS to be treated with mastectomy or with excision in an anatomic location (e.g., tail of the breast), which could compromise the performance of a future SLN biopsy, SLN biopsy may be considered. Endocrine therapy may be considered as a strategy to reduce the risk of ipsilateral breast cancer recurrence in women with ER-positive DCIS treated with breast-conserving therapy. The benefit of endocrine therapy for ER-negative DCIS is not established.

References

1. O'Neil M, Madan R, Tawfik OW, Thomas PA, Fan F. Lobular carcinoma in situ/atypical lobular hyperplasia on breast needle biopsies: does it warrant surgical excisional biopsy? A study of 27 cases. Ann Diagn Pathol. 2010;14:251–5.
2. College of American Pathologists. Protocols and guidelines. Available at: http://www.cap.org. Accessed 26 Feb 2018.
3. EORTC Breast Cancer Cooperative Group, EORTC Radiotherapy Group, Bijker N, Meijnen P, Peterse JL, Bogaerts J, Van Hoorebeeck I, Julien JP, et al. Breast-conserving treatment with or without radiotherapy in ductal carcinoma-in-situ: ten-year results of European Organisation for Research and Treatment of Cancer randomized phase III trial 10853--a study by the EORTC Breast Cancer Cooperative Group and EORTC Radiotherapy Group. J Clin Oncol. 2006;24:3381–7.
4. Gradishar WJ, Anderson BO, Balassanian R. Breast Cancer, version 4.2017, NCCN clinical practice guidelines in oncology. J Natl Compr Cancer Netw. 2018;16(3):310–20.
5. Leidenius M, Salmenkivi K, von Smitten K, Heikkilä P. Tumour-positive sentinel node findings in patients with ductal carcinoma in situ. J Surg Oncol. 2006;94:380–4.
6. Moore KH, Sweeney KJ, Wilson ME, Goldberg JI, Buchanan CL, Tan LK, et al. Outcomes for women with ductal carcinoma-in-situ and a positive sentinel node: a multi-institutional audit. Ann Surg Oncol. 2007;14:2911–7.
7. Meijnen P, Oldenburg HS, Loo CE, Nieweg OE, Peterse JL, Rutgers EJ. Risk of invasion and axillary lymph node metastasis in ductal carcinoma in situ diagnosed by core-needle biopsy. Br J Surg. 2007;94:952–6.
8. Yen TW, Hunt KK, Ross MI, Mirza NQ, Babiera GV, Meric-Bernstam F. Predictors of invasive breast cancer in patients with an initial diagnosis of ductal carcinoma in situ: a guide to selective use of sentinel lymph node biopsy in management of ductal carcinoma in situ. J Am Coll Surg. 2005;200:516–26.
9. Cody HS 3rd, Van Zee KJ. Point: sentinel lymph node biopsy is indicated for patients with DCIS. J Natl Compr Cancer Netw. 2003;1:199–206.
10. Silverstein MJ, Lagios MD, Groshen S, Waisman JR, Lewinsky BS, Martino S, et al. The influence of margin width on local control of ductal carcinoma in situ of the breast. N Engl J Med. 1999;340:1455–61.
11. Morrow M, Van Zee KJ, Solin LJ, Houssami N, Chavez-MacGregor M, Harris JR, et al. Society of Surgical Oncology-American Society for Radiation Oncology-American Society of Clinical Oncology consensus guideline on margins for breast-conserving surgery with whole-breast irradiation in ductal carcinoma in situ. J Clin Oncol. 2016;34:4040–6.
12. Shah C, Vicini F, Shaitelman SF, Hepel J, Keisch M, Arthur D, et al. The American Brachytherapy Society consensus statement for accelerated partial-breast irradiation. Brachytherapy. 2018;17(1):154–70.
13. ASBS: http://www.breastsurgeons.org/statements/apbi_statement_revised_100708.pdf.
14. ABS: http://www.americanbrachytherapy.org/recources/abs_breast_brachytherapy_taskgroup.Pdf.
15. Hughes LL, Wang M, Page DL, Gray R, Solin LJ, Davidson NE, et al. Local excision alone without irradiation for ductal carcinoma in situ of the breast: a trial of the eastern cooperative oncology group. J Clin Oncol. 2009;27:5319–24.
16. McCormick B, Winter K, Hudis C, Kuerer HM, Rakovitch E, Smith BL, et al. RTOG 9804: a prospective randomized trial for good-risk ductal carcinoma in situ comparing radiotherapy with observation. J Clin Oncol. 2015;33(7):709–15.
17. Smith B. When is good enough really good enough? Defining the role of radiation in low-risk ductal carcinoma in situ. J Clin Oncol. 2015;33(7):686–91.
18. Lagios MD, Silverstein MJ. Ductal carcinoma in situ: recent history and areas of controversy. Breast J. 2015;21:21–6.

19. Fisher B, Dignam J, Wolmark N, Mamounas E, Costantino J, Poller W, et al. Lumpectomy and radiation therapy for the treatment of intraductal breast cancer: findings from the National Surgical Adjuvant Breast and Bowel Project B-17. J Clin Oncol. 1998;16:441–52.
20. Julien JP, Bijker N, Fentiman IS, Peterse JL, Delledonne V, Rouanet P, et al. Radiotherapy in breast conserving treatment for ductal carcinoma in situ: first results of the EORCT randomized phase III trial 10853. Lancet. 2000;353:528–33.
21. UK Coordinating Committee on Cancer Research. Radiotherapy and tamoxifen in women with completely excised ductal carcinoma in situ of the breast in the UK, Australia, and New Zealand: randomized controlled trial. Lancet. 2003;362:95–102.
22. Fisher B, Land S, Mamounas E, Dignam J, Fisher ER, Wolmark N. Prevention of invasive breast cancer in women with ductal carcinoma in situ: An update of the national surgical adjuvant breast and bowel project experience. Semin Oncol. 2001;28:400–18.
23. Staley H, McCallum I, Bruce J. Postoperative Tamoxifen for ductal carcinoma in situ: Cochrane systematic review and meta-analysis. Breast. 2014;23:546–51.
24. Forbes F, Sestak I, Howell A, Bonanni B, Bundred N, Levy C, et al. Anastrozole versus tamoxifen for the prevention of locoregional and contralateral breast cancer in postmenopausal women with locally excised ductal carcinoma in situ (IBIS-II DCIS): a double-blind, randomised controlled trial. Lancet. 2016;387:866–73.

Chapter 13
Surgical Approach in Invasive Breast Cancer

Hasan Karanlik and Abdullah Igci

Historical Background

Beginning in the twentieth century, breast cancer was thought to arise in the breast and progress to other sides centrifugally. At that time more extensive procedures were performed to prevent disease spread to distant sites. Halsted radical mastectomy was the primary surgery with demonstrated improvements in survival. The procedure included removal of breast tissue with the overlying skin, underlying pectoral muscle and regional lymph nodes along the axillary vein. Halsted radical mastectomy remained the mainstay of breast surgical therapy until the 1970s. The modern era brought the hypothesis of both centrifugal spread to adjacent structures and lymphatic and blood vessel spread to distant sites, as many patients continued to suffer disease despite such large resections.

Breast cancer treatment now includes local and regional approaches together with medical therapies designed to treat systemic disease. The combination of multimodality treatment options has brought improvements in survival rates.

Planning Surgery

Before surgical treatment, the initial stage is to diagnose the disease. The primary choice for diagnosis is core biopsy. Excisional biopsy should be reserved for lesions

H. Karanlik
Istanbul University, Institute of Oncology, Department of Surgical Oncology, Istanbul, Turkey

A. Igci (✉)
General Surgery, Istanbul Medical Faculty, Department of Surgery,
Istanbul University, Istanbul, Turkey
e-mail: aigci@istanbul.edu.tr

A. Aydiner et al. (eds.), *Breast Cancer*, https://doi.org/10.1007/978-3-319-96947-3_13

that are not amenable to core biopsy. Fine needle aspiration (FNA) is one choice but has high false-negative rates. In addition, FNA cannot distinguish invasive from in situ lesions with high reliability. The biopsy should provide information about the tumor type, histological grade, lymphovascular invasion and hormone receptor status (ER, PR, HER2). The history of the patient should be taken, and a proper physical examination should be performed. Adequate and appropriate imaging studies are necessary to establish the extent of disease and to assign clinical stage. Patients with abnormal blood tests or chest radiographs and patients with locally advanced or inflammatory breast cancer should undergo further investigation for distant metastases.

The choice of treatment strategy is based on the tumor features (location and size of tumor, number of lesions, extent of lymph node involvement) and biology (pathology including biomarkers and gene expression) and on the age, general health status, and personal preferences of the patient. Patients should be actively involved in all management decisions. The possibility of hereditary cancer should be explored, and if needed, prophylactic procedures should be discussed following appropriate genetic counseling and testing of the patient. In younger premenopausal patients, possible fertility issues should be discussed, and guidance on fertility-preservation techniques should be provided before initiation of treatment [1–11].

The primary aim of breast cancer surgery is to eradicate the tumor and any local disease to achieve local control. Well-defined procedures in breast surgery include the following (Figs. 13.1 and 13.2):

Mastectomy
Breast-conserving surgery (followed by radiotherapy)
Contralateral mastectomy
Axillary staging
Surgical approach after systemic therapy
Breast reconstruction

Mastectomy

Mastectomy is required for tumors that are large compared to breast size, concomitant with large microcalcifications on mammography, or large with a lack of clear margins and for patients with contraindications for radiotherapy. Patient preference for mastectomy and a desire not to receive radiotherapy are also acceptable indications for mastectomy. Contraindications for radiotherapy are previous breast or chest wall irradiation, active lupus or scleroderma at the skin and pregnancy.

Simple and modified radical mastectomy both include removal of the gland together with the nipple and areola. Complete axillary lymph node dissection is part of modified radical mastectomy. An elliptical incision is planned for proper closure of future skin flaps and to contain the nipple areola complex and previous biopsy scars. Skin flaps are prepared, and glandular tissue is relieved. Breast tissue is separated from the underlying pectoral muscle with the pectoral fascia left on the breast specimen. In case of modified radical mastectomy, dissection is continued towards the axilla, and the specimen involves level I and II axillary lymph nodes. Level I

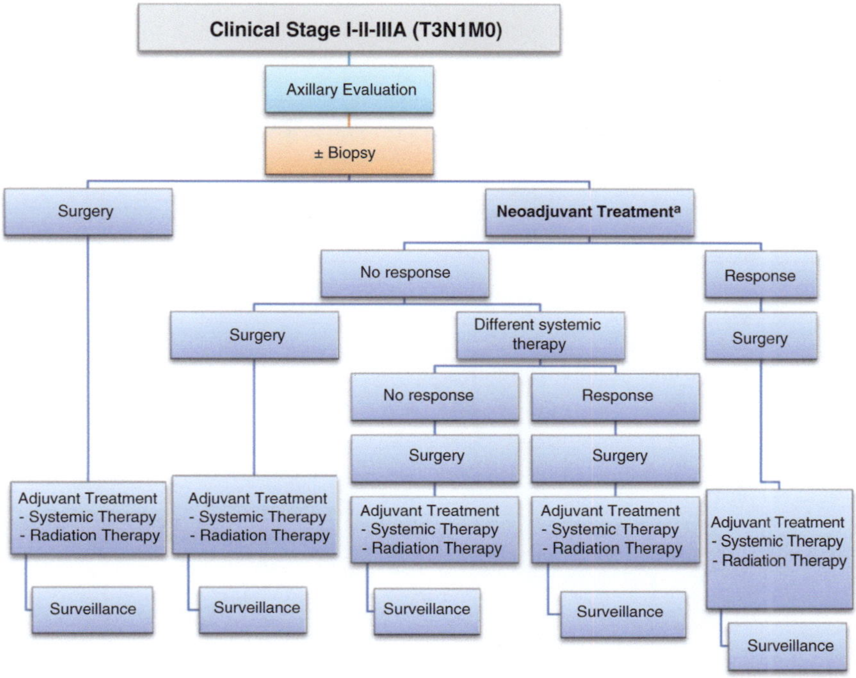

Fig. 13.1 Management of patients for stage I–II–IIIA (T3N1M0) breast cancer. [a]Neoadjuvant chemotherapy should be administered to T2 and T3 tumors (N0–N1) meeting BCS criteria except tumor diameter, or to triple negative and HER-2-positive patients

lymph nodes are inferior to the pectoralis minor muscle, whereas level II lymph nodes are posterior to the muscle.

If immediate reconstruction is planned, skin-sparing mastectomy may be performed. This procedure leaves the maximum skin possible by removing only the nipple areola complex with the breast tissue. If immediate reconstruction is not planned, sufficient skin is left for closure of the flaps. When performing prophylactic mastectomy, the nipple areola complex may be spared.

Breast-Conserving Surgery

Breast-conserving surgery (BCS) removes the tumor with clear margins, defined as no ink on tumor. More extensive procedures, such as quadrantectomy, that remove the tumor with wider margins have not been shown to improve survival. The removed specimen is oriented, and margins are inked prior to sectioning. Specimen mammogram is recommended if the tumor is not palpable or marked with a guide wire or if there is coexistence of microcalcifications. If margins are positive in perioperative pathological evaluation, re-excision should be performed to obtain clear margins. Wider excisions will lead to worse cosmetic outcomes. The defect is closed

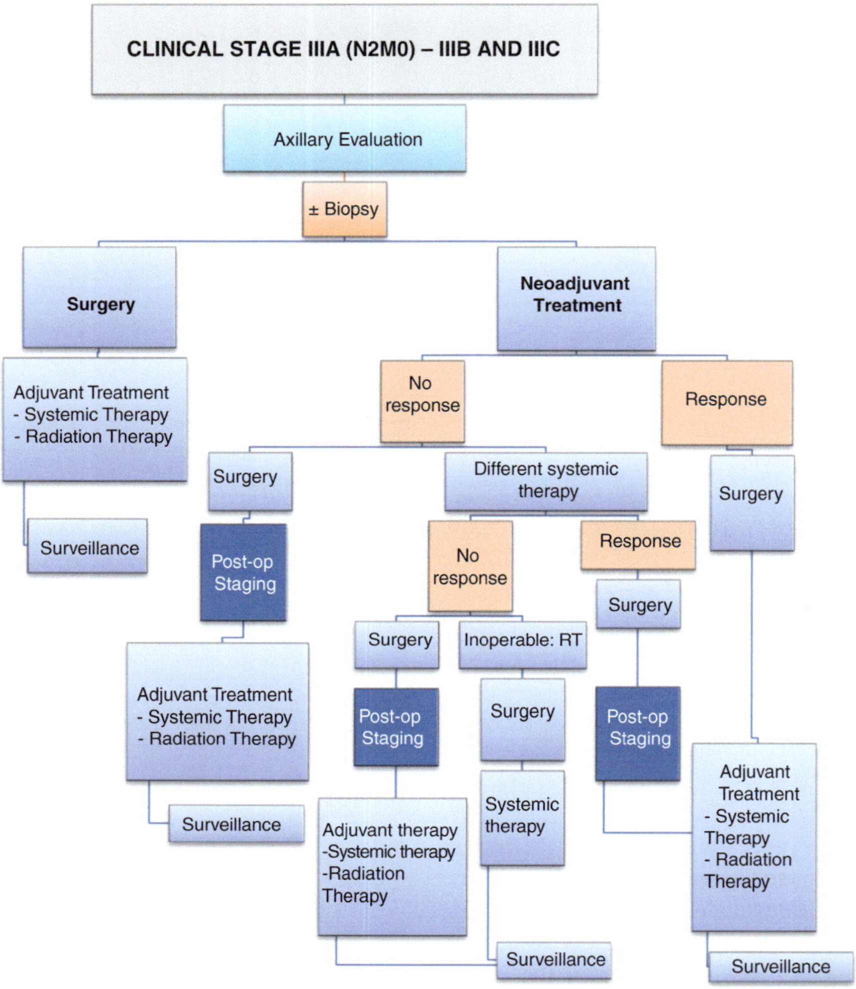

Fig. 13.2 Locoregional and adjuvant systemic treatment for clinical stage IIIA (N2M0)—IIIB and IIIC disease (non-inflammatory)

in a cosmetic fashion. There is an increasing trend of combining plastic surgery techniques with breast cancer surgery to maximize cosmetic results. This so-called "oncoplastic surgery" has been popularized to achieve the best aesthetic results with adequate oncologic margins. The primary aim is to preserve breast appearance and symmetry as much as possible. Several deformities may occur after BCS depending on the location of the tumor and the amount of excised tissue. The final aesthetic outcome may worsen with administration of radiotherapy, which may increase the deformity and make it more challenging to correct.

Axillary staging is usually performed through a separate incision. Sentinel lymph node biopsy is replacing axillary lymph node dissection in clinically node-negative patients. Axillary dissection is similar for those requiring modified radical mastectomy.

Breast-conserving therapy, axillary lymph node dissection, and whole-breast irradiation are equivalent to mastectomy with axillary lymph node dissection as the primary treatment for most women with stage I and stage II breast cancers *(Proposal 1)* [12–15]. Both procedures result in similar overall survival and disease-free survival.

Breast-conserving surgery is contraindicated for patients who are pregnant and would require radiotherapy during pregnancy; have diffuse disease that cannot be removed locally via a single incision with an acceptable cosmetic result; have widespread suspicious or malignant-appearing microcalcifications on mammography; or have positive pathologic margins after surgery. Patients with pathologically positive margins should generally undergo re-excision to achieve negative pathologic margins. If the margins remain positive after re-excision, mastectomy should be performed for optimal local control of the disease.

Relative contraindications to BCS include previous radiation therapy to the breast or chest wall; active connective tissue disease such as scleroderma and lupus involving the skin; tumors greater than 5 cm, and focally positive pathologic margins. Those patients with focally positive pathologic margins who do not undergo re-excision should be considered for a higher radiation boost dose to the tumor bed. To adequately assess margins following lumpectomy, surgical specimens should be oriented, and the pathologist should provide descriptions of the gross and microscopic margin status and the distance, orientation, and type of tumor in relation to the closest margin. Careful histological assessment of resection margins is essential, with no tumor at the inked margin required. Marking the tumor bed with clips facilitates accurate planning of the radiation boost field where appropriate. Acceptably low local recurrence rates remain the major quality assurance target. Current guidelines recommend local recurrence rates after wide excision and radiotherapy of <1% per year (with a target of <0.5%) and not exceeding 10% overall.

Women undergoing BCS plus radiotherapy have been shown to have better body self-image than those undergone mastectomy, but postoperative psychological well-being has not been shown to differ between these groups [16].

Recommendations

All patients with stage I or II breast cancer should be offered BCS or mastectomy *(Proposal 1)*.

The surgery type should be tailored to the individual patient, who should be informed of all options and made aware that radiotherapy is required following BCS and that further surgery is necessary in case of positive margins *(Proposal 1)*.

The patient should be aware of the advantages and harms of radiotherapy following BCS *(Proposal 1)*.

Mastectomy should be preferred to BCS in case of the following *(Proposal 1)*:

Inappropriate tumor-breast size ratio or tumor location interfering with cosmetic outcome after BCS;

Multifocal-multicentric disease that cannot be properly manipulated with acceptable cosmetic results after BCS;
Contraindication to radiotherapy

Due to adverse cosmetic outcomes, quadrantectomy is not recommended as BCS.

BCS should maintain total excision of the tumor with clear margins with acceptable cosmetic outcome following both surgery and radiotherapy.

A detailed pathological assessment should be made.

No ink on tumor should be assessed as clear margins.

Patients with positive margins should be considered for re-excision.

Categories indicate the strength of the supporting evidence rather than the importance of the recommendations.

Contralateral Mastectomy

Hereditary breast cancer is thought to represent only 5% of all breast cancer cases. Hereditary breast cancer is mainly caused by mutations in the BRCA1 and BRCA2 genes, which are located on chromosomes 17 and 13, respectively. Mutations in these genes predispose carriers to breast and ovarian cancer as well as melanoma and prostate, bile duct and pancreatic cancers. They are inherited in an autosomal dominant pattern and considered tumor suppressor genes. Rarer cases arise due to Li Fraumeni Syndrome (p53 mutation), Peutz-Jeghers Syndrome (STK11/LKB1 gene), Cowden Syndrome (PTEN gene), Hereditary Diffuse Gastric Cancer (HDGC; CDJ-1 gene) and Ataxia Telangiectasia (ATM gene) and consist of less than 1% of all breast cancer cases.

Both BRCA genes are very large, and more than one hundred different mutations have been reported, including for which clinical significance has not been established. Patients with these clinically unidentified significant mutations may or may not be at risk for cancer. In addition, not all mutations in certain sequences of BRCA1 and 2 are identified by screening methods. Technically, negative screening results do not exclude the possibility of the presence of a mutation. Consequently, several estimation models have been developed to aid clinicians in genetic counseling.

The complexity of genetic testing necessitates clinical guidance from a special health practitioner trained in and familiar with the field. A mutation is most likely to be identified in a family that includes patients who have already been diagnosed with breast or ovarian cancer. The screening method should be performed based on the patient with the youngest age of onset and who is less likely to have developed sporadic cancer. If a mutation is identified, the remaining relatives and offspring can be screened with high accuracy. Relatives found not to carry the mutation bear the same risk as the general population, whereas unaffected relatives with the mutation have a greater risk than the general population and require surveillance and prophylactic measures.

Prophylactic strategies consist of prophylactic mastectomy, salpingo-oophorectomy and chemoprevention.

Only limited data are available on the survival impact of contralateral mastectomy in unilateral breast cancer [17]. Women with breast cancer who are ≤35 years or premenopausal and carriers of a known BRCA1/2 mutation may be recommended additional risk-reduction strategies following appropriate risk assessment and counseling. The lifetime risk of breast cancer in a BRCA1 carrier is 80–85%, with a 10-year actuarial risk of contralateral breast cancer ranging from 25% to 31%. With bilateral mastectomy, the risks for both subsequent breast cancer incidence and mortality are reduced by 90–95%. The decision should be made with a multidisciplinary team before the surgery and should include a discussion of the risks associated with development of a contralateral breast cancer compared with the risks of recurrent disease from the primary cancer. Except as specifically outlined in some situations, prophylactic mastectomy of a breast contralateral to a known unilateral breast cancer treated with mastectomy is discouraged. The use of prophylactic mastectomy contralateral to a breast treated with breast-conserving surgery is very strongly discouraged in all patients.

Despite the overall trend toward breast conservation, increasing numbers of breast cancer patients are opting for bilateral mastectomy (incorporating contralateral risk-reducing surgery) in preference to breast conservation and mammographic surveillance of the irradiated breast. These patients should be counseled properly and should be informed of the finding that patients with early-stage breast cancer might have even better outcomes after breast-conserving therapy compared with after mastectomy.

Recommendations

Patients from high-risk families (multiple affected family members, male breast cancer, bilateral breast cancer, concomitant ovarian cancer, Ashkenazi Jewish, early onset of breast cancer) should be referred to genetic counseling.

Genetic counselling should be undertaken by physicians with specific training.

Patients with a family history of breast cancer or known BRCA1 or 2 gene mutations should be offered optional prophylactic mastectomy.

Prophylactic salpingo-oophorectomy should also be offered.

Axillary Staging

Axillary surgery is required for adequate staging and proper treatment of breast cancer. The primary aim is to eradicate local disease. Axillary surgery minimizes local recurrence and influences survival and prognosis by guiding adjuvant therapy. Axillary lymph node dissection (ALND) was a routine surgical procedure for breast cancer treatment. ALND provides useful information for staging of disease while eradicating local disease. The procedure involves removal of lymph nodes in the axillary fossa posterior to the pectoral minor muscle up to the axillary vein. The level of axillary lymph node dissection is defined as I, II or III according to the location of the lymph node basins removed relative to the pectoralis minor muscle. Unfortunately, ALND is associated with serious morbidities, such as placement of axillary drainage, longer hospitalization, recovery, postoperative pain and limitations in arm and shoulder movement due to lymphedema.

Sentinel lymph node biopsy (SLNB) was developed to reduce these morbidities associated with ALND while providing similar information on axillary status. The sentinel lymph node is defined as the first lymph node to which tumor cells are likely to spread from the primary breast tumor. Patients with positive SLNB may benefit from ALND, and negative patients that will avoid the morbidities of ALND. The sentinel lymph node is localized via lymph node mapping. Mapping may be performed with blue dye (methylene blue or isosulfan blue) or technetium-labeled sulfur colloid either alone or in combination. Several studies have demonstrated that the combination technique may result in lower false-negative rates. The mapping agents may be injected in the subdermal, periareolar or peritumoral region. The mapping agent(s) passes through the lymphatics and accumulates at the draining node. Then, the sentinel lymph node(s) are harvested if they are identified and then pathologically evaluated.

Preoperative lymphoscintigraphy may provide information on draining basins and sentinel lymph node number. The procedure may be performed the day prior to surgery or on the day of surgery. Peritumoral injection may provide an image of drainage to the axillary, internal mammillary, or both nodal basins. If subareolar or subdermal injection is used, only axillary drainage is revealed. A lack of lymph node detection on lymphoscintigraphy prior to operation does not preclude success of intraoperative detection. Preoperatively, blue dye is injected prior to incision in a volume of 3–5 ml, and massage is performed to facilitate drainage. A handheld gamma probe is used to detect radioactivity transcutaneously and guide incision. After the incision is made, the increased radioactivity and blue lymphatic channel guide the surgeon to the sentinel lymph node(s). After harvesting the node, the region is checked to confirm that the radioactivity has decreased. If not, the search continues to other sentinel lymph node(s).

Trained physicians have been reported to identify sentinel lymph nodes in 95% of cases with a less than 10% false-negative rate. Patients with clinically positive lymph nodes should be evaluated with ultrasound and FNA biopsy prior to surgery. In case of confirmed axillary metastasis, patients may be directed to ALND or considered for neoadjuvant chemotherapy. If no axillary metastasis is demonstrated, patients can proceed to SLNB.

Sentinel lymph node (SLN) mapping and surgical excision of clinically lymph node negative axilla are recommended to evaluate the pathologic status of the axillary lymph nodes in patients with stage I or stage II breast cancer [18–24]. This recommendation is supported by the results of randomized clinical trials showing decreased arm and shoulder morbidity such as pain, lymphedema and sensory loss in patients with breast cancer undergoing SLNB compared with patients undergoing standard ALND [24, 25]. An experienced SLN team is mandatory for the use of SLN mapping and excision [26, 27]. With appropriate training in the dual radiocolloid/blue dye or indocyanine green fluorescence technique, acceptably low false-negative rates and favorable axillary recurrence rates following SLNB are achievable. Women who have invasive breast cancer and do not have access to an experienced SLN team should be referred to an experienced SLN team for definitive surgical treatment of the breast and surgical axillary lymph node staging. Candidates for SLN mapping should have clinically negative axillary lymph nodes or a negative fine-needle aspiration (FNA) biopsy of any clinically suspicious axillary lymph nodes. There is no consensus for the pathologic assessment of SLNB. The significance of occult micrometastases in terms of surgical management and patient outcome appears to be negligible. Thus, routine IHC or PCR is not recommended for the evaluation of sentinel lymph nodes, and treatment decisions should be made based on H&E staining [28].

Multiple attempts have been made to identify cohorts of women with involved SLNs who have a sufficiently low risk of non-SLN involvement that complete axillary dissection might be avoided if the SLN is positive. None of the early studies identified a low-risk group of patients with positive SLN biopsies but consistently negative non-sentinel nodes [29–34]. Nonetheless, a randomized trial (ACOSOG Z0011) compared SLN resection alone with ALN dissection in women ≥18 years of age with T1/T2 tumors, fewer than 3 positive SLNs, and undergoing breast-conserving surgery and whole-breast irradiation. In this study, there was no difference in local recurrence, DFS, or OS between the two treatment groups. Only ER-negative status, age <50, and lack of adjuvant systemic therapy were associated with decreased OS. At a median follow-up of 9.3 years, 10-year locoregional recurrence did not differ significantly between the 2 groups. The 10-year OS was 86.3% in the SLND alone group and 83.6% in the ALND group ($p = 0.02$) [35]. In addition to this study, based on the results of the IBCSG 23–01 trial, further axillary treatment does not seem to be required when a sentinel node has micrometastasis (0.2–2 mm) [36]. Therefore, according to these results, patients with T1 or T2 tumors with 1–2 positive SLNs and undergoing BCS plus tangential breast irradiation may not require further axillary procedures. However, these results need to be confirmed and cannot be extended to patients with characteristics other than those of the trial's patient population.

Level I or II axillary dissection should be recommended when (1) patients have clinically positive nodes at the time of diagnosis that are confirmed by FNA or core biopsy or (2) sentinel nodes are not identified. Traditional level I and level II evaluation of axillary lymph nodes requires that at least 10 lymph nodes be removed for pathologic evaluation to accurately stage the axilla [37, 38]. Level III ALND should be performed only if gross disease is apparent in the level II nodes. Level I–II lymph node dissection should include tissue inferior to the axillary vein from the latissimus dorsi muscle laterally to the medial border of the pectoralis minor muscle.

Furthermore, without definitive data demonstrating superior survival with ALND or SLNB, these procedures may be considered optional in patients who have particularly favorable tumors, patients for whom the selection of adjuvant systemic therapy will not be affected by the results of the procedure, elderly patients, and patients with serious comorbid conditions. Patients with SLN metastasis and no

ALND or axillary lymph node irradiation are at increased risk for ipsilateral lymph node recurrence [39].

There are some unanswered questions regarding sentinel lymph node biopsy in early breast cancer:

accuracy in neoadjuvant chemotherapy;
accuracy in recurrent breast cancer;
the appropriate approach for non-axillary positive lymph nodes;
the optimal pathological method for evaluating sentinel nodes;
the role of intraoperative assessment and the proper method.

Recommendations

All patients with stage I or II breast cancer should be assessed for axillary lymph node status.

Axillary lymph node dissection should be offered for all patients with clinically positive lymph nodes, multifocal disease or non-successful SLNB.

Sentinel lymph node biopsy should be offered instead of ALND for all patients with clinically negative lymph nodes and stage I or II unifocal disease.

All patients should be informed of complications of ALND *(Proposal 1)*.

ALND should be performed in all women with more than 3 proven metastatic axillary lymph nodes.

Patients should be informed of probable unsuccessful SLNB or false-negative results and procedure consequences.

The SLNB procedure should be performed by appropriately trained and experienced physicians.

If available, preoperative lymphoscintigraphy combined with the intraoperative double technique (blue dye and radioisotope labeled tracers) should be performed.

If the double technique is not available, a single method is appropriate.

Sentinel lymph node evaluation should be definitive for proper tailoring.

Definitive histopathological analysis of SLNB should be performed to reduce the false-negative rate.

If the initial assessment of SLNB is negative, each 2-mm slice should be cut into 4 sections of 0.5-mm thickness, with 3 sections randomly evaluated with hematoxylin and eosin and one with cytokeratin immunohistochemistry.

Patients with positive non-axillary lymph nodes (internal mammillary, supra/infra clavicular) should be considered for appropriate radiotherapy.

Surgical Approach After Systemic Therapy

Neoadjuvant chemotherapy is recommended for patients with T4 tumors, axillary lymph node-positive T1–T3 tumors and axillary lymph node-negative T2–T3 tumors with triple-negative or HER2-positive tumors. In other cases, axillary lymph node positivity alone is not sufficient to make a decision regarding neoadjuvant treatment. In Luminal B tumors, chemotherapy can be considered a priority. Neoadjuvant hormone therapy alone may be considered to avoid mastectomy in node-negative select patients (i.e., patients with strong hormone receptor positivity, advanced age, or poor performance status) (Figs. 13.2 and 13.3). Patients with inoperable locally advanced breast cancer have large, fixed or erosive lesions that are not

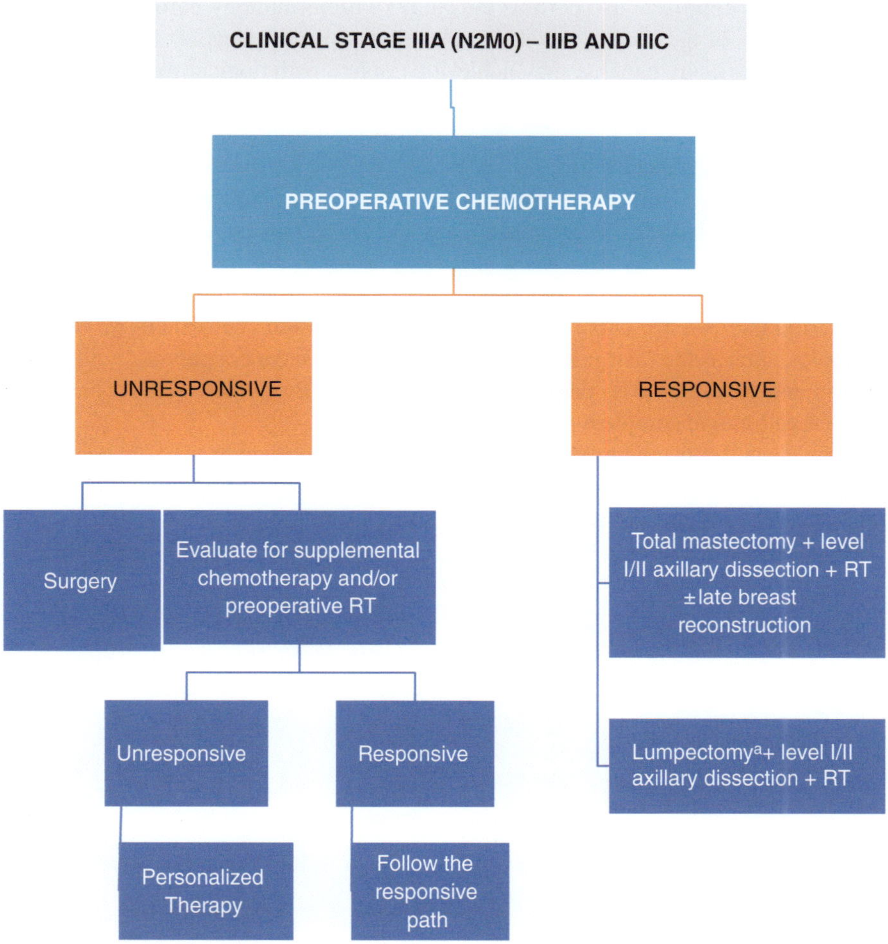

Fig. 13.3 Surgical approach after neoadjuvant systemic treatment for patients with clinical stage IIIA (N2M0)—IIIB and IIIC breast cancer. [a]After downstaging with systemic treatment, resection of the entire area of the original primary tumor is not necessary (if there is shrinkage in the tumor). MR imaging is recommended in patients who will undergo BCS after neoadjuvant therapy. Clinical examination and radiological imaging modalities (USG, MMG, MR imaging) are used to evaluate the tissue to be excised (shrinking or patching). However, if the tumor response is patchy, the original tumor area should be removed with clean surgical margins. If diffuse live tumor cells are observed in the excised lumpectomy specimen after neoadjuvant chemotherapy, re-excision should be performed, even if there is no surgical margin involvement

amenable to mastectomy; advanced nodal disease with arm edema due to fixed lymph nodes at the axilla; and inflammatory breast cancer. Systemic chemotherapy or hormonal therapy can result in breast tumor size reduction in nearly 80% of patients with locally advanced breast cancer. Systemic therapy can convert inoperable tumors to operable ones and convert the need for a surgical procedure from mastectomy to breast-conserving surgery, which will enable favorable cosmesis. Clinical trials are reporting better aesthetic results in early-stage breast cancer patients. This approach also permits the study of tumor biology before surgery and the evaluation of the tumor response to chemotherapy regimens. At the end of systemic therapy, many patients may achieve complete pathological response in both clinical examination and imaging studies. Consequently, the primary tumor site should be marked with a metallic clip prior to the initiation of chemotherapy to indicate the original tumor site.

Preoperative systemic chemotherapy trials have gathered some informative definitions and knowledge of breast cancer in recent years. This knowledge has revealed tumor and patient characteristics that can predict the response to therapy. Consequently, patients can be better defined and selected for appropriate drug regimens, and patients are obtaining greater benefit from the chemotherapy. Targeted therapies, such as the treatment of HER2-positive breast cancer patients with trastuzumab and pertuzumab in combination with chemotherapy, have led to increased rates of pathologic complete response.

Primary systemic chemotherapy (preoperative chemotherapy) should be considered for women with large clinical stage IIA, stage IIB, and T3N1 tumors who meet the criteria for breast-conserving therapy except for tumor size and who wish to undergo breast-conserving therapy (Figs. 13.1 and 13.4). In patients anticipated to

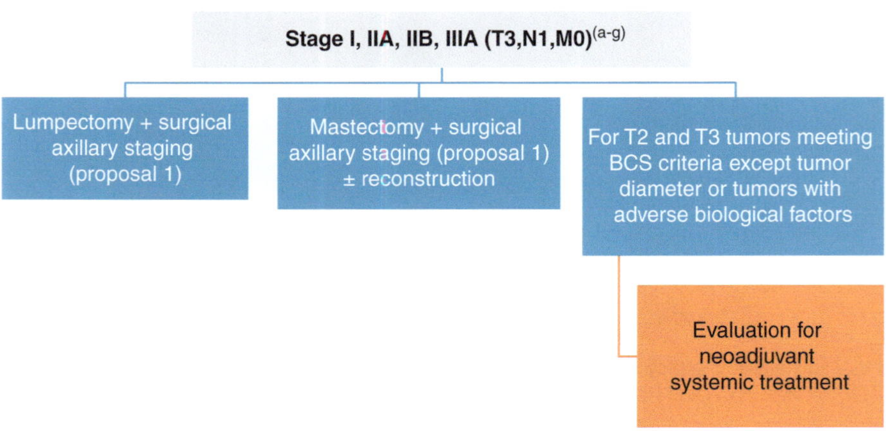

Fig. 13.4 Surgical treatment of patients with clinical stage I, II or IIIA (T3N1M0) disease[a–g]. [a]Absolute contraindications to breast-conserving surgery (BCS) include diffuse suspicious microcalcifications, widespread disease, and persistent positive pathological margins. Relative contraindications include tumor size >5 cm, prior radiation therapy, active connective tissue disease, focally positive margins, and a known or suspected genetic predisposition to breast cancer. Nipple-conserving surgery can be performed in patients with hereditary BRCA1/2 mutations if the

retroareolar tissue is determined to be clean by a pathologist. [b]In women undergoing BCS for invasive BC and proceeding to standard RT and adjuvant systemic therapy, the minimum acceptable surgical margin is “no ink on invasive tumor”. Tumor biology or patient age (<40) does not change the minimum acceptable surgical margins. [c]For BCS: If adjuvant whole-breast RT and systemic treatment will be given to the patient with macrometastasis in 1–2 sentinel lymph nodes, complete axillary dissection may not be performed regardless of tumor biology. [d]For mastectomy: Complete axillary dissection should be performed in patients with macrometastases in 1–2 sentinel lymph nodes if adjuvant RT is not planned. However, there is no complete consensus regarding the omission of axillary dissection in patients for whom RT has been planned. [e]Positive margins (ink on invasive carcinoma or ductal carcinoma in situ) were associated with a twofold increase in the risk of ipsilateral breast tumor recurrence (IBTR) compared with negative margins. This increased risk was not mitigated by favorable biology, endocrine therapy, or a radiation boost. More widely clear margins than no ink on tumor do not significantly decrease the rate of IBTR compared with “no ink on tumor”. No evidence indicates that more widely clear margins reduce IBTR in young patients or in those with unfavorable biology, lobular cancers, or cancers with an extensive intraductal component. The use of “no ink on tumor” is the standard for adequate margins in invasive cancer but not in DCIS. During the operation, it is best to perform the incision macroscopically 1 cm around the tumor. Postoperative MR imaging is appropriate for patients with tumors in close proximity to the surgical margin. In cases undergoing BCS, a surgical margin of 2 mm or greater is considered safe only in those with DCIS. If the invasive tumor is <1 mm in DCIS, the surgical border safety is evaluated according to DCIS. If the invasive focus is >1 mm in DCIS, the surgical margin width should be evaluated according to the invasive cancer. An adequate surgical margin should be decided by clinical, radiological and pathological evaluation. A “sufficient surgical margin” should be decided according to findings such as radiological additional foci (multifocal disease, microcalcification), invasive lobular carcinoma, multiple surgical margin involvement and persistent proximity of surgical margins in re-excision. [f]Neoadjuvant chemotherapy is recommended for patients with axillary lymph node-positive T1–T3 tumors and axillary lymph node-negative T2–T3 tumors with triple-negative or HER2-positive tumors. In other cases, axillary lymph node positivity alone is not sufficient to make a decision regarding neoadjuvant treatment. In Luminal B tumors, chemotherapy can be considered a priority. Neoadjuvant hormone therapy alone may be considered to avoid mastectomy in node-negative select patients (i.e., patients with strong hormone receptor positivity, advanced age, or poor performance status). Neoadjuvant hormonotherapy should last for 6–8 months, as long as the patient responds. The addition of hormonal agents to neoadjuvant chemotherapy can be made with a low level of evidence. Importantly, the guidelines emphasize that addition of endocrine therapy is not based on direct evidence. Additionally, they provide no reason why endocrine therapy should be delayed until completion of cytotoxic treatment. Tamoxifen as endocrine therapy should not be given with chemotherapy. When neoadjuvant chemotherapy is given, the use of chemotherapy in high-risk patients with very strong hormone-receptor positivity, aromatase inhibitors in the postmenopausal stage, and medical oophorectomy in the premenopausal stage [± aromatase inhibitor, especially in HER2-positive patients] may be considered (proposal 3). [g]In a patient who is clinically node positive (N1) at presentation and is downstaged after chemotherapy, sentinel lymph node (SLN) biopsy is appropriate. Marking of positive axillary nodes with a clip in the beginning of the chemotherapy should be considered to permit verification that the biopsy-positive lymph node has been removed at the time of definitive surgery. Among in these subgroup of patients, SLNB has a >10% false-negative rate when performed after preoperative systemic therapy. This false negative rate can be improved by marking biopsied lymph nodes to document their removal, using dual tracer, and by removing more than 2 sentinel nodes. If SLN is positive, axillary lymph node dissection must be performed. After downstaging, resection of the entire area of the original primary tumor is not necessary (if there is shrinkage in the tumor). MR imaging is recommended in patients who will undergo BCS after neoadjuvant therapy. Clinical examination and radiological imaging modalities (USG, MMG, MR imaging) are used to evaluate the tissue to be excised (shrinking or patching). However, if the tumor response is patchy, the original tumor area should be removed with clean surgical margins. If diffuse live tumor cells are observed in the excised lumpectomy specimen after neoadjuvant chemotherapy, re-excision should be performed, even if there is no surgical margin involvement

receive preoperative systemic therapy, core biopsy of the breast tumor and placement of image-detectable marker should be considered to demarcate the tumor bed for any future post-chemotherapy surgical management. Clinically positive ALN should be sampled by FNA or core biopsy, and positive nodes can be removed following preoperative systemic therapy at the time of definitive operation. Patients with clinically negative ALNs should undergo axillary ultrasound prior to neoadjuvant treatment. For those with clinically suspicious ALNs, core biopsy or FNA of these nodes is indicated [40].

Sentinel node biopsy or level I/II dissection can be performed as axillary staging after preoperative systemic therapy. Level I/II dissection should be performed when patients are proven node positive prior to neoadjuvant therapy. The false-negative rate of SLNB in either the pre- or post-chemotherapy settings is low [41–44]. Nevertheless, a pathologic complete response (pCR) following chemotherapy is possible in lymph node metastases previously undetected by clinical exam. An SLN excision can be considered before administering preoperative systemic therapy because it provides additional information to guide local and systemic treatment decisions. Close communication between members of the multidisciplinary team, including the pathologist, is particularly important when any treatment strategy involving preoperative systemic therapy is planned.

Because complete or near-complete clinical responses are common, the use of percutaneously placed clips in the breast under mammographic or ultrasound guidance aids post-chemotherapy resection of the original area of the tumor and is encouraged. Breast conservation rates are higher after preoperative systemic therapy [45].

Local therapy following a complete or partial response to preoperative systemic therapy is usually breast-conserving surgery if possible along with surgical axillary staging. If breast-conserving surgery is not possible or progressive disease is confirmed, mastectomy is performed along with surgical axillary staging with or without breast reconstruction. Surgical axillary staging may include SLN biopsy or level I/II dissection. If SLN biopsy was performed before administering preoperative systemic therapy and the findings were negative, then further ALN staging is not necessary. If an SLN procedure was performed before administering preoperative systemic therapy and the findings were positive, then a level I/II ALN dissection should be performed.

Patients with stage III disease may be further divided into (1) those in whom an initial surgical approach is unlikely to successfully remove all disease or to provide long-term local control; and (2) those in whom a reasonable initial surgical approach is likely to achieve pathologically negative margins and provide long-term local control. Thus, stage IIIA patients are divided into those with clinical T3N1 disease and those who have clinical T anyN2M0 disease based on evaluation by a multidisciplinary team.

In patients with inoperable, locally advanced non-inflammatory disease, anthracycline-based preoperative systemic therapy is standard therapy. Local therapy following a clinical response to preoperative systemic therapy usually consists of mastectomy or breast-conserving surgery with level I/II ALN dissection [45–47]. Delayed breast reconstruction can be considered in mastectomy patients.

Patients with a clinical/pathologic diagnosis of inflammatory breast cancer (IBC) should always be treated with preoperative chemotherapy [48, 49]. Primary surgery and SLN dissection is not a reliable approach in patients with IBC [50]. Breast-conserving surgery is not recommended in IBC patients due to poor cosmesis and higher local recurrence rates compared with mastectomy.

The use of breast-conserving surgery in patients with IBC has been associated with poor cosmesis, and limited data suggest that rates of local recurrence may be higher compared with mastectomy. Breast-conserving therapy is not recommended for patients with IBC.

Mastectomy with level I/II ALN dissection is the recommended surgical procedure for patients who respond to neoadjuvant chemotherapy. Delayed breast reconstruction is an option for patients with IBC who have undergone a modified radical mastectomy. Early/immediate reconstruction after mastectomy may compromise post-mastectomy radiotherapy outcomes [51].

For patients with IBC who do not respond to preoperative systemic therapy, mastectomy is not generally recommended. Additional systemic chemotherapy and/or preoperative radiation should be considered for these patients, and patients responding to this secondary therapy should undergo mastectomy and subsequent treatment as described above.

Breast Reconstruction

Breast reconstruction may be an option for any woman receiving surgical treatment for breast cancer. Therefore, all women undergoing breast cancer treatment should be educated about breast reconstructive options adapted to their individual clinical situation. However, breast reconstruction should not interfere with the appropriate surgical management of the cancer.

Breast reconstruction consists of several surgical techniques utilizing either prosthesis or tissue from elsewhere in the body to rebuild breast shape. The use of implants, pedicled flaps or free flaps are the most commonly applied procedures. Breast reconstruction can be immediate at the time of primary surgery or delayed to allow time to recover from the primary surgery and subsequent adjuvant treatments.

The decision regarding the type of reconstruction involves patient preference, body habitus, smoking history, comorbidities, plans for irradiation, and expertise and experience of the reconstruction team. Reconstruction is an optional procedure that does not impact the probability of recurrence or death but is associated with an improved quality of life for many patients. It is sometimes necessary to perform surgery on the contralateral breast (e.g., breast reduction, implantation) to achieve optimal symmetry between the ipsilateral reconstructed breast and the contralateral breast.

The loss of the breast for cosmetic, body image, and psychosocial issues may be partially overcome through the performance of breast reconstruction. Reconstruction can be performed either immediately following mastectomy and under the same anesthetic or in a delayed fashion following mastectomy. Breast reconstruction usually involves a staged approach requiring more than one procedure.

Many factors must be considered in decision making about breast reconstruction following mastectomy. Several different types of breast reconstruction, such as autogenous tissues, implants, or both, can be performed following mastectomy [52–54]. Reconstruction with implants can be performed either by immediate placement of a permanent subpectoral implant or initial placement of a subpectoral expander followed by replacement of the expander with a permanent implant. At 1 year after mastectomy, patients who underwent autologous reconstruction were more satisfied with their breasts and had greater psychosocial and sexual well-being than those who underwent implant reconstruction. Although satisfaction with breasts was equal to or greater than baseline levels, physical well-being was not fully restored [54]. Autogenous tissue methods of reconstruction use various combinations of donor sites (e.g., abdomen, buttock) that may be brought to the chest wall with their original blood supply or as free flaps with microvascular anastomoses to supply blood from the chest wall/thorax. Several procedures using autologous tissue are available, including transverse rectus abdominis myocutaneous flap, latissimus dorsi flap, and gluteus maximus myocutaneous flap reconstruction. Composite reconstruction techniques use implants in combination with autogenous tissue reconstruction to provide volume and symmetry. Patients with underlying diabetes or who smoke tobacco have increased rates of complications following autogenous tissue breast cancer reconstruction, presumably because of underlying microvascular disease.

Skin-Sparing Mastectomy

The possible advantages of skin-sparing mastectomy include improvements in breast cosmesis, body image, and nipple sensation following mastectomy, although the impact of this procedure on these quality-of-life issues has not been well studied [55–57]. There are limited data from surgical series with short follow-up suggesting that nipple-areolar complex (NAC)-sparing mastectomy in selected patients is associated with low rates of occult involvement of the NAC with breast cancer and local disease recurrence. NAC-sparing procedures may be an option in patients who are carefully selected by experienced multidisciplinary teams. Assessment of retroareolar margins is mandatory in patients considering an NAC-sparing procedure [56, 58, 59]. Retrospective studies validate the use of NAC-sparing procedures for patients with breast cancer with low rates of nipple involvement and low rates of local recurrence due to early-stage, biologically favorable tumors that are located >2 cm from the nipple [60, 61]. Contraindications for nipple preservation include findings of nipple involvement such as Paget's disease or bloody nipple discharge. Ongoing prospective trials to assess NAC-sparing mastectomy in the setting of malignancy will answer many questions, and participation in such trials is encouraged.

Although no randomized studies have been performed, the results of several retrospective studies have indicated that the risk of local recurrence is not increased among patients receiving skin-sparing mastectomies compared with those undergoing non-skin–sparing procedures. However, strong selection biases almost certainly exist in the identification of patients appropriate for skin-sparing procedures [62–66]. Reconstruction of the NAC may also be performed in a delayed fashion if desired by the patient. Reconstructed nipples are devoid of sensation. Skin-sparing mastectomy should be performed by an experienced breast surgery team working in a coordinated, multidisciplinary fashion to guide proper patient selection for skin-sparing mastectomy, determine optimal sequencing of the reconstructive procedure in relation to adjuvant therapies, and perform a resection that achieves appropriate surgical margins. Post-mastectomy radiation should still be applied for patients treated by skin-sparing mastectomy following the same selection criteria as for standard mastectomy.

Post-Mastectomy Radiation and Breast Reconstruction

The decision for post-mastectomy radiation therapy can affect reconstruction strategies because of the increased risk of complications, such as capsular contracture, following irradiation of the implant. Postmastectomy radiation therapy may also have a negative impact on breast cosmesis when autologous tissue is used in immediate breast reconstruction [67, 68]. Some studies, however, have not found a significant compromise in reconstruction cosmesis following irradiation [69]. While some experienced breast cancer teams have employed protocols in which immediate tissue reconstructions are followed by radiation therapy, it is generally preferred that radiation therapy precede the placement of autologous tissue because of reported loss of reconstruction cosmesis.

When implant reconstruction is planned in a patient requiring radiation therapy, a two-stage approach with immediate tissue expander placement followed by implant placement is recommended. Exchange of the tissue expanders with permanent implants can be performed prior to radiation or after completion of radiation therapy. The expansion of irradiated skin can result in an increased risk of malposition, capsular contracture, poor cosmesis, and implant exposure. The use of tissue expanders/implants is relatively contraindicated in patients who have been previously irradiated. Immediate placement of an implant in patients requiring postoperative radiation has an increased rate of complications such as capsular contracture, malposition, poor cosmesis, and implant exposure.

Recommendations

Breast reconstruction options should be offered for all patients undergoing mastectomy.

Immediate and delayed reconstruction should be discussed prior to mastectomy due to the importance of self-confidence and body image perception.

Breast Reconstruction Following BCS (Oncoplastic Approach)

The optimization of the cosmetic and oncologic outcomes of breast-conserving surgery has been addressed in recent years by the emergence of the field of oncoplastic surgery. The possible cosmetic outcome of lumpectomy should be evaluated prior to surgery. Oncoplastic techniques for breast conservation can extend breast-conserving surgical options in situations where the resection itself would likely yield an unacceptable cosmetic outcome [70]. The definition of oncoplastic surgery has been recently expanded to include a wide range of volume displacement or volume redistribution procedures performed by breast surgeons and general surgeons to optimize breast shape and breast volume following breast cancer surgery [71]. Oncoplastic volume displacement procedures combine the removal of generous regions of breast tissue with “mastopexy” techniques in which the remaining breast tissues are shifted together within the breast envelope to fill the resulting surgical defect, thus avoiding the creation of a significant breast deformity. Volume displacement techniques are generally performed during the same operative setting as the breast-conserving lumpectomy by the same surgeon who is performing the cancer resection [70–73].

The advantages of oncoplastic volume displacement techniques include the ability to remove larger regions of breast tissue, thus facilitating wider surgical margins around the cancer, while better preserving the natural shape and appearance of the breast compared to standard breast resections [73].

The limitations of oncoplastic volume displacement techniques include the lack of standardization among centers, performance at only a limited number of sites, and the possible need for subsequent mastectomy if pathologic margins are positive. Patients should be informed of the possibility of positive margins and the potential need for secondary surgery, which could include re-excision segmental resection or require mastectomy with or without loss of the nipple. Oncoplastic procedures can be combined with surgery on the contralateral unaffected breast to minimize long-term asymmetry.

Finally, it is important to note that the primary focus should be on treating the tumor and that such treatment should not be compromised when decisions regarding breast reconstruction are made. In the first international consensus conference on standardization of oncoplastic breast conserving surgery the panelists considered oncoplastic breast conserving surgery safe and effective for improving aesthetic outcomes and broadening the indication for breast conserving surgery towards larger tumors [74]. A slim majority believed that oncoplastic breast conserving surgery reduces the rate of positive margins; however, there was consensus that oncoplastic breast conserving surgery is associated with an increased risk of complications compared to conventional breast conserving surgery. The panel strongly endorsed patient-reported outcomes measurement, and recommended selected scales of the Breast-Q™-Breast Conserving Therapy Module for that purpose. The Clough bi-level classification was recommended for standard use in clinical practice for indicating, planning and performing oncoplastic breast conserving surgery, and the Hoffmann classification for surgical reports and billing purposes. Mastopexy and reduction mammoplasty were the only two recognized oncoplastic breast conserving surgery procedure categories supported by a majority of the panel. Finally, the experts unanimously supported the statement that every oncoplastic breast conserving surgery procedure should be tailored to each individual patient [74].

Surgery for Metastatic Breast Cancer

The primary treatment approach for women with metastatic breast cancer and an intact primary tumor is systemic therapy, with consideration of surgery after initial systemic treatment for those women requiring palliation of symptoms or with impending complications, such as skin ulceration, bleeding, fungation, and pain [75]. Generally, such surgery should be undertaken only if complete local clearance of the tumor may be obtained and if other sites of disease are not immediately threatening to life. Radiation therapy may be considered as an alternative to surgery. Surgery often requires collaboration between the breast surgeon and the reconstructive surgeon to provide optimal cancer control and wound closure.

Retrospective studies suggest a potential survival benefit from complete excision of the primary tumor in select patients with metastatic breast cancer [76–81]. Substantial selection biases exist in all of these studies and are likely to confound the study results. Two recent prospective, randomized studies assessed whether or not surgery on the primary tumor in the breast is necessary for women who are diagnosed with metastatic breast cancer. The results from both studies were similar and showed that surgical treatment of primary tumors in woman presenting with stage IV disease does not produce an increase in OS in general [82, 83]. However, a survival advantage for primary tumor excision was observed only in patients with solitary bone metastasis in the Turkish study [83].

Randomized clinical trials addressing the advantages and disadvantages of local therapy for patients with stage IV disease while eliminating selection biases are necessary. Patient enrollment in such trials is encouraged.

Conclusion

The use of no ink on the tumor as the standard for an adequate margin in invasive cancer in the era of multidisciplinary therapy is associated with low rates of IBTR and has the potential to decrease re-excision rates, improve cosmetic outcomes, and decrease health care costs. Patients without sentinel lymph node (SLN) metastases should not receive axillary lymph node dissection (ALND). Patients with one to two metastatic SLNs planning to undergo breast-conserving surgery with whole-breast radiotherapy should not undergo ALND (in most cases). Patients with SLN metastases who will undergo mastectomy should be offered ALND according to randomized controlled studies. Patients with operable breast cancer and multicentric tumors, with ductal carcinoma in situ (DCIS) who will undergo mastectomy, who previously underwent breast and/or axillary surgery, or who received preoperative/neoadjuvant systemic therapy may be offered SLN biopsy. Women who have large or locally advanced invasive breast cancer (tumor size T3/T4), inflammatory breast cancer, or DCIS (when breast-conserving surgery is planned) or are pregnant should not undergo SLN biopsy. All women undergoing breast cancer treatment should be educated about breast reconstructive options, as adapted to their individual clinical situation. These recommendations are based on cohort studies and/or informal consensus.

References

1. Fourquet A, Campana F, Zafrani B, Mosseri V, Vielh P, Durand JC. Prognostic factors of breast recurrence in the conservative management of early breast cancer: a 25-year follow-up. Int J Radiat Oncol Biol Phys. 1989;17:719–25.
2. Komoike Y, Akiyama F, Iino Y, Ikeda T, Akashi-Tanaka S, et al. Ipsilateral breast tumor recurrence (IBTR) after breast-conserving treatment for early breast cancer: risk factors and impact on distant metastases. Cancer. 2006;106:35–41.
3. Pierce LJ, Griffith KA, Buys S, Gaffney DK, Moran MS, Haffty BG, et al. Outcomes following breast conservation versus mastectomy in BRCA1/2 carriers with early-stage breast cancer [abstract]. J Clin Oncol. 2008;26(Suppl 15):536.
4. Zhou P, Gautam S, Recht A. Factors affecting outcome for young women with early stage invasive breast cancer treated with breast-conserving therapy. Breast Cancer Res Treat. 2007;101:51–7.
5. Golshan M, Miron A, Nixon AJ, Garber JE, Cash EP, Iglehart JD, et al. The prevalence of germline BRCA1 and BRCA2 mutations in young women with breast cancer undergoing breast-conservation therapy. Am J Surg. 2006;192:58–62.
6. Kroman N, Holtveg H, Wohlfahrt J, Jensen MB, Mouridsen HT, Blichert-Toft M, et al. Effect of breast-conserving therapy versus radical mastectomy on prognosis for young women with breast carcinoma. Cancer. 2004;100:688–93.
7. Cruz MR, Prestes JC, Gimenes DL, Fanelli MF. Fertility preservation in women with breast cancer undergoing adjuvant chemotherapy: a systematic review. Fertil Steril. 2010;94:138–43.
8. Dunn L, Fox KR. Techniques for fertility preservation in patients with breast cancer. Curr Opin Obstet Gynecol. 2009;21:68–73.
9. Oktay K, Harvey BE, Partridge AH, Quinn GP, Reinecke J, Taylor HS, et al. Fertility preservation in patients with cancer: ASCO clinical practice guideline update. J Clin Oncol. 2018;36(19):1994–2001.
10. Redig AJ, Brannigan R, Stryker SJ, Woodruff TK, Jeruss JS. Incorporating fertility preservation into the care of young oncology patients. Cancer. 2011;117:4–10.
11. Lee S, Ozkavukcu S, Heytens E, Moy F, Oktay K. Value of early referral to fertility preservation in young women with breast cancer. J Clin Oncol. 2010;28:4683–6.
12. Arriagada R, Le MG, Rochard F, Contesso G. Conservative treatment versus mastectomy in early breast cancer: patterns of failure with 15 years of follow-up data. Institut Gustave-Roussy Breast Cancer Group. J Clin Oncol. 1996;14:1558–64.
13. Clarke M, Collins R, Darby S, Davies C, Elphinstone P, Evans V, et al. Effects of radiotherapy and of differences in the extent of surgery for early breast cancer on local recurrence and 15-year survival: an overview of the randomised trials. Lancet. 2005;366:2087–106.

14. Fisher B, Anderson S, Bryant J, Margolese RG, Deutsch M, Fisher ER, et al. Twenty-year follow-up of a randomized trial comparing total mastectomy, lumpectomy, and lumpectomy plus irradiation for the treatment of invasive breast cancer. N Engl J Med. 2002;347:1233–41.
15. Veronesi U, Cascinelli N, Mariani L, Greco M, Saccozzi R, Luini A, et al. Twenty-year follow-up of a randomized study comparing breast-conserving surgery with radical mastectomy for early breast cancer. N Engl J Med. 2002;347:1227–32.
16. National Breast Cencer Centre. Clinical practice guidelines for the management of early breast cancer. 2nd ed. Camperdown: National Health and Medical Research Council (NHMRC); 2001.
17. Recht A. Contralateral prophylactic mastectomy: caveat emptor. J Clin Oncol. 2009;27:1347–9.
18. Lyman GH, Somerfield MR, Bosserman LD, Perkins CL, Weaver DL, Giuliano AE. Sentinel lymph node biopsy for patients with early-stage breast cancer: American Society of Clinical Oncology clinical practice guideline update. J Clin Oncol. 2017;35(5):561–4.
19. Bass SS, Lyman GH, McCann CR, Ku NN, Berman C, Durand K, et al. Lymphatic mapping and sentinel lymph node biopsy. Breast J. 1999;5:288–95.
20. Cox CE, Nguyen K, Gray RJ, Salud C, Ku NN, Dupont E, et al. Importance of lymphatic mapping in ductal carcinoma in situ (DCIS): why map DCIS? Am Surg. 2001;67:513–9.
21. Krag D, Weaver D, Ashikaga T, Moffat F, Klimberg VS, Shriver C, et al. The sentinel node in breast cancer—a multicenter validation study. N Engl J Med. 1998;339:941–6.
22. Krag DN, Anderson SJ, Julian TB, Brown AM, Harlow SP, Costantino JP, et al. Sentinel-lymph-node resection compared with conventional axillary-lymph-node dissection in clinically node-negative patients with breast cancer: overall survival findings from the NSABP B-32 randomised phase 3 trial. Lancet Oncol. 2010;11:927–33.
23. Kuehn T, Vogl FD, Helms G, Pueckler SV, Schirrmeister H, Strueber R, et al. Sentinel-node biopsy for axillary staging in breast cancer: results from a large prospective German multi-institutional trial. Eur J Surg Oncol. 2004;30:252–9.
24. Veronesi U, Paganelli G, Viale G, Luini A, Zurrida S, Galimberti V, et al. A randomized comparison of sentinel-node biopsy with routine axillary dissection in breast cancer. N Engl J Med. 2003;349:546–53.
25. Mansel RE, Fallowfield L, Kissin M, Goyal A, Newcombe RG, Dixon JM, et al. Randomized multicenter trial of sentinel node biopsy versus standard axillary treatment in operable breast cancer: the ALMANAC trial. J Natl Cancer Inst. 2006;98:599–609.
26. Cox CE, Salud CJ, Cantor A, Bass SS, Peltz ES, Ebert MD, et al. Learning curves for breast cancer sentinel lymph node mapping based on surgical volume analysis. J Am Coll Surg. 2001;193:593–600.
27. Dupont E, Cox C, Shivers S, Salud C, Nguyen K, Cantor A, et al. Learning curves and breast cancer lymphatic mapping: institutional volume index. J Surg Res. 2001;97:92–6.
28. Giuliano AE, Hawes D, Ballman KV, Whitworth PW, Blumencranz PW, Reintgen DS, et al. Association of occult metastases in sentinel lymph nodes and bone marrow with survival among women with early-stage invasive breast cancer. JAMA. 2011;306:385–93.
29. Ozmen V, Karanlik H, Cabioglu N, Igci A, Kecer M, Asoglu O, et al. Factors predicting the sentinel and non-sentinel lymph node metastases in breast cancer. Breast Cancer Res Treat. 2006;95(1):1–6.
30. Houvenaeghel G, Nos C, Giard S, Mignotte H, Esterni B, Jacquemier J, et al. A nomogram predictive of non-sentinel lymph node involvement in breast cancer patients with a sentinel lymph node micrometastasis. Eur J Surg Oncol. 2009;35:690–5.
31. Katz A, Smith BL, Golshan M, Niemierko A, Kobayashi W, Raad RA, et al. Nomogram for the prediction of having four or more involved nodes for sentinel lymph node-positive breast cancer. J Clin Oncol. 2008;26:2093–8.
32. Scow JS, Degnim AC, Hoskin TL, Reynolds C, Boughey JC. Assessment of the performance of the Stanford online calculator for the prediction of nonsentinel lymph node metastasis in sentinel lymph node-positive breast cancer patients. Cancer. 2009;115:4064–70.

33. van la Parra RFD, Ernst MF, Bevilacqua JLB, Mol SJ, Van Zee KJ, Broekman JM, et al. Validation of a nomogram to predict the risk of nonsentinel lymph node metastases in breast cancer patients with a positive sentinel node biopsy: validation of the MSKCC breast nomogram. Ann Surg Oncol. 2009;16:1128–35.
34. Werkoff G, Lambaudie E, Fondrinier E, Levêque J, Marchal F, Uzan M, et al. Prospective multicenter comparison of models to predict four or more involved axillary lymph nodes in patients with breast cancer with one to three metastatic sentinel lymph nodes. J Clin Oncol. 2009;27:5707–12.
35. Giuliano AE, Ballman KV, McCall L, Beitsch PD, Whitworth PW, Blumencranz PW, et al. Effect of axillary dissection vs no axillary dissection on 10-year overall survival among women with invasive breast cancer and sentinel node metastasis: the ACOSOGZ0011 (Alliance) randomized clinical trial. JAMA. 2017;318(10):918–26.
36. Galimberti V, Cole BF, Zurrida S, Viale G, Luini A, Veronesi P, et al. Axillary dissection versus no axillary dissection in patients with sentinel-node micrometastases (IBCSG 23-01): a phase 3 randomised controlled trial. Lancet Oncol. 2013;14:297–305.
37. Axelsson CK, Mouridsen HT, Zedeler K. Axillary dissection of level I and II lymph nodes is important in breast cancer classification. The Danish Breast Cancer Cooperative Group (DBCG). Eur J Cancer. 1992;28A:1415–8.
38. Kiricuta CI, Tausch J. A mathematical model of axillary lymph node involvement based on 1446 complete axillary dissections in patients with breast carcinoma. Cancer. 1992;69:2496–501.
39. Fisher B, Redmond C, Fisher ER, Bauer M, Wolmark N, Wickerham DL, et al. Ten-year results of a randomized clinical trial comparing radical mastectomy and total mastectomy with or without radiation. N Engl J Med. 1985;312:674–81.
40. Alkuwari E, Auger M. Accuracy of fine-needle aspiration cytology of axillary lymph nodes in breast cancer patients: a study of 115 cases with cytologic-histologic correlation. Cancer. 2008;114:89–93.
41. Classe JM, Bordes V, Campion L, Mignotte H, Dravet F, Leveque J, et al. Sentinel lymph node biopsy after neoadjuvant chemotherapy for advanced breast cancer: results of Ganglion Sentinelle et Chimiotherapie Neoadjuvante, a French prospective multicentric study. J Clin Oncol. 2009;27:726–32.
42. Hunt KK, Yi M, Mittendorf EA, Guerrero C, Babiera GV, Bedrosian I, et al. Sentinel lymph node surgery after neoadjuvant chemotherapy is accurate and reduces the need for axillary dissection in breast cancer patients. Ann Surg. 2009;250:558.
43. Kuehn T, Bauerfeind I, Fehm T, Fleige B, Hausschild M, Helms G, et al. Sentinel-lymph-node biopsy in patients with breast cancer before and after neoadjuvant chemotherapy (SENTINA): a prospective, multicentre cohort study. Lancet Oncol. 2013;14:609–18.
44. Boughey JC, Suman VJ, Mittendorf EA, Ahrendt GM, Wilke LG, Taback B, et al. Sentinel lymph node surgery after neoadjuvant chemotherapy in patients with node-positive breast cancer: the ACOSOG Z1071 (Alliance) clinical trial. JAMA. 2013;310:1455–61.
45. Fisher B, Bryant J, Wolmark N, Mamounas E, Brown A, Fisher ER, et al. Effect of preoperative chemotherapy on the outcome of women with operable breast cancer. J Clin Oncol. 1998;16:2672–85.
46. Bear HD, Anderson S, Smith RE, Geyer CE Jr, Mamounas EP, Fisher B, et al. Sequential preoperative or postoperative docetaxel added to preoperative doxorubicin plus cyclophosphamide for operable breast cancer: National Surgical Adjuvant Breast and Bowel Project Protocol B-27. J Clin Oncol. 2006;24:2019–27.
47. Hudis C, Modi S. Preoperative chemotherapy for breast cancer: miracle or mirage? JAMA. 2007;298:2665–7.
48. Dawood S, Cristofanilli M. What progress have we made in managing inflammatory breast cancer? Oncology. 2007;21:673–9.
49. Kell MR, Morrow M. Surgical aspects of inflammatory breast cancer. Breast Dis. 2005;22:67–73.

50. Stearns V, Ewing CA, Slack R, Penannen MF, Hayes DF, Tsangaris TN. Sentinel lymphadenectomy after neoadjuvant chemotherapy for breast cancer may reliably represent the axilla except for inflammatory breast cancer. Ann Surg Oncol. 2002;9:235–42.
51. Motwani SB, Strom EA, Schechter NR, Butler CE, Lee GK, Langstein HN, et al. The impact of immediate breast reconstruction on the technical delivery of postmastectomy radiotherapy. Int J Radiat Oncol Biol Phys. 2006;66:76–82.
52. Ahmed S, Snelling A, Bains M, Whitworth IH. Breast reconstruction. BMJ. 2005;330:943–8.
53. Edlich RF, Winters KL, Faulkner BC, Bill TJ, Lin KY. Advances in breast reconstruction after mastectomy. J Long-Term Eff Med Implants. 2005;15:197–207.
54. Pusic AL, Matros E, Fine N, Buchel E, Gordillo GM, Hamill JB, et al. Patient-reported outcomes 1 year after immediate breastreconstruction: results of the mastectomy reconstruction outcomes consortium study. J Clin Oncol. 2017;35(22):2499–506.
55. Garcia-Etienne CA, Cody Iii HS, Disa JJ, Cordeiro P, Sacchini V. Nipple-sparing mastectomy: initial experience at the Memorial Sloan-Kettering Cancer Center and a comprehensive review of literature. Breast J. 2009;15:440–9.
56. Petit JY, Veronesi U, Orecchia R, Rey P, Martella S, Didier F, et al. Nipple sparing mastectomy with nipple areola intraoperative radiotherapy: one thousand and one cases of a five years experience at the European institute of oncology of Milan (EIO). Breast Cancer Res Treat. 2009;117:333–8.
57. Yueh JH, Houlihan MJ, Slavin SA, Slavin SA, Lee BT, Pories SE, et al. Nipple-sparing mastectomy: evaluation of patient satisfaction, aesthetic results, and sensation. Ann Plast Surg. 2009;62:586–90.
58. Chung AP, Sacchini V. Nipple-sparing mastectomy: where are we now? Surg Oncol. 2008;17:261–6.
59. Gerber B, Krause A, Dieterich M, Kundt G, Reimer T. The oncological safety of skin sparing mastectomy with conservation of the nipple-areola complex and autologous reconstruction: an extended follow-up study. Ann Surg. 2009;249:461–8.
60. Piper M, Peled AW, Foster RD, Moore DH, Esserman LJ. Total skin-sparing mastectomy: a systematic review of oncologic outcomes and postoperative complications. Ann Plast Surg. 2013;70:435.
61. Mallon P, Feron JG, Couturaud B, Fitoussi A, Lemasurier P, Guihard T, et al. The role of nipple-sparing mastectomy in breast cancer: a comprehensive review of the literature. Plast Reconstr Surg. 2013;131:969–84.
62. Foster RD, Esserman LJ, Anthony JP, Hwang ES, Do H. Skin-sparing mastectomy and immediate breast reconstruction: a prospective cohort study for the treatment of advanced stages of breast carcinoma. Ann Surg Oncol. 2002;9:462–6.
63. Downes KJ, Glatt BS, Kanchwala SK, Mick R, Fraker DL, Fox KR, et al. Skin-sparing mastectomy and immediate reconstruction is an acceptable treatment option for patients with high-risk breast carcinoma. Cancer. 2005;103:906–13.
64. Carlson GW, Styblo TM, Lyles RH, Jones G, Murray DR, Staley CA, et al. The use of skin sparing mastectomy in the treatment of breast cancer: the Emory experience. Surg Oncol. 2003;12:265–9.
65. Newman LA, Kuerer HM, Hunt KK, Kroll SS, Ames FC, Ross MI, et al. Presentation, treatment, and outcome of local recurrence afterskin-sparing mastectomy and immediate breast reconstruction. Ann Surg Oncol. 1998;5:620–6.
66. Medina-Franco H, Vasconez LO, Fix RJ, Heslin MJ, Beenken SW, Bland KI, et al. Factors associated with local recurrence after skin-sparing mastectomy and immediate breast reconstruction for invasive breast cancer. Ann Surg. 2002;235:814–9.
67. Kronowitz SJ, Robb GL. Radiation therapy and breast reconstruction: a critical review of the literature. Plast Reconstr Surg. 2009;124:395–408.
68. Tran NV, Chang DW, Gupta A, Kroll SS, Robb GL. Comparison of immediate and delayed free TRAM flap breast reconstruction in patients receiving postmastectomy radiation therapy. Plast Reconstr Surg. 2001;108:78–82.

69. Mehta VK, Goffinet D. Postmastectomy radiation therapy after TRAM flap breast reconstruction. Breast J. 2004;10:118–22.
70. Clough KB, Kaufman GJ, Nos C, Buccimazza I, Sarfati IM. Improving breast cancer surgery: a classification and quadrant per quadrant atlas for oncoplastic surgery. Ann Surg Oncol. 2010;17:1375–91.
71. Anderson BO, Masetti R, Silverstein MJ. Oncoplastic approaches to partial mastectomy: an overview of volume-displacement techniques. Lancet Oncol. 2005;6:145–57.
72. Huemer GM, Schrenk P, Moser F, Wagner E, Wayand W. Oncoplastic techniques allow breast-conserving treatment in centrally located breast cancers. Plast Reconstr Surg. 2007;120:390–8.
73. Kaur N, Petit J-Y, Rietjens M, Maffini F, Luini A, Gatti G. Comparative study of surgical margins in oncoplastic surgery and quadrantectomy in breast cancer. Ann Surg Oncol. 2005;12:539–45.
74. Weber WP, Soysal SD, El-Tamer M, Sacchini V, Knauer M, Tausch C, et al. First international consensus conference on standardization of oncoplastic breast conserving surgery. Breast Cancer Res Treat. 2017;165(1):139–49.
75. Hortobagyi GN. Multidisciplinary management of advanced primary and metastatic breast cancer. Cancer. 1994;74:416–23.
76. Babiera GV, Rao R, Feng L, Meric-Bernstam F, Kuerer HM, Singletary SE, et al. Effect of primary tumor extirpation in breast cancer patients who present with stage IV disease and an intact primary tumor. Ann Surg Oncol. 2006;13:776–82.
77. Khan SA, Stewart AK, Morrow M. Does aggressive local therapy improve survival in metastatic breast cancer? Surgery. 2002;132:620–6.
78. Rao R, Feng L, Kuerer HM, Singletary SE, Bedrosian I, Hunt KK, et al. Timing of surgical intervention for the intact primary in stage IV breast cancer patients. Ann Surg Oncol. 2008;15:1696–702.
79. Rapiti E, Verkooijen HM, Vlastos G, Fioretta G, Neyroud-Caspar I, Sappino AP, et al. Complete excision of primary breast tumor improves survival of patients with metastatic breast cancer at diagnosis. J Clin Oncol. 2006;24:2743–9.
80. Morrow M, Goldstein L. Surgery of the primary tumor in metastatic breast cancer: closing the barn door after the horse has bolted? J Clin Oncol. 2006;24:2694–6.
81. Olson JA, Marcom PK. Benefit or bias? The role of surgery to remove the primary tumor in patients with metastatic breast cancer. Ann Surg. 2008;247:739–40.
82. Badwe R, Hawaldar R, Nair N, Nair N, Kaushik R, Siddique S, et al. Locoregional treatment versus no treatment of the primary tumour in metastatic breast cancer: an open-label randomised controlled trial. Lancet Oncol. 2015;16(13):1380–8.
83. Soran A, Ozmen V, Ozbas S, Karanlik H, Muslumanoglu M, Igci A, et al. Randomized trial comparing resection of primary tumor with no surgery in stage IV breast cancer at presentation: protocol MF07-01. Ann Surg Oncol. 2018. https://doi.org/10.1245/s10434-018-6494-6.

Chapter 14
Evaluation of Axillary Nodes

Mahmut Muslumanoglu

Introduction

Recent studies have demonstrated that the tumor biological characteristics of tumors are more important in determining treatment plans and prognosis than other factors, such as tumor diameter and axillary involvement. Clinical staging is still used to determine the tumor load. Tumor diameter and axillary involvement were used for a long time, and it is difficult for clinicians to abandon these customs. Consequently, tumor diameter and axillary involvement are still considered important major prognostic factors for predicting survival and selecting adjuvant treatment. Although axillary evaluation [sentinel lymph node (SLN), axillary lymph node dissection (ALND)] does not have a profound effect on overall survival (OS), the removal of metastatic lymph nodes from the axilla may contribute to locoregional control and improve quality of life. In the past, axillary staging with ALND was used in clinically node-negative early-stage breast cancer patients; however, this method carries the risk of some arm and shoulder morbidity without any survival benefit. SLN biopsy (SLNB) is equivalent to ALND in clinically node-negative patients in terms of staging, accuracy, disease-free survival (DFS), and OS. Consequently, ALND is not currently advised for patients able to undergo SLNB. SLNB examines the first lymph nodes because the lymphatics of the breast drain to these lymph nodes, which therefore are the site most likely to be reached by tumor cells. If there is no cancer metastasis in the SLN, the other lymph nodes are considered clear (not containing cancer cells); thus, the ALND technique has been abandoned.

M. Muslumanoglu (✉)
Istanbul University, Istanbul Medical Faculty, Department of General Surgery, Istanbul, Turkey
e-mail: mahmutm@istanbul.edu.tr

A. Aydiner et al. (eds.), *Breast Cancer*, https://doi.org/10.1007/978-3-319-96947-3_14

Lymphatic Drainage of the Breast

The lymphatics of the breast comprise interconnected superficial and deep lymphatic vessels. The subdermal plexus in the retroareolar space, which is called *Sappey's plexus*, drains the lymphatics of the areola and nipple. The lymphatics of the interlobular connective tissue of the breast and the lymphatics of the walls of the lactiferous channels also drain to this plexus. Efferent lymphatic channels leaving this plexus trace along the lateral border of the major pectoral muscle, penetrate the clavipectoral fascia, and enter the axilla. Axillary lymph nodes collect nearly 75% of the lymphatic drainage of the breast. The remaining lymphatics drain into the internal mammary (parasternal) lymph nodes (IMLNs) accompanying perforated branches of the internal mammary artery; this group generally receives drainage from the medial part of the breast.

Sentinel Lymph Node Biopsy

Sentinel means "sentry," and the SLN is the first lymph node at which cancer cells arrive via lymphatic channels starting from the primary tumor; multiple SLNs may exist. Because these lymph nodes are located on the lymphatic drainage course in breast cancer, they contain cancer cells when lymphatic metastasis has occurred. If metastasis is not detected in the pathological examination of the removed SLNs, the axilla is considered clear, and ALND is not performed.

Radioactive colloid and/or blue dye can be used to detect the SLN. Recently, iron oxide nanoparticles and indocyanine green have been developed for SLNB using the same technique. SLNs that are identified by scintigraphic imaging in the preoperative phase can be detected intraoperatively using a gamma probe and/or by injecting blue dye into the breast tissue; the dyed channel and lymph node can then be detected and removed surgically. There are different practices regarding the choice of agents used (blue dye, radioactive substance, or both) and location of injection (periareolar, subareolar, peritumoral). Extra-axillary lymph node (internal mammary group) excision is advised if it is identified as the first draining site by lymphoscintigraphy.

Indications for SLNB

SLNB has been accepted as a standard treatment approach in all clinically node-negative (with physical examination and imaging techniques) early stage (Figs. 14.1 and 14.2) breast cancer cases, regardless of tumor size (uni- or multiple) and location (central, inner or outer part of the breast).

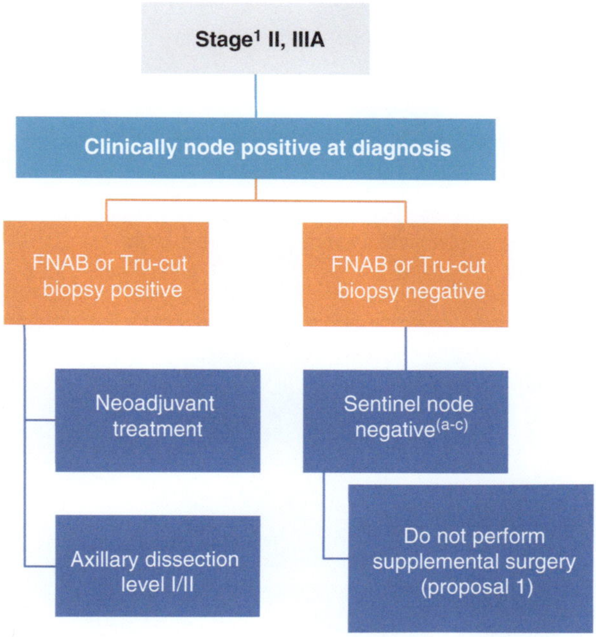

Fig. 14.1 Axillary management of patients with clinical node-positive stages II or IIIA. *FNAB* fine-needle aspiration biopsy, *SLN* sentinel lymph node, *BCS* breast-conserving surgery. [1]Clinical STAGE II (T0, N1, M0; T1, N1, M0; T2, N1, M0); STAGE IIIA (T3, N1, M0). [a]For BCS: In patients with micro/macrometastases in 1–2 sentinel lymph nodes, if there is no neoadjuvant therapy, complete axillary dissection can be safely omitted when "segmental resection with RT" is performed. [b]For mastectomy: In patients with macrometastases in 1–2 sentinel lymph nodes, complete axillary dissection must be performed when no adjuvant RT is planned; however, in patients for whom RT is planned, and if there is no neoadjuvant therapy, no consensus exists for omitting axillary dissection. [c]In patients with T1 or T2 tumors with BCS and 1–2 positive SLNs, if there is *no neoadjuvant chemotherapy* and whole-breast irradiation is planned, axillary dissection is not needed. Axillary dissection is recommended for SLN-positive patients with triple-negative breast cancer

Contraindications for SLNB

SLNB is contraindicated whenever a metastatic lymph node is clinically identified in the axilla [1]. This increases the false-negative rate. Diffuse blockage of lymphatic channels in locally advanced breast cancers manifesting as inflammatory breast cancer and dermal edema are also contraindications for SLNB.

Approximately 40% of node-positive patients can be detected with preoperative ultrasonography and needle biopsy [2]. Classically ALND should be performed directly in this case, or neoadjuvant chemotherapy may be recommended. However, in the near future, axillary tumor load (one or multiple cortical asymmetries or cortical enlargement of the LNs versus multiple gross positive LNs) will become important for deciding further ALND. During surgery, whenever any suspicious lymph nodes (hard) (non-SLNs) are palpated in SLNB-negative patients, excision

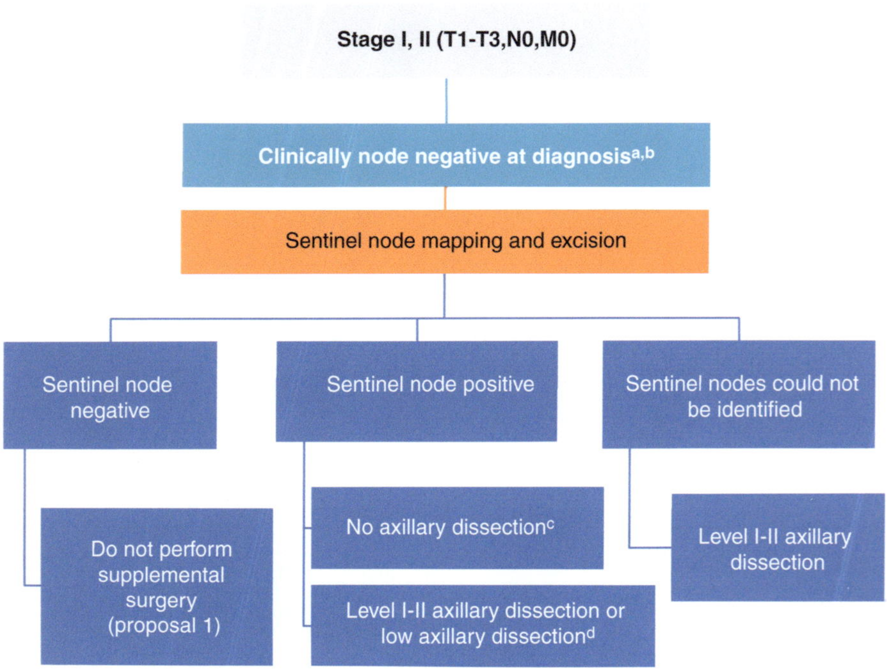

Fig. 14.2 Axillary management of patients with clinical node-negative stage I-II. *FNAB* fine-needle aspiration biopsy, *SLN* sentinel lymph node, *BCS* breast-conserving surgery. [a]For BCS: In patients with micro/macrometastases in 1–2 sentinel lymph nodes, complete axillary dissection can be safely omitted when "conservative resection with RT" is performed. [b]For mastectomy: In patients with macrometastases in 1–2 sentinel lymph nodes, complete axillary dissection must be performed when 'no adjuvant RT is planned'; however, in patients for whom RT is planned, no consensus exists for omitting axillary dissection. [c]In patients with T1 or T2 tumors with BCS and 1–2 positive SLNs, if there is no neoadjuvant chemotherapy and whole-breast irradiation is planned, axillary dissection is not needed. Axillary dissection is recommended for SLN-positive patients with triple-negative breast cancer. [d]Consider axillary dissection according to preoperative imaging results (mammography, ulrasonoghrapy and PET/CT)

must be considered, especially for those patients in whom core biopsy of the primary tumor was not performed. Sometimes, core biopsy can cause enlargement and stiffness in some of the axillary nodes, which may cause unnecessary LN excision together with SLNB. If metastasis is detected in SLNs or non-SLNs during paraffin section examinations, ALND or radiation therapy is decided in a multidisciplinary meeting for each patient according to all factors affecting locoregional recurrence risks and the benefits of adjuvant therapies.

Blue dye allergic reactions are observed in approximately 1–3% of cases and can cause serious anaphylactic reactions [3]. Blue dye is not used during pregnancy due to its potentially fatal effects [4]. Some studies have indicated that radioactive substances in low doses can be safely used during pregnancy [5–7].

SLNB in Specific Cases

Ductal Carcinoma In Situ

Metastasis is observed in 1–2% of DCIS cases, suggesting that some DCIS cases can indeed be invasive and that failure to diagnose metastasis is due to a pathologic sampling error [8, 9]. Because invasive foci can be detected in paraffin sections and SLNB is not associated with extensive complications, SLNB should be performed in DCIS patients who have signs on palpation (tumor mass) or a large area of DCIS (calcified areas >2–3 cm) [4]. SLNB is also recommended for patients planning to undergo mastectomy [10].

Multicentric and Multifocal Breast Cancer

In multifocal and multicentric breast cancer cases, SLNB can be safely performed. However, an increase in the false-negative rate has been reported in some studies. Performing the procedure using a radioactive substance may increase the accuracy of SLN [11–14].

SLNB for Patients with Previous Axillary and Breast Surgery

Studies have demonstrated that SLNs can be detected if superficial and deep lymphatic channels are not disrupted via excisional biopsy (particularly together with a large skin incision at the upper-lateral quadrant and if the deep pectoral fascia is not affected). However, in patients who have undergone breast-conserving surgery (BCS) and radiotherapy or have undergone ALND, lymphatic flow to the internal mammary glands and contralateral axilla is observed, and these areas are considered the second region for SLNs. The detection of axillary SLNs for the second time in patients who previously underwent SLNB is possible [15–18]. SLNB can be performed after aesthetic interventions and even mastectomy [19–21]. Using tandem methods (blue dye lymphoscintigraphy) during SLNB in patients with previous operations increases the success rate [15].

Male Breast Cancer

Breast cancer in males is rare and constitutes 1% of all breast cancer cases. SLNB should be performed in clinically node-negative male breast cancer to avoid unnecessary ALND. SLNB has the same identification and false-negative rates in males as in females [22–24].

Elderly and Overweight Patients

Although studies report high success rates of SLN detection in elderly and overweight patients, we have observed that this patient group is more problematic in practice; it is particularly difficult to detect SLNs using blue dye alone. The utilization of lymphoscintigraphy along with blue dye in elderly and overweight patients increases the success rate.

Axillary Staging in Patients Treated with Neoadjuvant Chemotherapy

The axilla is clinically negative in approximately 40–50% of patients who are planned to receive neoadjuvant chemotherapy. In cases with a positive axillary node, axillary downstaging occurs at a rate of 30–40% with treatment [25–27]. Research to identify an approach that avoids unnecessary ALND in these two patient groups is ongoing, and the method and timing of axillary staging remain controversial. In clinically axilla-negative cases, SLNB can be performed prior to neoadjuvant chemotherapy, and the need for ALND can be determined after treatment [25].

The opinion that alterations of the breast and lymphatic channels due to chemotherapeutic agents decrease the success rate of SLNB performed after chemotherapy and increase the false-negative rate has essentially been abandoned. In the NSABP-B27 trial, the SLN detection rate after neoadjuvant chemotherapy was 84.8%, and the false-negative rate was 10.6% [28]. Recent trials have shown that the use of radiocolloid alone or together with blue dye significantly enhances accuracy and that SLNB is possible after neoadjuvant chemotherapy [29, 30, 28]. ALND should be performed whenever the SLN cannot be detected.

SLNB Technique

Utilization of Radiocolloid and Lymphoscintigraphy

Lymphoscintigraphy is based on the detection of lymph nodes following drainage of the injected radiopharmaceutical agent to the regional lymph nodes via the lymphatic current. Regional lymphatic tracts are mapped using this method and whether an SLN is identified as axillary or extra-axillary using preoperative imaging techniques; during the operation, the SLN is detected by a gamma probe [31].

The most frequently used radiopharmaceuticals are 99mTc-sulfur colloid, 99mTc-nanocolloid, and 99mTc-antimony trisulfide colloid.

Technique During the operation, the tumor mass, including the primary site of injection, is excised first to perform the count correctly and minimize background activity. While the gamma probe is scanned over the skin of the axilla, the site producing the highest activity count is determined, and a small incision is made to enter the axilla. The gamma probe is inserted through the incision, and the lymph node yielding the highest activity count is excised together with its surrounding fat tissue by fine dissection. The activity count of the excised tissue is assessed in a separate location, and after confirming that it is the SLN, the axilla is reevaluated using the probe. If there are any remaining sites producing high activity counts, other SLNs are excised until the activity count is less than 10% of that of the initial node.

Vital Stain

Blue dye injection is another method for visualizing the SLN. The vital stains used for this purpose include patent blue V, isosulfan blue (1% lymphazurin), and methylene blue. Isosulfan blue is the most frequently used agent; however, following injection, reactions ranging from a simple rash to serious anaphylaxis are observed with an incidence ratio of 1:1.1% [32, 33]. Methylene blue is a less expensive alternative that does not bind to plasma proteins and causes fewer anaphylactic reactions. However, methylene blue can cause skin necrosis when intradermally administered, and a dilution ratio of 1:2 is recommended [34]. Studies have yielded similar mapping results using both dyes.

Technique During the operation, approximately 2–5 ml of blue dye is injected by the subareolar routes, and the area is massaged toward the axilla for 2–5 min. Then, the axilla is entered using a 2- to 3-cm transverse incision 2–3 cm below the axillary hairline. After opening the clavipectoral fascia, the lateral thoracic vein, which extends toward the tail of the breast, is identified. The SLN is generally located where the intercostal nerve crosses this region (axilla, level 1). The blue-stained tract is identified via dissection. When traced either to the axilla or to the breast, a blue-stained lymph node or nodes can be observed. The blue-stained lymph node is removed together with the surrounding thin fat tissue. The results obtained with blue dye are similar to those obtained using radioactive substances [35].

Combination of Vital Stains and Radioisotopic Methods

Many studies have reported that blue staining and radiocolloid use are complementary methods that enable the detection of additional SLNs when used together. Moreover, the addition of blue dye to the radiocolloid prevents unnecessary dissections. The SLN detection rate is 95–98% using the radioisotope method [35, 36] and is improved to 95–100% using the combined method. Both methods have high success rates when performed alone, but combined methods should be used in select cases (elderly, overweight, patients who are undergoing SLNB for the second time). We use blue dye (isosulfan blue) in routine practice in our clinic. Lymphoscintigraphy has the advantage of showing extra axillary drainage [19].

Determining the Site of Injection

Studies suggest that SLN detection is more successful via the intradermal or subareolar/periareolar routes; however, most studies indicate that the location of injection does not have an effect on SLN detection [35–39]. Each clinic should perform the technique that they have found successful. We prefer subareolar injections.

Number of SLNs

Frequently, one SLN is removed from the axilla. The false-negative rate drops to 1% when three or more SLNs are removed. However, no benefit is observed when more than four to five SLNs are removed [40, 41]. When more than one blue ganglion is detected, removing all of the lymph nodes decreases the false-negative rate.

Behavior of Micrometastases

Detailed SLN examination (multiple sections with several ganglia) has enabled the detection of smaller metastases. Metastases smaller than 0.2 mm are defined as submicro-isolated tumor cells, metastases that are 0.2–2 mm in size are classified as micrometastases, and those >2 mm are macrometastases. When isolated tumor cells are detected, the axilla is considered negative. When micrometastasis is detected in SLNs, the rate of metastasis in non-SLNs is 10–40%. In macrometastasis, this rate is even higher. Patients with micrometastases in SLNs who did not undergo ALND in BCS and who received radiation therapy were investigated in a randomized trial in Z0011 [42]. This trial followed 446 patients who underwent SLNB and 445 patients who underwent SLNB + ALND. The proportion of patients who had three or more positive LNs was 5% in the SLNB group and 17.6% in the SLNB + ALND group ($p < 0.001$). After an average follow-up of 9.3 years, the 10-year DFS was 80.2% in the SLNB-alone group and 78.2% in the ALND group. The OS rate was 86.3% in the SLNB-alone group and 83.6% in the ALND group. At 5 years, 1 nodal recurrence was observed in the SLNB-alone group vs none in the ALND group. Ten-year regional recurrence did not differ significantly between the two groups [42]. According to this study, which was terminated due to difficulties in patient accrual and low recurrence rates, there was no benefit for the patients in the ALND group.

The detection of minimal disease (micrometastasis) in SLNs may be sufficient to initiate adjuvant therapy. In all valid protocols used today, these patients receive adjuvant therapy similar to that used in axilla+ disease (N1a). Therefore, treatment for these patients is not incomplete.

The only difficulty in treating micrometastatic disease is determining the irradiation area for axillary and peripheral lymphatics. The number of involved axillary lymph nodes is a critical component of this decision. Given the availability of effective adjuvant treatment options and the very low axillary recurrence rates (as in ALND), conservative decisions are now made on behalf of the patient when selecting a radiotherapy area; irradiating wide areas, as is done in Nx, appears to be overtreatment.

Internal Mammary Lymph Node Biopsy (IMLNB)

A small percentage (10%) of lymphatics drain into the IMLNs, particularly in centrally and medially located tumors. IMLNB may alter the treatment plan in 0.1% of breast cancer patients and thus is regarded as unnecessary. However, according to the new staging system, only IMLN positivity is classified as N1c; therefore, IMLNB could change the stage for this group of patients. IMLN detection and sampling are necessary to make a decision regarding the adjuvant treatment policy in axilla-negative patients and to determine if IMLNs will be irradiated. For this reason, we recommend performing IMLNB when the axilla is negative in centrally or medially located tumors.

The only method demonstrating lymphatic drainage to this region is lymphoscintigraphy with the utilization of gamma probes. Usually, the second to third intercostal space is explored in selected axilla-negative cases.

Locally Advanced Breast Cancer

In locally advanced breast cancer (LABC), the utilization of axilla-effective systemic treatment modalities (taxane, trastuzumab, etc.) in routine practice has led to increases in complete response rates (breast + axilla) from approximately 10% to 39–70%; for some specific patient groups (ER negative, PR negative, HER2 positive), higher rates of complete response have been achieved. ALND following chemotherapy was the standard axillary approach for LABC, but SLNB is now recommended in patients with axilla positive prior to chemotherapy to obtain a complete clinical response after chemotherapy. According to the results of prospective randomized trials, if two to three lymph nodes are removed using both blue dye and lymphoscintigraphy, the false-negative rate is 14%, and the detection rate is 98% [25–27, 42, 43].

In cases with a positive axillary node, axillary downstaging occurs at a rate of 30–40% with treatment, and this rate is even higher in triple-negative and Her2-positive patients (Table 14.1) [25–27, 44]. The identification rate of SLNB may decrease in patients whose axilla become clinically negative after neoadjuvant therapy, and the false-negative rate may increase depending on case selection. The biology of the cancer is also an important factor predicting the response rate.

In a prospective study, after neoadjuvant therapy (n = 195) nodal pCR rates were: overall 49%; "ER+/HER2−" 21%; "ER+/HER2+" 70%; "ER−/HER2+" 97% and "ER−/HER2−" 47% [27]. The luminal A group has the lowest complete response rate. With neo-adjuvant CT, axillary dissection can be avoided in up to 48% of patients [27]. ALND should be performed whenever the SLN cannot be detected (Figs. 14.3 and 14.4).

Table 14.1 Nodal pCR after neoadjuvant therapy

	N	Nodal pCR[a] (%)
ACOSOG Z1071 [26]	694	41
FNAC [21]	145	35
Mamtani [1]	195	49

[a]Nodal pCR ranges from 21% in Er+/HER2- to 97% in ER-/HER2+ patients

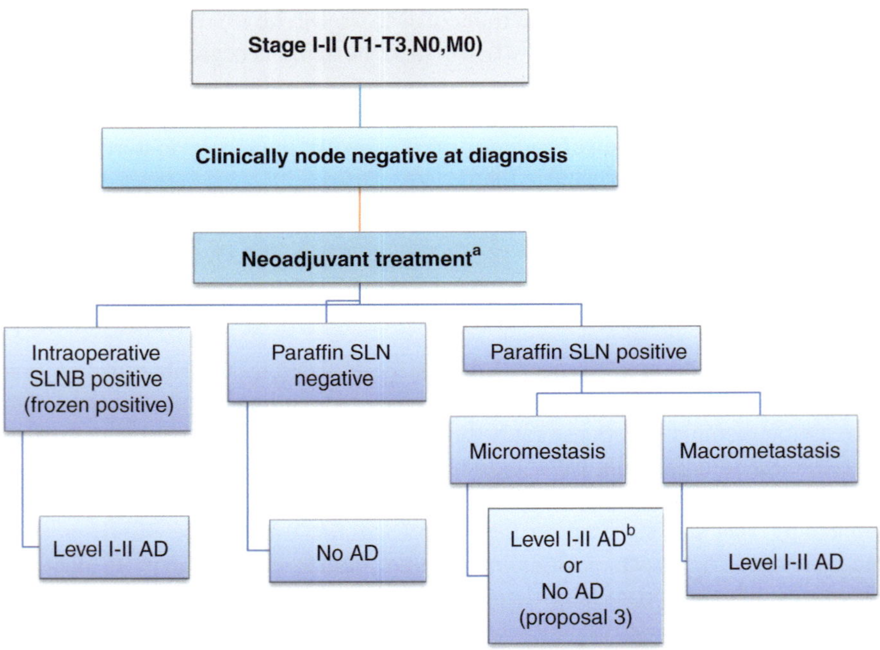

Fig. 14.3 Axillary management of patients with clinical node-negative stages I or II invasive breast cancer. *FNAB* fine-needle aspiration biopsy, *SLN* sentinel lymph node biopsy, *AD* axillary dissection. [a]Neoadjuvant chemotherapy is recommended for patients with axillary axillary lymph node-negative T2–T3 tumors with triple-negative or HER2-positive tumors. In Luminal B tumors, neoadjuvant chemotherapy can be considered. [b]Low-volume disease in the SLN after NAC is not an indicator of a low risk of additional positive axillary nodes. These tumor cells are potentially drug resistant and may be an indication of ALND, even when not detected on intraoperative frozen section

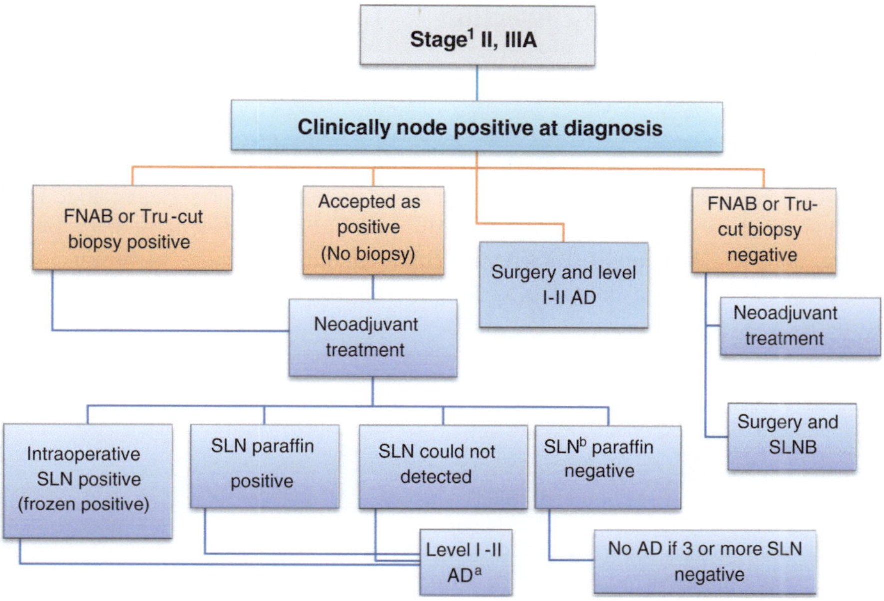

Fig. 14.4 Axillary management of patients with clinical node-positive stage II or IIIA invasive breast cancer. *FNAB* fine-needle aspiration biopsy, *SLN* sentinel lymph node biopsy, *AD* axillary dissection. [1]Clinical STAGE II (T0, N1, M0; T1, N1, M0; T2, N1, M0); STAGE IIIA (T3, N1, M0). [a]After neoadjuvant therapy, if the SLN is positive in frozen or paraffin sections, level I–II axillary dissection is recommended. [b]At least 3 SLNs should be assessed in patients receiving neoadjuvant treatment

Examination of the SLN

Paraffin blocks are prepared, and slices are obtained in numbers and thicknesses defined by the laboratory protocol; these sections are then evaluated using hematoxylin and eosin (H&E) and immunohistochemical staining methods. Intraoperative evaluation of the SLN in clinical axilla-negative patients lost its importance following the Z0011 trial based on the equivalent long-term results of ALND versus radiation therapy in axilla 1–2 micro/macro-positive SLNs [42].

False Negativity

False negativity is defined as the detection of negative SLNs when axillary metastasis is indeed present. SLNs should be detected in at least 85% of patients using the method of choice, and the false-negative rate should be less than 5% [11]. Use of the blue dye and radiocolloid techniques in combination is recommended for surgeons in training to allow them to become familiar with the anatomy and decrease false-negative results.

Axillary Lymph Node Dissection

Indications

ALND was once routinely practiced in breast cancer cases, but the indications for ALND have been revised as SLNB has become standard in early-stage (stage I, II) clinically N0 cases. Today, ALND is performed in clinical N+ early-stage breast cancer and N+ LABC post CT. General attitudes about early-stage N+ breast cancer have changed. Neoadjuvant CT is advised to achieve complete pathologic response to perform SLNB to preserve the axilla. ALND should also be performed when SLN cannot be detected.

Anatomy of the Axilla

Lymph node groups are categorized into three levels according to their orientation to the minor pectoral muscle for the surgeon's convenience. *Level 1* contains the lateral border of the minor pectoral muscle. The central and interpectoral groups, which are located between the medial and lateral borders of the minor pectoral muscle, form *level 2*. The subclavicular group, which is located medially or superiorly to the upper border of the minor pectoral muscle, is categorized as *level 3*.

Axillary Structure

The intercostal brachial and *intercostal thoracic nerves* are sensory nerves; they innervate the skin at the medial part of the upper arm and the posterior part of the axilla. Injury will result in sensory loss at the corresponding skin area.

The long thoracic nerve, which innervates the serratus anterior muscle, originates from C5 to C7, extends inferiorly over the thoracic wall, and branches at the level of the fourth to fifth intercostal. Its injury causes a winged scapula defect.

The thoracodorsal nerve, which innervates the latissimus dorsi, originates from C6 to C8. Preservation of this nerve during dissection is important for subsequent reconstructive interventions.

The Rotter ganglia are in contact with the lateral pectoral pedicle, which is located posteriorly to the major pectoral muscle.

The lateral pectoral nerve, which is located in this pedicle, innervates the medial part of the major pectoral muscle. Its injury results in atrophy of the major pectoral muscle.

The medial pectoral is located anteriorly to the minor pectoral muscle at a distance of 1–2 cm, and the lateral nerve is located more laterally. It originates from the medial chord of the brachial plexus (C8–T1). Its injury results in the atrophy of both muscles.

Atrophy of the pectoral muscles does not cause problems at the early stage but results in cosmetic issues at the chest wall in the long term.

ALND Technique

It is now known that extended lymphatic resection does not provide any benefit for patient survival. Therefore, in routine ALND, only level 1 and level 2 lymph nodes are removed. When lymph nodes are confirmed as positive by preoperative examinations or detected intraoperatively via palpation, level 3 lymph nodes are also included in the dissection. With efficient extraction, level 3 lymph nodes can be removed without sacrificing the minor pectoral muscle.

The incision should be made below the hairline to permit subsequent epilation and should not continue beyond the pectoral muscle anteriorly and the latissimus dorsi muscle posteriorly. Oblique transverse incisions, U-shaped incisions with the gap facing up, and reverse S incisions provide good exposure.

When started medially, the major pectoral muscle is elevated with a retractor. Anterior to the minor pectoral muscle below, the medial pectoral pedicle can be observed 1–2 cm medial of its border. This pedicle should be preserved to avoid atrophy of the major pectoral muscle.

The lateral border of the minor pectoral muscle is freed from the chest wall. This incision is extended upward until the axillary vein is exposed. In most cases, intercostal brachial nerves are sacrificed; however, with fine dissection at T2 and T3 above, the nerves can be separated from the axillary tissue and preserved.

Then, the long thoracic nerve is again identified over the serratus anterior muscle but located deeper (more posterior) than these sensory nerves. At the level of the third intercostal nerve below, it can be found by caressing the serratus anterior muscle with an index finger. It is located inside the fascia of the muscle and should always be preserved. After its exposure, the axillary tissue is dissected laterally from the chest wall. By retracting the major pectoral muscle, palpable lymph nodes are identified in the interpectoral region (Rotter ganglion). The few lymph nodes found here are removed without damaging the lateral pectoral pedicle, which extends anteriorly toward the major pectoral muscle.

There is no need to resect the minor pectoral muscle for a level 3 dissection. For a level 2 dissection, the surgeon should begin from the highest point posterior to the minor pectoral muscle. The surgeon should not extend the incision above the axillary vein; resection of the overlying fatty tissue increases the risk for lymphedema. Below the axillary vein, fatty tissue is skimmed off inferiorly from the chest wall. The dissection is continued inferiorly and laterally, and small branches emanating from the axillary vein are ligated. The lateral thoracic vein (thoracoepigastric vein), which originates from the direction of the axillary vein and enters the axillary tissue, is ligated. The thoracodorsal vein originates distally and posteriorly to the axillary vein and laterally to the lateral thoracic vein. The thoracodorsal nerve occasionally enters more medially, extends more deeply, and distally joins the thoracodorsal vessels.

The thoracodorsal nerve can also be observed as a single pedicle adhered to the thoracodorsal vessels. However, it always enters the latissimus dorsi muscle from the medial side.

Fatty tissue between the long thoracic nerve and the thoracodorsal pedicle is skimmed off inferiorly from the axillary vein, and the subscapular muscle is exposed behind. Then, by placing an index finger on the long thoracic nerve, the nerve is traced until its entry site into the serratus anterior muscle (finger dissection). Laterally, the thoracodorsal pedicle is traced until its entry site into the latissimus dorsi muscle; the small venous branches are ligated, and the specimen is removed during this procedure.

While approaching the axilla laterally to medially, the latissimus dorsi muscle is traced upward from its border; at the site where it becomes tendinous, the axillary vein is exposed. Dissection should be continued below to where the latissimus dorsi muscle joins the serratus anterior muscle. Following removal of the tissue, a suction drain is placed in the axillary cavity near the incision.

Complications of ALND

SLNB is now the method of choice to avoid short- and long-term morbidities caused by ALND. Unfortunately, ALND must still be performed in many cases.

Neurovascular Injury

The long thoracic nerve: Injury of this nerve is caused by cutting, traction, or thermal damage; however, it is damaged in less than 1% of cases. Winged scapula defect caused by its injury results in cosmetic problems.

The thoracodorsal nerve: Because this does not cause a significant neurological deficit, this nerve can be excised to obtain a clean axilla if it is invaded by metastatic lymph nodes.

The intercostal brachial nerve: This nerve transverses the axilla and is generally cut during ALND, causing paresthesia at the medial half of the upper arm and adversely affecting quality of life in women.

Injury to *the medial pectoral nerve* does not cause short-term problems but results in cosmetic problems due to atrophy of the major pectoral muscle.

The brachial plexus is located superior to the axillary vein; thus, there is no risk of injury as long as one does not extend the dissection above the axillary vein.

Seroma

Seroma forms in nearly all cases to some extent and is thus not considered a surgical complication. However, prolonged seroma increases the risk of infection and delays adjuvant treatment. A low-pressure suction drain is placed during the operation to inhibit seroma formation. Because prolonged seroma following removal of the drain is a source of infection, it should be emptied via percutaneous aspiration. One effective method is delaying exercise and complete shoulder movements until after the fifth day following the operation. However, some arm and shoulder exercises should be started in the early stage to prevent shoulder problems due to a limited range of movement.

Chronic Pain and Limited Range of Movement

More than 50% of women experience neuropathic pain, which is sometimes severe and interferes with sleep; this pain increases with movement; is localized to the chest wall, axilla, arm, and shoulder regions; and can continue after the third month postoperatively. These pains are thought to be due to nerve injury and to the addition of radiotherapy and/or chemotherapy to treatment [45]. Patients who experience more pain with movement generally limit their shoulder movements, leading to frozen shoulder syndrome. Starting arm movements at the early period postoperatively with the aid of adequate analgesia prevents these complications.

Lymphedema

Lymphatic fluid, which originates in small lymphatic channels, first drains into regional lymph nodes; it is then carried to the systemic circulation via efferent lymphatic channels and the main lymphatic duct. Any obstruction in these channels results in the development of lymphedema in the tissue that could not be drained. Irradiation of the peripheral lymphatics is another factor that increases lymphedema. Recurrent attacks of lymphangitis and cellulitis also increase the risk for lymphedema in the arm. Lymphedema of up to 1–2 cm is considered mild and is observed in 20–30% of patients with level 1–2 ALND. Larger swelling is considered a serious lymphedema and is observed in less than 5% of patients. The risk of lymphedema in patients with level 3 ALND is 30%, and therefore level 3 ALND is not performed without a valid reason. Mild lymphedema can be observed in 5% of patients following SLNB. The aims are to educate patients and prevent lymphedema before it develops. Patients who have undergone ALND should be advised not to strain the affected arm, not to suspend the arm while working, and to avoid procedures that could increase the risk of lymphangitis (skin injury due to manicure, etc.); patients are also recommended not to gain weight.

When lymphedema develops, its severity is first assessed as follows:

Stage 0: There is only dullness in the arm.

Stage 1: There is pitting edema (recoverable stage because there is no fibrosis).

Stage 2: The arm is stretched, and there is fibrosis.

Stage 3: Elephantiasis is present, with skin signs such as fibrosis, sclerosis, and keratosis.

Treatment and Prevention

Regular trunk cleaning and massage, which is called manual lymphatic drainage, are applied to patients by trained physiotherapists, and bandaging is applied. If no response is obtained using these procedures and if fibrosis has begun in the arm, laser therapy (low-level laser therapy) can be attempted. Laser therapy resolves fibrotic scar tissue by acting on fibroblasts and stimulates lymphatic drainage. This method was demonstrated to have a lymphedema-reducing effect in 52% of cases [45, 46].

The detection and preservation of lymphatics of the arm in the axilla using the injection of blue dye into the upper arm is called reverse axillary mapping. Research on this subject is ongoing [45].

Conclusion

SLNB is equivalent to ALND in clinically node-negative patients in terms of staging, accuracy, DFS, and OS. ALND has been considered mandatory in sentinel node-positive patients, but recent data with 10 years of follow-up have demonstrated that BCS and radiotherapy are equivalent to ALND of micro/macro-metastatic SLNs. This approach will reduce the morbidity of dissection without decreasing OS. SLNB is also beginning to be used in LABC patients treated with neo-adjuvant chemotherapy. In these cases, axilla can be saved, as in early breast cancer. With neo-adjuvant CT, axillary dissection can be avoided in up to half of patients. ALND should be performed whenever the SLN cannot be detected.

References

1. Filippakis GM, Zografos G. Contraindications of sentinel lymph node biopsy: are there any really? World J Surg Oncol. 2007;5:10.
2. Deurloo EE, Tanis PJ, Gilhuijs KG, Muller SH, Kröger R, Peterse JL, et al. Reduction in the number of sentinel lymph node procedures by preoperative ultrasonography of the axilla in breast cancer. Eur J Cancer. 2003;39:1068–73.
3. Raut CP, Hunt KK, Akins JS, Daley MD, Ross MI, Singletary SE, et al. Incidence of anaphylactoid reactions to isosulfan blue dye during breast carcinoma lymphatic mapping in patients treated with preoperative prophylaxis: results of a surgical prospective clinical practice protocol. Cancer. 2005;104:692–9.
4. Cheng G, Kurita S, Torigian DA, Alavi A. Current status of sentinel lymph node biopsy in patients with breast cancer. Eur J Nucl Med Mol Imaging. 2011;38(3):562–75.
5. Vogt H, Schmidt M, Bares R, Brenner W, Grünwald F, Kopp J, et al. Procedure guideline for sentinel node diagnosis. Nuklearmedizin. 2010;49:167–72.

6. Gentilini O, Cremonesi M, Toesca A, Colombo N, Peccatori F, Sironi R, et al. Sentinel lymph node biopsy in pregnant patients with breast cancer. Eur J Nucl Med Mol Imaging. 2010;37:78–83.
7. Spanheimer PM, Graham MM, Sugg SL, Scott-Conner CE, Weigel RJ. Measurement of uterine radiation exposure from lymphoscintigraphy indicates safety of sentinel lymph node biopsy during pregnancy. Ann Surg Oncol. 2009;16:1143–7.
8. Sakr R, Bezu C, Raoust I, Antoine M, Ettore F, Darcourt J, et al. The sentinel lymph node procedure for patients with preoperative diagnosis of ductal carcinoma in situ: risk factors for unsuspected invasive disease and for metastatic sentinel lymph nodes. Int J Clin Pract. 2008;62:1730–5.
9. Sakr R, Antoine M, Barranger E, Dubernard G, Salem C, Darai E, et al. Value of sentinel lymph node biopsy in breast ductal carcinoma in situ upstaged to invasive carcinoma. Breast J. 2008;14:55–60.
10. Ansari B, Ogston SA, Purdie CA, Adamson DJ, Brown DC, Thompson AM. Meta- analysis of sentinel node biopsy in ductal carcinoma in situ of the breast. Br J Surg. 2008;95:547–54.
11. Lyman GH, Somerfield MR, Bosserman LD, Perkins CL, Weaver DL, Giuliano AE. Sentinel lymph node biopsy for patients with early-stage breast cancer: American Society of Clinical Oncology clinical practice guideline update. J Clin Oncol. 2017;35(5):561–4.
12. Kumar R, Jana S, Heiba SI, Dakhel M, Axelrod D, Siegel B, et al. Retrospective analysis of sentinel node localization in multifocal, multicentric, palpable or nonpalpable breast cancer. J Nucl Med. 2003;44:7–10.
13. Knauer M, Konstantiniuk P, Haid A, Wenzl E, Riegler-Keilb M, Postlberger S, et al. Multicentric breast cancer: a new indication for sentinel node biopsy a multi-institutional validation study. J Clin Oncol. 2006;24:3374–80.
14. Goyal A, Newcombe RG, Mansel RE, Chetty U, Ell P, Fallowfield L, ALMANAC Trialists Group, et al. Sentinel lymph node biopsy in patients with multifocal breast cancer. Eur J Surg Oncol. 2004;30:475–9.
15. D'Eredita G, Giardina C, Ingravallo G, Rubini G, Lattanzio V, Berardi T. Sentinel lymph node biopsy in multiple breast cancer using subareolar injection of the tracer. Breast. 2007;16:316–22.
16. Port ER, Garcia-Etienne CA, Park J, Fey J, Borgen PI, Cody HS 3rd. Reoperative sentinel lymph node biopsy: a new frontier in the management of ipsilateral breast tumor recurrence. Ann Surg Oncol. 2007;14:2209–14.
17. Luini A, Galimberti V, Gatti G, Arnone P, Vento AR, Trifiro G, et al. The sentinel node biopsy after previous breast surgery: preliminary results on 543 patients treated at the European Institute of Oncology. Breast Cancer Res Treat. 2005;89:159–63.
18. Intra M, Trifiro G, Galimberti V, Gentilini O, Rotmensz N, Veronesi P. Second axillary sentinel node biopsy for ipsilateral breast tumor recurrence. Br J Surg. 2007;94:1216–9.
19. Koizumi M, Koyama M, Tada K, Nishimura S, Miyagi Y, Makita M, et al. The feasibility of sentinel node biopsy in the previously treated breast. Eur J Surg Oncol. 2008;34:365–8.
20. Rodriguez Fernandez J, Martella S, Trifiro G, Caliskan M, Chifu C, Brenelli F, et al. Sentinel node biopsy in patients with previous breast aesthetic surgery. Ann Surg Oncol. 2009;16:989–92.
21. Karam A, Stempel M, Cody HS 3rd, Port ER. Reoperative sentinel lymph node biopsy after previous mastectomy. J Am Coll Surg. 2008;207:543–8.
22. Boughey JC, Bedrosian I, Meric-Bernstam F, Ross MI, Kuerer HM, Akins JS, et al. Comparative analysis of sentinel lymph node operation in male and female breast cancer patients. J Am Coll Surg. 2006;203:475–80.
23. Gentilini O, Chagas E, Zurrida S, Intra M, De Cicco C, Gatti G, et al. Sentinel lymph node biopsy in male patients with early breast cancer. Oncologist. 2007;12:512–5.

24. Synn LW, Park J, Patil SM, Cody HS 3rd, Port ER. Sentinel lymph node biopsy is successful and accurate in male breast carcinoma. J Am Coll Surg. 2008;206:616–21.
25. Boughey JC, Suman VJ, Mittendorf EA, Ahrendt GM, Wilke LG, Taback B, et al. Sentinel lymph node surgery after neoadjuvant chemotherapy in patients with node-positive breast cancer: the ACOSOG Z1071 (Alliance) clinical trial. JAMA. 2013;310:1455–61.
26. Boileau JF, Poirier B, Basic M, Holloway MB, Gaboury L, Sideris L, et al. Sentinel node biopsy after neoadjuvant chemotherapy in biopsy proven node-positive breast cancer: the SN FNAC study. J Clin Oncol. 2015;33(3):258–64.
27. Mamtani A, Barrio AV, King TA, Zee KJV, Plitas G, Pilewskie M, et al. How often does neoadjuvant chemotherapy avoid axillary dissection in patients with histologically confirmed nodal metastases? Results of prospective study. Ann Surg Oncol. 2016;23(11):3467–74.
28. Mamounas EP, Brown A, Anderson S, Smith R, Julian T, Miller B, et al. Sentinel node biopsy after neoadjuvant chemotherapy in breast cancer: results from National Surgical Adjuvant Breast and Bowel Project Protocol B-27. J Clin Oncol. 2005;23:2694–702.
29. Xing Y, Foy M, Cox DD, Kuerer HM, Hunt KK, Cormier JN. Meta-analysis of sentinel lymph node biopsy after preoperative chemotherapy in patients with breast cancer. Br J Surg. 2006;93:539–46.
30. Kelly AM, Dwamena B, Cronin P, Carlos RC. Breast cancer sentinel node identification and classification after neoadjuvant chemotherapy-systematic review and meta-analysis. Acad Radiol. 2009;16:551–63.
31. Sherman AI, Ter-Pogossian M. Lymph-node concentration of radioactive colloidal gold following interstitial injection. Cancer. 1953;6:1238–40.
32. Sayman HB. In: Uras C, Aydogan F, editors, Sentinel Lenf Nodu Biopsisi, 1.Baskı, İstanbul Medical Yayıncılık, Sentinel lenf nodu biyopsisinde nükleer tıp teknikleri. Istanbul; 2007. p. 45–53.
33. Albo D, Wayne JD, Hunt KK, Rahlfs TF, Singletary SE, Ames FC, et al. Anaphylactic reactions to isosulphane blue during sentinel lymph node biopsy for breast cancer. Am J Surg. 2001;182:393–8.
34. Stradling B, Aranha G, Gabram S. Adverse skin reactions after methylene blue injections for sentinel lymph node localization. Am J Surg. 2002;184:350–2.
35. Kargozaran H, Shah M, Li Y, Beckett L, Gandour-Edwards R, Schneider PD, et al. Concordance of peritumoral technetium 99m colloid and subareolar blue dye injection in Breast cancer sentinel lymph node biopsy. J Surg Res. 2007;143:126–9.
36. Rodier JF, Velten M, Wilt M, Martel P, Ferron G, Vaini-Elies V, et al. Prospective multicentric randomized study comparing periareolar and peritumoral injection of radiotracer and blue dye for the detection of sentinel lymph node in breast sparing procedures: FRANSENODE trial. J Clin Oncol. 2007;25:3664–9.
37. Derossis AM, Fey J, Yeung H, Yeh SD, Heerdt AS, Petrek J, et al. A trend analysis of the relative value of blue dye and isotope localization in 2000 consecutive cases of sentinel node biopsy for breast cancer. J Am Coll Surg. 2001;193:473–8.
38. Bauer TW, Spitz FR, Callans LS, Alavi A, Mick R, Weinstein SP, et al. Subareolar and peritumoral injection identify similar sentinel nodes for breast cancer. Ann Surg Oncol. 2002;9:169–76.
39. Pelosi E, Baiocco C, Ala A, Gay E, Bello M, Varetto T, et al. Lymphatic mapping in early stage breast cancer: comparison between periareolar and subdermal injection. Nucl Med Commun. 2003;24:519–23.
40. Goyal A, Newcombe RG, Mansel RE, Axillary Lymphatic Mapping Against Nodal axillary Clearance (ALMANAC) Trialists Group. Clinical relevance of multiple sentinel nodes in patients with breast cancer. Br J Surg. 2005;92:438–42.
41. Goyal A, Newcombe RG, Chhabra A, Mansel RE, ALMANAC Trialists Group. Factors affecting failed localization and false-negative rates of sentinel node biopsy in breast cancer: results of the ALMANAC validation phase. Breast Cancer Res Treat. 2006;99:203–8.

42. Giuliano AE, Ballman KV, McCall L, Beitsch PD, Brennan MB, Kelemen PR, et al. Effect of axillary dissection vs no axillary dissection on 10-year overall survival among women with invasive breast cancer and sentinel node metastasis: The ACOSOG Z0011 (Alliance) Randomized Clinical Trial. JAMA. 2017;318:918–26.
43. Cserni G, Amendoeira I, Apostolikas N, Bellocq JP, Bianchi S, Bussolati G, et al. Pathological work-up of sentinel lymph node breast in cancer. Review of current data to be considered fort the formulation of guidelines. Eur J Cancer. 2003;39:1654–67.
44. Kuehn T, Bauerfeind I, Fehm T, Fleige B, Hausschild M, Helms G, et al. Sentinel-lymph-node biopsy in patients with breast cancer before and after neoadjuvant chemotherapy (SENTINA): a prospective, multicentre cohort study. Lancet. 2013;14:609–18.
45. Couceiro TC, Menezes TC, Valênça MM. Post mastectomy pain syndrome: the magnitude of the problem. Rev Bras Anestesiol. 2009;59:358–65.
46. Dirican A, Andacoglu O, Johnson R, McGuire K, Mager L, Soran A. The short-term effects of low-level laser therapy in the management of breast-cancer-related lymphedema. Support Care Cancer. 2011;19:685–90.

Part VI
Adjuvant Systemic Therapy for Breast Cancer

Chapter 15
Adjuvant Chemotherapy for HER2-Negative Early-Stage Breast Cancer

Leyla Ozer and Adnan Aydiner

Introduction

Breast cancer is the most frequent cause of cancer death in women in developing countries. Fortunately, the outcomes of patients with early breast cancer have improved with the use of adjuvant systemic treatments [1]. Long-term follow-up from the Oxford overview demonstrated absolute benefit from chemotherapy, regardless of age and estrogen receptor (ER) status [2]. However, breast cancer is a heterogeneous disease that is composed of several biological subtypes with distinct behaviors and responses to therapy. Consequently, chemotherapy does not offer the same magnitude of benefit for all breast cancer subtypes. Thus far, clinicopathological parameters have guided decisions for adjuvant systemic chemotherapy, but recently genomic tests have been integrated, especially for the intermediate-risk group. However, the selection of patients, timing, and dosing and the scheduling of the optimal chemotherapy regimen for the appropriate patient may be challenging. This chapter evaluates the evolution and recent advances in adjuvant systemic chemotherapy for human epidermal growth factor receptor 2 (HER2)-negative breast cancer (Figs. 15.1, 15.2, 15.3, 15.4, and 15.5).

L. Ozer
Internal Medicine, Department of Medical Oncology, Mehmet Ali Aydinlar University Hospital, Istanbul, Turkey

A. Aydiner (✉)
Internal Medicine, Medical Oncology, Istanbul Medical Faculty, Department of Medical Oncology, Institute of Oncology, Istanbul University, Istanbul, Turkey

A. Aydiner et al. (eds.), *Breast Cancer*, https://doi.org/10.1007/978-3-319-96947-3_15

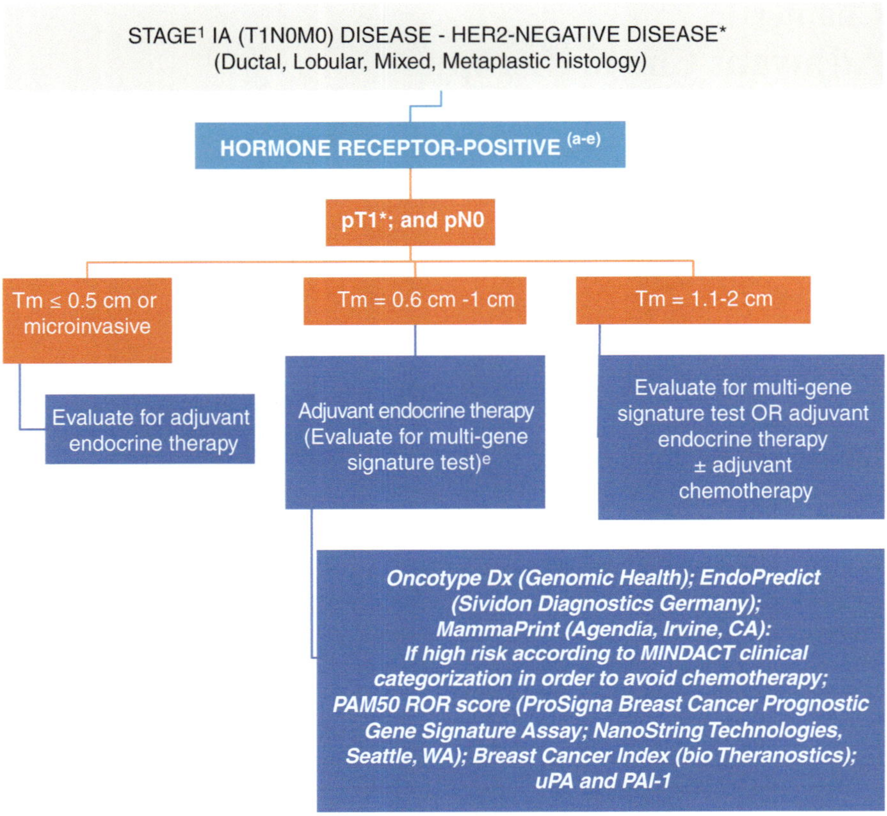

Fig. 15.1 Adjuvant systemic therapy for stage IA—hormone receptor-positive and HER2-negative disease. *In early-stage breast cancer, there are biomarkers that can be used to decide adjuvant systemic treatment administration. In the 8th version of the American Joint Commission of Cancer (AJCC) for breast cancer, prognostic gene signatures will be integrated into the staging scheme as prognostic staging: For patients with hormone receptor-positive, HER2-negative, and lymph node-negative tumors, prognostic gene signatures with a low risk score regardless of T size place the tumor in the same prognostic category as T1a–T1b N0M0, and the tumor is staged using the AJCC prognostic stage group table as stage I. Based on multigene signature tests, chemotherapy may be omitted for patients with Luminal B-like (HER2 negative) disease with a low Oncotype Dx® score, MammaPrint® low-risk status, low PAM50 ROR score, or EndoPredict® low-risk status. The situations in which multigene tests may be particularly helpful can be summarized as follows: tumor size between 1 and 3 cm *and* ER/PR positive *and* HER2 negative *and* node negative or N_{mi} *and* Grade 2 *and* Ki-67 between 15% and 35%. In hormone receptor-positive T1c N0 (1–2 cm) tumors, grade 3 disease with a high Ki-67 value (e.g., above 35%) and PgR <20% may be considered adequate for chemotherapy indication. In cases where multigene tests cannot be performed, the risk factors can be determined using web-based formulas, and an indication for chemotherapy administration can be established. [a]There is no absolute age limit. Rather, treatment depends on the disease, the presence of comorbidities, the patient's life expectancy, and patient preferences. Treatment should be individualized for patients >70 years of age. [b]Chemotherapy and endocrine therapy as adjuvant therapy should be given sequentially, with endocrine therapy following chemotherapy. The available data suggest that sequential or concurrent endocrine therapy with radiation therapy is acceptable. [c]Fertility preservation (e.g., by ovarian tissue or oocyte conservation) should be offered to women <40 years of age. Ovarian function suppression with LHRHa during chemotherapy should be offered for HR-negative disease. [d]Consider adjuvant bisphosphonate therapy in postmenopausal (natural or induced) patients receiving adjuvant therapy. [e]Evaluate for multi-gene signature test, especially for Luminal B-like, high Ki67, or grade III tumors

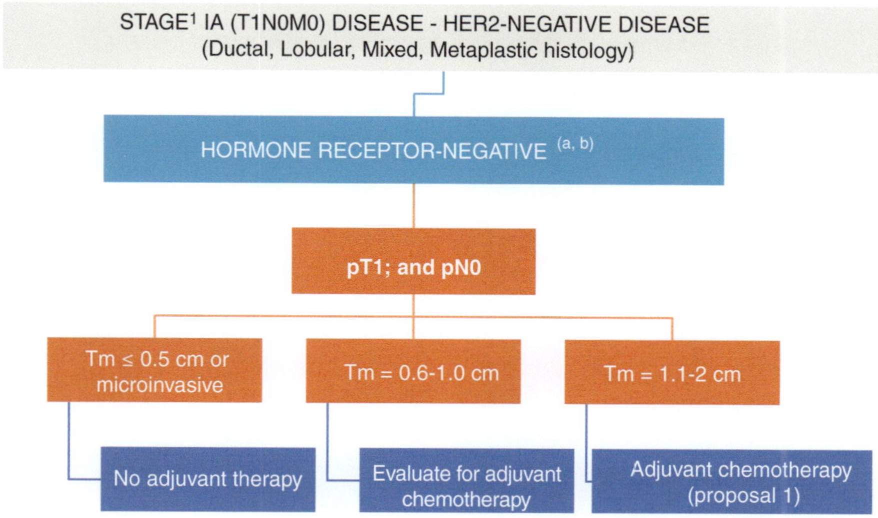

Fig. 15.2 Adjuvant systemic therapy for stage IA—hormone receptor-negative and HER2-negative disease. [a]There is no absolute age limit. Rather, treatment depends on the disease, the presence of comorbidities, the patient's life expectancy, and patient preferences. Treatment should be individualized for patients >70 years of age. [b]Fertility preservation (e.g., by ovarian tissue or oocyte conservation) should be offered to women <40 years of age. Ovarian function suppression with LHRHa during chemotherapy should be offered for HR-negative disease

Indications for Adjuvant Chemotherapy

Adjuvant cytotoxic chemotherapy is generally administered while relying on clinicopathological factors such as receptor status (expression of estrogen [ER] and/or progesterone [PR] receptors, human epidermal growth factor receptor [HER2]), tumor size, nodal involvement, histology, grade, age, comorbidities and patient preference. Standard pathological features may not be sufficient to avoid overtreatment, especially for luminal breast cancer patients with weaker ER expression and intermediate proliferation scores. In such situations, the absolute benefit expected from systemic adjuvant cytotoxic therapies could be estimated by either sophisticated gene expression assays or more historical clinical tools such as Adjuvant! Online (www.adjuvantonline.com) and some immunohistochemical tests.

Tumor Size

For patients with node-negative breast cancer, tumor size is a known independent prognostic factor [3]. Pathological tumor size (>2 cm) is associated with both distant disease-free survival (hazard ratio [HR] for recurrence 1.61, 95% CI 1.14–2.25) and overall survival (HR for mortality 1.68, 95% CI 1.12–2.52) [4]. The role of adjuvant therapy and long-term outcomes for patients with small (<1 cm),

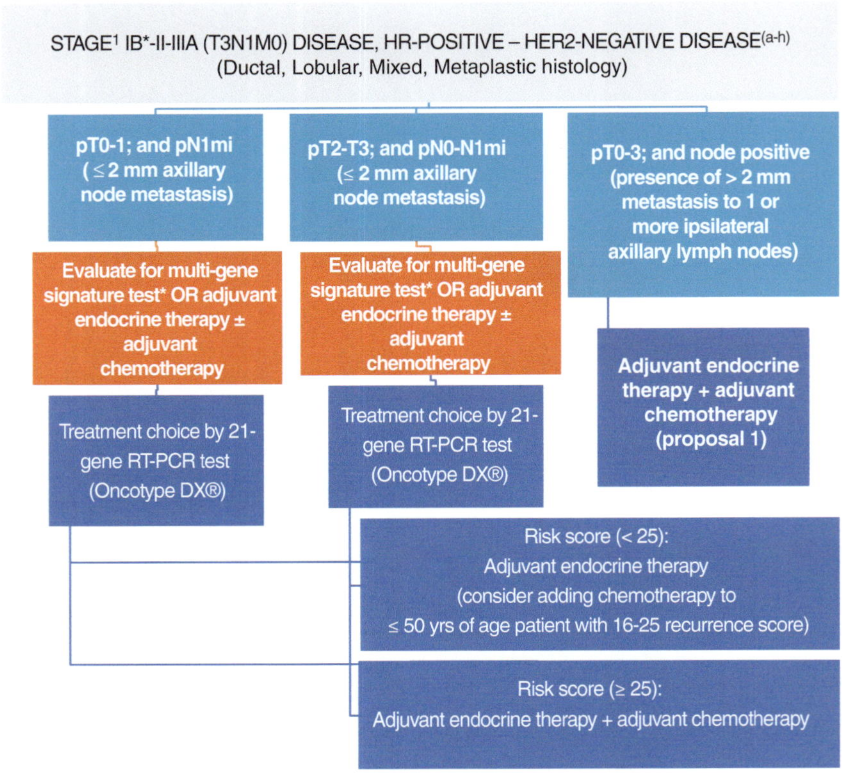

Fig. 15.3 Adjuvant systemic therapy for stage IB, II, IIIA—hormone receptor-positive and HER2-negative disease. *For patients with hormone receptor-positive, HER2-negative, and lymph node-negative tumors, prognostic gene signatures with a low risk score regardless of T size place the tumor in the same prognostic category as T1a–T1b N0 M0, and the tumor is staged using the AJCC prognostic stage group table as stage I (8th version). [a]There is no absolute age limit. The choice of treatment depends on disease, co-morbidities, life expectancy and patient preferences. In patients over 70 years of age, treatment should be individualized. A meta-analysis showed that dose-intensive treatment increased overall survival in hormone receptor-negative and hormone receptor-positive patients (EBTCG, San Antonio BCS, 2017). [b]In patients with Luminal A-like tumors and 1–3 positive lymph nodes (with the evaluation of other factors such as grade, age, or multigene signature test results), “adjuvant endocrine therapy alone” may be an option. [c]Factors that are relative indications for the inclusion of adjuvant cytotoxic chemotherapy include the following: histological grade 3 tumor, 4 or more positive nodes, high Ki67, extensive lymphovascular invasion, and low hormone receptor staining. [d]The Luminal A phenotype is less responsive to chemotherapy. In node-negative disease, chemotherapy should not be added based on the T size. A combination of the biological properties of the tumor (such as Ki67, LVI, grade, and multigene signature) must be used to assess whether to provide chemotherapy. Chemotherapy should be added in high-risk patients based on the involvement of 4 or more lymph nodes. [e]Based on immunohistochemistry (IHC), in Luminal B-like (HER2-negative) tumors, chemotherapy may be omitted in some low-risk patients (based on combinations of certain prognostic factors such as low tumor mass, low grade, low Ki67, an absence of LVI, and older age). [f]Based on multigene signature tests, chemotherapy may be omitted for patients with Luminal B-like (HER2-negative) disease with a low Oncotype Dx® score, MammaPrint® low-risk status, low PAM50 ROR score or EndoPredict® low-risk status. MammaPrint can be used in node-positive patients. In the TAILORx ClinicalTrial (ASCO Congress 2018), adjuvant endocrine therapy and chemoendocrine therapy had similar efficacy in women with hormone-receptor-positive, HER2-negative, axillary node-negative breast cancer who had a

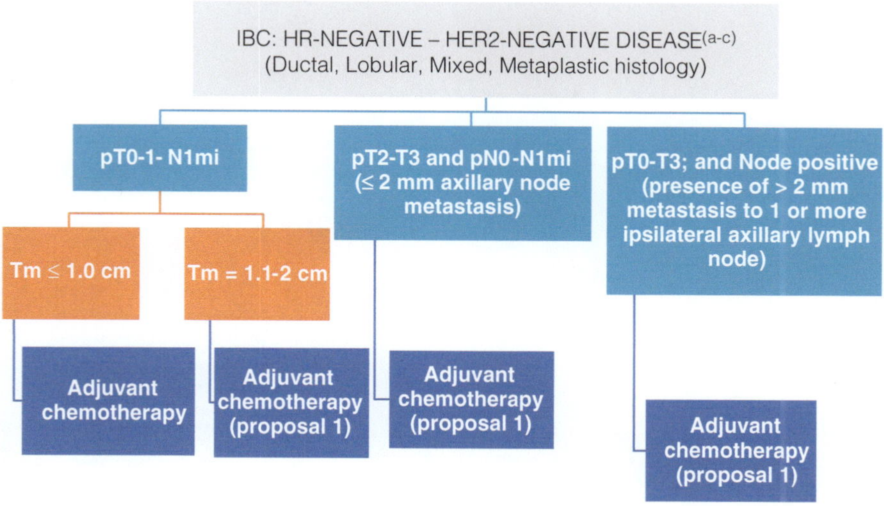

Fig. 15.4 Adjuvant systemic therapy for stage IB, II, IIIA (T3N1M0)—hormone receptor-negative and HER2-negative disease. [a]There is no absolute age limit. Rather, treatment depends on the disease, the presence of comorbidities, the patient's life expectancy, and patient preferences. For patients >70 years of age, treatment should be individualized. Regardless of the size of the invasive tumor, adjuvant chemotherapy may be recommended in the presence of $N1_{mi}$. [b]Fertility preservation (e.g., by ovarian tissue or oocyte conservation) should be offered to women <40 years of age. Ovarian function suppression with LHRHa during chemotherapy should be offered for receptor-negative disease. [c]In triple-negative breast cancer (TNBC), the regimen should include anthracyclines and taxanes. Although the data are insufficient, a platinum-based regimen may be considered only when a BRCA mutation has been identified. Anthracyclines followed by taxanes represent an acceptable regimen for BRCA-mutant TNBC. Dose-dense chemotherapy requiring growth factor support may also be an option. The preference of dose-intensive treatment in these patients was not recommended in St. Gallen 2017 (37% yes, 55% no). However, a meta-analysis showed that dose-intensive treatment improved overall survival in hormone receptor-negative and hormone receptor-positive patients (EBTCG, San Antonio BCS, 2017). Neoadjuvant treatment should be considered in triple-negative patients with stage II and III disease. Treatment with platinum or alkylating agents may be considered in neoadjuvant chemotherapy (71% yes, 15% no). Provision of platinum-based treatment for all patients was voted as 10% 'yes' and 86% 'no' at St Gallen 2017. A platinum-based regimen may be recommended, particularly when a BRCA mutation is detected (voted as 47% 'yes' and 43% 'no' at St Gallen 2017). The administration of capecitabine after anthracycline and taxane treatment reduces recurrence in patients with TNBC. Capecitabine reduces the recurrence rate in patients with residual tumors after neoadjuvant therapy

midrange 21-gene recurrence score. However, the chemotherapy benefit for invasive disease-free survival varied with the combination of recurrence score and age (P = 0.004), with some benefit of chemotherapy found in women 50 years of age or younger with a recurrence score of 16–25. MammaPrint (Agendia, Irvine, CA): In patients with 1–3 positive lymph nodes, tests can be performed to avoid adjuvant chemotherapy if the patient is at high clinical risk group in the MINDACT categorization (however, the patient should be informed that there may be an additional benefit of chemotherapy with multiple LN positivity). [g]For Luminal B-like (HER2-negative) tumors, the regimen, if given, should contain anthracyclines and taxanes. A high-risk group might exist for which dose-dense therapy with G-CSF may also be preferred. [h]Consider adjuvant bisphosphonate therapy in postmenopausal (natural or induced) patients receiving adjuvant therapy

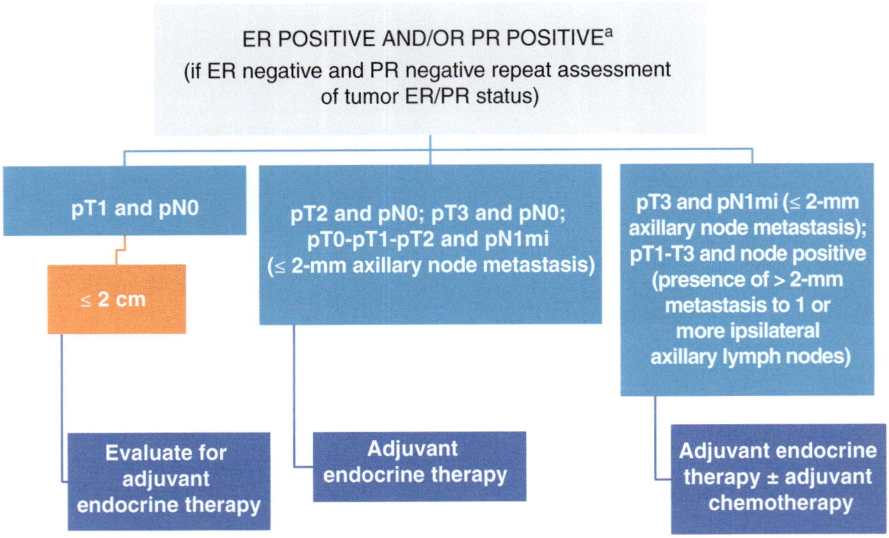

Fig. 15.5 Adjuvant systemic therapy for stage IB, II, IIIA (T3N1M0)—tubular and mucinous carcinoma. [a]Consider adjuvant bisphosphonate therapy in postmenopausal (natural or induced) patients receiving adjuvant therapy

node-negative breast cancer remain elusive. Clearly, triple-negative tumors have a worse prognosis compared to their ER-positive counterparts, even with a very small tumor size. This worse prognosis was supported by a study involving 421 breast cancer patients with <T1b tumors, of which 29 (7%) were triple negative [5]. The recurrence rate was 11.1, and 7 percent among triple-negative, ER-positive and HER2-positive patients, respectively. Thus, tumor size is not always an unfavorable risk factor; HER2-positive and triple-negative tumors have a higher recurrence rate despite a small tumor size, as expected.

Nodal Involvement

The rate of breast cancer recurrence is higher in patients with pathologically involved lymph nodes. The presence of isolated tumor cells is also defined as node-negative disease but is clinically insignificant. However, micrometastases carry a modest negative impact on breast outcomes and are treated as pathologically node-positive breast cancer. Compared to patients with disease confined to the breast only, those with disease spread to the lymph nodes have a lower rate of survival at 5 years (84% versus 99%, respectively) [6]. However, for luminal disease, one to three positive nodes is not a clear indication for adjuvant chemotherapy, especially in the setting of strong hormone receptor expression, low grade and low proliferation markers such as Ki67.

Tumor-Infiltrating Lymphocytes

Immune system activation has clear effects on the survival of breast cancer patients. Previously, lymphocytic infiltration was linked to high proliferation, and the presence of tumor-infiltrating lymphocytes (TILs) was associated with improved pathological response rates, disease-free survival (DFS) and overall survival (OS) for triple-negative breast cancer (TNBC) and HER2-positive breast cancer subtypes [7, 8]. The combined analysis of TNBC patients included in the ECOG 2197 and ECOG 1199 trials confirmed the independent prognostic value of TILs for DFS, OS and distant recurrence-free survival [9].

Intrinsic Subtypes and Genomic Tests

Gene-profiling techniques have confirmed biological heterogeneity for breast cancer with at least 6 major subtypes: luminal A and luminal B; HER2-enriched; basal-like; normal breast-like; and the claudin-low or mesenchymal-like subtype [10, 11]. Uncertainty about the optimal treatment usually arises in the case of the luminal subtype. Luminal A tumors are characterized by the expression of estrogen-regulated genes, transcription factors and luminal cytokeratins, whereas luminal B tumors are characterized by a higher genomic grade, lower ER levels, and varying degrees of HER2 gene cluster expression [11, 12]. 'Luminal A-like' disease is the preferred clinicopathological surrogate for the Luminal A subtype, which is described as ER and PgR positive, HER2-negative, and low Ki67.

Ki67 is a marker of proliferation that is expressed exclusively during active phases of the cell cycle [13]. It is commonly assessed by immunohistochemistry (IHC) in clinical settings and has been correlated with survival [14]. Ki67 scoring is moderately reproducible when manual scoring methods are used, and there is currently no consensus on the optimal Ki67 cut-off point for either molecular subtyping or the prediction of prognosis [15]. The 2013 St Gallen guidelines offer a level of <14% for the best correlation with the gene-expression definition of Luminal A; however, with this cut-off point, a high rate (25%) of misclassification was noted [16]. Due to the considerable disagreement at St Gallen 2013 about the optimal Ki67 cut-off, it was revised up to 20%. However, more recent guidelines suggest that Ki67 scores should be evaluated according to local institutional values [17]. If the median Ki67 score in receptor-positive disease for a given laboratory is 20%, values of 30% or above could be considered high and those of 10% or less as low. An international study has proposed that after calibrating to a common scoring method via a web-based tool, laboratories can achieve high inter-laboratory reproducibility in Ki67 scoring on centrally stained tissue microarray slides [18]. However, the lack of standardization of preanalytical and analytical features for IHC limits the utility of this method for clinical decision-making.

The level of progesterone receptor expression is also utilized to discriminate the 'Luminal A-like' and 'Luminal B-like' subtypes. Prat et al. [19] offered a cut-off of ≥20% as best corresponding to the Luminal A subtype. Lower or absent PgR correlates with Luminal B disease and poorer outcomes but may not add to Ki67 in differentiating Luminal A from B [20].

When adequate reproducibility is not achieved with either IHC technique, gene expression signatures may be preferred to identify low-risk patients who can be spared from chemotherapy. Multiparameter molecular tests such as PAM50 or MammaPrint/BluePrint can be used to determine the intrinsic subtypes [21, 22]. The PAM50 test, which is based on a qRT-PCR assay, classifies ER-positive and ER-negative breast cancer patients into subtypes that can predict outcomes [23, 24]. It measures the expression of 50 classifier genes and 5 control genes, categorizes tumors into the 4 intrinsic subtypes (luminal A, luminal B, HER2-enriched, and basal-like), and provides a risk of recurrence (ROR) score to estimate the probability of relapse at 5 years. The MammaPrint assay is a 70-gene signature test that classifies tumors into groups that are associated with good or poor prognosis on the basis of the risk of distant recurrence at 5 and 10 years [25]. A prospective, randomized phase III study (MINDACT) evaluated whether patients with high-risk clinical features and a low-risk gene-expression profile could be spared from chemotherapy safely [26]. Avoidance of chemotherapy on the basis of gene signature results led to a 5-year rate of distant metastasis-free survival (DMFS) (94.7%) that was 1.5% points lower than the rate obtained with chemotherapy (95% confidence interval [CI] 92.5–96.2%), thus achieving the primary objective of the study. The trial included both node-negative and node-positive patients, and similar rates of survival without distant metastasis were reported for both groups. An expert panel reviewed the results of the MINDACT study and recommended the MammaPrint assay for use in patients with one to three positive nodes and a high clinical risk (determined according to Adjuvant! Online) to inform decisions on withholding adjuvant systemic chemotherapy. However, patients, particularly those with more than one metastatic lymph node, should be informed that a benefit from chemotherapy cannot be excluded [27].

Other multigene assays that may assist in discriminating Luminal B-like breast cancer patients who would potentially benefit from chemotherapy include Oncotype Dx® and Endopredict®. Oncotype Dx is a 21-gene expression assay that estimates the 10-year risk of distant recurrence in patients with hormone receptor-positive (HR+), HER2 (−) and axillary lymph node-negative disease. The results of the test are reported as a *recurrence score (RS)* ranging from 0 to 100, divided into low-risk (<18), intermediate-risk (18–30), and high-risk (≥31) categories. However, the prospective validation trial of OncotypeDx (TAILORx) utilized different boundaries to minimize the potential for undertreatment of the participants involved (clinicaltrials.gov). The low-risk group was defined as those with RS ≤ 10, the intermediate-risk group as those with RS = 11–25, and the high-risk group as RS ≥ 26. For the low-risk population who received endocrine therapy alone, the invasive disease-free survival (IDFS) rate was 93.8%, and the overall survival (OS) rate was 98% at 5 years [28]. Approximately 30% of this group included patients with tumor size ≥2 cm, and 66% had intermediate or high histological grades and would otherwise be recommended to receive chemotherapy on the basis of clinicopathological features. The survival outcomes of the intermediate-risk group, which constituted the majority (67%) of the patients in this trial, had been reported in ASCO 2018 congress. In the TAILORx ClinicalTrial, adjuvant endocrine therapy and chemoendocrine therapy had similar efficacy in women with hormone-receptor-positive, HER2-negative, axillary node-negative breast cancer who had a midrange 21-gene recurrence score RS = 11–25. However, the chemotherapy benefit for invasive disease-free survival varied with the combination of recurrence score and age ($P = 0.004$), with some benefit of chemotherapy found in women 50 years of age or younger with a recurrence score of 16–25. Retrospective single-institution follow-up data from a similar set of patients with RS = 11–25 demonstrated a 5-year IDFS rate of 92.6%, which was comparable between those who received chemotherapy and those who did not. However, a benefit of chemotherapy in the intermediate-risk group cannot be ruled out based solely on the results of this analysis due to the small number of patients, short follow-up time, lack of events and retrospective nature of the trial. The utility of OncotypeDx for node-positive patients is not clear. The ongoing RxPONDER trial is currently evaluating the benefit of chemotherapy for patients with node-positive, HR-positive and HER2-negative disease with RS ≤ 25. The results of this study are supposed to guide treatment decisions for node-positive patients.

EndoPredict (EP) is another multigene assay including 8 genes associated with tumor proliferation and hormone receptor activity and 4 reference genes but not ER, PR and HER2 status. An EP score of 0–15 stratifies ER-positive, HER2-negative breast cancer patients into high- and low-risk groups. The assay was initially utilized to estimate distant recurrence risk among luminal breast cancer patients treated with adjuvant endocrine therapy alone [29]. EPclin is a combined score of clinical risk factors (tumor size and nodal status) that was compared with purely clinical risk classifications and found to be strikingly superior to known prognosticators such as St. Gallen, German S3 and NCCN [30].

The St Gallen 2017 guidelines recommend gene expression assays to guide the decision on adjuvant chemotherapy, mainly for patients with tumors between 1 and 3 cm, zero to two or three positive lymph nodes, and an intermediate proliferative fraction. The Panel has not endorsed a specific multigene assay but has suggested that none of the tests should be the only factor considered in making a decision to proceed with or avoid chemotherapy [31]. NCCN guidelines have additionally recommended OncotypeDx for select patients with one to three involved lymph nodes to guide chemotherapy decisions based on a retrospective analysis of a prospective study (www.nccn.org. version 1.2018). According to the NCCN panel, other prognostic multigene assays may be considered for prognostic purposes but not for predicting response to chemotherapy.

Rare Histological Subtypes

More than 90% of invasive breast carcinomas consist of infiltrating ductal, lobular or mixed histological subtypes. The rest, including mucinous (colloid), tubular, medullary, papillary, adenoid cystic, micropapillary, apocrine and metaplastic breast cancer, constitute less than 10% of cases [6]. Within these subtypes, tubular and mucinous carcinomas are characterized by better prognosis compared with infiltrating ductal carcinomas [32]. Thus, for tubular and mucinous cancers, the treatment decision is based on tumor size and ALN status. Since the majority of tubular cancer is ER positive and HER2-negative, the accuracy of the ER and/or HER2 determination should be reviewed if a tubular breast cancer is ER negative and/or HER2-positive. If a tubular or mucinous cancer is confirmed as ER negative, then the tumor should be treated according to the guidelines for usual histology, ER-negative breast cancers (Fig. 15.5).

Pure mucinous carcinoma is composed of nests of tumor cells floating in mucin, whereas the mixed form also contains common infiltrating ductal carcinoma NST (*no special type*) [33, 34]. There is no definite threshold for the percentage of mucinous component for discriminating between pure and mixed mucinous carcinoma. However, pure mucinous carcinomas are generally composed of more than 90% mucin [35]. The mucin component represents less than 50% in ductal carcinoma with a mucinous component. Pure mucinous carcinoma is generally diagnosed at older ages; the median age at diagnosis was 71 years according to a retrospective report [36].

Medullary carcinoma is characterized by high nuclear grade, lymphocytic infiltration and a pushing tumor border. Most of the cases present with triple-negative features in addition to cytokeratin 5/6 positivity [37]. The prognosis for pure medullary carcinomas appears to be more favorable than that of infiltrating ductal carcinomas despite an aggressive histological appearance. However, data regarding the potential for metastasis are conflicting; there is evidence suggesting that the risk of metastasis is equal to that of other high-grade carcinomas, even for cases that meet all pathological criteria for typical medullary carcinoma. In addition, many cases classified as medullary carcinoma do not have all pathological features on subsequent pathological review. Since there is concern that patients may be undertreated if a high-grade infiltrating ductal carcinoma is misclassified as typical medullary carcinoma, it is often recommended that medullary carcinoma be treated like other infiltrating ductal carcinomas based on tumor size, grade, and lymph node status.

Adenoid cystic carcinoma of the breast is a rare entity accounting for less than 1% of breast cancers. Morphologically, these cancers resemble adenoid cystic carcinomas of the salivary glands, with low mitotic activity and good prognosis [38, 39]. They are usually HR (−) and HER-2 (−), but in contrast to the common invasive ductal type triple-negative breast cancer, the 10-year overall survival rates generally exceed 90%.

Juvenile carcinoma or secretory breast carcinoma is a triple-negative subtype of breast cancer that usually presents at an earlier age [40, 41]. These cancers are also characterized by low Ki67 expression and good prognosis. Rarely, late metastatic or recurrent cases are reported [42]. Both adenoid cystic carcinomas and secretory carcinomas are generally triple-negative and are categorized in the good-prognosis group with an indolent course, even in the presence of recurrence and metastasis. Thus, adjuvant cytotoxic chemotherapy is generally not recommended in the case of node negativity, but due to the scarcity of data about these rare types of tumors, there is no strong scientific evidence in favor of adjuvant chemotherapy.

In contrast to adenoid cystic and secretory carcinomas, metaplastic breast cancer represents a poorly differentiated subtype with high Ki67 and p53 positivity [43]. The prognosis is usually poorer than that of triple-negative infiltrating ductal carcinoma [44]. Survival is generally less than 1 year in the setting of metastatic disease [45]. The clinical behavior of metaplastic breast cancer may resemble sarcomas or squamous cell carcinomas, depending on the specific metaplastic differentiation of cells. Although previous studies have demonstrated poor response to neoadjuvant chemotherapy, NCCN guidelines recommend that metaplastic breast carcinoma be evaluated as ductal or lobular carcinoma and treated accordingly [46].

Chemotherapy Schedule

The chemotherapy schedule, time and number of cycles depend on the tumor characteristics and patient factors, such as biological age, performance status, comorbid diseases and patient preference. If cytotoxic chemotherapy is to be administered, it should start within 2–6 weeks after surgery since delays of more than 12 weeks may compromise outcomes significantly. A study by Gagliato et al. [47] confirmed the unfavorable effect of delay in the initiation of adjuvant chemotherapy, particularly for triple-negative and HER2-positive breast cancer subtypes. Patients with TNBC and HER2-positive tumors treated with trastuzumab who started chemotherapy ≥61 days after surgery had significantly worse survival compared with those who initiated treatment in the first 30 days after surgery.

The survival benefit of polychemotherapy regimens in the adjuvant setting for breast cancer was demonstrated long ago in several randomized trials and meta-analyses. Although initial studies were conducted among patients with higher risk and node-positive disease, subsequent trials encompassing lower-risk groups have extended the spectrum of patients who might benefit from adjuvant chemotherapy. For instance, the 2005 Early Breast Cancer Trialists' Collaborative Group (EBCTCG) analysis reviewing polychemotherapy versus no adjuvant chemotherapy confirmed significant reductions in both recurrence and mortality rates for early breast cancer [5].

The type of adjuvant chemotherapy (CT) administered has evolved in the last two decades. The 2005 review by EBCTCG also included an indirect comparison of adjuvant cyclophosphamide, methotrexate, fluorouracil (CMF) and anthracycline-based (doxorubicin or epirubicin) chemotherapy and found no significant differences in proportional risk reductions in recurrence or breast cancer mortality between the two CT arms. However, the analysis included quite heterogeneous chemotherapy schemes with varying durations of 6, 9 or 12 months of treatment. In the 2011 EBCTCG meta-analysis, adjuvant chemotherapy using an anthracycline-based regimen was compared to no treatment; the use of an anthracycline-based regimen provided absolute improvements of 8% and 5% in the risk of recurrence and overall mortality, whereas the use of CMF was associated with absolute reductions of 10.2% and 4.7% in the risk of recurrence and overall mortality, respectively, at 10 years [48]. Although indirect comparisons of the two types of regimens did not indicate an obvious difference in efficacy, directly randomized comparisons in at least two National Surgical Adjuvant Breast and Bowel Project trials (NSABP-15 and NSABP-23) revealed that four cycles of doxorubicin and cyclophosphamide (AC) was equal to 6 months of the classic CMF regimen [49, 50]. In addition, for node-positive disease, cyclophosphamide, epirubicin and 5-fluorouracil (CEF) treatment was superior to classical CMF in terms of overall and disease-free survival [51]. Due to the convenience of a shorter duration of treatment and fewer hospital visits, most clinicians prefer anthracycline-based regimens based on collective experience.

Chemotherapy regimens have evolved during the last two decades, particularly with the introduction of taxanes to early breast cancer treatment. Cancer and Leukemia Group B (CALGB) 9344 was the first randomized trial incorporating sequential paclitaxel therapy for women receiving four cycles of AC chemotherapy [52]. Sequential paclitaxel was associated with improved disease-free and overall survival rates. Although not all of the randomized trials were able to demonstrate an overall survival benefit of the incorporation of taxanes in anthracycline-based regimens, generally there was a modest DFS benefit, particularly for node-positive disease [53, 54]. The efficacy of adjuvant taxanes for node-negative disease was initially evaluated in the Spanish Breast Cancer Research Group (GEICAM) 9805 trial; patients with node-negative breast cancer and at least one high-risk factor for recurrence were assigned to the docetaxel, doxorubicin, cyclophosphamide (TAC) or fluorouracil, doxorubicin, cyclophosphamide (FAC) arms [55]. High-risk factors were defined as tumor size >2 cm, negative results on tests for expression of ER and PgR, tumor histological grade 2 or 3, and age <35 years. Despite significant toxicity, the TAC regimen significantly reduced the risk of recurrence regardless of hormone-receptor status, menopausal status or the number of high-risk factors. Meta-analyses further confirmed that the addition of taxanes to the adjuvant treatment of high-risk early breast cancer significantly reduced the risk of death and relapse [56, 57]. It was unknown whether the benefit provided by the addition of taxane would obviate the need for anthracyclines. While confirmation in larger prospective trials is necessary, one randomized trial supported the use of a non-anthracycline regimen. US Oncology Trial 9735 assigned stage I-III breast cancer patients to AC or docetaxel/cyclophosphamide (TC) arms. The study indicated significantly higher DFS and OS with the TC regimen (81% vs 75% and 87% vs 82%, respectively) [58]. A recent meta-analysis of three adjuvant trials comparing TC for 6 cycles to different AC and taxane combination regimens did not meet the noninferiority criteria, with a 2.5% 4-year IDFS advantage for the AC and taxane combinations. A difference in survival was only evident for triple-negative and node-positive breast cancer patients [59].

Given the lack of more prospective randomized data in this setting, an anthracycline- and taxane-based CT regimen is recommended for most women with higher risk factors, but CMF and TC are acceptable alternatives for those with contraindications to anthracyclines.

Dose-dense treatment, which refers to the administration of drugs with shortened intervals, is based on observations in experimental models that a given dose always kills a certain fraction rather than a certain number of exponentially growing cancer cells [60]. Since human cancer cells in general are supposed to grow by nonexponential Gompertzian kinetics, regrowth of cancer cells between cytoreductive cycles is more rapid than in exponential models, and thus frequent administration of cytotoxic therapy with G-CSF support is assumed to be more effective against residual tumor cells. The concept of dose density has been addressed in several trials. The CALGB 9741 trial evaluated concurrent versus sequential chemotherapy (doxorubicin followed by paclitaxel followed by cyclophosphamide versus doxorubicin plus cyclophosphamide followed by paclitaxel) given either every 2 weeks with G-CSF support or every 3 weeks [61]. There was no difference between the sequential or concomitant arms, but the dose-dense (every-2-week) arm was associated with a reduction in the risk of recurrence and death. Another four-arm study by Budd et al. [62] also demonstrated that AC every 2 weeks followed by paclitaxel every 2 weeks conferred an OS benefit when compared with the other arms, despite no significant difference in DFS. The difference in OS seemed to be confined specifically to the triple-negative subgroup. In contrast to these studies, some trials failed to demonstrate a survival benefit with dose-dense regimens [63, 64]. More recently, an Italian phase 3 trial randomized node-positive breast cancer patients to four treatment arms that included 5-FU and EC followed by paclitaxel or EC followed by paclitaxel given in 2- or 3-weekly intervals [65]. The study suggested a DFS advantage for dose-dense regimens compared with standard interval chemotherapy protocols; in addition, there was no benefit of adding fluorouracil to sequential EC and paclitaxel.

A meta-analysis comparing dose-dense regimens with conventional regimens noted that in some trials, dose-dense treatment was associated with improvements in both OS and DFS (hazard ratio [HR]: 0.83, 95% Confidence Interval [CI] 0.73–0.94; HR: 0.84, 95%CI 0.72–0.98, respectively), but modified doses or regimens also provided improvement in DFS and OS (HR: 0.81, 95% CI 0.73–0.88; HR: 0.85, 95% CI 0.75–0.96, respectively) [66]. However, the benefit was evident in ER-negative disease rather than ER-positive disease. Thus, dose-dense strategies appear feasible with G-CSF support and have a modest impact on outcomes in an unselected patient cohort, but emerging data suggest that specific subtypes, such as triple-negative breast cancer, may obtain more benefit from intensification of CT [67].

Novel Strategies

Unfortunately, trials incorporating agents other than anthracyclines and taxanes in the adjuvant setting have not revealed consistently promising results. Capecitabine has yielded improved outcomes for some subgroups of patients, but overall benefit was limited. For instance, the phase III FinXX trial integrated capecitabine with sequential docetaxel (T) followed by CEF [68]. Although the interim analysis suggested an increase in recurrence-free survival (RFS) with capecitabine, the final results failed to demonstrate an improvement in RFS for the whole patient group [69]. However, in an exploratory subgroup analysis, capecitabine combined with sequential docetaxel followed by CEX (cyclophosphamide, epirubicin and capecitabine) was more effective than T+CEF in the subset of patients with TNBC (HR, 0.53).

Similarly, another trial performed among high-risk patients incorporated capecitabine with sequential AC followed by docetaxel. The study failed to meet its primary endpoint, DFS, whereas OS was improved with the addition of capecitabine [70]. Recently, a phase III trial evaluated the addition of adjuvant capecitabine for patients with residual breast cancer after neoadjuvant chemotherapy with anthracycline, taxane or both. At 5 years, overall survival was longer in the capecitabine group than the control group (89.2% vs 83.6%). Among patients with TNBC, the survival benefit was more evident [71]. Due to the positive findings in the FinXX and CREATE-X trials, the St Gallen 2017 guidelines recommend considering adjuvant capecitabine combined with anthracyclines and taxanes in the adjuvant setting and for residual cancer after neoadjuvant chemotherapy for the TNBC subtype [31].

All of these studies have pointed at an exceptional status for TNBC patients regarding novel therapies in the adjuvant setting. Most germline mutant BRCA1-associated breast cancers are TNBC, and some TNBC patients have somatic loss of BRCA1 function due to downregulated BRCA1 transcription or translation [72]. Since BRCA1-associated tumors are deficient in the genes that encode proteins critical in DNA repair, an increased susceptibility to DNA-damaging agents is expected. In preclinical models of BRCA1-deficient breast cancers, platinum agents have shown increased cytotoxicity through induction of double-strand breaks [73]. The data for carboplatin and cisplatin in TNBC predominantly emerge from small studies and retrospective analyses in the neoadjuvant or metastatic setting [74]. Although the St Gallen 2017 guidelines recommend platinum-based neoadjuvant chemotherapy for TNBC patients, there is no such recommendation for the adjuvant setting.

Integration of targeted agents has also failed to demonstrate survival advantage in the adjuvant setting, similar to colon cancer. The BEATRICE trial randomized TNBC patients to receive a minimum of four cycles of chemotherapy either alone or with bevacizumab [75]. After a median follow-up of 56 months, the five-year invasive disease-free survival (IDFS) and OS did not differ between arms. In addition, biomarker analysis did not point at a specific subgroup who may benefit from anti-VEGF therapy.

Treatment of Pregnant Patients

The majority of breast cancers during pregnancy are invasive ductal carcinomas of relatively advanced stage, particularly in those diagnosed while lactating [76].

Physical examination is hampered by hypertrophy, engorgement and indistinct nodularity in the pregnant patient's breast, and densities or nodularities of the gland are often ascribed to benign proliferative changes. These factors often cause a delay in diagnosis and advanced stage presentation.

The indications for systemic chemotherapy are the same in the pregnant patient as in the non-pregnant breast cancer patient, although chemotherapy should not be administered at any point during the first trimester of pregnancy due to high risk of fetal malformation. The evidence suggests that the incidence of congenital malformations is low (approximately 1.3%) if chemotherapy is administered to women in the second or third trimester, after the major period of organogenesis. The estimated risk of fetal malformation during first-trimester exposure to chemotherapeutics is 15–20% [77].

The largest experience to date has been with anthracyclines and alkylating agents [78, 79]. Anthracyclines are mutagenic and carcinogenic in vitro and in animals [80]. However, only low concentrations of anthracyclines have been detected in fetal tissues, probably for several reasons. First, the molecular weight of anthracyclines is greater than 500 Da, which results in incomplete transfer across the human placenta. Second, anthracyclines are products of p-glycoprotein, which is a placental drug-transporting glycoprotein that further limits fetal penetration and results in only barely detectable drug concentrations in the fetus. In a retrospective review from a single institution, 81 pregnant breast cancer patients were treated with FAC in the adjuvant or neoadjuvant setting; most of the children exposed to chemotherapy in utero grew normally without any significant exposure-related toxicity or health problems [81]. Three children were born with congenital abnormalities: one each with Down syndrome, ureteral reflux or clubfoot. The rate of congenital abnormalities in the cohort was similar to the national average of 3%. Moreover, as a general rule, breastfeeding during chemotherapy is contraindicated due to the excretion of cyclophosphamide and doxorubicin in breast milk [82]. Methotrexate is also avoided during pregnancy due to its abortifacient effect and teratogenic potential.

Currently, there are no data encouraging the safe administration of dose-dense AC with or without taxanes. A systematic review of taxane administration during pregnancy identified twenty-three publications describing a total of 40 women [83]. No spontaneous abortions or intrauterine deaths were reported. In two cases of exposure to paclitaxel, acute respiratory distress was possibly related to prematurity [84, 85]. The only malformation possibly related to taxanes was a case of pyloric stenosis in a neonate whom mother had received multiagent chemotherapy (doxorubicin, cyclophosphamide, paclitaxel, and docetaxel). Since the safety of taxanes is less well documented than that of anthracyclines, in some situations an additional cycle of anthracycline-based chemotherapy during pregnancy and completion of taxane-based chemotherapy after delivery can be considered [86]. According to the limited published data, the major cause of undesirable fetal outcome appears to be premature delivery rather than any direct effect of chemotherapy. Follow-up of children with specialized assessment, including detailed physiological and neurological functions, is necessary (Fig. 15.6).

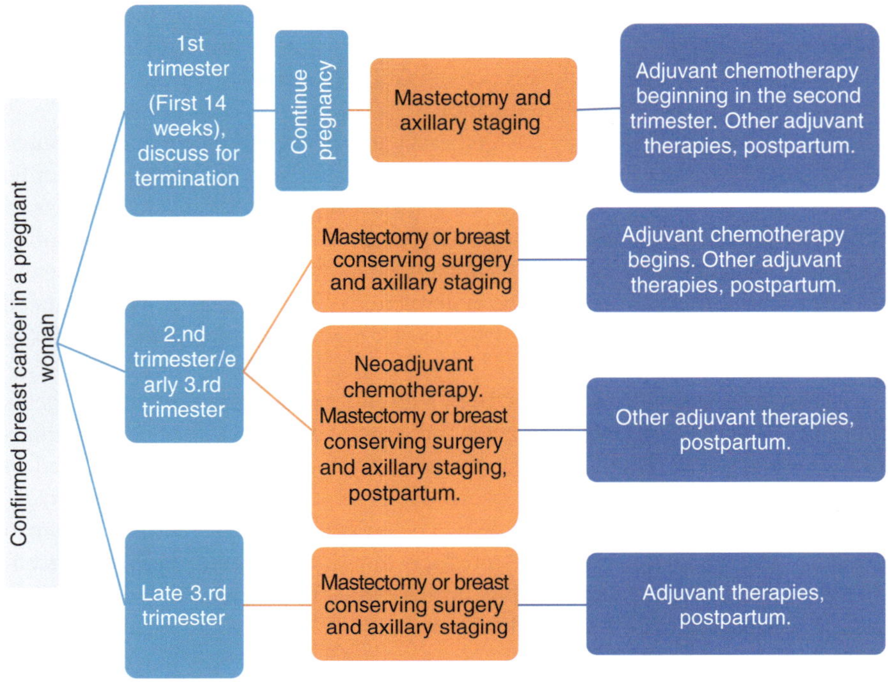

Fig. 15.6 Breast cancer management during pregnancy. [a]Pregnancy should be terminated in patients who become pregnant during tamoxifen treatment. The risk of malformation is high in the first trimester for tamoxifen use. Adjuvant trastuzumab is not recommended in pregnancy. However, the pregnancy can be continued by informing the patient because there are no sufficient data regarding the risk of malformation in women who become pregnant under trastuzumab treatment. Trastuzumab should be discontinued. [b]Premature delivery should be avoided. In patients receiving chemotherapy, the last chemotherapy cycle should not be given for a period of 1 month prior to the estimated date of birth (due to the risk of neutropenia in the baby). Breast conserving surgery can be performed in pregnancy, but the patient should be informed about the risk of local recurrence since RT will be performed after delivery (if RT cannot be started within 6 months after surgical operation). Blue dye is not used as the SLNB method. The radionuclide method in SLNB can be used as of the second trimester. Adjuvant RT, endocrine therapy and trastuzumab are administered after delivery when adjuvant therapy is indicated. Doxorubicin, 5-fluorouracil, and cyclophosphamide (FAC) can be used as chemotherapy (or AC). Ondansetron is preferred for nausea. Although there are no sufficient data yet, weekly paclitaxel can be given after the first trimester if there is a clinical indication (e.g., progression under neoadjuvant treatment with anthracycline)

Toxicity

Anthracyclines are believed to cause immediate damage to cardiac myocytes via several mechanisms. By activating calcium channels, intracellular calcium overload is triggered, and cardiac contractility may be reduced [87]. Generation of reactive oxygen species that induce sarcomere degeneration, mitochondrial dysfunction, DNA damage and alteration of gene expression can cause apoptotic and necrotic cell death [88, 89]. Trastuzumab for HER2-positive disease and adjuvant radiotherapy further contribute to cardiac dysfunction. The most common serious clinical cardiac complications that have been reported are arrhythmias, myocardial necrosis causing dilated cardiomyopathy, and vaso-occlusion or vasospasm resulting in angina or myocardial infarction. Reported heart failure rates associated with epirubicin range from 0.6% at a cumulative dose of 550 mg/m^2 to 14.5% at a cumulative dose of 1000 mg/m^2 [90]. A report of 630 patients treated with doxorubicin alone in three controlled trials estimated that as many as 26% of patients receiving a cumulative doxorubicin dose of 550 mg/m^2 would develop heart failure [91]. Based upon these observations, it has been generally recommended that cumulative doses be limited to 450–500 mg/m^2 for doxorubicin and 900 mg/m^2 for epirubicin in adults. The incidence of heart failure associated with taxanes according to retrospective analysis is relatively low, with a range of 2.3–8% for docetaxel [92]. For patients undergoing adjuvant chemotherapy, baseline cardiovascular examination should include management of risk factors such as hypertension and hyperlipidemia to avoid further cardiac damage.

A frustrating late side effect of alkylating agents is myelodysplasia (MDS) and bone marrow neoplasms. In 2003, the National Surgical Adjuvant Breast and Bowel Project (NSABP) reported a 0.27% eight-year cumulative incidence of MDS and/or acute myelogenous leukemia (AML) among patients with breast cancer treated with doxorubicin and cyclophosphamide [93]. Two genetic variants of therapy-related AML have been described: one after anthracyclines and/or topoisomerase inhibitors with a median latent period of 1–3 years and another after alkylating agents with median latency of 4–6 years, often preceded by MDS [94]. A recent study of bone marrow neoplasms following adjuvant chemotherapy for breast cancer revealed a slightly higher incidence (0.4–0.5% at 10 years) that was slightly higher than previously described. The effect of G-CSF was not evaluated, and taxane use did not increase myeloid neoplasms [95].

The most common side effect encountered due to taxanes is neurotoxicity. In a recent study, upon completion of docetaxel chemotherapy, 23% of patients reported grade 2–4 peripheral neuropathy (PN), and one third of these patients reported persistent symptoms 1–3 years later [96]. Among those without PN initially, 10% developed PN 1–3 years after. In 2014, the American Society of Clinical Oncology published a clinical practice guideline on chemotherapy-induced peripheral neuropathy (CIPN); no agent was offered for the prevention of CIPN due to a lack of consistent evidence [97]. However, for the treatment of CIPN, the guidelines recommend duloxetine, based on efficacy data from a large randomized placebo-controlled trial [98]. Patients who received duloxetine reported a significant decrease in pain, numbness and tingling symptoms compared with placebo. Exploratory subgroup analysis suggested that duloxetine may be more efficacious for oxaliplatin-induced than for paclitaxel-induced painful neuropathy.

Recommended Adjuvant Chemotherapy

Regimens

There is no single standard adjuvant chemotherapy protocol for the treatment of breast cancer. Commonly used regimens are listed below:

Non-Taxane Regimens

1. AC chemotherapy *(preferred)*
   Doxorubicin 60 mg/m^2 IV day 1
   Cyclophosphamide 600 mg/m^2 IV day 1
   (Cycled every 21 days for 4 cycles.)
   (in dose dense, every 14 days for 4 cycles with myeloid growth factor support)
2. EC chemotherapy
   Epirubicin 100 mg/m^2 IV day 1
   Cyclophosphamide 830 mg/m^2 IV day 1
   (Cycled every 21 days for 8 cycles.)
   (With myeloid growth factor support)
3. CMF chemotherapy
   Cyclophosphamide 100 mg/m^2 (PO) days 1–14
   Methotrexate 40 mg/m^2 IV days 1 and 8
   5-Fluorouracil 600 mg/m^2 IV days 1 and 8
   (Cycled every 28 days for 6 cycles.)

Taxane Regimens

1. Dose dense AC followed by paclitaxel chemotherapy *(preferred)*
   Doxorubicin 60 mg/m^2 IV day 1
   Cyclophosphamide 600 mg/m^2 IV day 1
   (Cycled every 14 days for 4 cycles)
   Followed by paclitaxel 175 mg/m^2 by 3-h IV infusion day 1
   (Cycled every 14 days for 4 cycles) (All cycles with myeloid growth factor support)
2. Dose-dense AC followed by weekly paclitaxel chemotherapy *(preferred)*
   Doxorubicin 60 mg/m^2 IV day 1
   Cyclophosphamide 600 mg/m^2 IV day 1
   (Cycled every 14 days for 4 cycles)
   (All cycles with myeloid growth factor support)
   Followed by paclitaxel 80 mg/m^2 by 1-h IV infusion weekly for 12 weeks.

3. TC chemotherapy *(preferred)*
   Docetaxel 75 mg/m^2 IV day 1
   Cyclophosphamide 600 mg/m^2 IV day 1
   (Cycled every 21 days for 4 cycles)
   (All cycles with myeloid growth factor support)
4. TAC chemotherapy
   Docetaxel 75 mg/m^2 IV day 1
   Doxorubicin 50 mg/m^2 IV day 1
   Cyclophosphamide 500 mg/m^2 IV day 1
   (Cycled every 21 days for 6 cycles)
   (All cycles with myeloid growth factor support)
5. AC followed by docetaxel chemotherapy
   Doxorubicin 60 mg/m^2 IV on day 1
   Cyclophosphamide 600 mg/m^2 IV day 1
   Cycled every 21 days for 4 cycles.
   Followed by docetaxel 100 mg/m^2 IV on day 1
   (Cycled every 21 days for 4 cycles.)
   (Docetaxel with myeloid growth factor support)
6. FEC followed by docetaxel chemotherapy
   5-Fluorouracil 500 mg/m^2 IV day 1
   Epirubicin 100 mg/m^2 IV day 1
   Cyclophosphamide 500 mg/m^2 IV day 1
   (Cycled every 21 days for 3 cycles.)
   Followed by docetaxel 100 mg/m^2 IV day 1
   (Cycled every 21 days for 3 cycles.)
   (All cycles with myeloid growth factor support)
7. FEC followed by weekly paclitaxel
   5-Fluorouracil 600 mg/m^2 IV day 1
   Epirubicin 90 mg/m^2 IV day 1
   Cyclophosphamide 600 mg/m^2 IV day 1
   (Cycled every 21 days for 4 cycles.)
   Followed by paclitaxel 100 mg/m^2 IV infusion weekly for 8 weeks.
8. FAC followed by weekly paclitaxel
   5-Fluorouracil 500 mg/m^2 IV days 1 and 8 or days 1 and 4
   Doxorubicin 50 mg/m^2 IV day 1
   (or by 72-h continuous infusion)
   Cyclophosphamide 500 mg/m^2 IV day 1
   (Cycled every 21 days for 6 cycles.)
   Followed by paclitaxel 80 mg/m^2 by 1-h IV infusion weekly for 12 weeks.

Conclusion

Optimizing adjuvant chemotherapy depends not only on determining the intrinsic subtypes and prognosis but also on defining the subgroup of patients for whom cytotoxic treatment is of no use or adjuvant hormone therapy is inadequate. Thus, treatment-oriented classification of subgroups of breast cancer is essential. For triple-negative breast cancer, adjuvant cytotoxic chemotherapy is recommended for tumors ≥5 mm. Without markers of lower endocrine responsiveness (Luminal A-like) disease, chemotherapy may be considered if four or more nodes are involved. Thus, with high ER/PR expression and clearly low Ki67, adjuvant endocrine therapy is usually adequate for tumors up to 5 cm (T1 and T2) with low or absent nodal involvement. For low ER/PR expression, high proliferation markers and high tumor burden (Luminal B-like) or multiparameter molecular tests suggesting an 'unfavorable prognosis', cytotoxic chemotherapy is recommended. Extensive nodal involvement, histological grade 3, extensive lymphovascular invasion, and larger T size (T3) are also considered indications for adjuvant chemotherapy. Anthracyclines and taxanes are the mainstay of adjuvant cytotoxic chemotherapy, although platinums can be considered for TNBC patients with known BRCA mutations. Adjuvant capecitabine for residual cancer after neoadjuvant chemotherapy may confer a survival benefit. Dose-dense regimens should be reserved mainly for patients with triple-negative breast cancer and extensive nodal involvement. Prevention and treatment of early and late side effects of chemotherapy requires life-long follow-up and detailed evaluation of each treatment and patient-related factors.

References

1. Berry DA, Cronin KA, Plevritis SK, Fryback DG, Clarke L, Zelen M, Cancer Intervention and Surveillance Modeling Network (CISNET) Collaborators, et al. Effect of screening and adjuvant therapy on mortality from breast cancer. N Engl J Med. 2005;353:1784–92.
2. Clarke M. Meta-analyses of adjuvant therapies for women with early breast cancer: the Early Breast Cancer Trialists' Collaborative Group overview. Ann Oncol. 2006;17(Suppl 10):x59–62.
3. Denduluri N, Chavez-MacGregor M, Telli ML, Eisen A, Graff SL, Hassett MJ, et al. Selection of optimal adjuvant chemotherapy and targeted therapy for early breast cancer: ASCO clinical practice guideline focused update. J Clin Oncol. 2018;36. https://doi.org/10.1200/JCO.2018.78.8604.
4. van der Hage JA, Mieog JS, van de Velde CJ, et al. Impact of established prognostic factors and molecular subtype in very young breast cancer patients: pooled analysis of four EORTC randomized controlled trials. Breast Cancer Res. 2011;13:R68.
5. Early Breast Cancer Trialists' Collaborative Group (EBCTCG). Effects of chemotherapy and hormonal therapy for early breast cancer on recurrence and 15-year survival: an overview of the randomised trials. Lancet. 2005;365:1687–717.
6. Li CI, Uribe DJ, Daling JR. Clinical characteristics of different histologic types of breast cancer. Br J Cancer. 2005;93:1046.
7. Denkert C, Loibl S, Noske A, Roller M, Müller BM, Komor M, et al. Tumor associated lymphocytes as an independent predictor of response to neoadjuvant chemotherapy in breast cancer. J Clin Oncol. 2010;28:105–13.
8. Loi S, Sirtaine N, Piette F, Salgado R, Viale G, Van Eenoo F, et al. Prognostic and predictive value of tumor-infiltrating lymphocytes in a phase III randomized adjuvant breast cancer trial in node-positive breast cancer comparing the addition of docetaxel to doxorubicin with doxorubicin-based chemotherapy: BIG 02-98. J Clin Oncol. 2013;31:860–7.

9. Adams S, Gray RJ, Demaria S, Goldstein L, Perez EA, Shulman LN, et al. Prognostic value of tumor-infiltrating lymphocytes in triple-negative breast cancers from two phase III randomized adjuvant breast cancer trials: ECOG 2197 and ECOG 1199. J Clin Oncol. 2014;32:2959–66.
10. Prat A, Parker JS, Karginova O, Fan C, Livasy C, Herschkowitz JI, et al. Phenotypic and molecular characterization of the claudin-low intrinsic subtype of breast cancer. Breast Cancer Res. 2010;12:R68.
11. Perou CM, Sørlie T, Elsen MB, van de Rijn M, Jeffrey SS, Rees CA, et al. Molecular portraits of human breast tumours. Nature. 2000;406:747–52.
12. Sørlie T. Molecular portraits of breast cancer: tumour subtypes as distinct disease entities. Eur J Cancer. 2004;40:2667–75.
13. Bullwinkel J, Baron-Luhr B, Ludemann A, Wohlenberg C, Gerdes J, Scholzen T. Ki67 protein is associated with ribosomal RNA transcription in quiescent and proliferating cells. J Cell Physiol. 2006;206:624–35.
14. Urruticoechea A, Smith IE, Dowsett M. Proliferation marker Ki67 in early breast cancer. J Clin Oncol. 2005;23(28):7212–20.
15. Polley MY, Leung SC, McShane LM, Gao D, Hugh JC, Mastropasqua MG, et al. An international Ki67 reproducibility study. J Natl Cancer Inst. 2013;105:1897–906.
16. Cheang MC, Chia SK, Voduc D, Gao D, Leung S, Snider J, et al. Ki67 index, HER2 status, and prognosis of patients with luminal B breast cancer. J Natl Cancer Inst. 2009;101(10):736e50.
17. Coates AS, Winer EP, Goldhirsch A, Gelber RD, Gnant M, Piccart-Gebhart M, Thürlimann B, Senn HJ, Panel Members. Tailoring therapies-improving the management of early breast cancer: St Gallen International Expert Consensus on the Primary Therapy of Early Breast Cancer 2015. Ann Oncol. 2015;26(8):1533–46.
18. Polley MY, Leung SC, Gao D, Mastropasqua MG, Zabaglo LA, Bartlett JM, et al. An international study to increase concordance in Ki67 scoring. Mod Pathol. 2015;28:778–86.
19. Prat A, Cheang MC, Martin M, Parker JS, Carrasco E, Caballero R, et al. Prognostic significance of progesterone receptor positive tumor cells within immunohistochemically defined luminal A breast cancer. J Clin Oncol. 2013;31:203–9.
20. Cancello G, Maisonneuve P, Rotmensz N, Viale G, Mastropasqua MG, Pruneri G, et al. Progesterone receptor loss identifies Luminal B breast cancer subgroups at higher risk of relapse. Ann Oncol. 2013;24(3):661e8.
21. Loi S, Haibe-Kains B, Desmedt C, Lallemand F, Tutt AM, Gillet C, et al. Definition of clinically distinct molecular subtypes in estrogen receptor-positive breast carcinomas through genomic grade. J Clin Oncol. 2007;25:1239–46.
22. Sorlie T, Tibshirani R, Parker J, Hastie T, Marron JS, Nobel A, et al. Repeated observation of breast tumor subtypes in independent gene expression data sets. Proc Natl Acad Sci U S A. 2003;100(14):8418–23.
23. Perou CM, Jeffrey SS, van de Rijn M, Rees CA, Eisen MB, Ross DT, et al. Distinctive gene expression patterns in human mammary epithelial cells and breast cancers. Proc Natl Acad Sci U S A. 1999;96:9212–7.
24. Sorlie T, Perou CM, Tibshirani R, Aas T, Geisler S, Johnsen H, et al. Gene expression patterns of breast carcinomas distinguish tumor subclasses with clinical implications. Proc Natl Acad Sci U S A. 2001;98:10869–74.
25. van de Vijver MJ, He YD, van 't Veer LJ, Dai H, Hart AA, Voskuil DW, et al. A gene-expression signature as a predictor of survival in breast cancer. N Engl J Med. 2002;347:1999–2009.
26. Cardoso F, van't Veer LJ, Bogaerts J, Slaets L, Viale G, Delaloge S, MINDACT Investigators, et al. 70-gene signature as an aid to treatment decisions in early-stage breast cancer. N Engl J Med. 2016;375:717–29.
27. Krop I, Ismailia N, Andre F, Bast RC, Barlow W, Collyar DE, et al. Use of biomarkers to guide decisions on adjuvant systemic therapy for women with early-stage invasive breast cancer: American Society of Clinical Oncology clinical practice guideline focused update. J Clin Oncol. 2017;35:2838–47.

28. Sparano JA, Gray RJ, Makover DF, Pritchard KI, Albain KS, et al. Prospective validation of a 21-gene expression assay in breast cancer. N Engl J Med. 2015;373:2005–14.
29. Filipits M, Rudas M, Jakesz R, Dubsky P, Fitzal F, Singer CF, et al. A new molecular predictor of distant recurrence in ER-positive, HER2-negative breast cancer adds independent information to conventional clinical risk actors. Clin Cancer Res. 2011;17(18):6012–20.
30. Dubsky P, Filipits M, Jakesz R, Rudas M, Singer CF, Greil R, et al. EndoPredict improves the prognostic classification derived from common clinical guidelines in ER-positive, HER2-negative early breast cancer. Ann Oncol. 2013;24:640–7.
31. Curigliano G, Burstein HJ, Winer EP, Gnant M, Dubsky P, Loibl S, et al. De-escalating and escalating treatments for early-stage breast cancer: the St. Gallen International Expert Consensus Conference on the Primary Therapy of Early Breast Cancer 2017. Ann Oncol. 2017;28:1700–12.
32. Thurman SA, Schnitt SJ, Connolly JL, Gelman R, Silver B, Harris JR, et al. Outcome after breast-conserving therapy for patients with stage I or II mucinous, medullary, or tubular breast carcinoma. Int J Radiat Oncol Biol Phys. 2004;59:152.
33. Capella C, Eusebi V, Mann B, Azzopardi JG. Endocrine differentiation in mucoid carcinoma of the breast. Histopathology. 1980;4:613–30.
34. Clayton F. Pure mucinous carcinomas of breast: morphologic features and prognostic correlates. Hum Pathol. 1986;17:34–8.
35. Tan PH, Tse GMK, Bay BH. Mucinous breast lesions: diagnostic challenges. J Clin Pathol. 2008;61:11–9.
36. Di Saverio S, Gutierrez J, Avisar E. A retrospective review with long term follow-up of 11,400 cases of pure mucinous breast carcinoma. Breast Cancer Res Treat. 2008;111:541–54.
37. Vu-Nishino H, Tavassoli FA, Ahrens WA, Haffty BG. Clinicopathologic features and long-term outcome of patients with medullary breast carcinoma managed with breast-conserving therapy (BCT). Int J Radiat Oncol Biol Phys. 2005;62:1040–7.
38. Thompson K, Grabowski J, Saltzstein SL, Sadler GR, Blair SL. Adenoid cystic breast carcinoma: is axillary staging necessary in all cases? Results from the California Cancer Registry. Breast J. 2011;17:485–9.
39. Ghabach B, Anderson WF, Curtis RE, Huycke MM, Lavigne JA, Dores GM. Adenoid cystic carcinoma of the breast in the United States (1977 to 2006): a population-based cohort study. Breast Cancer Res. 2010;12:R54.
40. Ozguroglu M, Tascilar K, Ilvan S, Soybir G, Celik V. Secretory carcinoma of the breast: case report and review of the literature. Oncology. 2005;68:263–8.
41. Vieni S, Cabibi D, Cipolla C, Fricano S, Graceffa G, Latteri MA. Secretory breast carcinoma with metastatic sentinel lymph node. World J Surg Oncol. 2006;4:88.
42. Herz H, Cooke B, Goldstein D. Metastatic secretory breast cancer. Non-responsiveness to chemotherapy: case report and review of the literature. Ann Oncol. 2000;11:1343–7.
43. Arpino G, Clark GM, Mohsin S, Bardou VJ, Elledge RM. Adenoid cystic carcinoma of the breast: molecular markers, treatment, and clinical outcome. Cancer. 2002;94:2119–27.
44. Aydiner A, Sen F, Tambas M, Ciftci R, Eralp Y, Saip P, Karanlik H, et al. Metaplastic breast carcinoma versus triple-negative breast cancer: survival and response to treatment. Medicine (Baltimore). 2015;94(52):e2341.
45. Tse GM, Tan PH, Putti TC, Lui PC, Chaiwun B, Law BK. Metaplastic carcinoma of the breast: a clinicopathological review. J Clin Pathol. 2006;59:1079–83.
46. Chen IC, Lin CH, Huang CS, Lien HC, Hsu C, Kuo WH, et al. Lack of efficacy to systemic chemotherapy for treatment of metaplastic carcinoma of the breast in the modern era. Breast Cancer Res Treat. 2011;130:345–51.
47. Gagliato Dde M, Gonzalez-Angulo AM, Lei X, Theriault RL, Giordano SH, Valero V, et al. Clinical impact of delaying initiation of adjuvant chemotherapy in patients with breast cancer. J Clin Oncol. 2014;32:735–44.
48. Early Breast Cancer Trialists' Collaborative Group (EBCTCG), Peto R, Davies C, Godwin J, Gray R, Pan HC, et al. Comparisons between different polychemotherapy regimens for early breast cancer: meta-analyses of long-term outcome among 100,000 women in 123 randomised trials. Lancet. 2012;379:432–44.

49. Fisher B, Brown AM, Dimitrov NV, Poisson R, Redmond C, Margolese RG, et al. Two months of doxorubicin-cyclophosphamide with and without interval reinduction therapy compared with 6 months of cyclophosphamide, methotrexate, and fluorouracil in positive-node breast cancer patients with tamoxifen-nonresponsive tumors: results from the National Surgical Adjuvant Breast and Bowel Project B-15. J Clin Oncol. 1990;8:1483–96.
50. Fisher B, Anderson S, Tan-Chiu E, Wolmark N, Wickerham DL, Fisher ER, et al. Tamoxifen and chemotherapy for axillary nodenegative, estrogen receptor-negative breast cancer: findings from National Surgical Adjuvant Breast and Bowel Project B-23. J Clin Oncol. 2001;19:931–42.
51. Levine M, Pritchard K, Bramwell V, Shepherd LE, Tu D, Paul N, et al. Randomized trial comparing cyclophosphamide, epirubicin, and fluorouracil with cyclophosphamide, methotrexate, and fluorouracil in premenopausal women with node-positive breast cancer: update of National Cancer Institute of Canada Clinical Trials Group Trial MA5. J Clin Oncol. 2005;23:5166–70.
52. Henderson I, Berry D, Demetri G, Cirrincione CT, Goldstein LJ, Martino S, et al. Improved outcomes from adding sequential Paclitaxel but not from escalating Doxorubicin dose in an adjuvant chemotherapy regimen for patients with node-positive primary breast cancer. J Clin Oncol. 2003;21:976–83.
53. Mamounas E, Bryant J, Lembersky B, Fehrenbacher L, Sedlacek SM, Fisher B, et al. Paclitaxel after doxorubicin plus cyclophosphamide as adjuvant chemotherapy for node-positive breast cancer: results from NSABP B-28. J Clin Oncol. 2005;23:3686–96.
54. Buzdar AU, Singletary SE, Valero V, Booser DJ, Ibrahim NK, Rahman Z, et al. Evaluation of paclitaxel in adjuvant chemotherapy for patients with operable breast cancer: preliminary data of a prospective randomized trial. Clin Cancer Res. 2002;8:1073–9.
55. Martín M, Seguí MA, Antón A, Ruiz A, Ramos M, Adrover E, et al. Adjuvant docetaxel for high-risk, node-negative breast cancer. N Engl J Med. 2010;363:2200–10.
56. De Laurentiis M, Cancello G, D'Agostino D, Giuliano M, Giordano A, Montagna E, et al. Taxane-based combinations as adjuvant chemotherapy of early breast cancer: a meta-analysis of randomized trials. J Clin Oncol. 2008;26:44–53.
57. Jacquin JP, Jones S, Magné N, Chapelle C, Ellis P, Janni W, et al. Docetaxel containing adjuvant chemotherapy in patients with early stage breast cancer. Consistency of effect independent of nodal and biomarker status: a meta-analysis of 14 randomized clinical trials. Breast Cancer Res Treat. 2012;134:903–13.
58. Jones S, Holmes FA, O'Shaughnessy J, Blum JL, Vukelja SJ, McIntyre KJ, et al. Docetaxel with cyclophosphamide is associated with an overall survival benefit compared with doxorubicin and cyclophosphamide: 7-year follow-up of US Oncology Research Trial 9735. J Clin Oncol. 2009;27:1178–83.
59. Blum JL, Flynn PJ, Yothers G, Asmar L, Geyer CE Jr, Jacobs SA, et al. Anthracyclines in early breast cancer: the ABC Trials-USOR 06-090, NSABP B-46-I/USOR 07132, and NSABP B-49 (NRG Oncology). J Clin Oncol. 2017;35:2647–55.
60. Skipper HE. Laboratory models: some historical perspectives. Cancer Treat Rep. 1986;70:3–7.
61. Citron ML, Berry DA, Cirrincione C, Hudis C, Winer EP, Gradishar WJ, et al. Randomized trial of dose-dense versus conventionally scheduled and sequential versus concurrent combination chemotherapy as postoperative adjuvant treatment of node-positive primary breast cancer: first report of Intergroup Trial C9741/Cancer and Leukemia Group B Trial 9741. J Clin Oncol. 2003;21:1431–9.
62. Budd GT, Barlow WE, Moore HC, Hobday TJ, Stewart JA, Isaacs C, et al. SWOG S0221: a phase III trial comparing chemotherapy schedules in high-risk early-stage breast cancer. J Clin Oncol. 2015;33:58–64.
63. Therasse P, Mauriac L, Welnicka-Jaskiewicz M, Bruning P, Cufer T, Bonnefoi H, et al. Final results of a randomized phase III trial comparing cyclophosphamide, epirubicin, and fluorouracil with dose-intensified epirubicin and cyclophosphamide plus filgrastim in locally advanced breast cancer. An EORTC-NCIC-SAKK multicenter study. J Clin Oncol. 2003;21:843–50.
64. Fountzilas G, Dafni U, Gogas H, Linardou H, Kalofonos HP, Briasoulis E, et al. Post-operative dose dense sequential chemotherapy with epirubicin, paclitaxel and CMF in patients with high-risk breast cancer: a Hellenic Cooperative Oncology Group randomized phase III trial HE 10/00. Ann Oncol. 2008;19:853–60.

65. Del Mastro L, De Placido S, Bruzzi P, De Laurentiis M, Boni C, Cavazzini G, Gruppo Italiano Mammella (GIM) Investigators, et al. Fluorouracil and dose-dense chemotherapy in adjuvant treatment of patients with early-stage breast cancer: an open-label, 2 × 2 factorial, randomised phase 3 trial. Lancet. 2015;385(9980):1863–72.
66. Bonilla L, Ben-Aharon I, Vidal L, Gafter-Gvili A, Leibovici L, Stemmer SM, et al. Dose-dense chemotherapy in nonmetastatic breast cancer: a systematic review and meta-analysis of randomized controlled trials. J Natl Cancer Inst. 2010;102:1845–54.
67. Bayraktar S, Arun B. Dose dense chemotherapy for breast cancer. Breast J. 2012;18:261–6.
68. Joensuu H, Kellokumpu-Lehtinen PL, Huovinen R, Jukkola-Vuorinen A, Tanner M, Asola R, et al. Adjuvant capecitabine in combination with docetaxel and cyclophosphamide plus epirubicin for breast cancer: an open-label, randomised controlled trial. Lancet Oncol. 2009;10:1145–51.
69. Joensuu H, Kellokumpu-Lehtinen PL, Huovinen R, Jukkola-Vuorinen A, Tanner M, Kokko R, et al. Adjuvant capecitabine in combination with docetaxel, epirubicin, and cyclophosphamide for early breast cancer: the randomized clinical FinXX trial. JAMA Oncol. 2017;3(6):793–800.
70. O'Shaughnessy J, Paul D, Stokoe C. First efficacy results of a randomized, open-label, phase II study of adjuvant doxorubicin plus cyclophosphamide, followed by docetaxel with or without capecitabine, in high-risk early breast cancer. In: 33rd annual san antonio breast cancer symposium 2010, San Antonio, TX, December 8-12 (abstr S4-2).
71. Masuda N, Lee SJ, Ohtani S, Im YH, Lee ES, Yokota I, et al. Adjuvant capecitabine for breast cancer after preoperative chemotherapy. N Engl J Med. 2017;376(22):2147–59.
72. Husain A, He G, Venkatraman ES, Spriggs DR. BRCA1 up-regulation is associated with repair-mediated resistance to cis-diamminedichloroplatinum(II). Cancer Res. 1998;58:1120–3.
73. Byrski T, Gronwald J, Huzarski T, Grzybowska E, Budryk M, Stawicka M, et al. Response to neo-adjuvant chemotherapy in women with BRCA1-positive breast cancers. Breast Cancer Res Treat. 2009;115:359–63.
74. Silver DP, Richardson AL, Eklund AC, Wang ZC, Szallasi Z, Li Q, et al. Efficacy of neoadjuvant cisplatin in triple-negative breast cancer. J Clin Oncol. 2010;28:1145–53.
75. Bell R, Brown J, Parmar M, Toi M, Suter T, Steger GG, et al. Final efficacy and updated safety results of the randomized phase III BEATRICE trial evaluating adjuvant bevacizumab-containing therapy in triple-negative early breast cancer. Ann Oncol. 2016;28(4):754–60.
76. Parente JT, Amsel M, Lerner R, Chinea F. Breast cancer associated with pregnancy. Obstet Gynecol. 1998;71:861–4.
77. Ring AE, Smith IE, Jones A, Shannon C, Galani E, Ellis PA. Chemotherapy for breast cancer during pregnancy: an 18-year experience from five London teaching hospitals. J Clin Oncol. 2005;23:4192–7.
78. Germann N, Goffinet F, Goldwasser F. Anthracyclines during pregnancy: embryo-fetal outcome in 160 patients. Ann Oncol. 2004;15:146–50.
79. Hahn KM, Johnson PH, Gordon N, Kuerer H, Middleton L, Ramirez M, et al. Treatment of pregnant breast cancer patients and outcomes of children exposed to chemotherapy in utero. Cancer. 2006;107(6):1219–26.
80. Marquardt H, Philips FS, Sternberg SS. Tumorigenicity in vivo and induction of malignant transformation and mutagenesis in cell cultures by adriamycin and daunomycin. Cancer Res. 1976;36:2065–9.
81. Murthy RK, Theriault RL, Barnett CM, Hodge S, Ramirez MM, Milbourne A, et al. Outcomes of children exposed in utero to chemotherapy for breast cancer. Breast Cancer Res. 2014;16(6):500.
82. Briggs GG, Freeman RK, Yaffe SJ. Drugs in pregnancy and lactation. 8th ed. Philadelphia: Lippincott Williams & Wilkins; 2008.
83. Mir O, Berveiller P, Goffinet F, Treluyer JM, Serreau R, Goldwasser F, et al. Taxanes for breast cancer during pregnancy: a systematic review. Ann Oncol. 2010;21:425–6.
84. Garcia-Gonzalez J, Cueva J, Lamas MJ, Curiel T, Graña B, López-López R. Paclitaxel and cisplatin in the treatment of metastatic non-small-cell lung cancer during pregnancy. Clin Transl Oncol. 2008;10:375–6.

85. Bader AA, Schlembach D, Tamussino KF, Pristauz G, Petru E. Anhydramnios associated with-administration of trastuzumab and paclitaxel for metastatic breast cancer during pregnancy. Lancet Oncol. 2007;8:79–81.
86. Amant F, Deckers S, Van Calsteren K, Loibl S, Halaska M, Brepoels L, et al. Breast cancer in pregnancy: recommendations of an international consensus meeting. Eur J Cancer. 2010;46:3158–68.
87. Ferlay J, Héry C, Autier P, Sankaranarayanan R. Global burden of breast cancer. In: Li C, editor. Breast cancer epidemiology. New York: Springer; 2010. p. 1–19.
88. Menna P, Gonzalez Paz O, Chello M, Covino E, Salvatorelli E, Minotti G. Anthracycline cardiotoxicity. Expert Opin Drug Saf. 2012;11:21–36.
89. Roca-Alonso L, Pellegrino L, Castellano L, Stebbing J. Breast cancer treatment and adverse cardiac events: what are the molecular mechanisms. Cardiology. 2012;122:253–9.
90. Maxwell CB, Jenkins AT. Drug-induced heart failure. Am J Health Syst Pharm. 2011;68:1791–804.
91. Swain SM, Whaley FS, Ewer MS. Congestive heart failure in patients treated with doxorubicin: a retrospective analysis of three trials. Cancer. 2003;97:2869–79.
92. Gharib MI, Burnett AK. Chemotherapy-induced cardiotoxicity: current practice and prospects of prophylaxis. Eur J Heart Fail. 2002;4:235–42.
93. Smith RE, Bryant J, DeCillis A, Anderson S. Acute myeloid leukemia and myelodysplastic syndrome after doxorubicin-cyclophosphamide adjuvant therapy for operable breast cancer: the National Surgical Adjuvant Breast and Bowel Project Experience. J Clin Oncol. 2003;21:1195–204.
94. Vardiman JW, Thiele J, Arber DA, Brunning RD, Borowitz MJ, Porwit A. The 2008 revision of the World Health Organization (WHO) classification of myeloid neoplasms and acute leukemia: rationale and important changes. Blood. 2009;114:937–51.
95. Wolff AC, Blackford AL, Visvanathan K, Rugo HS, Moy B, Goldstein LJ, et al. Risk of marrow neoplasms after adjuvant breast cancer therapy: the national comprehensive cancer network experience. J Clin Oncol. 2015;33:340–8.
96. Eckhoff L, Knoop A, Jensen MB, Ewertz M. Persistence of docetaxel-induced neuropathy and impact on quality of life among breast cancer survivors. Eur J Cancer. 2015;51:292–300.
97. Hershman DL, Lacchetti C, Dworkin RH, Lavoie Smith EM, Bleeker J, Cavaletti G, et al. Prevention and management of chemotherapy-induced peripheral neuropathy in survivors of adult cancers: American Society of Clinical Oncology clinical practice guideline. J Clin Oncol. 2014;32(18):1941–67.
98. Smith EM, Pang H, Cirrincione C, Fleishman S, Paskett ED, Ahles T. Effect of duloxetine on pain, function, and quality of life among patients with chemotherapy-induced painful peripheral neuropathy: a randomized clinical trial. JAMA. 2013;309:1359–67.

Chapter 16
Adjuvant Therapy for HER2-Positive Early-Stage Breast Cancer

Soley Bayraktar and Adnan Aydiner

Introduction

Breast cancer remains one of the leading causes of cancer-related death worldwide [1]. Although chemotherapy has improved outcomes for patients, the marginal benefits achieved with cytotoxic agents seem to have reached a plateau. Fortunately, technological advances have enabled the characterization of the molecular subtypes [2, 3] of breast cancer, which has, in turn, facilitated the development of molecularly targeted therapeutics for this disease. One subtype is distinguished by amplification of the gene encoding human epidermal growth factor receptor 2 (HER2). This subtype accounts for approximately 20–30% of invasive breast cancers, and until the discovery of effective anti-HER2 therapies (the first of which was trastuzumab), was associated with reduced disease-free survival (DFS), increased risk of metastasis and shorter overall survival (OS) [4, 5]. By 2005, the natural history of this breast cancer subtype in the adjuvant setting was forever changed with the release of the findings of first-generation adjuvant trials that combined trastuzumab with chemotherapy, concomitantly or sequentially.

HER2 is a member of the ErbB family of receptor tyrosine kinases (RTKs), which includes HER1 (epidermal growth factor receptor [EGFR]), HER3, and HER4. HER2-mediated signal transduction is believed to depend largely on heterodimerization with other family members [5]. Trastuzumab is a humanized monoclonal antibody that targets the extracellular portion of HER2. This was the first HER2-targeted agent to be approved by the United States Food and Drug Administration (FDA) for the treatment of both early-stage and metastatic HER2-overexpressing (HER2+)

S. Bayraktar
Department of Medical Oncology, Memorial Hospital, Istanbul, Turkey

A. Aydiner (✉)
Internal Medicine, Medical Oncology, Istanbul Medical Faculty, Department of Medical Oncology, Institute of Oncology, Istanbul University, Istanbul, Turkey

A. Aydiner et al. (eds.), *Breast Cancer*, https://doi.org/10.1007/978-3-319-96947-3_16

breast cancer [6, 7]. Subsequently, lapatinib, an orally bioavailable small-molecule dual HER2- and EGFR/HER1-specific tyrosine kinase inhibitor (TKI), received FDA approval in combination with capecitabine for patients with advanced HER2+ breast cancer [8]. Pertuzumab in 2012 and ado-trastuzumab emtansine in 2013 were subsequently approved in the US and elsewhere based on evidence showing an improvement in survival outcomes in patients with mostly trastuzumab-naïve or trastuzumab-exposed metastatic disease [9, 10]. The clinical benefit demonstrated by those drugs in advanced disease has triggered several adjuvant and neoadjuvant trials testing them in combination with chemotherapy but also without conventional chemotherapy, using single or dual HER2-targeting drugs. In this chapter, we review the current data on the therapeutic management of HER2-positive early-stage breast cancer in the adjuvant and neoadjuvant settings.

Defining HER2-Positive Breast Cancer

A key first step in appropriately deciding on the use of HER2-targeted therapy is the accurate determination of HER2 overexpression either by immunohistochemistry (IHC) or fluorescence in situ hybridization (FISH). The 2013 American Society of Clinical Oncology (ASCO)/College of American Pathologists (CAP) guidelines define HER2 positivity as 3+ on IHC (defined as uniform intense membrane staining of >10% of invasive tumor cells) or amplified on FISH (a HER2:chromosome enumeration probe [CEP]17 ratio of >2.0, or <2.0 plus average HER2 copy number >6 signals/cell) [11]. Recently updated 2018 ASCO/CAP HER2 testing guidelines addressed specific testing strategies to better define and distinguish HER2 status of tumors. Specifically, the draft update recommends: the addition of IHC testing in the same laboratory or institution performing ISH as part of the evaluation of less common patterns observed with dual-probe ISH testing. In cases where the recommended testing strategy does not resolve the clinical concerns, the draft update currently states that pathologists may obtain second opinions. The draft update no longer recommends alternative probe testing in the guideline algorithm for dual probe ISH testing.

Although a detailed discussion of HER2 testing is beyond the scope of this chapter, we would like to note that if a patient's HER2 expression is ultimately deemed to be equivocal on both IHC and FISH, the oncologist can still consider HER2-targeted therapy based on the patient's history, prognosis, and comorbidities.

Anti-HER-2 Therapy for Early-Stage Breast Cancer

In this section, we summarize all the relevant phase III and some phase II clinical trials that constitute the theoretical framework to support our daily practice. We subdivide this section according to the 2 clinical settings: adjuvant and neoadjuvant (Figs. 16.1, 16.2, 16.3, and 16.4).

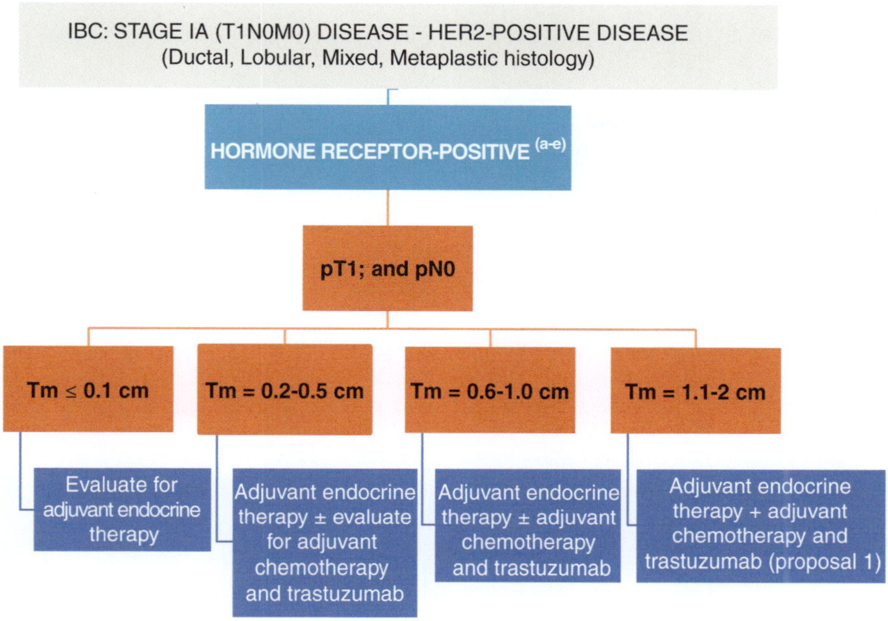

Fig. 16.1 Adjuvant systemic therapy for stage IA (T1N0M0)—hormone receptor-positive and HER2-positive disease. [a]There is no absolute age limit. Instead, treatment depends on the disease, the presence of comorbidities, the patient's life expectancy, and patient preferences. Treatment should be individualized for patients >70 years of age. [b]Chemotherapy and endocrine therapy as adjuvant therapy should be given sequentially, with endocrine therapy following chemotherapy. The available data suggest that sequential or concurrent endocrine therapy with radiation therapy is acceptable. [c]Assuming that HER2 positivity is determined according to the ASCO/CAP guidelines, most patients with T1b disease and all patients with T1c disease require anti-HER2 therapy. The chemotherapy regimen for these patients may contain anthracyclines. If provided in stage I and if the tumor diameter is <1 to 2 cm, the combination of paclitaxel and trastuzumab is the preferred regimen. Trastuzumab or chemotherapy is not recommended for microinvasive disease (invasive tumor ≤1 mm). [d]Fertility preservation (e.g., by ovarian tissue or oocyte conservation) should be offered to women <40 years of age. [e]Consider adjuvant bisphosphonate therapy in postmenopausal (natural or induced) patients receiving adjuvant therapy

Adjuvant Setting

Published results from adjuvant trials have described anti-HER2 therapy use in concomitant and sequential combination with anthracycline and non-anthracycline chemotherapy regimens (Table 16.1). The monoclonal antibody trastuzumab is the first and only targeted agent approved for the adjuvant treatment of early-stage HER2-positive breast cancer. Trastuzumab binds to the extracellular domain of HER2, thereby suppressing its signaling activity and inducing antibody-dependent cell-mediated cytotoxicity (ADCC).

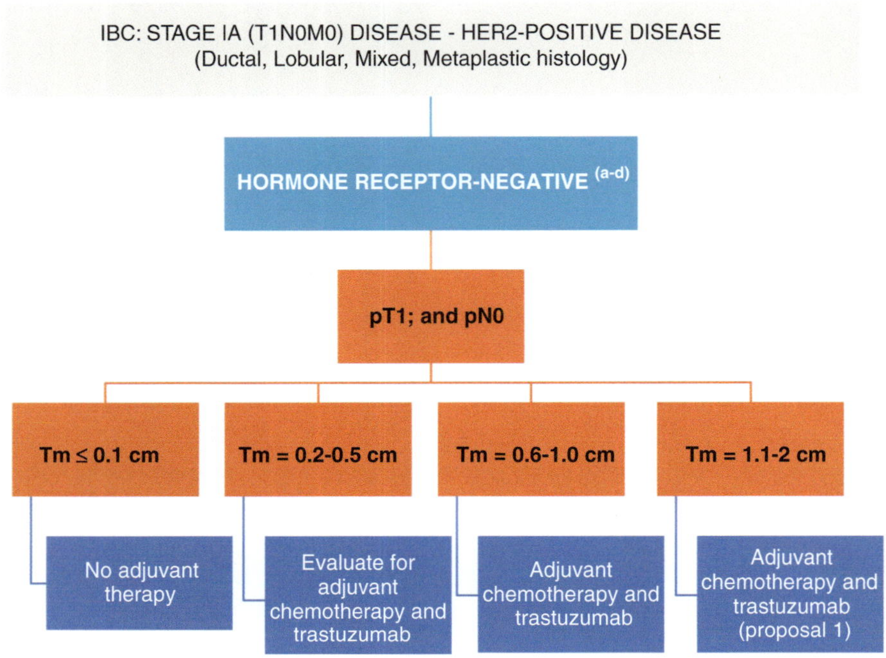

Fig. 16.2 Adjuvant systemic therapy for stage IA (T1N0M0)—hormone receptor-negative and HER2-positive disease. [a]There is no absolute age limit. Instead, treatment depends on the disease, the presence of comorbidities, the patient's life expectancy, and patient preferences. Treatment should be individualized for patients >70 years of age. [b]Assuming that HER2 positivity is determined according to the ASCO/CAP guidelines, most patients with T1b disease and all patients with T1c disease require anti-HER2 therapy. The chemotherapy regimen for these patients may contain anthracyclines. If provided in stage I and if the tumor diameter is ≤1 cm, the combination of paclitaxel and trastuzumab is the preferred regimen. For patients in stage I with a tumor diameter >1, anthracyclines followed by taxanes and trastuzumab may be preferred, although paclitaxel-trastuzumab may also be an option in select patients. Trastuzumab or chemotherapy is not recommended for microinvasive disease (invasive tumor ≤1 mm). [c]Fertility preservation (e.g., by ovarian tissue or oocyte conservation) should be offered to women <40 years of age. [d]Consider adjuvant bisphosphonate therapy in postmenopausal (natural or induced) patients receiving adjuvant therapy

Concomitant Chemotherapy/Trastuzumab

While initially designed as 2 separate trials, the National Surgical Adjuvant Breast and Bowel Project (NSABP) B-31 and North Central Cancer Treatment Group (NCCTG) N9831 trials were jointly analyzed in 2005 due to their similar eligibility criteria and to allow an earlier evaluation of clinical outcomes. The studies had similar patient populations, although N9831 also included women with high-risk node-negative disease defined as tumors ≥2 cm and positive for hormone receptors or tumors larger than 1 cm with negative hormone receptors. NSABP B-31 compared four cycles of doxorubicin and cyclophosphamide (AC) followed by four cycles of

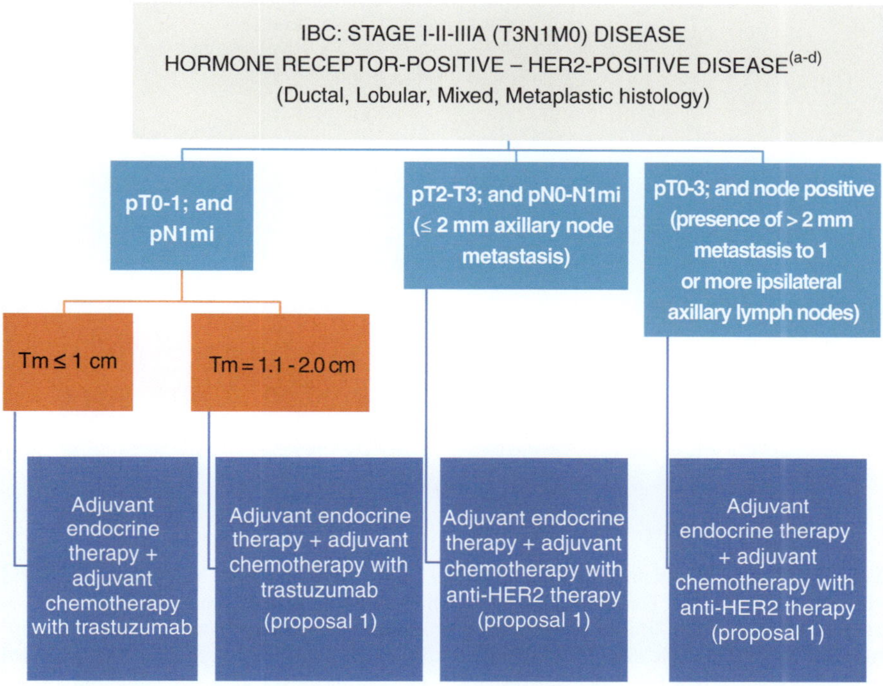

Fig. 16.3 Adjuvant systemic therapy for stage I, II, IIIA—hormone receptor-positive and HER2-positive disease. [a]There is no absolute age limit. Rather, treatment depends on the disease, the presence of comorbidities, the patient's life expectancy, and patient preferences. Treatment should be individualized for patients >70 years of age. [b]Neoadjuvant therapy is recommended in HER2-positive stage II and III patients. Trastuzumab and pertuzumab are recommended in neoadjuvant therapy. The St Gallen panel did not support dual HER2 blockade with pertuzumab or lapatinib in the postoperative adjuvant treatment. According to the APHINITY study, which published the early results, adjuvant trastuzumab + pertuzumab treatment prolonged disease-free survival in HER2-positive patients. This benefit was particularly evident in high-risk patients who were hormone receptor negative and node positive. According to a randomized controlled trial, 1-year neratinib use after 1-year administration of trastuzumab reduced the recurrence rate. This benefit was especially evident in ER-positive, Her-2-positive disease. However, diarrhea was an important adverse effect. After 1 year of trastuzumab administration in hormone receptor-positive patients, 1 year of neratinib can be used. [c]In high-risk premenopausal patients, "LHRH-agonist + aromatase inhibitor" may be the preferred adjuvant endocrine therapy. In postmenopausal patients, aromatase inhibitors may be preferred over tamoxifen. [d]Chemotherapy and endocrine therapy as adjuvant therapy should be given sequentially, with endocrine therapy following chemotherapy. The available data suggest that sequential or concurrent endocrine therapy with radiation therapy is acceptable

paclitaxel (AC-T) every 3 weeks to the same regimen plus trastuzumab given for 52 weeks starting concurrently with paclitaxel (AC-TH). NCCTG N9831 randomized patients to receive 4 cycles of AC followed by weekly paclitaxel for 12 cycles with or without trastuzumab administered concurrently or sequentially with paclitaxel for 52 weeks (AC-T-H vs AC-TH). In a joint analysis that included patients similarly treated in the control (AC-T) and concomitant (AC-TH) arms of N9831 and the NSABP B-31 trials, a significant improvement in DFS (HR: 0.52, $P < 0.001$)

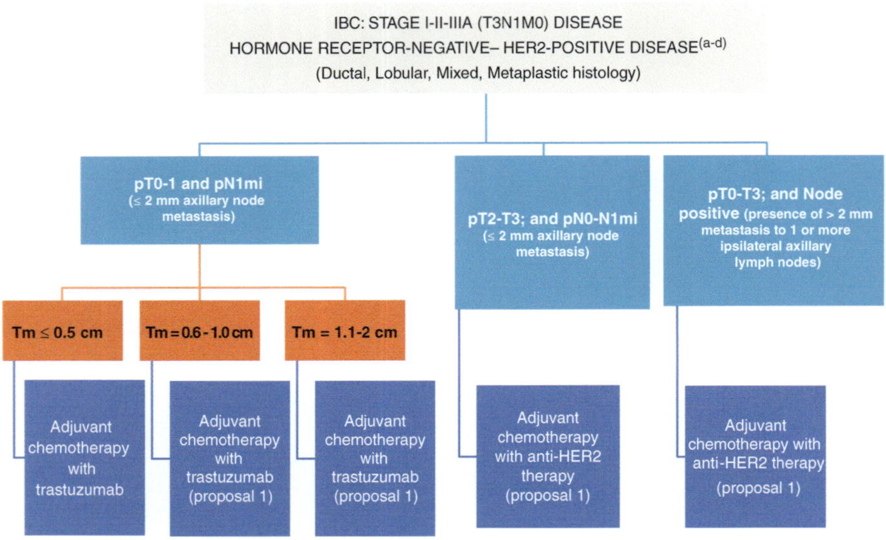

Fig. 16.4 Adjuvant systemic therapy for stage IB, II, IIIA—hormone receptor-negative and HER2-positive disease. [a]There is no absolute age limit. The choice of treatment choice depends on disease, co-morbidities, life expectancy and patient preferences. Neoadjuvant therapy is recommended in HER2-positive stage II and III patients. Trastuzumab and pertuzumab are recommended in neoadjuvant therapy. For patients >70 years of age, treatment should be individualized. [b]AC—paclitaxel and trastuzumab (± pertuzumab); TCH ± pertuzumab (pertuzumab given to patients with greater than or equal to T2 or greater than or equal to N1, HER2-positive, early-stage breast cancer) can be recommended. According to the early results of the APHINITY study, the authors concluded that pertuzumab can be considered as adjuvant therapy in patients with node-positive or locally advanced tumors. [c]In patients with HER2-positive, stage 2 disease, chemotherapy should always be provided to patients who require anti-HER2 therapy. The chemotherapy regimen for these patients should preferably contain anthracyclines and taxanes. Anti-HER2 therapy should be initiated concurrently with taxane therapy. [d]Consider adjuvant bisphosphonate therapy in post-menopausal (natural or induced) patients receiving adjuvant therapy

and a reduction of death by 39% (OS, HR: 0.61, $P < 0.001$) were observed with the addition of trastuzumab starting with paclitaxel versus chemotherapy only [12]. The efficacy of concurrent vs sequential administration of trastuzumab showed a trend toward improvement in DFS in the concurrent arm; however, sequential was still better than placebo ($P < 0.001$).

Sequential Chemotherapy/Trastuzumab

Another pivotal adjuvant trial also first reported at the 2005 Annual Meeting of the American Society of Clinical Oncology was the HERA trial [13], which tested adding 1 or 2 years of trastuzumab after completion of various standard adjuvant chemotherapy regimens. HERA randomly assigned 5102 patients to begin adjuvant trastuzumab versus no adjuvant trastuzumab after chemotherapy (median time from

Table 16.1 Selected clinical trials in the adjuvant setting for human epidermal growth factor receptor-2-positive breast cancer

Study name	Population included	No. of patients	Comparison	Median follow-up	DFS (5 year)	OS (5 year)	Drop LVEF
Trastuzumab							
NCCTG N9831 [12]	LN+ or high-risk LN (−)	1087 949 954	AC → T vs AC → T → H (52 weeks) vs AC → TH (H then 40 weeks more)	72 months	71.8% 80.1% 84.4%	88.4% 89.7% 91.9%	0% 7% 3.6%
HERA [13]	LN+ or high-risk LN (−)	1552 1553 1697	Std QT → H (52 weeks) vs Std QT → H (40 weeks) vs Std QT → Observation	96 months	75.9% 76.5% 70.0%	86.9% 88.7% 84.5%	7.2% 4.1% 0.9%
BCIRG006 [15]	LN+ or high-risk LN (−)	1073 1074 1075	AC → Docetaxel vs AC → Docetaxel + H vs TCH	65 months	75% 84% 81%	87% 92% 91%	11.2% 18.6% 9.4%
PACS04 [16]	LN+	260 268	FE100C or ED75 → Obser vs FE100C or ED75 → H	62 months	77.9% 80.9%	96% 95%	14.2% 35.4%
FINHER [17]	LN+ or high-risk LN (−)	58 58 54 61	Docetaxel → FEC vs Vinorelbine → FEC vs Docetaxel + H → FEC vs Vinorelbine + H → FEC	62 months	74.1% 72% 92.5% 75.2%	82% 82.8% 94.4% 88.4%	10.5% (QT only) 6.8% (QT + H)
PHARE [18]	HER2+ early breast cancer	1690 1690	Std QT → H (26 weeks) vs Std QT → H (52 weeks)	42.5 months	91.1% 93.8%	96.1% 94.5%	5.7% (both) 1.9% (both)
Lapatinib							
TEACH [19]	Stage I–III H naive	1230 1260	Std QT → L (52 weeks) Std QT → Observation	47.4 months	87% 83%	94% 94%	3% 3%
ALTTO [20]	Stage I–III H naive	8381	Trastuzumab vs Trastuzumab → Lapatinib vs Trastuzumab + Lapatinib	53 months	86% 87% 88%	94% 95% 95%	3% 3% 3%

Abbreviations: *LN* lymph nodes, *AC → T* adriamycin cyclophosphamide paclitaxel, *FEC* 5-FU epirubicin cyclophosphamide, *ED* epirubicin docetaxel, *Std QT* standard chemotherapy, *OS* overall survival, *DFS* disease-free survival, *LVEF* left ventricular ejection fraction

diagnosis, 8 months). Patients with HER2-positive disease were eligible if node-positive or node-negative with tumor >1 cm (T1c). At a median follow-up of 4 years, one year of adjuvant trastuzumab led to a 24% reduction in recurrence (HR: 0.76, P < 0.0001). However, partly due to the significant crossover (65%) from the observation arm to trastuzumab after the first results were released, the OS benefit from trastuzumab in HERA became apparent when evaluated after 4 years (HR: 0.85, P = 0.11) [14]. A recent update after a median follow-up of 8 years confirmed the DFS (HR: 0.76, P < 0.0001) and OS benefit (HR: 0.76, P = 0.0005) from one year of trastuzumab [13]. However, there was no incremental benefit from a longer duration of trastuzumab (2 years), and more cardiac events were observed.

Cardiotoxicity is the most important adverse effect of treatment with trastuzumab and is worsened when combined with anthracyclines. Therefore, there has been a special interest in studying anthracycline-free regimens to minimize the cardiotoxicity risk. The BCIRG 006 [15] study was designed to provide information on this issue. Patients received AC followed by docetaxel (AC → T), AC followed by docetaxel with 1 year of trastuzumab (AC → TH), or docetaxel plus carboplatin and trastuzumab followed by trastuzumab to complete 1 year of therapy (TCH). After 65 months of follow-up, DFS was significantly improved with the addition of trastuzumab to chemotherapy (AC → T: 75%, AC → TH: 84%, and TCH 81%; HR for AC-TH was 0.64 (P < 0.001) and for TCH was 0.75 (P = 0.04) with a significant improvement in OS (AC → T: 87% vs AC → TH: 92%; HR: 0.63, P < 0.001), and TCH 91% (HR: 0.77, P = 0.038). However, despite the apparent numerical advantage of AC → TH over TCH, the study was not designed to directly compare these two arms. To confirm that one regimen is better than the other, further evidence is required. Additionally, the incidence of cardiac toxicity was five times greater with ACTH (2%) compared with TCH (0.4%). Reductions in LVEF of greater than 10% from basal measurements were more frequently associated with AC → TH than with TCH (18.6 vs 9.4%; P < 0.001). In addition, the rate of symptomatic congestive heart failure favored treatment with TCH (P < 0.001).

The only trial that did not show a survival benefit from adjuvant trastuzumab was FNCLCC-PACS-04 [16]. A total of 3010 patients with early-stage breast cancer were randomly assigned to adjuvant treatment with anthracycline-based chemotherapy with or without docetaxel. Patients with HER-2 over-amplified tumors (n = 528) were subsequently randomized to receive trastuzumab sequentially every 3 weeks. The primary endpoint was DFS. Treatment with trastuzumab resulted in a nonsignificant 14% reduction in the risk of relapse (P = 0.41), and there was no difference in OS. However, 10% of the patients assigned to trastuzumab were never treated, and 25% of patients discontinued before the 16th cycle. In addition, sequential use seemed to be inferior to concurrent use of trastuzumab and chemotherapy.

Shorter Duration of Trastuzumab

The duration of adjuvant treatment in HER2-positive breast cancer is a current topic of discussion. Based on the previously analyzed HERA trial, 2 years of treatment with trastuzumab is not superior to 1 year. There is a special interest in investigating whether treatment duration could be shortened due to concerns about cardiotoxicity. In the early 2000s, the Finland Herceptin (FinHER) trial [17] aimed to determine the role of vinorelbine compared to docetaxel in the adjuvant setting in patients with node-positive and high-risk node-negative breast cancer and tested a shorter course of trastuzumab. A total of 1010 patients were randomized to treatment with vinorelbine or docetaxel for 3 cycles followed by three cycles of 5-FU, epirubicin and cyclophosphamide. A group of 232 patients with HER-2-amplified tumors were again randomized to receive nine weekly cycles of trastuzumab concurrently with docetaxel or vinorelbine. The primary endpoint was distant DFS, and with a median follow-up of 62 months, it favored treatment with docetaxel over vinorelbine ($P = 0.010$). OS also tended to be better in patients treated with docetaxel compared to vinorelbine (39 vs 55 deaths, respectively; $P = 0.086$). In HER-2-positive patients, the trastuzumab arms had favorable recurrence-free survival irrespective of the chemotherapy regimen (80% vs 73%; $P = 0.12$). This benefit was maintained when adjusted for nodal involvement and in patients treated with docetaxel over vinorelbine. The main limitation of this trial is the small number of patients with HER-2-positive tumors that were included, which reduced the power of the study to detect a statistically significant benefit with trastuzumab. In addition, even though the results suggested a benefit in patients treated with trastuzumab in combination with chemotherapy, the short course of treatment might have underestimated the real efficacy of the drug in this population.

The PHARE trial [18] is a noninferiority study designed to evaluate adjuvant treatment length with trastuzumab for 6 months compared to 1 year. A total of 1691 patients were treated with trastuzumab for 12 months and 1693 for 6 months after receiving at least 4 cycles of adjuvant chemotherapy. Patients were stratified according to sequential or concurrent treatment and estrogen-receptor (ER) status. The primary endpoint was DFS, and with a median follow-up of 42.5 months, the 2-year DFS was 93.8% for the 12-month group and 91.1% for the 6-month group (HR: 1.28; 95% CI: 1.05–1.56), indicating that 6 months of treatment did not reach the noninferiority criteria. However, cardiac events were more common in the 12-month treatment arm (5.7% vs 1.9%; $P < 0.001$), and further analysis is still required.

FinHER investigators are now comparing 9 weeks of trastuzumab plus docetaxel and FEC with the same regimen followed by 1 year of trastuzumab therapy in the SOLD study (NCT00593697). SHORT-HER (NCT00629278) is testing 9 weeks versus 12 months of trastuzumab. Two other studies in progress are testing 6 versus 12 months of trastuzumab, including PERSEPHONE (NCT00712140) and a trial by the Hellenic Oncology Research Group (NCT00615602). On the basis of current available evidence, 12 months of adjuvant treatment with trastuzumab remains the standard of care.

Lapatinib

Lapatinib is currently approved for metastatic disease, but its use has also been evaluated in the adjuvant setting due to its oral bioavailability. The TEACH trial [19] studied the efficacy of lapatinib in trastuzumab-naïve patients as adjuvant treatment. A total of 3147 patients were randomized to treatment with lapatinib or placebo for 12 months or until progression. DFS was non-significantly prolonged in patients treated with lapatinib (87% vs 83%; P = 0.09). In patients with centrally confirmed HER-2 status, the HR was 0.92 (P = 0.94). In the ALTTO trial (Adjuvant Lapatinib and/or Trastuzumab Treatment Optimisation) [20], the investigators hypothesized that in the adjuvant setting, two HER2-targeted agents would be superior to trastuzumab alone in preventing breast cancer recurrences. It was the largest-ever adjuvant clinical trial in HER2-positive breast cancer, involving 8381 women from 946 centers in 44 countries. Patients were randomly assigned to 1 year of adjuvant therapy with trastuzumab (T), lapatinib (L), their sequence (T → L), or their combination (L + T). In 2011, due to futility to demonstrate noninferiority of L versus T, the L arm was closed, and patients free of disease were offered adjuvant T. The primary endpoint was disease-free survival (DFS), with 850 events required for 80% power to detect a hazard ratio (HR) of 0.8 for L + T versus T. At a median follow-up of 4.5 years, dual targeting—either concurrently or sequentially—was associated with slight numerical reductions in disease recurrences, but the differences were not statistically significant vs trastuzumab alone. The disease-free survival rates at 4 years were 86% with trastuzumab, 88% with concurrent HER2-directed treatment, and 87% in the sequential T arm (555 DFS events; HR: 0.84; 97.5% CI: 0.70–1.02; P = 0.048). Median overall survival rates were 94%, 95%, and 95%, respectively (HR: 0.96; 97.5% CI: 0.80–1.15; P = 0.61). Updated 10-year results from the phase III ALTTO trial presented at the ASCO 2017 annual meeting showed a stronger benefit of the dual HER2 agents in patients with ER-negative breast cancer. The HRs for this updated analysis were similar to those from the primary analysis, and the event rate remains lower than anticipated (705 vs 850 planned) [21]. This analysis suggests that HER2+/ER− tumors may have a different biology than HER2+/ER+ and may benefit more from dual HER2 blockade. Lapatinib was also associated with significant increases in adverse events—diarrhea, skin rash or erythema, and hepatobiliary problems. In conclusion, lapatinib either as a single agent or in combination with trastuzumab seems to be quite ineffective and more toxic in the adjuvant setting.

Adjuvant Therapy for Tumors Smaller than 1 cm

Data on the role of trastuzumab in small node-negative tumors remain scarce. Retrospective institutional series from MD Anderson Cancer Center (MDACC) [22] and Milan [23] suggest that small HER2-positive tumors prognostically have a poor long-term outcome compared to their HER2-negative counterparts. Subgroup analyses from several randomized trials have shown a benefit of adjuvant trastuzumab irrespective of tumor size [24], though its actual absolute benefit in small stage 1 tumors (such as those with T1a up to 0.5 cm disease) remains unknown. A large, retrospective European study [25] compared the outcomes of patients with T1a/b node-negative tumors who either received adjuvant trastuzumab-based chemotherapy or did not and demonstrated a statistically significant 2–3% improvement in recurrence-free survival in the trastuzumab arm after a multivariate analysis. Hormone receptor (HR) status was also notable, as larger differences were seen in patients with high-risk features such as HR-negative or positive lymphatic vascular invasion. Therefore, it stands to reason that we could treat these tumors with adjuvant trastuzumab, especially if they are T1b or have other poor risk features.

A single-arm multicenter trial [26] included breast cancer patients with node-negative tumors up to 3 cm. Patients received weekly treatment with paclitaxel and trastuzumab for 12 weeks, followed by 9 months of trastuzumab monotherapy. The primary endpoint was survival free from invasive disease. The 3-year rate of survival free from invasive disease was 98.7% (95% CI: 97.6–99.8). The results suggest a low risk of cancer recurrence (less than 2% at 3 years) with a regimen in which the rate of serious toxic effects was low (with an incidence of heart failure that was only 0.5%). At the ASCO 2017 annual meeting, an updated analysis with 7-year DFS was provided [27]. The 7-year DFS was 93.3% (95% CI: 90.4–96.2); 7-year DFS was 94.6% for ER+ pts (95% CI: 91.8–97.5) and 90.7% for ER− pts (95% CI: 84.6–97.2). Moreover, 7-year recurrence-free interval (RFI) was 97.5% (95% CI: 95.9–99.1); 7-year breast cancer-specific survival (BCSS) was 98.6% (95% CI: 97.0–100); and 7-year OS was 95.0% (95% CI: 92.4–97.7). These data suggest that TH as adjuvant therapy for node-negative HER2+ breast cancer was associated with few recurrences and only 4 distant recurrences with longer follow-up. In the absence of randomized data, this regimen might become an option for patients with small node-negative HER2-positive disease in clinical scenarios where there is concern about potential toxicity from established regimens.

Ongoing Adjuvant Trials

Several drugs are under intensive study for use in the adjuvant therapy of HER2-positive breast cancer: trastuzumab, pertuzumab (Perjeta), ado-trastuzumab emtansine (formerly known as T-DM1 [Kadcyla]), and the investigational tyrosine kinase inhibitor neratinib (Table 16.2).

The BETH trial is evaluating the blockade of both the HER2 and vascular endothelial growth factor (VEGF) pathways by combining trastuzumab with the anti-VEGF monoclonal antibody bevacizumab, based on preclinical data showing a correlation between HER2 and VEGF expression [28, 29]. In the BETH trial [30], more than 3000 patients were treated with docetaxel plus carboplatin (TC) with trastuzumab versus TC with trastuzumab and bevacizumab, and targeted therapy was given for one year in both arms. The researchers found that after a median of 38 months of follow-up, DFS was 92% for both arms of the TCH cohort. In addition, the results of the trial were negative for any benefit of adding bevacizumab to adjuvant therapy for HER2-positive breast cancer. This lack of benefit may have occurred because 92% of the patients in the TCH control arm remained disease-free after a median follow-up of 38 months. This trial also demonstrated that it is not necessary to include an anthracycline as part of the treatment regimen, even for large tumors or node-positive disease.

Table 16.2 Ongoing adjuvant phase III trials

Study name	Estimated sample size	Study design	Primary endpoint	Estimated primary completion date[a]
BETH[b] [30]	3509	Trastuzumab + carboplatin + docetaxel → trastuzumab vs Bevacizumab + trastuzumab + docetaxel + carboplatin → trastuzumab + bevacizumab	IDFS	March 2016
APHINITY [33]	4800	Pertuzumab + trastuzumab + CT[c] Placebo + trastuzumab + CT[c]	IDFS	November 2023
KATHERINE[d] [34]	1484	Ado-trastuzumab emtansine	IDFS	March 2023
Neratinib [35]	2821	Trastuzumab containing adjuvant CT → trastuzumab vs neratinib for 12 months	IDFS	November 2016

Abbreviations: *IDFS* invasive disease-free survival, *CT* chemotherapy
[a]Date is defined as final data collection date for primary outcome measure
[b]Included patients with node-positive or high-risk node-negative HER2-positive breast cancer
[c]Chemotherapy can be either non-anthracycline-based or anthracycline-based.
[d]Patients must be HER2-positive with residual tumor in the breast or axillary lymph nodes following preoperative therapy

Data from metastatic trials of pertuzumab [31] and ado-trastuzumab emtansine [32] have now led to ongoing adjuvant trials, one of which is the APHINITY trial (NCT01358877), which compares standard chemotherapy (non-anthracycline or anthracycline-based) plus trastuzumab with or without pertuzumab. The results of the APHINITY trial were presented at the ASCO 2017 Annual meeting [33]. In this phase III clinical trial of 4805 women with HER2-positive breast cancer, the addition of pertuzumab to trastuzumab reduced the chance of developing invasive breast cancer by 19% compared to trastuzumab alone. At a median follow-up of almost 4 years, 171 patients (7.1%) in the pertuzumab group had developed invasive breast cancer, compared to 210 patients (8.7%) in the placebo group. At 3 years, an estimated 94.1% of patients in the pertuzumab group were free of invasive breast cancer, compared to 93.2% of patients in the placebo group. The rates of serious side effects were low and similar in both groups—heart failure or heart-related death occurred in 0.7% of patients in the pertuzumab group and 0.3% of patients in the placebo group. Severe diarrhea was more common with pertuzumab, occurring in 9.8% of patients compared to 3.7% of those who received placebo. The results of APHINITY trial led to full FDA approval. Based on the phase III APHINITY data, ASCO updated their recommendations in 2018 stating that 1 year of pertuzumab may be offered in addition to trastuzumab and combination chemotherapy for patients with high-risk, early-stage breast cancer, such as those with node-positive disease. 2018 ASCO updated guidelines stressed that APHINITY data showed no clinically meaningful benefit among patients with node-negative breast cancer and the first planned interim analysis did not show an OS benefit. Importantly, there are no data to guide the duration of pertuzumab treatment in patients who received neoadjuvant pertuzumab and achieved a pathologic complete response.

The KATHERINE trial (NCT01772472) [34] is comparing 14 cycles of ado-trastuzumab emtansine versus 14 cycles of trastuzumab in patients with HER2-positive disease and less than a pathologic complete response (pCR) after preoperative therapy with a trastuzumab-based regimen. Fifty-percent of planned enrollment is completed. The primary endpoint of the study is DFS.

Neratinib is an irreversible pan-HER tyrosine kinase inhibitor with clinical efficacy in trastuzumab pre-treated HER2-positive (HER2+) metastatic breast cancer. The ExteNET study examined sequential therapy with 1 year of trastuzumab followed by 1 year of neratinib in stage 2–3c Her2+ breast cancer patients who had received the last dose of trastuzumab within the last 1 year before enrollment in the clinical trial [35]. In this study, eligible women with stage 1–3c (modified to stage 2–3c in February 2010) operable breast cancer who had completed neoadjuvant and adjuvant chemotherapy plus trastuzumab with no evidence of disease recurrence or metastatic disease at study entry were randomly assigned according to hormone receptor status (ER-positive vs ER-negative), nodal status (0 vs 1–3 vs or ≥4 positive nodes), and trastuzumab adjuvant regimen (given sequentially vs concurrently with chemotherapy), followed by 1 year of oral neratinib 240 mg/day or matching placebo. After a median follow-up of 5.2 years (IQR 2.1–5.3), patients in the neratinib group had significantly fewer invasive DFS events than those in the placebo group (116 vs 163 events; stratified hazard ratio 0.73, 95% CI: 0.57–0.92, P = 0.0083). Five-year invasive disease-free survival was 90.2% (95% CI: 88.3–91.8) in the neratinib group and 87.7% (85.7–89.4) in the placebo group. Without diarrhea prophylaxis, the most common grade 3–4 adverse events in the neratinib group compared with the placebo group were diarrhea (561 [40%] grade 3 and one [<1%] grade 4 with neratinib vs 23 [2%] grade 3 with placebo), vomiting (grade 3: 47 [3%] vs five [<1%]), and nausea (grade 3: 26 [2%] vs two [<1%]). Treatment-emergent serious adverse events occurred in 103 (7%) women in the neratinib group and 85 (6%) women in the placebo group. No evidence of increased risk of long-term toxicity or long-term adverse consequences of neratinib-associated diarrhea were identified with neratinib compared with placebo. This study led to FDA approval of 1 year of extended adjuvant therapy with neratinib on July 17, 2017, to follow adjuvant trastuzumab-based therapy. ASCO 2018 guidelines reported their recommendations about neratinib use in patients with HER2-positive early breast cancer. The expert panel emphasized that the observed benefit from neratinib was higher in hormone receptor-positive and node-positive patients, and no OS advantage has been observed thus far. Patients who began neratinib within 1 year of trastuzumab completion appeared to derive the greatest benefit. Currently there are no reported data on the incremental benefit offered by neratinib in patients who completed up to a year of pertuzumab in the neoadjuvant or adjuvant setting.

Neoadjuvant Setting

In the last decade, researchers have modernized trial design by using pCR as an endpoint, since pCR correlates with long-term outcome and is quicker than waiting,

Table 16.3 Selected clinical trials in the neoadjuvant setting for HER-2-positive breast cancer

Study name	Neoadjuvant chemotherapy	No. of patients	pCR%	Comments
Trastuzumab				
NOAH trial [36]	A + T → T → CMF vs A + T → T → CMF + H	117 HER2+ vs 118 HER2+	22% vs 43%	Not originally designed to test the efficacy of neoadjuvant trastuzumab use
Z1041 trial [37]	FEC → TH vs T + H → FEC + H	138 vs 142	56.5% vs 54.2%	Concurrent use of trastuzumab with anthracyclines is not better
HannaH trial [38]	Doc + H (SQ) → FEC + H vs Doc + H (IV) → FEC + H	260 vs 263	45.4% vs 40.7%	Trastuzumab can be administered subcutaneously
Lapatinib (L) ± H				
GeparQuinto trial [39]	ECH → TH vs ECL → TL	309 vs 311	30.3% vs 22.7%	Lapatinib is less effective than trastuzumab
NeoALTTO trial [40]	TH vs TL vs THL	149 vs 154 vs 152	29.5% vs 24.7% vs 51.3%	Suggested that combination trastuzumab and lapatinib could be quite effective
NSABP B-41 trial [41]	AC → TH vs AC → TL vs AC → THL	181 vs 174 vs 174	52.5% vs 53.2% vs 62%	Trastuzumab and lapatinib no better. All patients received anthracyclines
Pertuzumab				
NeoSphere trial [42]	Do + H vs Do + P + H vs Do + P vs P+H	107 vs 107 vs 107 vs 96	29% vs 45.8% vs 24% vs 16.8%	Combination P + H results in better pCR and improved survival rates
TRYPHAENA trial [43]	FEC + HP → Do + HP vs FEC → Do + HP vs TCH + P	223 patients in total	56% vs 57% vs 64%	TCH+P is an active combination, with left ventricular dysfunction occurring in 4% of patients

Abbreviations: *T* paclitaxel, *H* herceptin (trastuzumab), *L* lapatinib, *F* 5-FU, *E* epirubicin, *C* cyclophosphamide, *A* adriamycin, *M* methotrexate, *Do* docetaxel, *TC* docetaxel-cyclophosphamide

possibly for years, for data on recurrence or death. Consequently, researchers have examined the impact of HER2-targeted agents on pCR in the neoadjuvant setting (Table 16.3).

The results of the NOAH trial, a randomized phase III study, increased enthusiasm for this approach [36]. The study was originally designed to compare neoadjuvant chemotherapy plus trastuzumab followed by 1-year trastuzumab to neoadjuvant chemotherapy alone in patients with locally advanced or inflammatory HER-2 positive tumors. Among the 238 patients who were originally randomized to neoadjuvant treatment with or without trastuzumab, the addition of anti-HER-2 therapy improved pCR from 22% to 43% ($P < 0.001$). Trastuzumab also resulted in a 40% reduction of the risk of recurrence, progression or death compared to chemotherapy alone.

The value of overlapping anthracycline with trastuzumab in the neoadjuvant setting was explored in the American Z1041 trial [37], which randomized 282 women with HER-2-positive and ≥2-cm tumors to receive trastuzumab and paclitaxel concurrently with of after FEC-75. There was no difference in pCR for sequential versus overlapping anthracycline and trastuzumab (54% and 56%), but the concurrent use of anthracyclines and trastuzumab resulted in a greater drop in the cardiac ejection fraction (2.9% vs 0.8% at 12 weeks, respectively). Finally, similar rates of pCR were described in patients treated with chemotherapy and trastuzumab in the HannaH trial (41% and 45% for intravenous vs subcutaneous trastuzumab, respectively) [38]. A slightly higher incidence of serious AEs (SAEs), mainly due to infections, was reported with subcutaneous treatment; however, the differences were small and often based on rare events, with no observable pattern across reported events. An early analysis of DFS showed rates of 95% in both groups 1 year post-randomization.

In an attempt to improve pCR, some researchers have begun exploring the use of other anti-HER2 blockers alone or in combination with trastuzumab in the neoadjuvant setting. In the German GeparQuinto study [39], 620 patients received four cycles of epirubicin and cyclophosphamide (EC) followed by docetaxel and were randomized to either trastuzumab or lapatinib. All patients received standard-of-care trastuzumab for 1 year after surgical resection. The primary outcome was pCR, and trastuzumab yielded approximately 7% more complete responses than lapatinib (30.3% vs 22.7%; $P = 0.04$). Given these results and the significant number of adverse events described in this study, it is unlikely that lapatinib could replace trastuzumab in the neoadjuvant setting; dual HER-2 inhibition appears to be a better option.

In four trials examining combinations of trastuzumab with lapatinib or pertuzumab—including NeoALTTO (NCT00553358) and Neo-Sphere (NCT00545688)—dual blockade resulted in a higher pCR rate. NeoALTTO, an international, randomized, phase III study, compared the use of single-agent lapatinib, trastuzumab or the combination of both in addition to paclitaxel for neoadjuvant treatment [40]. Interestingly, the combination arm showed a remarkable improvement in pCR that nearly duplicated that in the two single-agent anti-HER2 arms (51% vs 29.5% trastuzumab vs 24.7% lapatinib; $P < 0.001$). As expected, the addition of lapatinib resulted in worse side effects, mainly related to diarrhea and rash. However, in contrast to NeoALTTO, the NSABP B-41 study showed no significant difference between the combination of trastuzumab and lapatinib and either drug used as a single agent [41]. Two issues warrant further discussion. First, even though the populations included in both trials were similar, the chemotherapy regimens were not. In the NSABP study, all patients received four cycles of AC and then were randomized to paclitaxel plus trastuzumab, lapatinib or both. Second, the rates of pCR in all three arms were unusually high (62% for the combination, 53% for trastuzumab and 52.5% for lapatinib).

The FDA has recently granted accelerated approval to pertuzumab for use before surgery when combined with trastuzumab and chemotherapy. This controversial decision was based on the results of two phase II clinical trials. The NeoSphere trial [42] was a multicenter, open-label, randomized phase II study in which 417 patients were randomized to one of four possible arms: pertuzumab (P) + trastuzumab (T) + docetaxel (Do); T + Do; P + Do or P + T alone. All eligible patients then underwent surgical resection followed by adjuvant FEC and 1 year of trastuzumab. The three-drug arm (P + T + Do) yielded the maximal rate of pCR (46%) and was significantly different from T + Do (29%; P = 0.014). Pertuzumab + docetaxel resulted in a 24% pCR, and the chemotherapy-free arm had a 17% pCR. In the T + Do and P + T + D0 arms, respectively, the 3-year survival rates were 85% and 92% for DFS (HR: 0.60, 95% CI: 0.28–1.27) and 86% and 90% for PFS (HR: 0.69, 95% CI: 0.34–1.40). Importantly, the addition of pertuzumab did not produce any significant drop in cardiac function (4–5% EF drop across all groups). An additional neoadjuvant phase II trial (TRYPHAENA) [43] was conducted in 225 patients with HER2-positive, locally advanced, operable, or inflammatory breast cancer and was designed primarily to assess the cardiac safety of pertuzumab in different neoadjuvant regimens. Patients were randomly allocated to receive one of three neoadjuvant regimens prior to surgery: three cycles of FEC followed by three cycles of docetaxel, all in combination with pertuzumab and trastuzumab (A); three cycles of FEC alone followed by three cycles of docetaxel and trastuzumab in combination with pertuzumab (B); or six cycles of docetaxel, carboplatin, and trastuzumab (TCH) in combination with pertuzumab (C). Following surgery, all patients received trastuzumab intravenously every 3 weeks to complete 1 year of therapy. The results suggest that all three arms achieved >55% pCR. During post-treatment follow-up, 2.8%, 4.0% and 5.4% patients in groups A-C had any-grade left ventricular systolic dysfunction; 11.1%, 16.0% and 11.8% patients experienced left ventricular ejection fraction declines ≥10% from baseline to <50. Currently, there are insufficient cardiac safety data to recommend concomitant administration of an anthracycline with pertuzumab and trastuzumab.

The I-SPY 2 trial (NCT01042379) is an ongoing multidrug, multicenter neoadjuvant phase II breast cancer trial to determine whether adding experimental agents to standard neoadjuvant medications increases the probability of pCR compared to standard neoadjuvant chemotherapy for each biomarker signature established at trial entry. A variety of agents are being investigated, both in combination with trastuzumab and alone, including T-DM1, pertuzumab, neratinib, pembrolizumab as well as AKT inhibitors. The findings reported at the San Antonio Breast Cancer Symposium included positive results for the PARP inhibitor veliparib, the first drug to complete testing in the trial. Although the estimated pCR rate for patients with triple-negative breast cancer was 52% after receipt of chemotherapy plus veliparib/carboplatin and standard paclitaxel followed by anthracycline-based chemotherapy vs 26% with control chemotherapy alone, in "signatures" other than triple-negative breast cancer, the combination was predicted to be far less successful. For the hormone receptor-positive/HER2-negative group, the estimated pathologic complete response rate was 14% for the combination and 19% for controls. The pCR rates for HER2+ group have not been reported yet.

The GeparSixto [44] study evaluated the benefit of adding carboplatin to paclitaxel plus pegylated liposomal doxorubicin given as a weekly regimen for 18 weeks to 595 patients. Added to this backbone were three targeted agents corresponding to tumor subtype: trastuzumab and lapatinib for HER2-positive patients and bevacizumab (Avastin) for triple-negative patients. Investigators compared the rates of pCR between paclitaxel/doxorubicin and paclitaxel/doxorubicin/carboplatin. The addition of carboplatin significantly increased the pathologic complete response rate, which was 37.2% in the control arm and 46.7% in the carboplatin arm ($P < 0.2$) for patients with triple-negative breast cancer. However, the HER2-positive subgroup did not benefit. Among HER2-positive patients, pathologic complete responses were achieved by 36.8% and 32.8% in the control arm and the carboplatin arm, respectively ($P = 0.581$; test for interaction $P = 0.015$).

Optimizing Therapy for Hormone Receptor–Coexpressing Disease

At least half of HER2-positive breast cancer coexpresses one or both hormone receptors, and this coexpression may serve as a pathway for resistance to HER2-targeted therapy. However, HER2-targeted therapy is not necessarily inactive in hormone receptor-positive breast cancer. In fact, analyses from the AC/trastuzumab and AC/T arms of the BCIRG-00651 and B-3153 trials have shown that the HRs for DFS are very similar for hormone receptor-positive (HR, 0.65 and 0.61 for BCIRG-006 and B-31, respectively) and hormone receptor-negative (HR, 0.64 and 0.62 for BCIRG-006 and B-31, respectively) disease. This also holds true for OS. Subset analysis of the HERA study at 11 years of follow-up also demonstrated long-term trastuzumab benefit for all patients, regardless of HR status [45]. Although trastuzumab imparts DFS and OS benefit, regardless of hormone receptor status, the presence of ER may indicate more indolent, luminal-like tumor behavior. For example, Kaplan–Meier curves from HERA indicate that although the long-term risk of recurrence is similar in hormone receptor-positive and hormone receptor-negative subtypes, patients with hormone receptor-negative disease have earlier recurrences, which is consistent with a more aggressive disease biology. Further evidence supporting the notion that disease behavior differs based on hormone receptor expression comes from neoadjuvant clinical trials, which have consistently shown that pCR rates are lower for hormone receptor-positive, HER2-positive breast cancer than for hormone receptor-negative disease [40, 41, 46, 47]. However, the longer follow-up of the NeoSphere trial indicates that patients with hormone receptor coexpression have numerically higher PFS than those with tumors lacking hormone receptors (5-year PFS for patients who achieved pCR: 90% if hormone receptor positive, 84% if hormone receptor negative; 5-year PFS for patients who did not achieve pCR: 80% if hormone receptor positive, 72% if hormone receptor negative). Thus, patients with hormone receptor-positive tumors may do better in the long run. Intriguing biomarker analyses from HERA suggest that although ER-positive tumors with a high level of HER2 amplification (by FISH ratio) derive clear benefit from trastuzumab, those with a low level of HER2 amplification may not receive benefit from trastuzumab-based therapy [48].

Several clinical trials aiming to evaluate co-targeting of hormone receptor and HER2 have been conducted. The first of these, TBCRC-006, evaluated 12 weeks of neoadjuvant lapatinib plus trastuzumab (with letrozole for ER-positive tumors)

[49]. pCR (breast) for HER2-positive/hormone receptor-positive tumors was 21% in this proof-of-concept study, indicating that a relatively well-tolerated chemotherapy-free regimen might be highly effective for patients if accurate biomarkers for selection can be identified.

Trastuzumab emtansine has also been evaluated in the neoadjuvant and adjuvant settings. The WGS-ADAPT study compared four cycles of T-DM1, either alone or in combination with endocrine therapy, to trastuzumab plus endocrine therapy for hormone receptor-positive, HER2-positive patients [50]. This relatively short course of T-DM1 was associated with an impressive pCR rate (breast and lymph nodes) of 41%, which was considerably higher than that achieved with trastuzumab plus endocrine therapy.

Although neither of these relatively small studies has changed the standard of care, the intriguing results should encourage the investigation of whether similar, less-toxic regimens might be beneficial for selected patient populations.

In December 2016, the results of the NSABP B-52 trial were presented. This study was designed to evaluate whether the addition of an aromatase inhibitor to standard chemotherapy plus HER2-targeted therapy (TCHP) would improve pCR rates for hormone receptor-positive/HER2-positive breast cancer and to test whether endocrine therapy is antagonistic in combination with chemotherapy [51]. Although the addition of endocrine therapy to TCHP did not lead to a statistically notable improvement in pCR (41% for TCHP vs. 46% for TCHP plus endocrine therapy), it did not appear to be antagonistic, leaving room for future studies to test less toxic chemotherapy regimens concurrently with hormone therapy approaches.

In summary, in just over a decade, the management of early-stage HER2-positive breast cancer has changed drastically because of the development of highly effective biologically targeted therapies. The therapeutic options available to the patient in both the neoadjuvant and adjuvant settings are now nearly countless, making the choice of optimal therapy somewhat difficult at times. Our pursuit to provide patients with the safest and most effective therapies for their particular disease requires us to design carefully selected clinical trials with attention toward the discovery of molecular drivers of disease biology and markers of response to therapy.

Resistance to Trastuzumab and Lapatinib

Although HER2-targeted therapies have had a significant impact on patient outcomes, resistance to these agents is common. In clinical trials, 74% of patients with HER2+ metastatic breast cancer did not have a tumor response to first-line trastuzumab monotherapy [52], and 50% did not respond to trastuzumab in combination with chemotherapy [6]. These examples illustrate the problem that inherent (de novo) resistance to HER2-targeted agents poses for the effective treatment of HER2+ BC. Moreover, only approximately one quarter of patients with HER2+ metastatic breast cancer who were previously treated with trastuzumab achieved a response with lapatinib plus capecitabine [8]. These limitations have led to efforts to better understand the molecular determinants of resistance to these agents to improve the selection of patients who are most likely to benefit from specific therapies and to develop new agents that can overcome resistance. Here, we discuss new strategies that are mostly being investigated in metastatic breast cancer, although some are being studied in adjuvant and neoadjuvant settings.

Afatinib

Afatinib is an oral small molecule that irreversibly inhibits HER-1, 2 and 4 [53]. In a phase II study, 4 of 35 patients with trastuzumab-resistant metastatic breast cancer showed partial responses [53]. Adverse events included diarrhea and rash. However, the recently published LUX-Breast 1 [54] trial was a negative trial for afatinib. This was a phase III study comparing vinorelbine plus trastuzumab or afatinib plus vinorelbine for metastatic patients who progressed to one chemotherapy regimen containing trastuzumab. Recruitment was stopped on April 26, 2013, after a benefit-risk assessment by the independent data monitoring committee was unfavorable for the afatinib group. Patients on afatinib plus vinorelbine had to switch to trastuzumab plus vinorelbine.

Neratinib

Neratinib is also an oral, irreversible inhibitor of HER-1,-2 and -4 [55]. A phase II trial evaluated neratinib in 136 HER-2-positive patients [55]. The median PFS was 22.3 and 39.6 weeks and the overall response rate (ORR) was 24% and 56% in pretreated and trastuzumab-naïve patients, respectively. Diarrhea was the most common grade 3/4 adverse effect. Another phase I–II trial combined neratinib plus trastuzumab in 45 metastatic, and trastuzumab-resistant patients showed an encouraging 27% ORR [56]. Finally, a phase I–II trial evaluated neratinib plus vinorelbine in trastuzumab- or lapatinib-pretreated patients (n = 77) [57]. ORR was 41% (no prior lapatinib) and 8% (prior lapatinib). A phase III trial (ExteNET) in the adjuvant setting is ongoing (NCT00878709) (Table 16.2).

MM-111

MM-11 is a bi-specific monoclonal antibody that reversibly targets the HER-2 and -3 heterodimer. A phase I–II study is currently evaluating its efficacy as a single agent in HER-2-positive advanced breast cancer patients who have received prior trastuzumab or lapatinib therapy (clinicaltrials.gov, NCT00911898). Another phase I trial is studying MM-111 plus trastuzumab in HER2-positive, heregulin-positive, advanced and refractory breast cancer (clinicaltrials.gov, NCT01097460).

Trastuzumab Deruxtecan

Trastuzumab deruxtecan (ds-8201a), a HER2-targeting antibody-drug conjugate, demonstrated significant clinical activity in heavily pretreated patients with HER2-expressing metastatic breast cancers who previously received ado-trastuzumab emtansine (T-DM1; Kadcyla). Whereas T-DM1 is a tubulin-targeting chemotherapy, trastuzumab deruxtecan is a topoisomerase 1 inhibitor. It is highly potent, with a drug-to-antibody ratio of 7.8, compared with 3.5 for T-DM1.

In an ongoing 2-part phase I study, the ORR to trastuzumab deruxtecan in 57 evaluable patients with HER2-positive tumors was 61.4%. In the HER2-positive cohort, the ORR was 56.4% (22 of 39) among those with ER-positive disease and 75.0% (12 of 16) among those with ER-negative disease. Notably, the ORR was 62.5% among the 50 patients in this cohort who had received prior pertuzumab treatment. The disease control rate (DCR) was 94.7% overall in the HER2-positive subset: 92.3% in the ER-positive group, 100.0% in the ER-negative group, and 94.0% among those who had received prior pertuzumab. Median PFS was not reached in the ER-positive group and was 10.3 months in the ER-negative group. Median PFS was 10.3 months in the HER2-positive cohort who had received prior pertuzumab, as reported by Shanu Modi, MD, at the 2017 San Antonio Breast Cancer Symposium. The main toxicity was grade 1/2 gastrointestinal toxicity. Grade 1/2 nausea was reported by 67.9%. Grade 3 and 4 events were hematological in nature. The rates of grade 3/4 anemia were 8.7% in the HER2-positive group and 0.9% in the HER2-low group. The rates of grade 3 decreases in neutrophil count and white blood cell count were each 10.4%. Across the study, 5 patients (4.3%) had a grade 4 decrease in neutrophil count.

In August 2017, trastuzumab deruxtecan received FDA breakthrough therapy designation for the treatment of patients with HER2-positive, locally advanced, or metastatic breast cancer who have been treated with trastuzumab and pertuzumab and have disease progression after T-DM1. An ongoing pivotal phase II trial called DESTINY-Breast01 is examining the efficacy and safety of trastuzumab deruxtecan in patients with HER2-positive unresectable and/or metastatic breast cancer who are resistant or refractory to T-DM1.

HER2-Targeted Vaccines

Cancer vaccines designed to induce specific anti-HER-2 immunity are being investigated. Different strategies include protein-based vaccines, plasmid DNA-based vaccines, and vaccines that deliver HER-2 in a viral vector. HER-2 peptide-based vaccines have been tested in patients with metastatic HER-2-positive breast cancer [58]. Immunized patients developed delayed-type hypersensitivity reactions and strong CD8+ cell responses specific for HER-2 [59]. A dendritic cell-based vaccine was also tested in a small group of patients with stage IV breast cancer [60]. One patient showed a partial response, and three had stable disease for ≥12 months.

Using a different strategy, cell-based GM-CSF secreting vaccines were tested in combination with trastuzumab [61].

Other Exploratory Anti-HER-2 Blocking Strategies

Ongoing trials combining anti-HER-2 agents with drugs blocking other signaling pathways hold the promise of further improvement. An auspicious approach is the combination of anti-HER-2 therapy with insulin growth factor receptor (IGFR-1)-blocking agents. IGFR-1 inhibition has been shown to restore sensitivity to trastuzumab in animal models [62]. Another potential combination is dual blockade of HER-2 and SRC, which was recently shown to work at a central node downstream of multiple trastuzumab-resistance mechanisms [63]. Finally, HER-3 is another strong activator of PI3K/Akt signaling pathway that has been demonstrated to be up-regulated after HER-2 blockade [64]. Although still in early phases of development, Rb disruption strategies and the use of CDK-4/6 inhibitors may be clinically useful [65]. Future studies of HER2-positive patients will be challenging because of the small window to improve outcome beyond what is achievable today.

Conclusion

The current available evidence supports the use of anti-HER2 drugs as a neoadjuvant treatment, and in terms of selecting the appropriate chemotherapy regimen, a couple of important points should be emphasized. First, dual blockade of the HER-2 receptor, even without chemotherapy, results in an at least 15% pCR (NeoSphere Trial), which suggests that 1 in 6 patients may not need chemotherapy. This certainly represents an attractive option for patients who cannot tolerate more than targeted agents. Second, the addition of chemotherapy leads to a more robust effect, with values of 40–50% when trastuzumab alone is used and >50% when dual blockade is applied. Moreover, anthracyclines appear to play a significant role in HER2-positive tumors; however, the results from the NeoALTTO and TRYPHAENA trials suggest that when dual blockade is used, anthracycline toxicity might be spared. Third, in all clinical trials available, pCR is markedly diminished in tumors expressing hormone receptors in addition to HER2. Finally, there is a need for predictors of which patients will most benefit from trastuzumab-containing therapies. Few markers are known, and confusion about some markers has emerged. For instance, p95, a truncated HER2 protein that had been associated with resistance to trastuzumab, was unexpectedly linked to a stronger response to the drug when tested in the GeparQuattro study [66].

Most likely, the most important question is how reliable is pCR as a valid surrogate for DFS and OS. A meta-analysis with 12900 patients enrolled in randomized neoadjuvant trials showed the strongest correlation between pCR and event-free survival (EFS) in patients with triple-negative breast cancer (TNBC) (EFS: HR 0.24, 95% CI: 0.18–0.33; OS: 0.16, 0.11–0.25) and in those with HER2-positive, hormone-receptor-negative tumors who received trastuzumab (EFS: 0.15, 0.09–0.27; OS: 0.08, 0.03, 0.22) [47]. Based on the phase III APHINITYdata, ASCO updated their recommendations in 2018 stating that 1 year of pertuzumab may be offered in addition to trastuzumab and combination chemotherapy for patients with high-risk, early-stage breast cancer, such as those with node-positive disease. Importantly, there are no data to guide the duration of pertuzumab treatment in patients who received neoadjuvant pertuzumab and achieved a pathologic complete response [67]. Neoadjuvant treatment with anti-HER-2 agents remains a valid and approved option, especially in those patients with locally advanced, unresectable tumors. Its use in small resectable cancer is probably appropriate but must be balanced with practical considerations and the patient's own preferences.

Adjuvant/Neoadjuvant Regimens in HER2-Positive Breast Cancer

AC followed by paclitaxel + trastuzumab
Doxorubicin 60 mg/m^2 IV day 1,
Cyclophosphamide 600 mg/m^2 IV day 1,
Cycled every 21 days for 4 cycles.
Followed by:
Paclitaxel 80 mg/m^2 day 1, 1 h IV infusion weekly for 12 weeks.
With*:
Trastuzumab 8 mg/kg IV with first dose of paclitaxel
Followed by:
Trastuzumab 6 mg/kg IV every 21 days to complete 1 year of treatment.
*Evaluate left ventricular ejection fraction prior to and every 3 months during treatment.

Dose dense AC (doxorubicin/cyclophosphamide) followed by paclitaxel trastuzumab
Doxorubicin 60 mg/m^2 IV day 1,
Cyclophosphamide 600 mg/m^2 IV day 1,
Cycled every 14 days for 4 cycles, all cycles are with GCSF support.
Followed by:
Paclitaxel 175 mg/m^2 day 1, 3 h IV infusion,
Cycled every 14 days for 4 cycles, all cycles are with GCSF support.
With*:
Trastuzumab 4 mg/kg IV with first dose of paclitaxel
Followed by:
Trastuzumab 2 mg/kg IV weekly to complete 1 year of treatment.
As an alternative, trastuzumab 6 mg/kg IV every 21 days may be used following the completion of paclitaxel, and given to complete 1 year of trastuzumab treatment.

*Evaluate left ventricular ejection fraction prior to and every 3 months during treatment.

AC (doxorubicin/cyclophosphamide) followed by weekly paclitaxel + trastuzumab + pertuzumab
Doxorubicin 60 mg/m^2 IV day 1,
Cyclophosphamide 600 mg/m^2 IV day 1,
Cycled every 21 days for 4 cycles.
Followed by*:
Pertuzumab 840 mg IV day 1 followed by 420 mg IV, every 21 days to complete 1 year of treatment,
Trastuzumab 8 mg/kg day 1 followed by 6 mg/kg IV, every 21 days to complete 1 year of treatment,
Paclitaxel 80 mg /m^2 day 1, 1 h IV infusion weekly for 12 weeks.
*Evaluate left ventricular ejection fraction prior to and every 3 months during treatment.

TCH (Docetaxel + carboplatin + trastuzumab)
Docetaxel 75 mg/m^2 IV day 1,
Carboplatin AUC 6 IV day 1,
Cycled every 21 days for 6 cycles.
Trastuzumab 4 mg/kg IV week 1
Followed by*:
Trastuzumab 2 mg/kg IV weekly for 17 weeks.
Followed by:
Trastuzumab 6 mg/kg IV cycled every 21 days to complete 1 year of trastuzumab treatment.
OR
Trastuzumab 8 mg/kg IV week 1
Followed by:
Trastuzumab 6 mg/kg IV cycled every 21 days to complete 1 year of trastuzumab treatment.
*Evaluate left ventricular ejection fraction prior to and every 3 months during treatment.

TCH (Docetaxel + carboplatin + trastuzumab) + pertuzumab
Docetaxel 75 mg/m^2 IV day 1,
Carboplatin AUC 6 IV day 1,
Cycled every 21 days for 6 cycles.
AND*
Pertuzumab 840 mg IV day 1
Trastuzumab 8 mg/kg IV day 1
Followed by:
Trastuzumab 6 mg/kg IV day 1
Pertuzumab 420 mg IV day 1
Cycled every 21 days to complete 1 year of therapy.

*Evaluate left ventricular ejection fraction prior to and every 3 months during treatment.

AC followed by docetaxel + trastuzumab

Cyclophosphamide 600 mg/m^2 IV day 1,
Doxorubicin 60 mg/m^2 IV day 1,
Cycled every 21 days for 4 cycles.
Followed by:
Docetaxel 100 mg/m^2 IV day 1, all cycles are with GCSF support.
Cycled every 21 days for 4 cycles.
With*:
Trastuzumab 8 mg/kg IV week 1
Followed by:
Trastuzumab 6 mg/kg IV cycled every 21 days to complete 1 year of trastuzumab therapy.
*Evaluate left ventricular ejection fraction prior to and every 3 months during treatment.

AC followed by docetaxel + trastuzumab + pertuzumab

Cyclophosphamide 600 mg/m^2 IV day 1,
Doxorubicin 60 mg/m^2 IV day 1,
Cycled every 21 days for 4 cycles.
Followed by*:
Pertuzumab 840 mg IV day 1 follewed by 420 mg IV
Trastuzumab 8 mg/kg IV day 1 followed by 6 mg/kg IV
Docetaxel 75–100 mg/m^2 IV day 1, with GCSF support.
Cycled every 21 days for 4 cycles.
Followed by:
Trastuzumab 6 mg/kg IV
Pertuzumab 420 mg IV day 1
Cycled every 21 days to complete 1 year of trastuzumab therapy.
*Evaluate left ventricular ejection fraction prior to and every 3 months during treatment.

Docetaxel + cyclophosphamid + trastuzumab

Docetaxel 75 mg/m^2 IV day 1,
Cyclophosphamide 600 mg/m^2 IV day 1
Cycled every 21 days for 4 cycles, all cycles are with GCSF support.
With*:
Trastuzumab 8 mg/kg IV week 1
Followed by:
Trastuzumab 6 mg/kg IV cycled every 21 days to complete 1 year of trastuzumab therapy.
*Evaluate left ventricular ejection fraction prior to and every 3 months during treatment.

Paclitaxel + trastuzumab

Paclitaxel 80 mg/m^2 day 1, 1 h IV infusion weekly for 12 weeks.

With:

Trastuzumab 4 mg/kg IV with first dose of paclitaxel

Followed by:

Trastuzumab 2 mg/kg IV weekly to complete 1 year of treatment.

As an alternative trastuzumab 6 mg/kg IV every 21 days may be used following the completion of paclitaxel, and given to complete 1 year of trastuzumab treatment.

*Evaluate left ventricular ejection fraction prior to and every 3 months during treatment.

References

1. Torre LA, Bray F, Siegel RL, Ferlay J, Lortet-Tieulent J, Jemal A. Global cancer statistics, 2012. CA Cancer J Clin. 2015;65(2):87–108.
2. Perou CM, Sorlie T, Eisen MB, van de Rijn M, Jeffrey SS, Rees CA, et al. Molecular portraits of human breast tumours. Nature. 2000;406(6797):747–52.
3. Sorlie T, Perou CM, Tibshirani R, Aas T, Geisler S, Johnsen H, et al. Gene expression patterns of breast carcinomas distinguish tumor subclasses with clinical implications. Proc Natl Acad Sci U S A. 2001;98(19):10869–74.
4. Slamon DJ, Clark GM, Wong SG, Levin WJ, Ullrich A, McGuire WL. Human breast cancer: correlation of relapse and survival with amplification of the HER-2/neu oncogene. Science. 1987;235(4785):177–82.
5. Yarden Y, Sliwkowski MX. Untangling the ErbB signalling network. Nat Rev Mol Cell Biol. 2001;2(2):127–37.
6. Slamon DJ, Leyland-Jones B, Shak S, Fuchs H, Paton V, Bajamonde A, et al. Use of chemotherapy plus a monoclonal antibody against HER2 for metastatic breast cancer that overexpresses HER2. N Engl J Med. 2001;344(11):783–92.
7. Romond EH, Perez EA, Bryant J, Suman VJ, Geyer CE Jr, Davidson NE, et al. Trastuzumab plus adjuvant chemotherapy for operable HER2-positive breast cancer. N Engl J Med. 2005;353(16):1673–84.
8. Geyer CE, Forster J, Lindquist D, Chan S, Romieu CG, Pienkowski T, et al. Lapatinib plus capecitabine for HER2-positive advanced breast cancer. N Engl J Med. 2006;355(26):2733–43.
9. Ryan Q, Ibrahim A, Cohen MH, Johnson J, Ko CW, Sridhara R, et al. FDA drug approval summary: lapatinib in combination with capecitabine for previously treated metastatic breast cancer that overexpresses HER-2. Oncologist. 2008;13(10):1114–9.
10. Blumenthal GM, Scher NS, Cortazar P, Chattopadhyay S, Tang S, Song P, et al. First FDA approval of dual anti-HER2 regimen: pertuzumab in combination with trastuzumab and docetaxel for HER2-positive metastatic breast cancer. Clin Cancer Res. 2013;19(18):4911–6.
11. Wolff AC, Hammond ME, Hicks DG, Dowsett M, McShane LM, Allison KH, et al. Recommendations for human epidermal growth factor receptor 2 testing in breast cancer: American Society of Clinical Oncology/College of American Pathologists clinical practice guideline update. J Clin Oncol. 2013;31(31):3997–4013.
12. Perez EA, Romond EH, Suman VJ, Jeong JH, Davidson NE, Geyer CE Jr, et al. Four-year follow-up of trastuzumab plus adjuvant chemotherapy for operable human epidermal growth factor receptor 2-positive breast cancer: joint analysis of data from NCCTG N9831 and NSABP B-31. J Clin Oncol. 2011;29(25):3366–73.

13. Goldhirsch A, Gelber RD, Piccart-Gebhart MJ, de Azambuja E, Procter M, Suter TM, et al. 2 years versus 1 year of adjuvant trastuzumab for HER2-positive breast cancer (HERA): an open-label, randomised controlled trial. Lancet. 2013;382(9897):1021–8.
14. Gianni L, Dafni U, Gelber RD, Azambuja E, Muehlbauer S, Goldhirsch A, et al. Treatment with trastuzumab for 1 year after adjuvant chemotherapy in patients with HER2-positive early breast cancer: a 4-year follow-up of a randomised controlled trial. Lancet Oncol. 2011;12(3):236–44.
15. Slamon D, Eiermann W, Robert N, Pienkowski T, Martin M, Press M, et al. Adjuvant trastuzumab in HER2-positive breast cancer. N Engl J Med. 2011;365(14):1273–83.
16. Spielmann M, Roche H, Delozier T, Canon JL, Romieu G, Bourgeois H, et al. Trastuzumab for patients with axillary-node-positive breast cancer: results of the FNCLCC-PACS 04 trial. J Clin Oncol. 2009;27(36):6129–34.
17. Joensuu H, Kellokumpu-Lehtinen PL, Bono P, Alanko T, Kataja V, Asola R, et al. Adjuvant docetaxel or vinorelbine with or without trastuzumab for breast cancer. N Engl J Med. 2006;354(8):809–20.
18. Pivot X, Romieu G, Debled M, Pierga JY, Kerbrat P, Bachelot T, et al. 6 months versus 12 months of adjuvant trastuzumab for patients with HER2-positive early breast cancer (PHARE): a randomised phase 3 trial. Lancet Oncol. 2013;14(8):741–8.
19. Goss PE, Smith IE, O'Shaughnessy J, Ejlertsen B, Kaufmann M, Boyle F, et al. Adjuvant lapatinib for women with early-stage HER2-positive breast cancer: a randomised, controlled, phase 3 trial. Lancet Oncol. 2013;14(1):88–96.
20. Piccart-Gebhart M, Holmes E, Baselga J, de Azambuja E, Dueck AC, Viale G, et al. Adjuvant lapatinib and trastuzumab for early human epidermal growth factor receptor 2-positive breast cancer: results from the randomized phase III adjuvant lapatinib and/or trastuzumab treatment optimization trial. J Clin Oncol. 2016;34:1034.
21. Moreno-Aspiti A, et al. J Clin Oncol. 2017;35(suppl; abstr 502).
22. Gonzalez-Angulo AM, Litton JK, Broglio KR, Meric-Bernstam F, Rakkhit R, Cardoso F, et al. High risk of recurrence for patients with breast cancer who have human epidermal growth factor receptor 2-positive, node-negative tumors 1 cm or smaller. J Clin Oncol. 2009;27(34):5700–6.
23. Curigliano G, Viale G, Bagnardi V, Fumagalli L, Locatelli M, Rotmensz N, et al. Clinical relevance of HER2 overexpression/amplification in patients with small tumor size and node-negative breast cancer. J Clin Oncol. 2009;27(34):5693–9.
24. Banerjee S, Smith IE. Management of small HER2-positive breast cancers. Lancet Oncol. 2010;11(12):1193–9.
25. Rodrigues MJ, Peron J, Frenel JS, Vano YA, Wassermann J, Debled M, et al. Benefit of adjuvant trastuzumab-based chemotherapy in T1ab node-negative HER2-overexpressing breast carcinomas: a multicenter retrospective series. Ann Oncol. 2013;24(4):916–24.
26. Tolaney SM, Barry WT, Dang CT, Yardley DA, Moy B, Marcom PK, et al. Adjuvant paclitaxel and trastuzumab for node-negative, HER2-positive breast cancer. N Engl J Med. 2015;372(2):134–41.
27. Tolaney S, et al. 2017 ASCO annual meeting. J Clin Oncol. 2017(suppl; abstr 511).
28. Yen L, You XL, Al Moustafa AE, Batist G, Hynes NE, Mader S, et al. Heregulin selectively upregulates vascular endothelial growth factor secretion in cancer cells and stimulates angiogenesis. Oncogene. 2000;19(31):3460–9.
29. Epstein M, Ayala R, Tchekmedyian N, Borgstrom P, Pegram M, Slamon D. HER2-overexpressing human breast cancer xenografts exhibit increased angiogenic potential mediated by vascular endothelial growth factor (VEGF). Breast Cancer Res Treat. 2002;76:S143.
30. Slamon DJ, Swain SM, Buyse M, et al. Primary results from BETH, a phase 3 controlled study of adjuvant chemotherapy and trastuzumab ± bevacizumab in patients with HER2-positive, node-positive or high risk node-negative breast cancer. 2013 San Antonio breast cancer symposium. Abstract S1-03. Presented 11 Dec 2013.
31. Baselga J, Cortes J, Kim SB, Im SA, Hegg R, Im YH, et al. Pertuzumab plus trastuzumab plus docetaxel for metastatic breast cancer. N Engl J Med. 2012;366(2):109–19.

32. Verma S, Miles D, Gianni L, Krop IE, Welslau M, Baselga J, et al. Trastuzumab emtansine for HER2-positive advanced breast cancer. N Engl J Med. 2012;367(19):1783–91.
33. von Minckwitz G, Procter M, de Azambuja E, Zardavas D, Benyunes M, Viale G, et al. Adjuvant pertuzumab and trastuzumab in early HER2-positive breast cancer. N Engl J Med. 2017;377(2):122–31.
34. A study of trastuzumab emtansine versus trastuzumab as adjuvant therapy in patients with HER2-positive breast cancer who have residual tumor in the breast or axillary lymph nodes following preoperative therapy (KATHERINE). ClinicalTrials.gov/show/NCT01772472. U.S. National Library of Medicine. Accessed 17 Jan 2016.
35. Martin M, Holmes FA, Ejlertsen B, Delaloge S, Moy B, Iwata H, et al. Neratinib after trastuzumab-based adjuvant therapy in HER2-positive breast cancer (ExteNET): 5-year analysis of a randomized, double-blind, placebo-controlled, phase 3 trial. Lancet Oncol. 2017;18(12):1688–700.
36. Gianni L, Eiermann W, Semiglazov V, Manikhas A, Lluch A, Tjulandin S, et al. Neoadjuvant chemotherapy with trastuzumab followed by adjuvant trastuzumab versus neoadjuvant chemotherapy alone, in patients with HER2-positive locally advanced breast cancer (the NOAH trial): a randomised controlled superiority trial with a parallel HER2-negative cohort. Lancet. 2010;375(9712):377–84.
37. Buzdar AU, Suman VJ, Meric-Bernstam F, Leitch AM, Ellis MJ, Boughey JC, et al. Fluorouracil, epirubicin, and cyclophosphamide (FEC-75) followed by paclitaxel plus trastuzumab versus paclitaxel plus trastuzumab followed by FEC-75 plus trastuzumab as neoadjuvant treatment for patients with HER2-positive breast cancer (Z1041): a randomised, controlled, phase 3 trial. Lancet Oncol. 2013;14(13):1317–25.
38. Jackisch C, Kim SB, Semiglazov V, Melichar B, Pivot X, Hillenbach C, et al. Subcutaneous versus intravenous formulation of trastuzumab for HER2-positive early breast cancer: updated results from the phase III HannaH study. Ann Oncol. 2015;26(2):320–5.
39. Untch M, Loibl S, Bischoff J, Eidtmann H, Kaufmann M, Blohmer JU, et al. Lapatinib versus trastuzumab in combination with neoadjuvant anthracycline-taxane-based chemotherapy (GeparQuinto, GBG 44): a randomised phase 3 trial. Lancet Oncol. 2012;13(2):135–44.
40. Baselga J, Bradbury I, Eidtmann H, Di Cosimo S, de Azambuja E, Aura C, et al. Lapatinib with trastuzumab for HER2-positive early breast cancer (NeoALTTO): a randomised, open-label, multicentre, phase 3 trial. Lancet. 2012;379(9816):633–40.
41. Robidoux A, Tang G, Rastogi P, Geyer CE Jr, Azar CA, Atkins JN, et al. Lapatinib as a component of neoadjuvant therapy for HER2-positive operable breast cancer (NSABP protocol B-41): an open-label, randomised phase 3 trial. Lancet Oncol. 2013;14(12):1183–92.
42. Gianni L, Pienkowski T, Im YH, Tseng LM, Liu MC, Lluch A, et al. 5-year analysis of neoadjuvant pertuzumab and trastuzumab in patients with locally advanced, inflammatory, or early-stage HER2-positive breast cancer (NeoSphere): a multicentre, open-label, phase 2 randomised trial. Lancet Oncol. 2016;17(6):791–800.
43. Schneeweiss A, Chia S, Hickish T, Harvey V, Eniu A, Waldron-Lynch M, et al. Long-term efficacy analysis of the randomised, phase II TRYPHAENA cardiac safety study: Evaluating pertuzumab and trastuzumab plus standard neoadjuvant anthracycline-containing and anthracycline-free chemotherapy regimens in patients with HER2-positive early breast cancer. Eur J Cancer. 2018;89:27–35.
44. von Minckwitz G, Schneeweiss A, Loibl S, Salat C, Denkert C, Rezai M, et al. Neoadjuvant carboplatin in patients with triple-negative and HER2-positive early breast cancer (GeparSixto; GBG 66): a randomised phase 2 trial. Lancet Oncol. 2014;15(7):747–56.
45. Cameron D, Piccart-Gebhart MJ, Gelber RD, Procter M, Goldhirsch A, de Azambuja E, et al. 11 years' follow-up of trastuzumab after adjuvant chemotherapy in HER2-positive early breast cancer: final analysis of the HERceptin Adjuvant (HERA) trial. Lancet. 2017;389(10075):1195–205.
46. Schneeweiss A, Chia S, Hickish T, Harvey V, Eniu A, Hegg R, et al. Pertuzumab plus trastuzumab in combination with standard neoadjuvant anthracycline-containing and anthracycline-

free chemotherapy regimens in patients with HER2-positive early breast cancer: a randomized phase II cardiac safety study (TRYPHAENA). Ann Oncol. 2013;24(9):2278–84.
47. Cortazar P, Zhang L, Untch M, Mehta K, Costantino JP, Wolmark N, et al. Pathological complete response and long-term clinical benefit in breast cancer: the CTNeoBC pooled analysis. Lancet. 2014;384(9938):164–72.
48. Loi S, Dafni U, Karlis D, Polydoropoulou V, Young BM, Willis S, et al. Effects of estrogen receptor and human epidermal growth factor receptor-2 levels on the efficacy of trastuzumab: a secondary analysis of the HERA trial. JAMA Oncol. 2016;2(8):1040–7.
49. Rimawi MF, Mayer IA, Forero A, Nanda R, Goetz MP, Rodriguez AA, et al. Multicenter phase II study of neoadjuvant lapatinib and trastuzumab with hormonal therapy and without chemotherapy in patients with human epidermal growth factor receptor 2-overexpressing breast cancer: TBCRC 006. J Clin Oncol. 2013;31(14):1726–31.
50. Harbeck N, Gluz O, Christgen M, et al. Efficacy of 12-weeks of neoadjuvant TDM1 with or without endocrine therapy in HER2- positive hormone-receptor-positive early breast cancer: WSG-ADAPT HER2+/HR+ phase II trial. J Clin Oncol. 2015;33(suppl; abstr 506).
51. Rimawi MF, Cecchini RS, Rastogi P, et al. A phase III trial evaluating pCR in patients with HR+, HER2-positive breast cancer treated with neoadjuvant docetaxel, carboplatin, trastuzumab, and pertuzumab (TCHP) +/- estrogen deprivation: NRG Oncology/NSABP B-52. Cancer Res. 2016;77(suppl; abstr S3-06).
52. Vogel CL, Cobleigh MA, Tripathy D, Gutheil JC, Harris LN, Fehrenbacher L, et al. Efficacy and safety of trastuzumab as a single agent in first-line treatment of HER2-overexpressing metastatic breast cancer. J Clin Oncol. 2002;20(3):719–26.
53. Lin NU, Winer EP, Wheatley D, Carey LA, Houston S, Mendelson D, et al. A phase II study of afatinib (BIBW 2992), an irreversible ErbB family blocker, in patients with HER2-positive metastatic breast cancer progressing after trastuzumab. Breast Cancer Res Treat. 2012;133(3):1057–65.
54. Harbeck N, Huang CS, Hurvitz S, Yeh DC, Shao Z, Im SA, et al. Afatinib plus vinorelbine versus trastuzumab plus vinorelbine in patients with HER2-overexpressing metastatic breast cancer who had progressed on one previous trastuzumab treatment (LUX-Breast 1): an open-label, randomised, phase 3 trial. Lancet Oncol. 2016;17:357.
55. Burstein HJ, Sun Y, Dirix LY, Jiang Z, Paridaens R, Tan AR, et al. Neratinib, an irreversible ErbB receptor tyrosine kinase inhibitor, in patients with advanced ErbB2-positive breast cancer. J Clin Oncol. 2010;28(8):1301–7.
56. Swaby R, Blackwell K, Jiang Z, Sun Y, Dieras V, Zaman K, Zacharchuk C, Powell C, Abbas R, Thakuria M. Neratinib in combination with trastuzumab for the treatment of advanced breast cancer: a phase I/II study. J Clin Oncol. 2009;27(15_suppl):1004.
57. Awada A, Dirix L, Manso Sanchez L, Xu B, Luu T, Dieras V, et al. Safety and efficacy of neratinib (HKI-272) plus vinorelbine in the treatment of patients with ErbB2-positive metastatic breast cancer pretreated with anti-HER2 therapy. Ann Oncol. 2013;24(1):109–16.
58. Disis ML, Gooley TA, Rinn K, Davis D, Piepkorn M, Cheever MA, et al. Generation of T-cell immunity to the HER-2/neu protein after active immunization with HER-2/neu peptide-based vaccines. J Clin Oncol. 2002;20(11):2624–32.
59. Knutson KL, Schiffman K, Cheever MA, Disis ML. Immunization of cancer patients with a HER-2/neu, HLA-A2 peptide, p369-377, results in short-lived peptide-specific immunity. Clin Cancer Res. 2002;8(5):1014–8.
60. Park JW, Melisko ME, Esserman LJ, Jones LA, Wollan JB, Sims R. Treatment with autologous antigen-presenting cells activated with the HER-2 based antigen Lapuleucel-T: results of a phase I study in immunologic and clinical activity in HER-2 overexpressing breast cancer. J Clin Oncol. 2007;25(24):3680–7.
61. Hamilton E, Blackwell K, Hobeika AC, Clay TM, Broadwater G, Ren XR, et al. Phase 1 clinical trial of HER2-specific immunotherapy with concomitant HER2 kinase inhibition [corrected]. J Transl Med. 2012;10:28.

62. Nahta R, Yuan LX, Zhang B, Kobayashi R, Esteva FJ. Insulin-like growth factor-I receptor/human epidermal growth factor receptor 2 heterodimerization contributes to trastuzumab resistance of breast cancer cells. Cancer Res. 2005;65(23):11118–28.
63. Zhang S, Huang WC, Li P, Guo H, Poh SB, Brady SW, et al. Combating trastuzumab resistance by targeting SRC, a common node downstream of multiple resistance pathways. Nat Med. 2011;17(4):461–9.
64. Garrett JT, Olivares MG, Rinehart C, Granja-Ingram ND, Sanchez V, Chakrabarty A, et al. Transcriptional and posttranslational up-regulation of HER3 (ErbB3) compensates for inhibition of the HER2 tyrosine kinase. Proc Natl Acad Sci U S A. 2011;108(12):5021–6.
65. Witkiewicz AK, Ertel A, McFalls J, Valsecchi ME, Schwartz G, Knudsen ES. RB-pathway disruption is associated with improved response to neoadjuvant chemotherapy in breast cancer. Clin Cancer Res. 2012;18(18):5110–22.
66. Untch M, Rezai M, Loibl S, Fasching PA, Huober J, Tesch H, et al. Neoadjuvant treatment with trastuzumab in HER2-positive breast cancer: results from the GeparQuattro study. J Clin Oncol. 2010;28(12):2024–31.
67. Denduluri N, Chavez-MacGregor M, Telli ML, Eisen A, Graff SL, Hassett MJ, et al. Selection of optimal adjuvant chemotherapy and targeted therapy for early breast cancer: ASCO clinical practice guideline focused update. J Clin Oncol. 2018;36:2433–43. https://doi.org/10.1200/JCO.2018.78.8604.

Chapter 17
Adjuvant Endocrine Therapy for Breast Cancer

Ibrahim Yildiz and Adnan Aydiner

Introduction

Adjuvant endocrine therapy is a pivotal component of treatment for women with hormone receptor-positive early-stage breast cancer and has been shown to delay local and distant relapse and prolong survival. Patients with estrogen receptor (ER)- and/or progesterone receptor (PR)-positive invasive breast cancers should be considered for adjuvant endocrine therapy, regardless of age, lymph node status, or adjuvant chemotherapy use. Adjuvant hormonal manipulation is achieved by blocking the ER in breast tumor tissues with tamoxifen in premenopausal and postmenopausal women, lowering systemic estrogen levels with luteinizing hormone-releasing hormone agonists in premenopausal women, or blocking estrogen biosynthesis in non-ovarian tissues with aromatase inhibitors in postmenopausal women. Features indicative of uncertain endocrine responsiveness include low levels of hormone receptor immunoreactivity, PR negativity, poor differentiation (grade 3), high Ki67 index, human epidermal growth factor receptor 2 overexpression, and high gene recurrence score (Figs. 17.1, 17.2, 17.3, 17.4, and 17.5).

I. Yildiz
Internal Medicine, Department of Medical Oncology, Acibadem Hospital, Istanbul, Turkey

A. Aydiner (✉)
Internal Medicine, Medical Oncology, Istanbul Medical Faculty, Department of Medical Oncology, Institute of Oncology, Istanbul University, Istanbul, Turkey

A. Aydiner et al. (eds.), *Breast Cancer*, https://doi.org/10.1007/978-3-319-96947-3_17

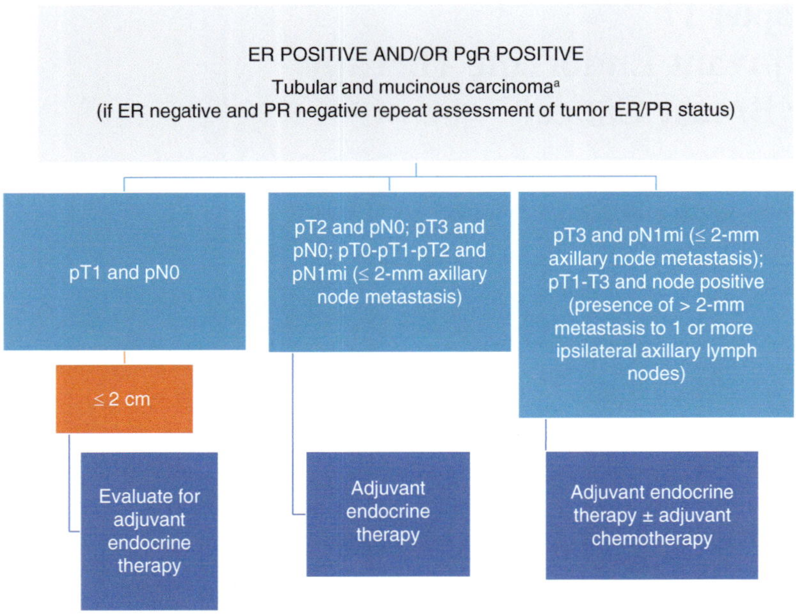

Fig. 17.1 Adjuvant systemic therapy for pure tubular and pure mucinous carcinoma. [a]Consider adjuvant bisphosphonate therapy in postmenopausal (natural or induced) patients receiving adjuvant therapy

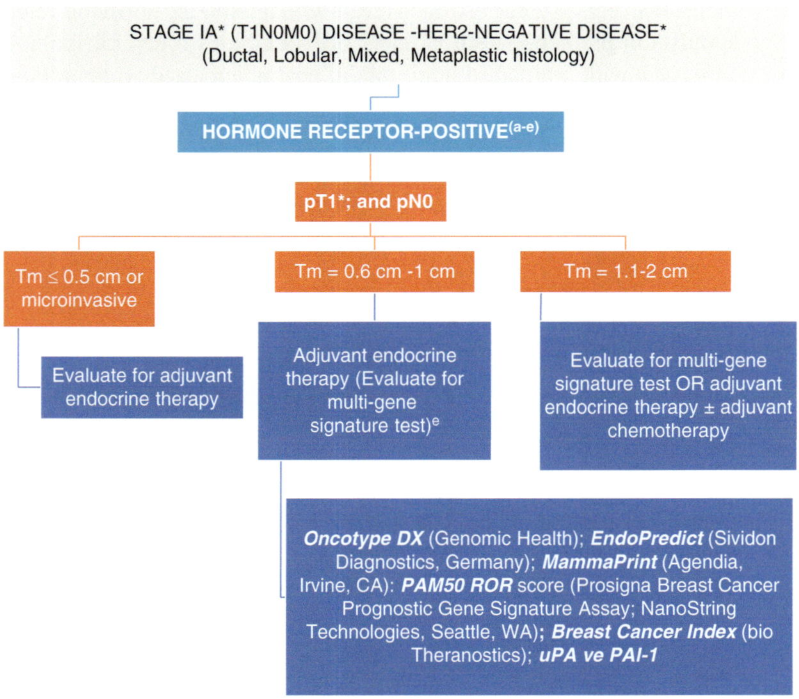

Fig. 17.2 Adjuvant systemic therapy for stage IA—hormone receptor-positive and HER2-negative disease. *In early-stage breast cancer, there are biomarkers that can be used to decide adjuvant

Principles of Adjuvant Endocrine Therapy

Adjuvant endocrine therapy (ET) is a major treatment modality for ER-positive breast cancer. Among early-stage breast cancer patients, approximately 60% require adjuvant ET after chemotherapy (CT), 20% require only ET, and 20% require only CT. ER-positive breast cancer is frequently associated with an older age and lower histological grade.

The current ETs modulate or disrupt estrogen production or ER function/expression in breast cancer cells. In premenopausal women, the ovarian follicles are the main source of estrogen production. Estrogen production by the ovary is regulated by the anterior pituitary gland, which produces luteinizing hormone (LH) and follicle-stimulating hormone (FSH). LH acts on thecal cells to stimulate androgen synthesis, whereas FSH acts upon granulosa cells to stimulate production of the enzyme aromatase, which converts testosterone and androstenedione to estradiol (E_2) and estrone, respectively, through aromatization. Pituitary LH and FSH production are, in turn, regulated by LH-releasing hormone (LHRH) (also known as

systemic treatment administration. In the 8th version of the American Joint Commission of Cancer (AJCC) for breast cancer, prognostic gene signatures will be integrated into the staging scheme as prognostic staging: For patients with hormone receptor-positive, HER2-negative, and lymph node-negative tumors, prognostic gene signatures (Oncotype DX) with a low risk score regardless of T size place the tumor in the same prognostic category as T1a–T1b N0 M0, and the tumor is staged using the AJCC prognostic stage group table as stage I. Based on multigene signature tests, chemotherapy may be omitted for patients with Luminal B-like (HER2 negative) disease with a low Oncotype Dx® score, MammaPrint® low-risk status, low PAM50 ROR score, or EndoPredict® low-risk status. In the TAILORx ClinicalTrial (ASCO Congress 2018), adjuvant endocrine therapy and chemoendocrine therapy had similar efficacy in women with hormone-receptor-positive, HER2-negative, axillary node-negative breast cancer who had a midrange 21-gene recurrence score (RS 11–25). However, the chemotherapy benefit for invasive disease-free survival varied with the combination of recurrence score and age ($P = 0.004$), with some benefit of chemotherapy found in women 50 years of age or younger with a recurrence score of 16–25. The situations in which multigene tests may be particularly helpful can be summarized as follows: tumor size between 1 and 3 cm *and* ER/PR positive *and* HER2 negative *and* node negative or N_{mi} *and* Grade 2 *and* Ki-67 between 15% and 35%. In hormone receptor-positive T1c N0 (1–2 cm) tumors, grade 3 disease with a high Ki-67 value (e.g., above 35%) and PgR <20% may be considered adequate for chemotherapy indication. In cases where multigene tests cannot be performed, the risk factors can be determined using web-based formulas, and an indication for chemotherapy administration can be established. [a]There is no absolute age limit. Rather, treatment depends on the disease, the presence of comorbidities, the patient's life expectancy, and patient preferences. Treatment should be individualized for patients >70 years of age. [b] Chemotherapy and endocrine therapy as adjuvant therapy should be given sequentially, with endocrine therapy following chemotherapy. The available data suggest that sequential or concurrent endocrine therapy with radiation therapy is acceptable. [c]Fertility preservation (e.g., by ovarian tissue or oocyte conservation) should be offered to women <40 years of age. Ovarian function suppression with LHRHa during chemotherapy should be offered for HR-negative disease. [d]Consider adjuvant bisphosphonate therapy in postmenopausal (natural or induced) patients receiving adjuvant therapy. [e]Evaluate for multi-gene signature test, especially for Luminal B-like, high Ki67, or grade III tumors

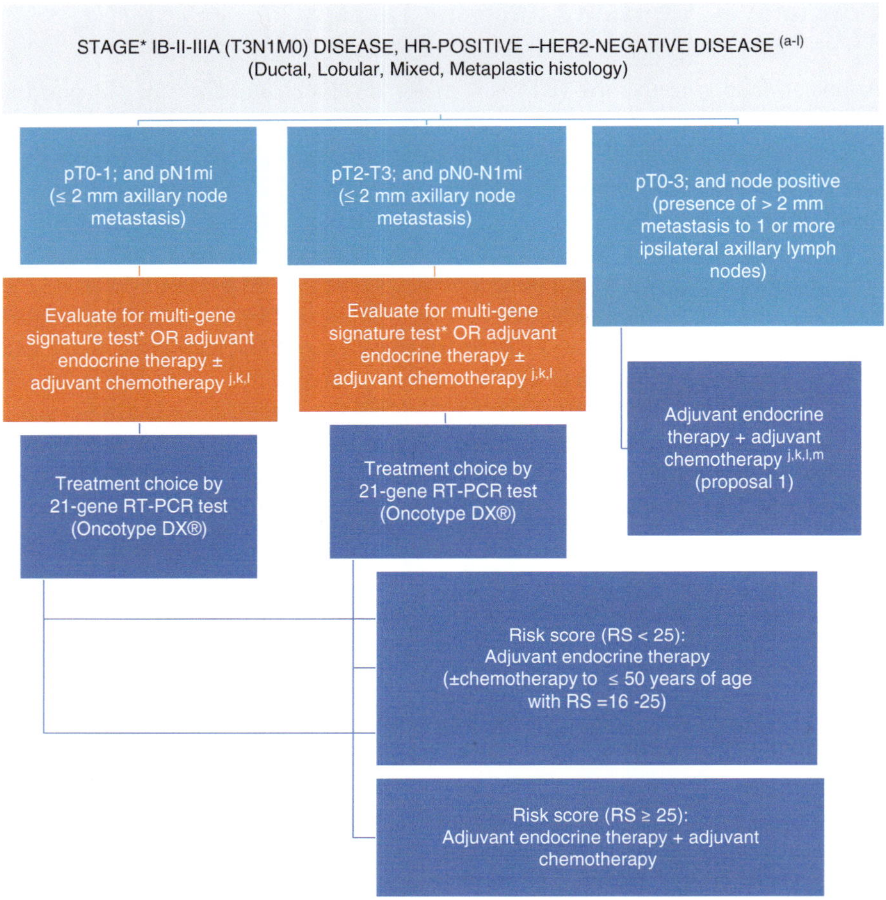

Fig. 17.3 Adjuvant systemic therapy for stage IB, II, IIIA—hormone receptor-positive and HER2-negative disease. *For patients with hormone receptor-positive, HER2-negative, and lymph node-negative tumors, prognostic gene signatures (Oncotype DX) with a low risk score regardless of T size place the tumor in the same prognostic category as T1a–T1b N0 M0, and the tumor is staged using the AJCC prognostic stage group table as stage I (8th version). [a]There is no absolute age limit. The choice of treatment depends on disease, co-morbidities, life expectancy and patient preferences. In patients over 70 years of age, treatment should be individualized. [b]The following factors are indications for including ovarian function suppression (OFS): age ≤35 years, premenopausal estrogen level following adjuvant chemotherapy, grade 3 disease, involvement of 4 or more nodes, and adverse multigene test results. The ASCO Guideline recommends OFS in premenopausal patients with stage II and III disease who have chemotherapy indications; however, this is not recommended for stage I disease. The optimal OFS duration is 5 years. [c]In high-risk premenopausal women, 'LHRH-agonist + aromatase inhibitor' may be the preferred adjuvant endocrine therapy. The following factors are indications for the use of OFS plus an aromatase inhibitor (AI) rather than OFS plus tamoxifen: age ≤35 years, grade 3 disease, involvement of 4 or more nodes, and adverse multigene test results. [d]In patients with Luminal A-like tumors and 1–3 positive lymph nodes (with the evaluation of other factors such as grade, age, or multigene signature test results), "adjuvant endocrine therapy alone" may be an option. [e]Some patients may be adequately treated with tamoxifen alone. In high-risk postmenopausal patients, AIs may be preferred over tamoxifen.

gonadotrophin-releasing hormone), which is produced in the hypothalamus. In postmenopausal women, estrogen production is dependent on peripheral aromatization, predominantly in the liver, adrenal glands, and adipose tissue. ET modulates or disrupts ER signaling by blocking pituitary LH/FSH production (LHRH agonists), blocking the ER (tamoxifen), degrading the ER (fulvestrant), or inhibiting peripheral estrogen production (aromatase inhibitors (AIs)). Given their different modes of action, menopausal status is important in ET selection.

ERs belong to a family of nuclear steroid receptors that includes thyroid hormone, vitamin D, and retinoids. ER phosphorylation upon estrogen binding induces a conformational change, resulting in receptor dimerization [1]. The receptor complex binds to specific estrogen response elements in target gene promoters, resulting in the up-regulation of target gene expression [1]. Two ERs, ERα and ERβ, have been described [2]. ERβ is broadly expressed in a variety of tissues, whereas ERα has a more restricted expression pattern (breast, ovary, uterus, and endometrium). The function and role of ERβ in breast cancer are not yet clear, so ER generally

The following factors support the inclusion of an AI at some point: lymph node involvement, grade 3 disease, high Ki67 proliferation index, or HER2 positivity. If an AI is used, it should be started upfront in patients at higher risk. The upfront AI can be switched to tamoxifen after 2 years in selected patients (e.g., those experiencing side effects of the AI). [f]After 5 years of adjuvant tamoxifen, continued AI (for postmenopausal estrogen levels at baseline or postmenopausal patients with premenopausal estrogen levels at baseline) or tamoxifen (for premenopausal or postmenopausal patients) for up to 10 years should be recommended to patients with node-positive disease, grade 3 disease, or high Ki-67. [g]After 5 years of adjuvant therapy involving a switch from tamoxifen to an AI (therefore assuming postmenopausal status at the 5-year time point and reasonable tolerance to endocrine therapy), patients may continue AI therapy for a cumulative total of 5 years. [h]After 5 years of continuous AI adjuvant therapy, we do not (yet) know whether to provide 3–5 years of tamoxifen, 3–5 years of AI, or no further endocrine treatment. AI can be considered for an additional 5 years. However, a randomized clinical trial failed to show a difference in survival between 2 and 5 years' use of additional AI. (San Antonio BCS, 2017). [i]The optimal OFS duration is 5 years. [j]The Luminal A phenotype is less responsive to chemotherapy. In node-negative disease, chemotherapy should not be added based on the T size. A combination of the biological properties of the tumor (such as Ki67, LVI, grade, and multigene signature) must be used to assess whether to provide chemotherapy. [k]Based on immunohistochemistry (IHC), in Luminal B-like (HER2-negative) tumors, chemotherapy may be omitted in some low-risk patients (based on combinations of certain prognostic factors such as low tumor mass, low grade, low Ki67, an absence of LVI, and older age). [l]Based on multigene signature tests, chemotherapy may be omitted for patients with Luminal B-like (HER2-negative) disease with a low Oncotype Dx® score, MammaPrint® low-risk status, low PAM50 ROR score or EndoPredict® low-risk status. In the TAILORx ClinicalTrial (ASCO Congress 2018), adjuvant endocrine therapy and chemoendocrine therapy had similar efficacy in women with hormone-receptor-positive, HER2-negative, axillary node-negative breast cancer who had a midrange 21-gene recurrence score (RS 11–25). However, the chemotherapy benefit for invasive disease-free survival varied with the combination of recurrence score and age ($P = 0.004$), with some benefit of chemotherapy found in women 50 years of age or younger with a recurrence score of 16–25. MammaPrint can be used in node-positive patients. MammaPrint (Agendia, Irvine, CA): In patients with 1–3 positive lymph nodes, tests can be performed to avoid adjuvant chemotherapy if the patient is at *high clinical risk* in the MINDACT categorization (however, the patient should be informed that there may be an additional benefit of chemotherapy with multiple LN positivity)

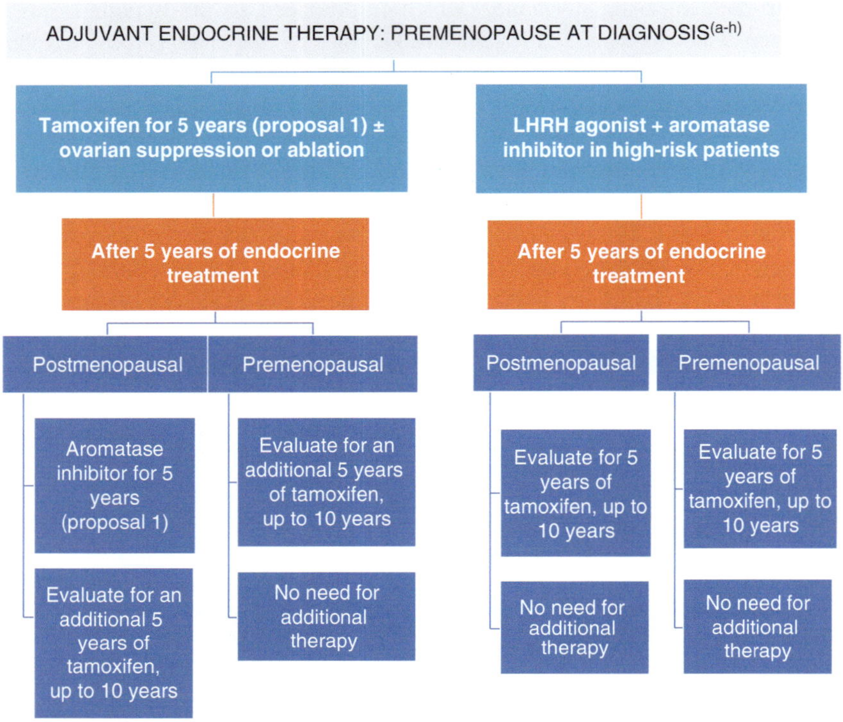

Fig. 17.4 Adjuvant endocrine therapy for premenopausal patients. [a]The following factors are indications for including ovarian function suppression (OFS): age ≤35 years, premenopausal estrogen levels following adjuvant chemotherapy, grade 3 disease, involvement of 4 or more nodes, and adverse multigene test results. The ASCO Guideline recommends OFS for pre-menopausal patients with stage II and III disease for whom chemotherapy has been indicated. By contrast, OFS is not recommended in stage I disease. [b]The optimal duration of OFS (with tamoxifen) may be 5 years. Its use for 5 years should be strongly recommended, especially in high-risk patients.[c]In high-risk premenopausal patients, 5 years of "LHRH-agonist plus aromatase inhibitor (AI)" may be the preferred adjuvant endocrine therapy. Exemestane, letrozole or anastrozole can be used as an AI. The following factors are indications for the use of OFS plus AI rather than OFS plus tamoxifen: age ≤35 years, grade 3 disease, high Ki67, node positivity, lobular histology, HER-2 positivity, and adverse multigene test results. Serum estrogen, follicle-stimulating hormone (FSH) and luteinizing hormone (LH) levels should be measured in the evaluation of menopausal status for the use of an aromatase inhibitor in premenopausal patients who have received chemotherapy. Estradiol levels should be checked at certain intervals. [d]After 5 years of continuous "LHRH-agonist plus AI" adjuvant therapy, we do not (yet) know whether to provide further endocrine treatment. [e]In patients with Luminal A-like tumors and 1–3 positive lymph nodes (with the evaluation of other factors such as grade, age or multigene signature test results), "adjuvant endocrine therapy alone" may be an option. [f]Adjuvant endocrine therapy should be completed in 10 years in stage II and III patients, especially those with moderate to high recurrence risk, but is not recommended for stage I patients. After 5 years of adjuvant tamoxifen, continued AI (for postmenopausal patients with premenopausal estrogen levels at baseline) or tamoxifen for up to 10 years should be recommended to patients with node-positive disease, grade 3 disease, or high Ki-67. [g]After 5 years of adjuvant therapy involving a switch from tamoxifen to an AI (therefore assuming postmenopausal status at the 5-year time point and reasonable tolerance to endocrine therapy), patients may continue AI therapy for a cumulative total of 5 years. This subject requires clarification. There was no difference in survival between 2 years and 5 years of AI in a randomized clinical trial. (San Antonio BCS, 2017). [h]Consider adjuvant bisphosphonate therapy in postmenopausal (natural or induced) patients receiving adjuvant therapy

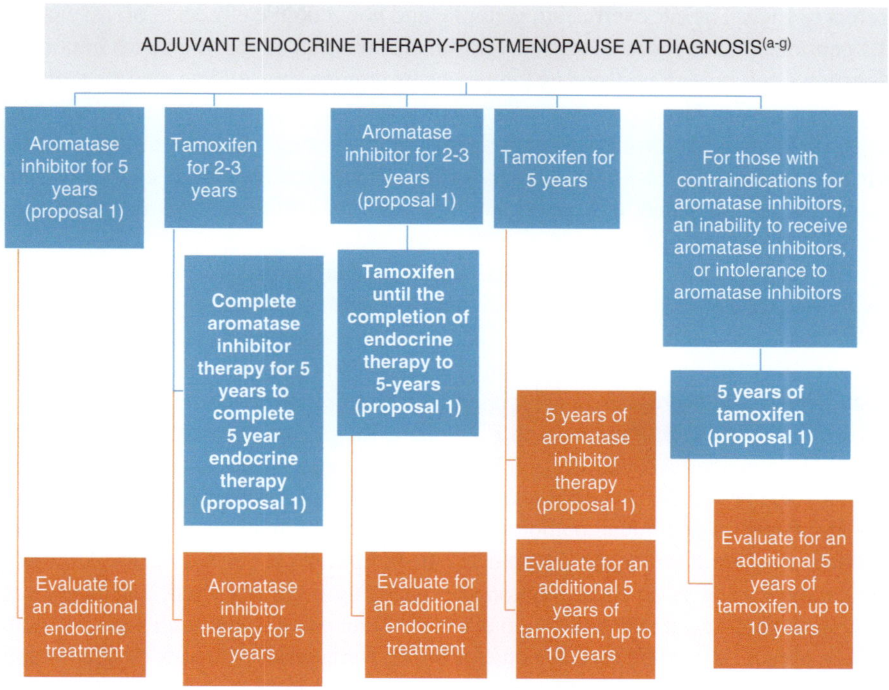

Fig. 17.5 Adjuvant endocrine therapy for postmenopausal patients. [a]In patients with Luminal A-like tumors and 1–3 positive lymph nodes (with the evaluation of other factors such as grade, age, or multigene signature test results), "adjuvant endocrine therapy alone" may be an option. [b]Some patients may be adequately treated with tamoxifen alone. In high-risk postmenopausal patients, aromatase inhibitors (AIs) may be preferred over tamoxifen. The following factors argue for the inclusion of an AI at some point: lymph node involvement, grade 3 disease, high Ki67 proliferation index, or HER2 positivity. If an AI is used, it should be started upfront in patients at higher risk. The upfront AI can be switched to tamoxifen after 2 years in selected patients (e.g., those experiencing side effects of the AI). [c]After 5 years of adjuvant tamoxifen, continued AI or tamoxifen (for patients with intolerance to AI therapy) for up to 10 years should be recommended to patients with node-positive disease, grade 3 disease, or high Ki-67. [d]After 5 years of adjuvant therapy involving a switch from tamoxifen to an AI (therefore assuming postmenopausal status at the 5-year time point and reasonable tolerance to endocrine therapy), patients may continue AI therapy for a cumulative total of 5 years. This subject requires clarification. [e]After 5 years of continuous AI adjuvant therapy, extension of treatment with an aromatase inhibitor may be recommended for 3–5 years. In a randomized study, no difference between the 2- and 5-year survival was observed (San Antonio BCS, 2017). In patients with moderate to high risk, adjuvant endocrine treatment should be increased to 10 years (in patients with stage II and III disease); this increase is not recommended for stage I patients. [f]The definition of menopause is important and can include natural menopause (no menses for 12 months before starting chemotherapy or hormone therapy) or menopause with ovarian ablation or suppression. Luteinizing hormone (LH), follicle-stimulating hormone (FSH), and serum estradiol (E2) levels should be at postmenopausal levels and should be measured before systemic treatment unless oophorectomy has been performed with hysterectomy in women aged 60 years or younger (Box 17.1). [g]Consider adjuvant bisphosphonate therapy in postmenopausal (natural or induced) patients receiving adjuvant therapy

refers to ERα. The ER exerts both genomic and nongenomic effects in breast cancer. Its genomic effects include the transcriptional activation of specific genes important for tumor cell growth and survival, whereas its nongenomic effects include the activation of growth factor pathways, such as human epidermal growth factor receptor-2 (HER2) and insulin-like growth factor receptor that enhance tumor growth. Growth factor receptor-linked kinases further activate the ER and its coactivators to augment ER-mediated transcriptional activity. This bidirectional crosstalk can cause ET resistance [3].

HR status is currently determined based on the immunohistochemical (IHC) expression of ER and PR. Tumors with any detectable ($\geq 1\%$) ER and/or PR expression are considered HR-positive. ER expression correlates with slower tumor growth, better differentiation, and longer natural history. By contrast, the absence of both ER and PR expression is associated with poorer prognosis and a reduced overall survival (OS) rate. Patients with ER- and/or PR-positive invasive breast cancers should be considered for adjuvant ET, regardless of age, lymph node status, or adjuvant CT use [4]. Endocrine-responsive breast cancer is a heterogeneous disease with a wide spectrum of clinical, pathological, and molecular features. There is no single marker that can identify the optimal ET to be used in a given patient. Although molecular typing is an ideal method for assessing recurrence risk and treatment response, routine genetic profiling has not yet been established in clinical practice. IHC typing is still considered the state of the art for assessing the risk of relapse and potential benefit of specific therapies. Features indicative of uncertain endocrine responsiveness include low levels of HR immunoreactivity, PR negativity, poor differentiation (grade 3), high proliferation index (Ki67), HER2 overexpression, and high gene recurrence score [5]. Patients with tumors of uncertain endocrine responsiveness are usually treated with a combination of ET and CT. The benefit of adjuvant endocrine therapy is very small in patients with hormone receptor-positive disease and those who have lymph node-negative cancers ≤0.5 cm or 0.6–1.0 cm in diameter with favorable prognostic features.

Gene expression profiling has shed light on the complex molecular background of this disease and holds the potential for more accurate prognostication and patient stratification for therapy [6–8]. A list of intrinsic genes is used to differentiate subtypes and includes ER, HER2, and proliferation-related genes as well as a unique cluster of genes called the basal cluster. The molecular subtypes include the following: (1) the luminal subtype (luminal A and B), which expresses genes associated with luminal epithelial cells of normal breast tissue and overlaps with ER-positive breast cancers as defined by clinical assays; (2) the HER2-enriched subtype, which represents the majority of clinically HER2-positive breast cancers; and (3) the ER-negative subtype, which expresses low levels of HR-related genes.

Several genomic tests have been developed with the aim of improving prognostic information beyond that provided by classic clinicopathological parameters [6–8]. Some of these tests are currently available in the clinic and are used to determine prognosis and, more importantly, to assist in determining the need for adjuvant chemotherapy, particularly in patients with ER-positive disease. The available data suggest that information generated from genomic tests has resulted in a change in decision making in approximately 25–30% of cases. Molecular signatures, such as the 21-gene recurrence score (RS; Oncotype DX®) [9], Amsterdam 70-gene prognostic profile (MammaPrint®) [10], and Rotterdam/Veridex 76-gene signature [11], increase the prognostic value of conventional indicators in predicting breast cancer outcomes and treatment response. Oncotype DX is the most widely used of these assays. Oncotype DX can be performed using formalin-fixed paraffin-embedded tissue, whereas the other tests require fresh or frozen tissue. The predictive value of Oncotype DX has been validated in both premenopausal and postmenopausal women, and its use in node-negative, ER-positive breast cancer patients is suggested in the American Society of Clinical Oncology (ASCO) guidelines.

Menopausal status is generally assessed using clinical features such as age, menstrual history, and menopausal symptoms and may be confirmed by the presence of serum FSH and E_2 levels within menopausal range. Elevated FSH and reduced E_2 levels generally confirm the clinical diagnosis of menopause. However, the use of these biomarkers has several limitations. The transition toward menopause is highly variable, thus making it difficult to define diagnostic cutoff values for FSH/E_2. Therefore, single-time-point testing of FSH/E_2 levels is insufficient to confirm menopause. Furthermore, FSH/estrogen levels are influenced by ETs. Tamoxifen has been reported to increase circulating estrogens and decrease the FSH levels [12]. AIs have been shown to profoundly decrease estrogen levels and increase FSH levels in postmenopausal patients [12]. CT can also cause significant changes in ovarian function by directly destroying remnant functional follicles or indirectly promoting the loss of functional follicles through induction of ovarian fibrosis. CT can also lead to amenorrhea by inducing primary or hypergonadotropic hypogonadism [13]. The risk of CT-induced *primary ovarian insufficiency* (POI) has been correlated with CT type, higher cumulative CT dose, and older age, with age >40 years being the strongest predictor of both chemotherapy-induced amenorrhea (CIA) and chemotherapy-induced menopause (CIM) [14, 15]. Therefore, in these clinical settings, FSH/E_2 levels are not reliable surrogate markers of menopause.

Assessment of ovarian function is important in hormone-sensitive breast cancer patients who are eligible to receive adjuvant ET (Box 17.1). Adjuvant AI treatment administered upfront or switching to tamoxifen has proved to be superior to tamoxifen alone in postmenopausal patients and therefore has become the standard of care in these patients. By contrast, adjuvant treatment with tamoxifen with or without ovarian suppression is recommended in premenopausal women. Tamoxifen can be safely given to premenopausal women; however, this is not the case for AIs. AIs interfere with androgen to estrogen conversion by blocking aromatase, thereby lowering E_2 levels in truly postmenopausal women. However, in the presence of functional ovaries, low levels of estrogen will enhance pituitary FSH production, thereby indirectly stimulating follicular aromatase production and subsequent E_2 production. Consequently, AI treatment in the absence of an LHRH agonist may be ineffective in postmenopausal women inaccurately classified as premenopausal. Moreover, in the case of CIA, AIs may promote recovery of ovarian function, leading to therapeutic failure and even to unwanted pregnancy.

Endocrine strategies in premenopausal women include estrogen receptor blockade with tamoxifen, temporary ovarian suppression with LHRH agonists, or permanent ovarian suppression with oophorectomy or radiotherapy. Tamoxifen is the mainstay of ET in premenopausal women. In patients receiving both tamoxifen and chemotherapy, chemotherapy should be given first, followed by sequential tamoxifen. Prospective randomized trials have demonstrated that 5 years of tamoxifen is more effective than 1–2 years of tamoxifen.

The 2011 EBCTCG meta-analysis, which compared 5 years of tamoxifen treatment to no ET in premenopausal and postmenopausal women, was instrumental in establishing the efficacy of adjuvant tamoxifen [16]. Tamoxifen treatment resulted in a 39% reduction in breast cancer recurrence compared with placebo (relative risk [RR] 0.61, 95% CI 0.57–0.65), which translated to a 15-year absolute reduction of 13% (33% vs. 46%). This outcome was observed in both node-negative and node-positive patients. Tamoxifen treatment also resulted in a 30% reduction in breast cancer mortality risk (RR 0.70, 95% CI 0.64–0.75), which translated to a 15-year absolute reduction of 9% (24% vs. 33%). The magnitude of benefit was similar between women <45 and 55–69 years of age. Tamoxifen also reduced the risk of local recurrence (RR 0.54; $P < 0.000001$) and contralateral breast cancer (RR 0.62; $P < 0.00001$).

Duration of Tamoxifen

For decades, tamoxifen for 5 years has been the standard ET for premenopausal women [17]. Tamoxifen for more than 5 years has not been shown to be more beneficial than tamoxifen for 5 years in two North American and Scottish trials [18, 19]. However, the results of the ATLAS (Adjuvant Tamoxifen-Longer Against Shorter) and Adjuvant Tamoxifen-To Offer More (aTTom) trials have recently changed this paradigm [20]. The ATLAS study, which randomized nearly 7000 ER-positive patients between 5 and 10 years tamoxifen, showed a benefit for continuing tamoxifen with an absolute benefit of 3.7% (21.4% vs 25.1%) for recurrence risk and an absolute mortality reduction of 2.8% (12.2% vs 15%). Remarkably, these benefits were mainly observed in the 10 years after treatment was ceased. This was attributed to a carryover effect, which is well known for tamoxifen. However, fewer than 20% of patients enrolled in ATLAS had low risk (i.e., node negative or tumor size <2 cm); therefore, it is difficult to determine the true benefit of extending tamoxifen therapy for these patients. Similar results were observed in the ATTOM trial [21]. Combining the results of the ATTOM and ATLAS trials enhanced the statistical significance of the benefits for recurrence ($P < 0.0001$), breast cancer mortality ($P = 0.002$), and OS ($P = 0.005$). Tamoxifen is associated with an increased risk of thromboembolic events (1–2% increased risk of deep venous thrombosis and threefold increased risk of pulmonary embolism), increased vaginal bleeding, and a threefold increased risk of endometrial cancer. However, the absolute increase in endometrial cancer is <1%, and almost all cancers that develop are stage I adenocarcinomas.

The expression of growth factor receptors, such as HER2, is associated with the development of tamoxifen resistance in breast cancer [22]. Studies suggest that PgR negativity in ER-positive tumors may be associated with increased growth factor expression, a more aggressive tumor phenotype, and tamoxifen resistance. By contrast, higher quantitative ER levels have been shown to predict greater tamoxifen benefits. Other factors that may contribute to tamoxifen resistance include variable expression of ERα and ERβ isoforms, interference with coactivator and corepressor binding, alternative splicing of ER mRNA variants, modulators of ER expression (e.g., epidermal growth factor and its receptors such as epidermal growth factor receptor-1 and HER2), and inherited drug-metabolizing CYP2D6 genotypes [23, 24]. Given the limited and conflicting evidence at this time, the NCCN Breast Cancer guideline does not recommend CYP2D6 testing as a tool to determine the optimal adjuvant endocrine strategy.

Ovarian Suppression

Ovarian ablation therapy is the oldest type of breast cancer therapy. The ovaries are the main site of estrogen production in premenopausal women. Therefore, ovarian ablation/suppression is an endocrine therapeutic option to consider in young women with ER-positive disease. In premenopausal women, cessation of ovarian function can be achieved on a temporary basis by pharmacological interventions that inhibit ovarian production of estrogen, such as gonadotropin-releasing hormone (LHRH) agonists, or permanently by surgery (oophorectomy) or pelvic radiation (ovarian ablation). Goserelin, leuprolide, and triptorelin are also used for chemical ovarian suppression; however, only goserelin has been approved by the FDA.

For premenopausal patients, monotherapy with tamoxifen was the standard therapy for a long time, with a possible benefit from ovarian suppression for patients 40 years of age and younger [25]. Recently, the results of the TEXT (Tamoxifen and Exemestane Trial) and SOFT (The Suppression of Ovarian Function Trial) trials revealed that for premenopausal patients, addition of ovarian function suppression should be considered for patients younger than 35 years (5-year breast cancer-free interval of 67.7% for tamoxifen vs 78.9% for tamoxifen plus OFS and 83.4% for exemestane plus OFS) or who received chemotherapy (5-year breast cancer-free interval 78% for tamoxifen vs 82.5% for tamoxifen plus OFS vs 85.7% for exemestane plus OFS) [26]. The OS data from these trials are still pending because overall follow-up is relatively short in the context of endocrine-sensitive disease.

In addition, randomized trials have shown that ovarian suppression with GnRH agonist therapy administered during adjuvant chemotherapy in premenopausal women with ER-negative tumors may preserve ovarian function and diminish the likelihood of chemotherapy-induced amenorrhea.

The abrupt interruption of ovarian function is a significant problem in young premenopausal patients. Adverse events may include severe menopause-related signs and symptoms, psychological distress, impaired quality of life, sexual dysfunction, changes in personal and family relationships, and bone loss.

The St Gallen International Breast Cancer Conference (2017) reviewed substantial new evidence on systemic therapies for early breast cancer. For premenopausal patients with endocrine responsive, the Panel endorsed the role of ovarian function suppression with either tamoxifen or exemestane for patients at higher risk. More generally, the Panel considered that the factors arguing for the inclusion of OFS were age 35 or less, persisting premenopausal estrogen levels after adjuvant chemotherapy; or the involvement of four or more axillary nodes. A lesser majority would add grade 3 disease or an adverse result from a multiparameter molecular marker test as indications for OFS. The panel noted the value an LHRH agonist given during chemotherapy for premenopausal women with ER-negative disease in protecting against premature ovarian failure and preserving fertility.

For premenopausal women, the evidence-based choices are tamoxifen for 5–10 years; tamoxifen for 5 years followed by AI for 5 years; and ovarian suppression with tamoxifen or AI, which should be considered for higher-risk patients (<35 years, premenopausal after chemotherapy and multiple positive axillary nodes). In low-risk hormone receptor-positive premenopausal breast cancer, OA is not beneficial, and tamoxifen remains the anti-hormone treatment of choice.

Adjuvant Endocrine Therapy for Postmenopausal Women

Approximately 75% of breast cancers are diagnosed in postmenopausal women, 80% of which are HR-positive [27]. Third-generation AIs, including anastrozole, letrozole, and exemestane, block estrogen synthesis by inhibiting aromatase. Because these AIs do not block ovarian estrogen production, their use is limited to postmenopausal women (Box 17.1) (Fig. 17.5).

A number of studies have compared AIs with tamoxifen in the adjuvant setting using either a head-to-head (i.e., randomly assigning patients to 5 years of either drug) or switch schedule approach (i.e., initial tamoxifen for 2–3 years followed by either an AI for 2–3 years or continued tamoxifen for a total of 5 years). The results of the ATAC, BIG 1-98 and TEAM trials clearly show that AI-containing adjuvant regimes, either as a monotherapy or as a switch scheme, are preferred over tamoxifen monotherapy. The use of AIs in either approach reduces breast cancer recurrence rates compared with tamoxifen alone; however, their effect on survival is less clear [28]. Randomized studies showed no significant difference in recurrence or survival between upfront and switching AI therapy [29–31]. The Early Breast Cancer Trialist's Cooperative Group (EBCTCG) meta-analysis also showed that 5-year adjuvant endocrine treatment including AIs was more effective than tamoxifen monotherapy in preventing recurrence and breast cancer death in either continuous or sequential regimens [32].

Hormone receptor-positive breast cancer is characterized by a very long natural history. As a consequence, some women remain at risk of late recurrence for years, fueling the discussion to prolong endocrine therapy beyond 5 years. The risk of breast cancer recurrence after 5 years of endocrine therapy was evaluated in a meta-analysis by the EBCTCG. In that meta-analysis, breast cancer recurrences occurred at a steady rate throughout the study period from 5 to 20 years, strongly correlated with the original tumor- and nodal status and tumor grade [33]. Several trials, including the large MA.17 trial and the smaller ABCSG 6 and NSABP B-33 trials, have also demonstrated that extended ET with 3–5 years of an AI following 5 years of tamoxifen decreases relapse rates and may affect survival, especially in women with nodal involvement [34–37] (Table 17.1). The MA.17 trial demonstrated that compared with placebo, extended letrozole therapy provided a survival advantage in women with axillary lymph node-positive but not in those with lymph node-negative ER-positive breast cancer [34]. The recently reported MA.17R trial randomized women who had already completed 5 years of aromatase inhibitor therapy with or without previous tamoxifen to a further 5 years of letrozole or placebo. DFS was significantly improved in the extended letrozole group, quality of life was similar, but bone fracture rates were higher. The 5-year DFS rate was 95% for the letrozole arm compared with 91% for the placebo arm [hazard ratio 0.66, 95% CI (0.48–0.91); $P < 0.01$] [35].

Several studies investigated the efficacy and safety of additional treatment with AIs after a sequential regimen of tamoxifen and an AI for 5 years [38–40]. However, results from NSABP-B42, the DATA trial, and the IDEAL trial have not confirmed the benefit on recurrence-free survival seen in MA17R. The NSABP B42 study investigated the efficacy of 5 years of letrozole after an initial 5-year of endocrine therapy including an AI. This could be either AI monotherapy, or sequenced with tamoxifen. In contrast to the findings of the MA.17R trial, the difference in DFS between the control and placebo groups did not reach statistical significance [7-year DFS 84.7 vs 81.3%, HR 0.85, $P = 0.048$, statistical significance level 0.0418]. For OS, a significant difference between the control and placebo groups was also not found [91.8 vs 92.3%, HR 1.15, $P = 0.22$]. However, patients under extended endocrine therapy were significantly less frequently affected by distant recurrence [HR 0.72, $P = 0.03$]; a risk reduction of 28% was observed. Furthermore, a significantly longer BC-free interval (BCFI), defined as time to recurrence or contralateral BC as the first event, could be observed in the letrozole group [incidence of BCFI events 6.7 vs 10.0%, HR 0.71, $P = 0.003$] [38].

The DATA trial presented at the San Antonio Breast Cancer Symposium in 2016 was designed to investigate the effect of extended AI therapy after TAM. In this multicenter phase III trial, 1660 postmenopausal women with HR-positive early breast cancer who underwent 2–3 years of TAM therapy, were randomized to 6 or 3 years of anastrozole daily. The 5-year adapted DFS did not differ significantly [83.1 vs 79.4%, HR 0.79, $P = 0.07$] [39]. The IDEAL trial is a multicenter phase III trial that included 1824 women with HR-positive breast cancer randomized between 2007 and 2011 with the intention to determine the optimal duration of extended adjuvant letrozole therapy. This study was presented at the San Antonio Breast Cancer Symposium in 2016. Patients had to complete 5 years of any commonly used endocrine therapy regimen and were subsequently randomized to extended

Table 17.1 Prospective randomized trials evaluating more than 5 years of endocrine therapy[a]

Trial	No. of patients	Pre-randomization therapy	Randomization	HR for DFS	HR for OS
ATLAS [20]	6846	5 ys TAM	TAM (5 ys)	0.84 (p = 0.002)	0.71 (p = 0.01)
			Control		
aTTom [21]	6953	5 ys TAM	TAM (5 ys)	0.86 (p = 0.003	0.91 (p = ns)
			Control		
MA.17 [34]	5187	5 ys TAM	Letrozole (5 ys)	0.57 (p < 0.0001)	0.76 (p = 0.25)
			Placebo		
NSABP B33 [37]	1598	5 ys TAM	Exemestane (5 ys)	0.68 (p = 0.07)	NA
			Placebo		
MA.17R [35]	1918	3–5 ys TAM-5 ys AI	Letrozole (5 ys)	0.66 (p = 0.01)	0.97 (p = ns)
			Placebo		
NSABP B42 [38]	3923	5 ys (or TAM sequenced to AI)	Letrozol (5 ys)	0.85 (p = ns)	1.15 (p = ns)
			Placebo		
IDEAL [40]	1824	5 ys AI or TAM or TAM sequenced to AI	Letrozol (5 ys)	0.92 (p = ns)	1.04 (p = ns)
			Letrozol (2.5 ys)		
DATA [39]	1660	2–3 ys TAM	Anastrazol (6 ys)	0.79 (p = 0.07)	0.91 (p = ns)
			Anastrazol (3 ys)		
SOLE [42]	4884	5 ys AI or TAM or TAM sequenced to AI	Letrozol (5 ys-cont)	1.08 (p = ns)	0.05 (p = ns)
			Letrozol (5 ys-int)		

[a]*TAM* tamoxifen, *ys* years, *AI* aromatase inhibitor, *NA* not available, *ns* non-significant

adjuvant letrozole therapy for either 2.5 years or 5 years. The median follow-up was 6.5 years. No significant difference in 5-year DFS was observed between patients with 2.5 years or 5 years of extended letrozole therapy [88.4 vs 87.9%, HR 0.96, P = 0.70]. The 5-year OS also did not differ significantly between those groups [93.5 vs 92.6%, HR 1.08, P = 0.59] [40]. In a recent meta-analysis on extended endocrine therapy, including the above mentioned trials, particularly women with a positive nodal status seemed to have more benefit of extended endocrine therapy (node positive HR 0.72 versus node negative HR 0.83). Similarly, a relative larger benefit was seen from extended endocrine therapy in women with a larger tumor size and for those with both ER and PR expression versus single receptor expression. A greater effect was also seen in patients who received adjuvant chemotherapy compared with those who did not [41].

Other trials have evaluated less intensive extended endocrine regimens and suggested their equivalence with extended therapy for an additional five years. For example, The SOLE phase III trial included 4884 postmenopausal women with HR^+, N^+ early-stage BC with the purpose of investigating the effect of a new therapeutic concept of letrozole [42]. The trial was designed to assess the role of continuous *versus* intermittent letrozole intake. After 5 years of adjuvant endocrine therapy, patients were randomized to 5 years of either continuous ($n = 2441$) or intermittent ($n = 2443$) letrozole administration, with mandatory 3-month treatment-free intervals. After 60 months of follow-up, similar 5-year DFS rates were observed in patients with intermittent and continuous letrozole administration [85.8 *vs* 87.5%, HR 1.08, P = 0.31].

Sequential rather than concurrent administration of cytotoxic and endocrine therapies should be used. The concurrent use of tamoxifen and anthracyclines has been shown to have detrimental effects, whereas the concurrent use of AIs and CT has not been investigated [7].

The prognostic significance of ER and PR levels, PR negativity, HER2 overexpression, Ki67 levels, and 21-gene RS has been examined. In the initial exploratory analysis of the ATAC trial, a greater benefit of anastrozole compared with tamoxifen in the PR-negative subgroup was suggested. The TEAM trial showed that, in patients receiving exemestane, the ER and PR expression levels predicted DFS. The relative risk of relapse increased with decreased ER and PR expression, and PR status did not predict treatment response. In the BIG 1-98 trial, more relapses occurred in the first 2 years in women who received tamoxifen followed by letrozole than in those who received letrozole alone (4.4% vs. 3.1%). This increased risk of relapse was particularly evident in women with >3 involved nodes ($P < 0.001$), tumors 2 cm in size ($P = 0.001$), or vascular invasion ($P = 0.02$). A retrospective analysis demonstrated that these factors in conjunction with ER and PR levels, Ki67 labeling index, and HER2 status may be useful in guiding the selection of letrozole or tamoxifen [43]. IHC analysis of the nuclear antigen Ki67 is used to estimate the proliferative activity of tumor cells. Studies have demonstrated the prognostic value of Ki67 in predicting response and clinical outcomes [44]. One small study suggested that analysis of Ki67 after short-term ET may be useful in selecting patients who are resistant to ET and may benefit from additional interventions [45]. However, these data require greater analytical and clinical validation.

Studies have consistently demonstrated that the use of third-generation AIs as initial adjuvant therapy, sequential therapy, or extended therapy lowers recurrence risk, including ipsilateral breast tumor recurrence, contralateral breast cancer, and distant metastatic disease, in postmenopausal women with HR-positive breast cancer. However, a direct comparison of these strategies is not possible given the differences in design and patient populations among studies. All three adjuvant strategies have shown similar antitumor efficacy and toxicity profiles in randomized studies. Although it has been shown that letrozole leads to more complete aromatase inhibition [46] and lower serum estrogen levels [47] compared to anastrozole, the clinical importance of these findings is unclear. To date, indirect comparisons between adjuvant trials suggest that letrozole, anastrozole, and exemestane have similar benefits when compared with tamoxifen. In addition, a neoadjuvant study showed that letrozole, anastrozole, and exemestane similarly suppress the proliferation marker Ki67 and preoperative endocrine prognostic index scores [48].

The St. Gallen Consensus Conference 2017 panel was almost unanimous that some postmenopausal patients can be treated with tamoxifen alone. Slightly more than half of the panelists believed that an aromatase inhibitor should be used at some point during the course of adjuvant therapy. Factors that favored the use of an aromatase inhibitor include node positivity, high Ki67, high grade, lobular histology, and HER2 positivity. The Panel recommended longer durations of therapy in women with moderate to high risk of recurrence, typically defined as stage II or III breast cancers [49].

Tamoxifen and AIs have different side effect profiles, although both can cause hot flashes, night sweats, and vaginal dryness. AIs are more commonly associated with musculoskeletal symptoms, osteoporosis, and increased rates of bone fracture, whereas tamoxifen is associated with an increased risk of uterine cancer and deep venous thrombosis. Osteoporosis/osteopenia, hypertriglyceridemia, vaginal bleeding, and hypercholesterolemia were less frequent on exemestane, whereas mild liver function abnormalities and rare episodes of atrial fibrillation were less frequent on anastrozole. Vasomotor and musculoskeletal symptoms were similar between arms. Compliance is a major issue for the use of all chronic medications, including adjuvant ET.

The current version (Version 1.2018) of the NCCN Guideline recommends the following adjuvant ET options for postmenopausal women with early breast cancer: 5 years of AI as initial adjuvant therapy (category 1); 2–3 years of AI followed by tamoxifen to complete 5 years of adjuvant ET (category 1); 2–3 years of tamoxifen followed by an AI to complete 5 years (category 1) or 5 years of AI alone (category 2B); or 5 years of tamoxifen followed by 5 years of AI (category 1) (https://www.nccn.org/professionals/physician_gls/pdf/breast.pdf. Breast Cancer, version 1.2018). Five years or longer use of tamoxifen alone is limited to postmenopausal women who decline AI treatment or have a contraindication to AIs. It is relevant that patients who experience intolerable adverse effects on initial adjuvant AI therapy and switch to tamoxifen after 2 years have similar outcomes to those who complete 5 years of AI therapy [30]. Switching to a different AI is reasonable because 39% of patients are able to tolerate an alternative AI [50]. In conclusion, AI use, either upfront or after 2–3 years of tamoxifen, should be recommended for the majority of breast cancer patients. When choosing between upfront and switch strategies, it is reasonable to weigh the potential added benefit of AIs in reducing early relapse in patients most likely to suffer tamoxifen and AI toxicities [51]. Support from prospective studies for the preferential use of upfront AI in patients with greater tumor burdens or more aggressive tumor biology would be extremely useful [43].

Conclusion

Adjuvant endocrine therapy should be administered to patients with ER-positive and/or PR-positive invasive breast cancer, regardless of HER2 status, patient age, or cytotoxic therapy provided. Endocrine therapy can be initiated either with or after radiotherapy. In high-risk patients with multiple poor prognostic factors, an aromatase inhibitor (AI) (plus OFS in premenopausal patients) may be the best treatment option.

Box 17.1
The definition of menopause. Menopause can be defined as natural menopause (no menses for 12 months before starting chemotherapy or hormone therapy) or as menopause with ovarian ablation or suppression. Luteinizing hormone (LH), follicle-stimulating hormone (FSH), and serum estradiol (E2) levels should be at postmenopausal levels and should be measured before systemic treatment unless oophorectomy has been performed with hysterectomy in women aged 60 years or younger.

The definition of menopause: "Prior bilateral oophorectomy" OR "Age ≥60 years" OR "Age <60 years" and amenorrheic for 12 or more months in the absence of chemotherapy, tamoxifen, toremifene, or ovarian suppression and follicle-stimulating hormone (FSH) and estradiol in the postmenopausal range OR "If taking tamoxifen or toremifene, and age <60 years, then FSH and plasma estradiol levels in postmenopausal ranges".

References

1. Osborne CK, Schiff R, Fuqua SA, Shou J. Estrogen receptor: current understanding of its activation and modulation. Clin Cancer Res. 2001;7:4338s–4342s; discussion 4411s–4412s.
2. Kumar R, Thompson EB. The structure of the nuclear hormone receptors. Steroids. 1999;64:310–9.
3. Shou J, Massarweh S, Osborne CK, Wakeling AE, Ali S, Weiss H, et al. Mechanisms of tamoxifen resistance: increased estrogen receptor-HER2/neu cross-talk in ER/HER2-positive breast cancer. J Natl Cancer Inst. 2004;96:926–35.
4. Tamoxifen for early breast cancer: an overview of the randomised trials. Early Breast Cancer Trialists' Collaborative Group. Lancet. 1998;351:1451–67.
5. Goldhirsch A, Ingle JN, Gelber RD, Coates AS, Thürlimann B, Senn HJ, Panel members. Thresholds for therapies: highlights of the St Gallen International Expert Consensus on the primary therapy of early breast cancer 2009. Ann Oncol. 2009;20:1319–29.
6. Perou CM, Sorlie T, Eisen MB, van de Rijn M, Jeffrey SS, Rees CA, et al. Molecular portraits of human breast tumours. Nature. 2000;406:747–52.
7. Goldhirsch A, Wood WC, Coates AS, Gelber RD, Thürlimann B, Senn HJ, Panel members. Strategies for subtypes—dealing with the diversity of breast cancer: highlights of the St. Gallen International Expert Consensus on the Primary Therapy of Early Breast Cancer 2011. Ann Oncol. 2011;22:1736–47.
8. Sorlie T, Perou CM, Tibshirani R, Aas T, Geisler S, Johnsen H, et al. Gene expression patterns of breast carcinomas distinguish tumor subclasses with clinical implications. Proc Natl Acad Sci U S A. 2001;98:10869–74.
9. Paik S, Shak S, Tang G, Kim C, Baker J, Cronin M, et al. A multigene assay to predict recurrence of tamoxifen-treated, node-negative breast cancer. N Engl J Med. 2004;351:2817–26.

10. van de Vijver MJ, He YD, van't Veer LJ, Dai H, Hart AA, Voskuil DW, et al. A gene-expression signature as a predictor of survival in breast cancer. N Engl J Med. 2002;347:1999–2009.
11. Wang Y, Klijn JG, Zhang Y, Sieuwerts AM, Look MP, Yang F, et al. Gene-expression profiles to predict distant metastasis of lymph-node-negative primary breast cancer. Lancet. 2005;365:671–9.
12. Rossi E, Morabito A, Di Rella F, Esposito G, Gravina A, Labonia V, et al. Endocrine effects of adjuvant letrozole compared with tamoxifen in hormone-responsive postmenopausal patients with early breast cancer: the HOBOE trial. J Clin Oncol. 2009;27:3192–7.
13. Bines J, Oleske DM, Cobleigh MA. Ovarian function in premenopausal women treated with adjuvant chemotherapy for breast cancer. J Clin Oncol. 1996;14:1718–29.
14. De Vos M, Devroey P, Fauser BC. Primary ovarian insufficiency. Lancet. 2010;376:911–21.
15. Torino F, Barnabei A, De Vecchis L, Appetecchia M, Strigari L, Corsello SM. Recognizing menopause in women with amenorrhea induced by cytotoxic chemotherapy for endocrine-responsive early breast cancer. Endocr Relat Cancer. 2012;19:R21–33.
16. Early Breast Cancer Trialists' Collaborative Group (EBCTCG), Davies C, Godwin J, Gray R, Clarke M, Cutter D, Darby S, et al. Relevance of breast cancer hormone receptors and other factors to the efficacy of adjuvant tamoxifen: patient-level meta-analysis of randomised trials. Lancet. 2011;378:771–84.
17. Lonning PE. Evolution of endocrine adjuvant therapy for early breast cancer. Expert Opin Investig Drugs. 2010;19(Suppl 1):S19–30.
18. Fisher B, Dignam J, Bryant J, DeCillis A, Wickerham DL, Wolmark N, et al. Five versus more than five years of tamoxifen therapy for breast cancer patients with negative lymph nodes and estrogen receptor-positive tumors. J Natl Cancer Inst. 1996;88:1529–42.
19. Stewart HJ, Forrest AP, Everington D, McDonald CC, Dewar JA, Hawkins RA, et al. Randomised comparison of 5 years of adjuvant tamoxifen with continuous therapy for operable breast cancer. the Scottish Cancer Trials Breast Group. Br J Cancer. 1996;74:297–9.
20. Davies C, Pan H, Godwin J, Gray R, Arriagada R, Raina V, et al. Long-term effects of continuing adjuvant tamoxifen to 10 years versus stopping at 5 years after diagnosis of oestrogen receptor-positive breast cancer: ATLAS, a randomised trial. Lancet. 2013;381:805–16.
21. Petrelli F, Coinu A, Cabiddu M, Ghilardi M, Lonati V, Barni S. Five or more years of adjuvant endocrine therapy in breast cancer: a meta-analysis of published randomised trials. Breast Cancer Res Treat. 2013;140:233–40.
22. Dowsett M, Allred C, Knox J, Quinn E, Salter J, Wale C, et al. Relationship between quantitative estrogen and progesterone receptor expression and human epidermal growth factor receptor 2 (HER-2) status with recurrence in the Arimidex, Tamoxifen, Alone or in Combination trial. J Clin Oncol. 2008;26:1059–65.
23. Regan MM, Leyland-Jones B, Bouzyk M, Pagani O, Tang W, Kammler R, et al. CYP2D6 genotype and tamoxifen response in postmenopausal women with endocrine-responsive breast cancer: the breast international group 1-98 trial. J Natl Cancer Inst. 2012;104:441–51.
24. Rae JM, Drury S, Hayes DF, Stearns V, Thibert JN, Haynes BP, et al. CYP2D6 and UGT2B7 genotype and risk of recurrence in tamoxifen-treated breast cancer patients. J Natl Cancer Inst. 2012;104:452–60.
25. LHRH-agonists in Early Breast Cancer Overview group, Cuzick J, Ambroisine L, Davidson N, Jakesz R, Kaufmann M, Regan M, et al. Use of luteinising-hormone-releasing hormone agonists as adjuvant treatment in premenopausal patients with hormone-receptor-positive breast cancer: a meta-analysis of individual patient data from randomised adjuvant trials. Lancet. 2007;369:1711–23.
26. Pagani O, Regan MM, Walley BA, Fleming GF, Colleoni M, Láng I, et al. Adjuvant exemestane with ovarian suppression in premenopausal breast cancer. N Engl J Med. 2014;371:107–18.
27. Anderson WF, Chatterjee N, Ershler WB, Brawley OW. Estrogen receptor breast cancer phenotypes in the Surveillance, Epidemiology, and End Results database. Breast Cancer Res Treat. 2002;76:27–36.
28. Dowsett M, Cuzick J, Ingle J, Coates A, Forbes J, Bliss J, et al. Meta-analysis of breast cancer outcomes in adjuvant trials of aromatase inhibitors versus tamoxifen. J Clin Oncol. 2010;28:509–18.

29. BIG 1-98 Collaborative Group, Mouridsen H, Giobbie-Hurder A, Goldhirsch A, Thürlimann B, Paridaens R, Smith I, et al. Letrozole therapy alone or in sequence with tamoxifen in women with breast cancer. N Engl J Med. 2009;361:766–76.
30. Regan MM, Neven P, Giobbie-Hurder A, Goldhirsch A, Ejlertsen B, Mauriac L, et al. Assessment of letrozole and tamoxifen alone and in sequence for postmenopausal women with steroid hormone receptor-positive breast cancer: the BIG 1-98 randomised clinical trial at 8.1 years median follow-up. Lancet Oncol. 2011;12:1101–8.
31. van de Velde CJ, Rea D, Seynaeve C, Putter H, Hasenburg A, Vannetzel JM, et al. Adjuvant tamoxifen and exemestane in early breast cancer (TEAM): a randomised phase 3 trial. Lancet. 2011;377:321–31.
32. Early Breast Cancer Trialists' Collaborative Group (EBCTCG). Aromatase inhibitors versus tamoxifen in early breast cancer: patient-level meta-analysis of the randomised trials. Lancet. 2015;386:1341–52.
33. Pan H, Gray R, Braybrooke J, Davies C, Taylor C, McGale P, et al. 20-year risks of breast-cancer recurrence after stopping endocrine therapy at 5 years. N Engl J Med. 2017;377(19):1836–46.
34. Goss PE, Ingle JN, Martino S, Robert NJ, Muss HB, Piccart MJ, et al. Randomized trial of letrozole following tamoxifen as extended adjuvant therapy in receptor-positive breast cancer: updated findings from NCIC CTG MA.17. J Natl Cancer Inst. 2005;97:1262–71.
35. Goss PE, Ingle JN, Pritchard KI, Robert NJ, Muss H, Gralow J, et al. Extending aromatase-inhibitor adjuvant therapy to 10 years. N Engl J Med. 2016;375(3):209–19.
36. Jakesz R, Greil R, Gnant M, Schmid M, Kwasny W, Kubista E, et al. Extended adjuvant therapy with anastrozole among postmenopausal breast cancer patients: results from the randomized Austrian Breast and Colorectal Cancer Study Group Trial 6a. J Natl Cancer Inst. 2007;99:1845–53.
37. Mamounas EP, Jeong JH, Wickerham DL, Smith RE, Ganz PA, Land SR, et al. Benefit from exemestane as extended adjuvant therapy after 5 years of adjuvant tamoxifen: intention-to-treat analysis of the National Surgical Adjuvant Breast And Bowel Project B-33 trial. J Clin Oncol. 2008;26:1965–71.
38. Mamounas EP, Bandos H, Lembersky BC. A randomized, double-blinded, placebo-controlled clinical trial of extended adjuvant endocrine therapy (tx) with letrozole (L) in postmenopausal women with hormone-receptor (+) breast cancer (BC) who have completed previous adjuvant tx with an aromatase inhibitor (AI): results from NRG Oncology/NSABP B-42. In: Presented at: 2016 San Antonio breast cancer symposium; December 6–10; San Antonio, TX, 2016.
39. Tjan-Heijnen VCG, van Hellemond IEG, Peer PGM, Swinkels ACP, Smorenburg CH, van der Sangen MJC, Dutch Breast Cancer Research Group (BOOG) for the DATA Investigators, et al. Extended adjuvant aromatase inhibition after sequential endocrine therapy (DATA): a randomised, phase 3 trial. Lancet Oncol. 2017;18:1502–11.
40. Blok EJ, Kroep JR, Meershoek-Klein Kranenbarg E, Duijm-de Carpentier M, Putter H, van den Bosch J, et al. IDEAL Study Group. Optimal duration of extended adjuvant endocrine therapy for early breast cancer; results of the IDEAL trial (BOOG 2006-05). J Natl Cancer Inst. 2018;110(1). https://doi.org/10.1093/jnci/djx134.
41. Goldvaser H, AlGorashi I, Ribnikar D, Seruga B, Templeton AJ, Ocana A, et al. Efficacy of extended adjuvant therapy with aromatase inhibitors in early breast cancer among common clinicopathologically-defined subgroups: a systematic review and meta-analysis. Cancer Treat Rev. 2017;60:53–9.
42. Colleoni M, Luo W, Karlsson P, Chirgwin J, Aebi S, Jerusalem G, SOLE Investigators, et al. Extended adjuvant intermittent letrozole versus continuous letrozole in postmenopausal women with breast cancer (SOLE): a multicentre, open-label, randomised, phase 3 trial. Lancet Oncol. 2018;19:127.
43. Viale G, Regan MM, Dell'Orto P, Mastropasqua MG, Maiorano E, Rasmussen BB, et al. Which patients benefit most from adjuvant aromatase inhibitors? Results using a composite measure of prognostic risk in the BIG 1-98 randomized trial. Ann Oncol. 2011;22:2201–7.
44. Dowsett M, Nielsen TO, A'Hern R, Bartlett J, Coombes RC, Cuzick J, et al. Assessment of Ki67 in breast cancer: recommendations from the International Ki67 in Breast Cancer working group. J Natl Cancer Inst. 2011;103:1656–64.

45. Dowsett M, Smith IE, Ebbs SR, Dixon JM, Skene A, A'Hern R, et al. Prognostic value of Ki67 expression after short-term presurgical endocrine therapy for primary breast cancer. J Natl Cancer Inst. 2007;99:167–70.
46. Geisler J, Haynes B, Anker G, Dowsett M, Lønning PE. Influence of letrozole and anastrozole on total body aromatization and plasma estrogen levels in postmenopausal breast cancer patients evaluated in a randomized, cross-over study. J Clin Oncol. 2002;20:751–7.
47. Dixon JM, Renshaw L, Young O, Murray J, Macaskill EJ, McHugh M, et al. Letrozole suppresses plasma estradiol and estrone sulphate more completely than anastrozole in postmenopausal women with breast cancer. J Clin Oncol. 2008;26:1671–6.
48. Ellis MJ, Suman VJ, Hoog J, Lin L, Snider J, Prat A, et al. Randomized phase II neoadjuvant comparison between letrozole, anastrozole, and exemestane for postmenopausal women with estrogen receptor-rich stage 2 to 3 breast cancer: clinical and biomarker outcomes and predictive value of the baseline PAM50-based intrinsic subtype—ACOSOG Z1031. J Clin Oncol. 2011;29:2342–9.
49. Curigliano G, Burstein HJ, Winer EP, Gnant M, Dubsky P, Loibl S, et al. De-escalating and escalating treatments for early-stage breast cancer: the St. Gallen International Expert Consensus Conference on the Primary Therapy of Early Breast Cancer 2017. Ann Oncol. 2017;28:1700–12.
50. Henry NL, Azzouz F, Desta Z, Li L, Nguyen AT, Lemler S, et al. Predictors of aromatase inhibitor discontinuation as a result of treatment-emergent symptoms in early-stage breast cancer. J Clin Oncol. 2012;30:936–42.
51. Aydiner A. Meta-analysis of breast cancer outcome and toxicity in adjuvant trials of aromatase inhibitors in postmenopausal women. Breast. 2013;22:121–9.

Chapter 18
Bone-Targeted Therapy in Early Breast Cancer

Ece Esin and Irfan Cicin

Introduction

Breast cancer is the most common malignancy in females worldwide, but it has a good prognosis if it is diagnosed in early stages. The estimated five-year overall survival rates exceed 89% following the initial diagnosis of early-stage breast cancer [1, 2]. Hence, the long-term toxicities of chemotherapeutics and other adjuvant therapies should be considered for breast cancer survivors.

Systemic therapies for treating early breast cancer can be associated with accelerated bone loss and an increased risk of osteoporotic fractures. Bone mineral density (BMD) can decrease as a result of a temporary or permanent suppression of ovarian function due to chemotherapy and/or the end organ effect of gonadotropin-releasing hormone (GnRH) agonists, aromatase inhibitors and tamoxifen.

This chapter focuses on the use of bone-targeted drugs for the preservation of BMD in adjuvant treatment, the long-term follow-up setting of early breast cancer, and the use of bone-targeted agents to aid adjuvant therapy to impact breast cancer outcomes.

E. Esin
Department of Medical Oncology, Dr. A. Y. Ankara Oncology Education and Research Hospital, Ankara, Turkey

I. Cicin (✉)
Department of Medical Oncology, Faculty of Medicine, Balkan Oncology Hospital, Trakya University of Medicine, Edirne, Turkey
e-mail: irfancicin@trakya.edu.tr

A. Aydiner et al. (eds.), *Breast Cancer*, https://doi.org/10.1007/978-3-319-96947-3_18

Breast Cancer-Associated Bone Loss

Epidemiology of Breast Cancer Treatment-Associated Bone Loss

Epidemiology in Premenopausal Women

Under normal conditions, estrogen plays a key role in maintaining bone integrity and density to ensure that a premenopausal woman's bones are healthy and strong. Premenopausal women face osteoporosis secondary to the effects of systemic therapies [3, 4]. Chemotherapeutics may result in temporary or permanent ovarian failure; tamoxifen alone or in conjunction with gonadotropin-releasing hormone antagonists (GnRHa) or supportive medicines such as glucocorticoids lead to a prematurely induced osteoporotic state that puts women with a history of breast cancer at risk of osteoporosis and osteoporotic complications.

A woman diagnosed with breast cancer in early life has an anticipated long life expectancy, which demands necessary measures to screen, diagnose and treat osteoporosis. Premenopausal women should be reviewed and assessed for the risk of bone loss, and a dual-energy X-ray absorptiometry (DEXA) scan can be offered. The risk of bone loss is related to the age of diagnosis, the age of initial treatment and the type of treatment. According to the results of observational studies, bone mineral density (BMD) decreases by 3–8% after 12 months of chemotherapy in the premenopausal stage [5, 6]. Tamoxifen has been shown to cause bone loss alone both in the adjuvant setting and with GnRHa [7–10]. The accelerated bone loss of early artificial menopause versus the delayed, longstanding bone loss that proceeds over years have not been formally compared, and the fracture risk of decreased BMD has not been proven. Finally, it is not yet clear how the DEXA value changes fracture effects.

Epidemiology in Postmenopausal Women

Postmenopausal women have a significantly increased risk of osteoporosis and skeletal events after the diagnosis of cancer. Preliminary studies have shown that postmenopausal women with breast cancer are at risk of osteoporosis due to chemotherapy [11]. Subgroup analyses of the Women Health Initiative Study revealed that in both the prospective and observational study groups, women faced increased BMD loss after the diagnosis of cancer as well as increased risks of falls and fractures [12–14]. Women receiving adjuvant chemotherapy may lose 1–10% of bone mass per year of chemotherapy [11].

Adjuvant hormonotherapy has been more thoroughly studied in postmenopausal women. It is well known that adjuvant aromatase inhibitors have a class effect of accelerated bone loss and promotion of fractures. By contrast, the end organ effect of tamoxifen as a selective estrogen receptor modulator may induce bone stabilization [7, 8, 15].

Prevention of Breast Cancer Treatment-Associated Bone Loss

Prevention in Premenopausal Women

The main preventive measures in premenopausal women are to avoid factors that increase bone loss by eliminating smoking, controlling thyroid hormone functions and optimizing vitamin D and calcium intake. If the osteoporosis risk is estimated to be high, pharmacologic intervention is required.

In premenopausal women, bisphosphonates are proven to preserve the bone reserve when used in patients with early secondary ovarian failure either due to chemotherapy or GnRHa use. Although BMD is preserved, there are less data on fracture prevention and the timing of bisphosphonate initiation and risk reduction. In premenopausal women with decreased BMD secondary to all causes, bisphosphonates could be started after necessary changes and measures are implemented [16].

There are some small-size studies of the use of medications in women with breast cancer. Clodronate, risedronate, pamidronate and zoledronic acid are among the bisphosphonates studied in premenopausal breast cancer patients [7, 9, 18, 19].

The CALGB 70809 (Cancer and Leukemia Group B) Trial 79809 enrolled early breast cancer patients requiring adjuvant chemotherapy who were at least 40 years old and investigated the efficacy of zoledronic acid on BMD [20]. Zoledronic acid was given either as an upfront therapy of 4 mg every 3 months for 2 years or delayed to begin 1 year after randomization. All participants were advised and self-reported to take daily intake of 400 IU of vitamin D with 1000 mg calcium. In 1 year, 150 of 439 women developed chemotherapy-induced secondary ovarian failure. Zoledronic acid was found to be associated with an increase in lumbar spine BMD, and delayed use was reported as the preferred sequence.

Results for zoledronic acid were reported in ABCSG (The Austrian Breast and Colorectal Cancer Study Group)-12 trial as a subgroup analysis [7]. This trial was a four-arm study in which tamoxifen with goserelin and anastrozole with goserelin were compared either with zoledronic acid or alone. Patients were given zoledronic acid 4 mg every 6 months. The results showed that BMD decreased significantly with endocrine therapy, but the decrease was highest with anastrozole. Zoledronic acid was significantly associated with the stabilization of BMD.

Prevention in Postmenopausal Women

Postmenopausal women are a population at high risk for osteoporosis due to age and gender. Adjuvant endocrine therapy is associated with additional loss of bone mass. Many postmenopausal women who are diagnosed with breast cancer receive chemotherapy and adjuvant endocrine hormonotherapy, which have been proven to decrease BMD further. These patients should be screened for vitamin D deficiency; BMD can be evaluated by DEXA, and if a risk of osteoporosis and fracture is found, bisphosphonates may be indicated [11, 12, 14, 21]. Denosumab is a fully humanized monoclonal antibody to the receptor activator of nuclear factor kappa-B (RANK) ligand. This ligand is responsible for osteoclastic differentiation; thereby, denosumab inhibits osteoclast differentiation and prevents bone loss. In the ABCSG-18 trial, denosumab 60 mg twice yearly was shown to decrease osteoporotic fractures in postmenopausal women associated with aromatase inhibitor therapy [17].

Impact of Bone-Targeted Treatment on Breast Cancer Outcomes

The Role of Adjuvant Bisphosphonates

Although there is a clear role of bisphosphonates in preventing osteoporosis and related bone fractures, the data supporting their use as adjuvant treatment in early breast cancer are continuously evolving.

Circulating tumor cells may stay dormant in body and can be attracted years later to surfaces within the bones. Binding of these cells to osteoblastic niches can result in the development of bone metastases [22]. The hypothesis of adjuvant bisphosphonate treatment developed from the fact that bisphosphonate has a negative effect on osteoclasts and affects T-cell function [23, 24]. Consequently, bisphosphonate can delay or prevent bone recurrences [25]. Thus, in addition to the use of bisphosphonate for osteoporosis prevention in postmenopausal women, Bisphosphonate can be added to adjuvant treatment for the prevention of bone recurrences. However, the data showing that bisphosphonates improve bone metastasis-free survival, disease-free survival and overall survival are controversial.

Oral clodronate and zoledronic acid were shown to be effective in some adjuvant trials [26–28]. However, in other trials, no significant benefit or some benefit was achieved only in postmenopausal or ovarian-suppressed [29–31]. In an individual data meta-analysis by EBCTCG (Early Breast Cancer Trialist' Collaborative Group), there was a definitive benefit of bisphosphonate in improving breast cancer-specific survival rates only in postmenopausal women [32]. The Cochrane analyses clearly determined overall survival and disease-free survival benefits for postmenopausal women [33]. However, current guidelines are generally in favor of the addition of bisphosphonates to adjuvant treatment: a European Panel consensus recommends zoledronic acid 4 mg iv twice yearly or oral clodronate 1600 mg daily for a period of 3–5 years, especially in ovarian-suppressed premenopausal women and postmenopausal women at intermediate-high risk [34]. By contrast, ASCO advises considering the addition of bisphosphonate when systemic adjuvant therapy is planned [35]. There are scarce data showing an advantage of one bisphosphonate over another. However, there is insufficient evidence on adjuvant alendronate or risedronate for improving breast cancer-specific survival rates. In the SWOG (Southwest Oncology Group) S0307 study, oral clodronate, oral ibandronate (50 mg oral daily) and zoledronic acid were compared in the adjuvant setting [36]. The SWOG S0307 results showed that oral therapy was preferred to iv zoledronic acid.

This study did not have a control arm; hence the data do not support bisphosphonate to improve survival outcomes. There is no clear evidence of the dose or duration of bisphosphonate treatment as adjuvant therapy in early breast cancer; the doses used in osteoporosis treatment (zoledronic acid. 4 mg twice yearly and oral clodronate 1600 mg per day) for a duration of 3–5 years are the preferred regimens.

The Role of Adjuvant Anti-Rank Ligand

Denosumab as an osteoclast differentiation inhibitor may have a role in preventing osteoporosis-related fractures and may increase breast cancer-specific survival rates; however, the data are not yet mature. EBCST-18 was a phase III, randomized study enrolling postmenopausal hormone receptor-positive breast cancer patients. In this study, patients were randomized one-to-one to either denosumab 60 mg twice yearly or placebo. The primary endpoint was to show a decrease in fractures, and PFS was a secondary endpoint. Patients who received denosumab experienced less fractures, and DFS was in favor of the denosumab arm in four-year follow-up. Further final results of denosumab studies are awaited to draw conclusions about its efficacy in the survival rates of early breast cancer (NCT01077154).

Toxicity Related to Bone-Targeted Therapy

Despite the overall beneficial effects of bisphosphonates and denosumab, these agents are not without adverse events and have some common relatively predictable toxicities. In general, they may result in acute-phase reactions, hypocalcemia, and osteonecrosis of the jaw (ONJ). Oral bisphosphonates may result in some degree of gastrointestinal irritation. Occasionally, subcutaneous local reactions are observed with denosumab [37, 38]. In randomized studies, both medications resulted in serious side effects at the same rates, and treatment discontinuation rates due to adverse events were similar for both agents [39]. Acute-phase reactions are flu-like symptoms, which usually occur within 3 days and may be observed in 10% of patients taking bisphosphonates or denosumab [40]. Paracetamol, nonsteroidal anti-inflammatories with caution for the glomerular filtration rate and antipyretics can be used for symptomatic treatment [41].

Bisphosphonates are excreted from the kidneys, and their metabolism is highly dependent on the glomerular filtration rate (GFR) and the applied dose. Among bisphosphonates, zoledronic acid is the most frequently reported cause of renal failure [42, 43]. The renal toxicity of zoledronic acid may be reversible, but pamidronate is associated with nephrotic syndrome, which may not be reversible [44, 45]. By contrast, denosumab is relatively safe in renal aspects compared to bisphosphonates. In patients with normal function as well as patients with a decreased GFR, denosumab can be safely administered without any dose change [35, 37, 38, 46]. To avoid bisphosphonate-induced nephrotoxicity, patients should be screened for GFR before each bisphosphonate application, and bisphosphonates should not be given if the GFR is below 30 ml/min.

Hypocalcemia is a shared toxicity of bisphosphonates and denosumab and is related to antiresorptive activities. The risk of hypocalcemia is higher if there is a pre-existing vitamin D deficiency, hypothyroidism or hypoparathyroidism. Bisphosphonates have a relatively lower risk of hypocalcemia development compared to denosumab [39]. The risk of denosumab-associated hypocalcemia is especially high if the GFR is below 30 ml/min; therefore, precautions should be taken, such as proper administration of supplemental calcium and vitamin D.

Osteonecrosis of the jaw is one of the most debilitating complications of bone targeting in malignancies and is well recognized. It is related to osteonecrosis of the mandible and/or maxilla. Apart from the use of bisphosphonates or denosumab, poor oral hygiene and preceding oral interventions such as tooth extraction has been defined as risk factors. The risk of ONJ increases continuously with repeated doses and lower intervals of bone-targeted agent use [47]. No statistically significant difference was observed in the ONJ rates between denosumab and bisphosphonates [47, 48]. Although there is a class-generated toxicity of ONJ in bisphosphonates, nitrogen-containing zoledronic acid is more responsible for ONJ than are pamidronate and ibandronate [49]. To avoid ONJ, preventive measures such as oral hygiene, regular dental care and avoiding dental procedures should be taken.

Conclusion

Systemic adjuvant chemotherapy and hormonotherapy may result in osteoporosis in both premenopausal and postmenopausal women diagnosed with early breast cancer. Bisphosphonates and denosumab have proven efficacy in the prevention and treatment of secondary osteoporosis associated with treatment modalities. Evidence supporting a survival benefit of bone-targeted agents is evolving but mainly involves postmenopausal patients. The toxicity of bone–targeted agents should be kept in mind, and the necessary precautions should be taken.

References

1. Iqbal J, Ginsburg O, Rochon PA, Sun P, Narod SA. Differences in breast cancer stage at diagnosis and cancer-specific survival by race and ethnicity in the United States. JAMA. 2015;313:165–73.
2. Howlader N, Cronin KA, Kurian AW, Andridge R. Differences in breast cancer survival by molecular subtypes in the United States. Cancer Epidemiol Biomark Prev. 2018;27:619.
3. Greep NC, Giuliano AE, Hansen NM, Taketani T, Wang HJ, Singer FR. The effects of adjuvant chemotherapy on bone density in postmenopausal women with early breast cancer. Am J Med. 2003;114:653–9.

4. Lustberg MB, Reinbolt RE, Shapiro CL. Bone health in adult cancer survivorship. J Clin Oncol. 2012;30:3665–74.
5. Shapiro CL, Manola J, Leboff M. Ovarian failure after adjuvant chemotherapy is associated with rapid bone loss in women with early-stage breast cancer. J Clin Oncol. 2001;19:3306–11.
6. Saarto T, Blomqvist C, Valimaki M, Makela P, Sarna S, Elomaa I. Chemical castration induced by adjuvant cyclophosphamide, methotrexate, and fluorouracil chemotherapy causes rapid bone loss that is reduced by clodronate: a randomized study in premenopausal breast cancer patients. J Clin Oncol. 1997;15:1341–7.
7. Gnant MF, Mlineritsch B, Luschin-Ebengreuth G, Grampp S, Kaessmann H, Schmid M, et al. Zoledronic acid prevents cancer treatment-induced bone loss in premenopausal women receiving adjuvant endocrine therapy for hormone-responsive breast cancer: a report from the Austrian Breast and Colorectal Cancer Study Group. J Clin Oncol. 2007;25:820–8.
8. Powles TJ, Hickish T, Kanis JA, Tidy A, Ashley S. Effect of tamoxifen on bone mineral density measured by dual-energy x-ray absorptiometry in healthy premenopausal and postmenopausal women. J Clin Oncol. 1996;14:78–84.
9. Delmas PD, Balena R, Confravreux E, Hardouin C, Hardy P, Bremond A. Bisphosphonate risedronate prevents bone loss in women with artificial menopause due to chemotherapy of breast cancer: a double-blind, placebo-controlled study. J Clin Oncol. 1997;15:955–62.
10. Vehmanen L, Elomaa I, Blomqvist C, Saarto T. Tamoxifen treatment after adjuvant chemotherapy has opposite effects on bone mineral density in premenopausal patients depending on menstrual status. J Clin Oncol. 2006;24:675–80.
11. Van Poznak CPM, D'Andrea G, Schott A, Griggs J, Fornier M, Smerage J, et al. Bone mineral density (BMD) changes at 1 year in postmenopausal women who are not receiving adjuvant endocrine therapy for breast cancer (BCA). In: San Antonio breast cancer conference, USA; 2009. Abstract no. 1066.
12. Chen Z, Maricic M, Pettinger M, Ritenbaugh C, Lopez AM, Barad DH, et al. Osteoporosis and rate of bone loss among postmenopausal survivors of breast cancer. Cancer. 2005;104:1520–30.
13. Chen Z, Maricic M, Bassford TL, Pettinger M, Ritenbaugh C, Lopez AM, et al. Fracture risk among breast cancer survivors: results from the Women's Health Initiative Observational Study. Arch Intern Med. 2005;165:552–8.
14. Chen Z, Maricic M, Aragaki AK, Mouton C, Arendell L, Lopez AM, et al. Fracture risk increases after diagnosis of breast or other cancers in postmenopausal women: results from the Women's Health Initiative. Osteoporos Int. 2009;20:527–36.
15. Love RR, Mazess RB, Barden HS, Epstein S, Newcomb PA, Jordan VC, et al. Effects of tamoxifen on bone mineral density in postmenopausal women with breast cancer. N Engl J Med. 1992;326:852–6.
16. Abraham A, Cohen A, Shane E. Premenopausal bone health: osteoporosis in premenopausal women. Clin Obstet Gynecol. 2013;56:722–9.
17. Gnant M, Pfeiler G, Dubsky PC, Hubalek M, Greil R, Jakesz R, et al. Adjuvant denosumab in breast cancer (ABCSG-18): a multicentre, randomised, double-blind, placebo-controlled trial. Lancet. 2015;386:433–43.
18. Fuleihan Gel H, Salamoun M, Mourad YA, Chehal A, Salem Z, Mahfoud Z, et al. Pamidronate in the prevention of chemotherapy-induced bone loss in premenopausal women with breast cancer: a randomized controlled trial. J Clin Endocrinol Metab. 2005;90:3209–14.
19. Vehmanen L, Saarto T, Elomaa I, Makela P, Valimaki M, Blomqvist C. Long-term impact of chemotherapy-induced ovarian failure on bone mineral density (BMD) in premenopausal breast cancer patients. The effect of adjuvant clodronate treatment. Eur J Cancer. 2001;37:2373–8.
20. Shapiro CL, Halabi S, Hars V, Archer L, Weckstein D, Kirshner J, et al. Zoledronic acid preserves bone mineral density in premenopausal women who develop ovarian failure due to adjuvant chemotherapy: final results from CALGB trial 79809. Eur J Cancer. 2011;47:683–9.
21. Reid DM, Doughty J, Eastell R, Heys SD, Howell A, McCloskey EV, et al. Guidance for the management of breast cancer treatment-induced bone loss: a consensus position statement from a UK Expert Group. Cancer Treat Rev. 2008;34(Suppl 1):S3–18.

22. Weilbaecher KN, Guise TA, McCauley LK. Cancer to bone: a fatal attraction. Nat Rev Cancer. 2011;11:411–25.
23. Thompson K, Roelofs AJ, Jauhiainen M, Monkkonen H, Monkkonen J, Rogers MJ. Activation of gammadelta T cells by bisphosphonates. Adv Exp Med Biol. 2010;658:11–20.
24. Roodman GD. Mechanisms of bone metastasis. N Engl J Med. 2004;350:1655–64.
25. Kanis JA, Powles T, Paterson AH, McCloskey EV, Ashley S. Clodronate decreases the frequency of skeletal metastases in women with breast cancer. Bone. 1996;19:663–7.
26. Gnant M, Mlineritsch B, Schippinger W, Luschin-Ebengreuth G, Postlberger S, Menzel C, et al. Endocrine therapy plus zoledronic acid in premenopausal breast cancer. N Engl J Med. 2009;360:679–91.
27. Powles T, Paterson A, McCloskey E, Schein P, Scheffler B, Tidy A, et al. Reduction in bone relapse and improved survival with oral clodronate for adjuvant treatment of operable breast cancer [ISRCTN83688026]. Breast Cancer Res. 2006;8:R13.
28. Diel IJ, Jaschke A, Solomayer EF, Gollan C, Bastert G, Sohn C, et al. Adjuvant oral clodronate improves the overall survival of primary breast cancer patients with micrometastases to the bone marrow: a long-term follow-up. Ann Oncol. 2008;19:2007–11.
29. von Minckwitz G, Mobus V, Schneeweiss A, Huober J, Thomssen C, Untch M, et al. German adjuvant intergroup node-positive study: a phase III trial to compare oral ibandronate versus observation in patients with high-risk early breast cancer. J Clin Oncol. 2013;31:3531–9.
30. Paterson AH, Anderson SJ, Lembersky BC, Fehrenbacher L, Falkson CI, King KM, et al. Oral clodronate for adjuvant treatment of operable breast cancer (National Surgical Adjuvant Breast and Bowel Project protocol B-34): a multicentre, placebo-controlled, randomised trial. Lancet Oncol. 2012;13:734–42.
31. Coleman R, Cameron D, Dodwell D, Bell R, Wilson C, Rathbone E, et al. Adjuvant zoledronic acid in patients with early breast cancer: final efficacy analysis of the AZURE (BIG 01/04) randomised open-label phase 3 trial. Lancet Oncol. 2014;15:997–1006.
32. Early Breast Cancer Trialists' Collaborative Group. Adjuvant bisphosphonate treatment in early breast cancer: meta-analyses of individual patient data from randomised trials. Lancet. 2015;386:1353–61.
33. O'Carrigan B, Wong MH, Willson ML, Stockler MR, Pavlakis N, Goodwin A. Bisphosphonates and other bone agents for breast cancer. Cochrane Database Syst Rev. 2017;10:CD003474.
34. Hadji P, Coleman RE, Wilson C, Powles TJ, Clezardin P, Aapro M, et al. Adjuvant bisphosphonates in early breast cancer: consensus guidance for clinical practice from a European Panel. Ann Oncol. 2016;27:379–90.
35. Dhesy-Thind S, Fletcher GG, Blanchette PS, Clemons MJ, Dillmon MS, Frank ES, et al. Use of adjuvant bisphosphonates and other bone-modifying agents in breast cancer: a Cancer Care Ontario and American Society of Clinical Oncology clinical practice guideline. J Clin Oncol. 2017;35:2062–81.
36. Gralow J, Barlow WE, Paterson AHG, Lew D, Stopeck A, Hayes DF, et al. SWOG S0307 phase III trial of bisphosphonates as adjuvant therapy in primary breast cancer: comparison of toxicities and patient-stated preference for oral versus intravenous delivery. J Clin Oncol. 2014;32:558.
37. Prommer E. Palliative oncology: denosumab. Am J Hosp Palliat Care. 2015;32:568–72.
38. Anghel R, Bachmann A, Beksac M, Brodowicz T, Finek J, Komadina R, et al. Expert opinion 2011 on the use of new anti-resorptive agents in the prevention of skeletal-related events in metastatic bone disease. Wien Klin Wochenschr. 2013;125:439–47.
39. Stopeck AT, Lipton A, Body JJ, Steger GG, Tonkin K, de Boer RH, et al. Denosumab compared with zoledronic acid for the treatment of bone metastases in patients with advanced breast cancer: a randomized, double-blind study. J Clin Oncol. 2010;28:5132–9.
40. Thiebaud D, Sauty A, Burckhardt P, Leuenberger P, Sitzler L, Green JR, et al. An in vitro and in vivo study of cytokines in the acute-phase response associated with bisphosphonates. Calcif Tissue Int. 1997;61:386–92.

41. Wark JD, Bensen W, Recknor C, Ryabitseva O, Chiodo J 3rd, Mesenbrink P, et al. Treatment with acetaminophen/paracetamol or ibuprofen alleviates post-dose symptoms related to intravenous infusion with zoledronic acid 5 mg. Osteoporos Int. 2012;23:503–12.
42. Tanvetyanon T, Stiff PJ. Management of the adverse effects associated with intravenous bisphosphonates. Ann Oncol. 2006;17:897–907.
43. Berenson JR, Vescio RA, Rosen LS, VonTeichert JM, Woo M, Swift R, et al. A phase I dose-ranging trial of monthly infusions of zoledronic acid for the treatment of osteolytic bone metastases. Clin Cancer Res. 2001;7:478–85.
44. Markowitz GS, Fine PL, Stack JI, Kunis CL, Radhakrishnan J, Palecki W, et al. Toxic acute tubular necrosis following treatment with zoledronate (Zometa). Kidney Int. 2003;64:281–9.
45. Markowitz GS, Fine PL, D'Agati VD. Nephrotic syndrome after treatment with pamidronate. Am J Kidney Dis. 2002;39:1118–22.
46. Domschke C, Schuetz F. Side effects of bone-targeted therapies in advanced breast cancer. Breast Care. 2014;9:332–6.
47. Campisi G, Fedele S, Fusco V, Pizzo G, Di Fede O, Bedogni A. Epidemiology, clinical manifestations, risk reduction and treatment strategies of jaw osteonecrosis in cancer patients exposed to antiresorptive agents. Future Oncol. 2014;10:257–75.
48. Wang X, Yang KH, Wanyan P, Tian JH. Comparison of the efficacy and safety of denosumab versus bisphosphonates in breast cancer and bone metastases treatment: a meta-analysis of randomized controlled trials. Oncol Lett. 2014;7:1997–2002.
49. Diel IJ. Bisphosphonates in breast cancer patients with bone metastases. Breast Care. 2010;5:306–11.

Part VII
Breast Cancer Radiotherapy

Chapter 19
Early-Stage Breast Cancer Radiotherapy

Kamuran Arslan Ibis, Makbule Tambas, and Seden Kucucuk

Introduction

In early breast cancer, the need for radiotherapy (RT) depends on the surgery type, lymph node (LN) status and T stage. In this chapter, RT for in situ disease and invasive disease, boost RT, accelerated partial-breast irradiation, hypofractionation, and regional lymphatic irradiation are discussed.

Radiotherapy in Ductal Carcinoma In Situ Disease

In ductal carcinoma in situ (DCIS), breast RT following surgery with clear margins has been shown to decrease in-breast relapse rates by approximately one half without a survival benefit or distant metastasis-free survival benefit in prospective randomized trials [1]. In a recently published systematic review and meta-analysis of 5 prospective and 21 retrospective studies including 9391 DCIS patients with ≥10 years follow-up, local recurrence was found 2.6%, 13.6%, 25.5%, and 27.8% for mastectomy, breast-conserving surgery (BCS) with RT, BCS without RT and biopsy only, respectively. In addition, the local recurrence rates were reduced with the addition of RT + tamoxifen (TAM) to BCS, with local recurrence rates of 9.7% for BCS + RT + TAM; 14.1% for BCS + RT; 24.7% for BCS + TAM; and 25.1% for BCS ($p < 0.0001$). Furthermore, triple treatment modalities including BCS, RT and TAM led to lower rates of local invasive relapse compared with BCS alone (odds ratio (OR): 2.61, $p < 0.0001$),

K. Arslan Ibis (✉) · S. Kucucuk
Istanbul Medical Faculty, Department of Radiation Oncology, Istanbul University, Institute of Oncology, Istanbul, Turkey

M. Tambas
Department of Radiation Oncology, University of Health Sciences, Okmeydanı Training and Research Hospital, Istanbul, Turkey

A. Aydiner et al. (eds.), *Breast Cancer*, https://doi.org/10.1007/978-3-319-96947-3_19

BCS + TAM (OR: 2.52, p = 0.001), and BCS + RT (OR: 1.59, p = 0.022). By contrast, breast cancer-related death rates were similar among the mastectomy, BCS ± RT (1.3–2%) and biopsy-only groups (2.7%) [2].

If total *mastectomy* is performed with negative margins, there is no need for adjuvant irradiation rates since total mastectomy provides local control rates equivalent to those of excision and breast RT [3–5]. In cases operated with nipple-sparing mastectomy and reconstruction, irradiation of the nipple-areola complex is not standard. Breast tissue that is inadvertently left under the skin flaps should not be an indication for postoperative RT.

In cases treated with *lumpectomy*, adjuvant RT using partial-breast irradiation (PBI) techniques is under investigation in randomized trials, and this approach is considered "suitable" for DCIS that meets all criteria (detected by screening, low to intermediate nuclear grade, size ≥2.5 cm, and negative margins at ≥3 mm) and "unsuitable" for DCIS with size >3 cm by the American Society for Radiation Oncology (ASTRO) and other groups [6–9]. Lumpectomy without RT has been investigated in prospective and randomized trials in patients who are considered to be at low risk of local recurrence [10, 11]. Common sense in such low-risk DCIS patients is to consider whole-breast RT by decision making with the patient while taking age, comorbidity, radiation risks, patient preference, and salvage options into account. To consider a patient as a low-risk DCIS case, the following criteria must be present: mammographic detection, no palpable mass, lesion size smaller than 2.5 cm, nuclear grade I or II, and clear surgical margins of at least 3 mm [12]. All other cases of DCIS treated with lumpectomy are candidates for whole-breast irradiation [4, 13–15].

The recently defined adequate *surgical margin* for DCIS is 2 mm for patients treated with BCS and whole-breast RT in the consensus guidelines of Society of Surgical Oncology (SSO), American Society of Clinical Oncology (ASCO), and ASTRO [16]. However, close margins at the chest wall or skin do not warrant re-excision for DCIS, but a higher boost dose can be given to the involved lumpectomy site. Boost to the tumor bed may be an indication particularly for patients ≤50 years of age with negative margins to minimize local recurrence [17].

The safety and efficacy of *hypofractionation* (40–42 Gy/15–16 fraction) and boost for DCIS compared with conventional fractionation were shown in a meta-analysis by Nelson et al. Patients with positive margins benefited from boost to the tumor bed in this analysis [18]. In addition, an increase in the 15-year local control rate was reported for DCIS patients who received boost treatment in a multicenter retrospective study presented during the ASCO annual meeting in 2016 (91.6% vs. 88.0%, p = 0.013) [19]. The results of ongoing randomized trials are pending to clarify the roles of hypofractionation (the TROG 07.01 trial) and boost RT (the TROG 07.01 trial (NCT00470236) and the Bonbis trial (NCT00907868)) in patients with DCIS.

Radiotherapy in Invasive Disease

Postmastectomy radiotherapy (PMRT) in patients with 4 or more LNs with metastatic involvement is the standard of care [20] (Figs. 19.1 and 19.2). However, the benefit of PMRT in patients with 1–3 involved nodes was more controversial until recently. Although some trials from the 1990s showed a benefit for PMRT in patients with involvement of 1–3 nodes, these trials were criticized for using substandard chemotherapy and having unusually high locoregional recurrence rates without PMRT compared to other studies [21–23]. A recent meta-analysis showed more evidence of a benefit of PMRT in 1–3 nodes involved patients [24]. In addition, indirect evidence from a Canadian randomized trial showed benefit (in terms of locoregional control and disease-free survival but not overall survival) for regional nodal and breast/chest wall irradiation in patients with less than 3 involved nodes [25]. PMRT has been shown to provide no benefit in pathologically node-negative patients with at least 1-mm negative surgical margins [24–26]. NSABP trials analyzed collectively showed no benefit of PMRT in T3N0MX patients [27].

Recently, ASCO, ASTRO and SSO updated the guidelines on PMRT. The panel recommended PMRT for patients with T1–2 breast cancer with 1–3 positive LNs, although it was stated that the benefit and potential toxicities should be discussed with low-risk older patients with a limited life expectancy. In addition, PMRT is recommended in patients with T1–2 tumors and positive SLNB who have not undergone completion ALND and in clinical stage I or II cancer patients with positive axillary LNs after neoadjuvant chemotherapy. Moreover, the inclusion of both the mammaria interna and supraclavicular-axillary apical nodes in the PMRT field is recommended in patients with T1–2 tumors with 1–3 positive axillary nodes [28].

After lumpectomy, whole-breast RT is still considered the standard of care [29–32] (Fig. 19.3). A meta-analysis showed a statistically significant increase in in-breast control and a decrease in breast cancer-specific deaths [33]. However, controversial results have been reported for accelerated partial-breast irradiation (APBI) in patients with a low risk of local recurrence. Two large randomized APBI trials showed higher in-breast recurrences in patients treated with APBI compared to treatment with whole-breast RT [34, 35]. By contrast, a recently published randomized, phase 3, non-inferiority trial found that 5-year local control and side effects were similar between APBI using sole interstitial multi catheter brachyther-

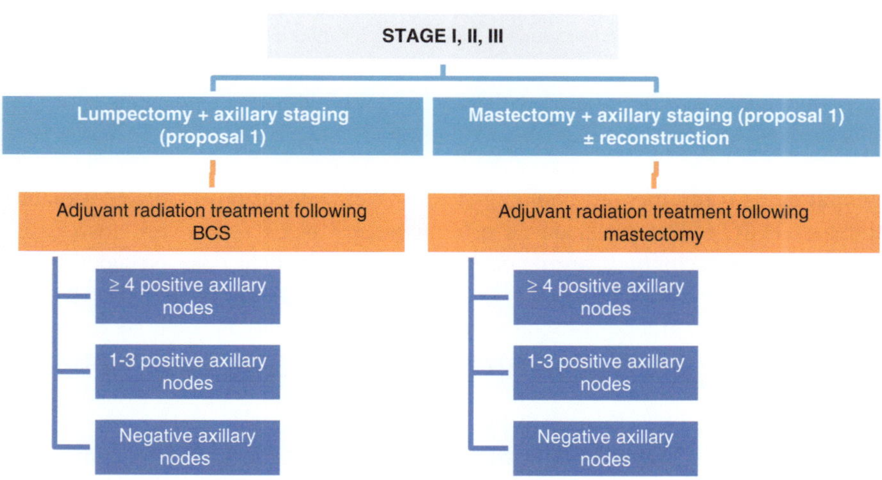

Fig. 19.1 Evaluation for adjuvant radiotherapy after breast-conserving surgery or mastectomy

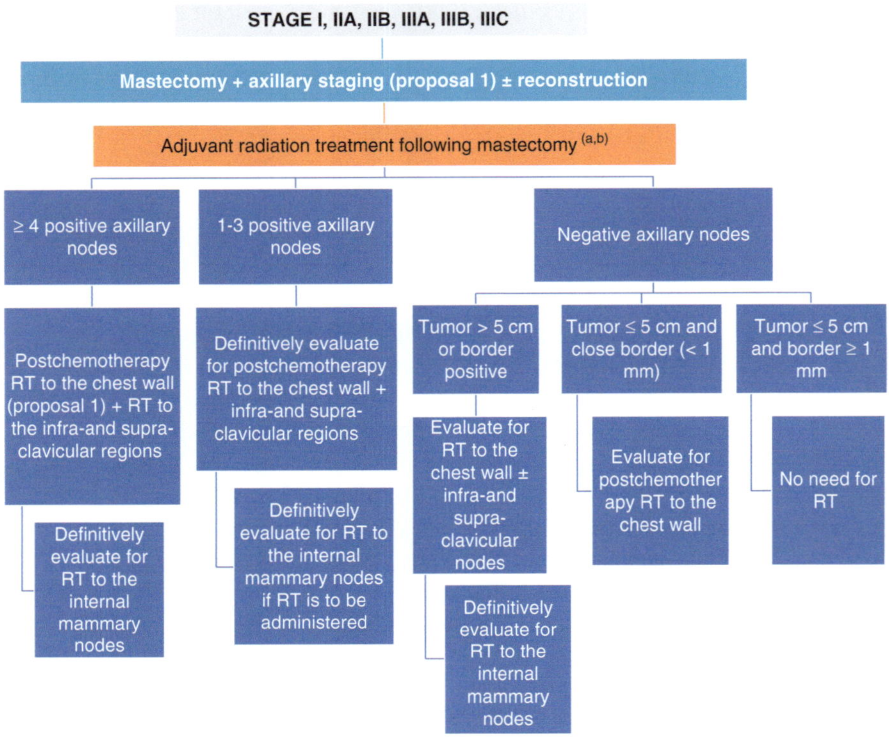

Fig. 19.2 Adjuvant radiotherapy (RT) after mastectomy. [a]RT following chemotherapy if chemotherapy is indicated. [b]Post-mastectomy RT is standard for patients who meet the following criteria: T size ≥5 cm (node negative); 1–3 nodes with adverse pathology [this is not the sole criterion in patients of young age (<40); 4 or more positive axillary LNs; and positive sentinel lymph node biopsy with no axillary dissection. The tumor biology should be considered together with tumor size and stage in the decision for RT after mastectomy. For pN1 low-risk findings, RT should be performed after having considered the toxicity risks after mastectomy, and doing so is more important if the patient is to undergo breast reconstruction. Patients with pT1–pT2, pN1 (1–3) and favorable biological features should be evaluated for omitting RT after mastectomy

apy and whole-breast irradiation with boost after breast-conserving surgery for low-risk invasive and in situ carcinoma of the female breast [36]. CT-based treatment planning should be used for target delineation. The most popular technique is tangential fields using forward planning (field-in-field) intensity-modulated radiation therapy (IMRT). The preferred dose homogeneity is ±7%. For left-sided cases, breath-holding techniques are recommended. The classical dose provided to the whole breast is 45-50.4 Gy in 25–28 fractions, with an additional boost dose of 10–16 Gy in 2 Gy fractions to the tumor bed. In patients older than 50 years with T1/T2N0 disease and clear surgical margins, hypofractionated whole-breast irradiation at 42.5 Gy/16 fractions should be considered for both convenience and effectiveness. Revised ASTRO guideline in 2018, doesn't take into account the age and previous adjuvant chemotherapy administration when considering hypofractionation for whole breast; recommended doses/fractions are 40Gy/15 or 42.5/16.

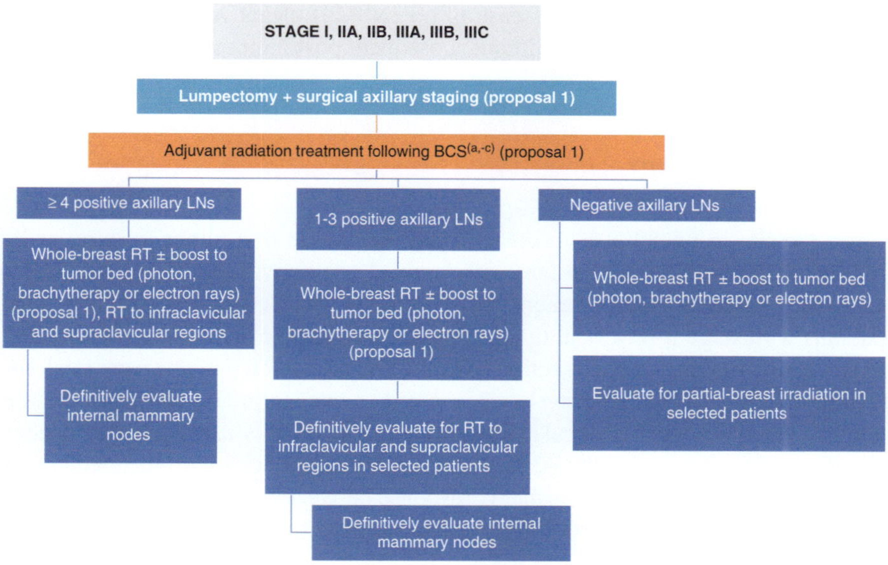

Fig. 19.3 Adjuvant radiotherapy (RT) after breast-conserving surgery (BCS). [a]RT following chemotherapy if chemotherapy is indicated. [b]Following BCS, hypofractionated whole-breast irradiation may be used in patients without prior chemotherapy or axillary lymph node involvement, in patients 50 years of age or older and in patients <50 years of age. According to the results of a clinical trial that randomized low-risk early-stage breast cancer patients, accelerated partial-breast RT was not inferior to standard whole-breast RT. Partial-breast RT can be performed in ASTRO/ESTRO "eligible" low-risk patients, although there are insufficient data in the literature (at St Gallen 2017: 67% yes, 24% no). Whole-breast RT should be performed in other patients. Boost therapy may not be performed in patients aged 60 years or older, patients with low-grade tumors having favorable tumor biology and/or patients who will receive adjuvant endocrine therapy. Regional node irradiation (RNI) prolongs disease-free survival in high-risk patients, but the risk of toxicity increases and may lead to complications during reconstruction surgery. At St. Gallen 2017, RNI was recommended in pN1 (1–3 positive lymph nodes) in the presence of unfavorable clinical features (40 years and younger, unfavorable tumor biology, low or negative estrogen-receptor status, high grade [grade 3], diffuse lymphovascular invasion, and positivity of more than 3 lymph nodes). According to the NCCN guidelines, axilla-negative patients should be evaluated for RNI for central/medial tumors or >2 cm tumors and the presence of other risk factors (young age or extensive lymphovascular invasion). [c]Studies are underway to evaluate the RT decision in patients with complete response after neoadjuvant chemotherapy. Patients must be evaluated individually. The decision for RT is determined according to the disease stage before neoadjuvant chemotherapy, but the disease stage may also be important for management after treatment. When the NSABP B-51 and Alliance A11202 studies are completed, they will provide information about the sufficiency of axillary staging and RT application

There are several different techniques for delivering APBI (such as external beam, intra-cavitary brachytherapy, interstitial brachytherapy, and intra-operative irradiation). It is suspected that not all of these techniques are capable of achieving adequate local control with low rates of side effects [37, 38]. The results of large randomized trials must be reported before APBI can be considered standard in some patients [7, 39]. Data are accumulating to consider some elderly (above the age of

65–70) patients with low-risk disease (T1/T2N0M0), negative margins, and hormone receptor-positive tumors without subsequent post lumpectomy RT [40, 41].

Boost Radiotherapy

Since the site in 65–80% of in-breast recurrence is the first tumor location or its immediate surroundings, two large randomized trials investigated whether boost can provide a local control benefit [42, 43]. The Lyon Boost Trial included 1024 patients with stage I–II (<3 cm tumor) breast cancer. After lumpectomy with negative margins + axillary LN dissection (ALND) and 50 Gy RT, patients were randomized to receive 10 Gy of electron boost or not. At a median follow-up of 5 years, the addition of boost reduced local failures (3.6 vs. 4.5%, $p = 0.04$). Despite a non-significant increase in grade 1–2 telangiectasia (12.4 vs 5.9%), no difference was observed in the self-assessed cosmetic response between the arms [42].

The second trial, the EORTC Boost Trial, randomized 5518 patients with Stage I/II breast cancer to 50 Gy RT vs. 50 Gy + 16 Gy boost following lumpectomy (negative invasive margins, DCIS margins ignored). At 10-year follow-up, local failure was decreased from 10.2% to 6.2% ($p < 0.0001$) in those with boost, and the largest benefit was observed in patients ≤40 years (local failure decreased from 23.9 to 13%) [43]. Additionally, the updated results of this study with a median follow-up of 17.2 years detected a significant 20-year risk reduction (from 16.4% to 12%). Again, the most obvious benefit was observed in patients ≤40 years of age (36% vs. 24.4%) at the expense of increased moderate/serious fibrosis rates (30.4 vs. 15%, $p < 0.0001$) [44]. Furthermore, the EORTC 22881 trial demonstrated no difference in local control between three different methods of boost application: photon, electron and interstitial brachytherapy [45].

Accelerated Partial-Breast Irradiation

Irradiating only the tumor-bearing quadrant of the breast after BCS instead of irradiating the whole breast has gained much popularity over the last decade. This type of breast RT is termed accelerated partial-breast irradiation (APBI). In this technique, the RT period is shortened considerably, and adjacent normal tissue and organs as well as parts of the breast distant to the tumor bed receive a minimal dose. One disadvantage of this technique, at least in theory, is that parts of the breast distant to the tumor bed that harbor occult tumor foci that do not receive therapeutic doses of RT may cause higher rates of in-breast recurrences or new primaries with longer follow-up.

As a result of increasing interest in this technique, many randomized trials have begun comparing APBI with whole-breast RT. The results of some of these randomized trials have been published recently with limited follow-up [34, 35].

A large multi-institutional trial from the US has completed accrual, and the results are pending [39]. Despite a lack of randomized and solid evidence for the safety and efficacy of APBI, the growing popularity of APBI has driven European and American RT societies to publish guidelines that may aid the selection of patients who are most suitable for APBI applications [7, 8]. Researchers including Holland, Vaidya, Faverly, Frazier, and Rosen investigated the presence of tumor foci in the other quadrants of the breast on operation specimens when a tumor mass was diagnosed in one site [46–50]. In 60% of the cases, invasive but occult tumor foci were identified in quadrants of the breast other than the quadrant that harbored the index tumor. These findings raised doubts about the efficacy of APBI. The irradiation period in APBI is shortened from 10 fractions in 5 days to a single fraction, which requires giving very high doses of RT in very few fractions over a very short time. This type of ultra-hypofractionation raises questions regarding the safety of APBI in terms of late sequelae and cosmesis [51, 52]. In addition, radiobiological concerns about the use of a single very high dose of irradiation and known mathematical models of radiobiological equivalence have been raised [51].

At this time, according to the updated guidelines published by larger RT societies, it is considered safer to use APBI in those who are ≥50 years of age and with hormone receptor-positive, BRCA 1/2-negative, T1 or Tis, node-negative disease without lymphovascular invasion that is removed surgically with clear margins (≥2 mm) or patients who have ≤2.5 cm, low to intermediate nuclear graded, screen-detected DCIS with negative margins of ≥3 mm. By contrast, patients who are ≤40 years of age with positive margins and DCIS ≥3 cm should be accepted as 'unsuitable candidates' for APBI. The results of the ongoing RTOG 0413/NSABP B39 trial comparing whole-breast RT and APBI in patients with <3 cm invasive or non-invasive tumors with 1–3 positive nodes will provide more accurate data about the safety and efficiency of APBI. The recommended dose regimens are 34 Gy in 10 fractions twice daily for brachytherapy or 38.5 Gy in 10 fractions twice daily for external beam RT [7, 8, 17].

Hypofractionation

The rationale for hypofractionation was demonstrated by a study by Yarnold et al. in which the α/β ratios for the tumor and late side effects for the breast were found to be 4 Gy and 3.6 Gy, respectively [53]. Four major randomized trials investigated whether hypofractionation is as effective and safe as conventional fractionation. The first one, the Canada Ontario Clinical Oncology Group (OCOG) trial, emphasized that a 42.5 Gy /16 Fr/22-day treatment schedule was similar to the 50 Gy/5 Fr/35-day treatment schedule with no boost in terms of 10-year local invasive recurrence rates (6.2 vs 6.7%) and good cosmetic results (69.8 vs 71.3%) among 1234 patients staged T1–2N0M0 who received BCS + level I–II ALND with no involved node or margin positivity. Although unconfirmed by other studies, an increase in local recurrence was detected in the high-grade tumor subgroup in the hypofractionation arm (15.5 vs. 4.7%, p = 0.01) [54].

Three additional randomized trials from England compared hypofractionation and conventional fractionation, all without boost treatment. A total of 1410 patients with T1-3N0M0 disease treated with BCS were randomized to three different dose schemas (50 Gy/25 Fr vs. 42.9 Gy/13 Fr vs. 39 Gy/13 Fr) with a total treatment time of 5 weeks in all groups. Ten-year recurrence rates were 12.1%, 9.6%, and 14.8%, respectively, and the difference between 42.9 Gy and 39 Gy was significant (p = 0.027) [55]. Furthermore, the other two randomized trials, START-A (n = 2236) and -B (n=2215) included T1-3N0-1M0 patients who were treated with either BCS or modified radical mastectomy (MRM) [55, 56]. Similar to the previous trial, patients were randomized to receive 50 Gy/25 Fr vs. 41.6 Gy/13 Fr vs. 39 Gy/13 Fr, all in 5 weeks in START-A whereas the randomization arms were 50 Gy/25 Fr in 5 weeks and 40 Gy/15 Fr in 3 weeks in the START-B trial. The three arms were similar in START-A, whereas a survival benefit in the hypofractionation group was demonstrated in the START-B trial (84 vs. 81%, p = 0.042) [55, 56].

Finally, more hypofractioned regimens (28.5 or 30 Gy in 5 weeks Fr vs. 50 Gy/25 Fr) were evaluated in the FAST trial, which included 729 patients aged ≥50 years with early-stage node-negative disease resected with negative margins. Three-year moderate/marked side effects were more common for 30 Gy (17.3 vs. 9.5%, p < 0.001) and 28.5 Gy (11.1 vs. 9.5%, p = 0.18) than 50 Gy/25 Fr [57].

Valle et al. compared standard fractionation and hypofractionated irradiation in 8189 patients undergoing BCS with stage T1–T2 and/or N1 breast cancer or DCIS in a recent systematic review and meta-analysis of 13 randomized controlled trials that included a highly selected group of patients who were node-negative, chemotherapy-naive, and without high-grade tumors. Local failure (n = 7 trials; RR 0.97; 95% CI 0.78–1.19, $I^2 = 0\%$), locoregional failure (n = 8 trials; RR 0.86; 95% CI 0.63–1.16, $I^2 = 0\%$), and survival (n = 4 trials; RR 1.00; 95% CI 0.85–1.17, $I^2 = 0\%$) were similar. The acute toxicity rate (n = 5 trials; RR 0.36; 95% CI 0.21–0.62, $I^2 = 20\%$) was lower in the hypofractionation arm, whereas no difference in late cosmesis was detected (RR 0.95; 95% CI 0.81–1.12, $I^2 = 54\%$). Similar conclusions were reached in two previous meta-analyses [58, 59].

Since the ratio of young patients was 25% in these randomized trials, hypofractionated regimes are recommend with additional doses in young patients and grade 3 disease by ASTRO [60]. However, the use of hypofractionation in patients <50 years of age with high-grade tumors and together with boost RT or pre- or post-RT chemotherapy is controversial. Ongoing trials will provide more evidence about the use of hypofractionation in DCIS, sequential and integrated additional dose administrations, chest wall and regional lymphatic RT and APBI. Until then, conventional fractionation is the standard treatment regimen in cases in whom dose inhomogeneity >7% exists or who require chemotherapy or regional lymphatic RT.

Regional Lymphatic Irradiation

The axillary LN involvement rate is 10–40% among clinically node-negative patients, depending on other prognostic factors [61]. Although the probability of involvement of level II LNs in the absence of level I nodes has been shown to be 1.2%, the risk of involvement of level II and other nodes increases up to 40% in the case of level I node metastasis [62]. Additionally, the second most common relapse site following the chest wall is the supraclavicular LN, and the reported recurrence rate in the supra- and infraclavicular region is as high as 14–17% in patients with axillary LN involvement and extracapsular extension [62]. By contrast, the supraclavicular fossa recurrence rate is approximately 1% in those with minimal (1–3 node) or without nodal involvement [63, 64]. The predictive factors for supraclavicular LN involvement are higher histological grade, >4 node involvement, level II or III involvement, and extracapsular extension [63, 65]. The frequency of supraclavicular LN metastasis is 4.4% in those with level I involvement and ≤4 node positivity and increases up to 15.1% in the case of level III involvement [66]. Locoregional recurrence has been found to be 15–20% in patients <50 years of age with 1–3 node positivity, grade III, or ER-negative disease, even if they received BCS, whole-breast RT and systemic therapy, thus emphasizing the importance of nodal irradiation in this group of patients [67].

Identified risk factors for "in breast LN" involvement are the presence of peritumoral vascular invasion in the primary tumor on histological examination (22.8%), axillary node metastases (21.9%) and >2 cm size of the primary tumor (16%), whereas the only factor affecting mammary interna node metastasis is peritumoral vascular invasion status in patients with negative axilla (16.4%) [68].

Randomized Trials of Nodal Irradiation

The inclusion criteria, number of patients, follow-up times, results, significant patient characteristics and results of important randomized trials investigating the role of nodal RT are summarized in Table 19.1.

1. *American College of Surgeons Oncology Group (ACOSOG) Z0011:* Patients with cT1–2, cN0, and 1 or 2 sentinel LN metastasis were randomized to BCS + sentinel lymph node dissection (SLND) + ALND + whole-breast RT (n = 446) versus BCS + SLND + whole-breast RT without ALND (n = 445). The incidences of ≥3 involved LNs were 17.6 vs. 5%, $p < 0.001$. Five-year in-breast recurrence (3.7 vs 2.1%, $p = 0.16$), nodal recurrence (0.6 vs 1.3%, $p = 0.44$), OS (91.9 vs 92.5%, $p = 0.24$) and DFS (82.2 vs 83.8%, $p = 0.13$) were similar between groups [69]. Although there was no difference between arms regarding the use of protocol-prohibited nodal fields, detailed RT records were available only for 228 patients. High tangents (cranial tangent border 2 cm from the

Table 19.1 Randomized trials investigating the role of regional nodal radiotherapy in patients with breast cancer

Trial	Randomization	Inclusion criteria	N	Follow up (years)	Characteristics/side effects	Locoregional control and survival
ACOSOG Z0011, 2010 [70]	SLND + ALND + WBRT vs SLND + WBRT	cN0, 1 or 2 SN met	446 vs 445	6.2	Median LN removed: 17 vs 2 ≥3 involved LN: 17.6 vs 5.0%($p < 0.001$)	5-year in-breast recurrence: 3.7 vs 2.1% ($p = 0.16$) 5-year nodal recurrence: 0.6 vs 1.3% ($p = 0.44$) 5-year OS: 91.9 vs 92.5% ($p = 0.24$) 5-year DFS: 82.2 vs 83.8% ($p = 0.13$)
IBCSG 23–01, 2013 [71]	SLND + ALND + WBRT vs SLND + WBRT	T: <5 cm, cN0, ≥1 SN micromet, ECE (–)	464 vs 467	5	Sensory neuropathy: 18 vs 12%, $p = 0.012$ Lymphoedema: 13 vs 3%, $p < 0.0001$ Motor neuropathy: 8 vs 3%, $p = 0.0004$	Events: 10.3% vs 10% 5-year DFS: 84.4 vs 87.8% ($p = 0.16$)
EORTC 10981-22023 AMAROS, 2014 [72]	SLND + ALND vs SLND + axillary RT	T1–2, cN0, SN positive	744 vs 681	6.1	SN macromet: 59% vs 62% Non-SN LN met: 33% (in ALND arm) Lymphedema: 1 year 28 vs 15%, $p < 0.001$ 3 years 23 vs 14%, $p = 0.003$ 5 years 23 vs 11%, $p < 0.0001$	5-year axillary relapse: 0.43 vs 1.19% 5-year DFS: 86.9 vs 82.7%, $p = 0.18$ 5-year OS: 93.3 vs 92.5% ($p = 0.34$)

EORTC 22922/10925, 2010 [73]	WBRT/CWRT + nodal RT (medial supra + MI) vs WBRT/CWRT	– Stage I, II, or III (centrally/medially located tumor ± ALN positivity) – ALN involvement (externally located) – Mastectomy/ BCS±ALND	2002 vs 2002	10.9	pT ≤ 5 cm: 96 vs 95.8% pN0: 44.4 vs 45.4% pN1a: 42.9 vs 43.3 Pulmonary fibrosis: 4.4 vs 1.7%, p < 0.001 Cardiac fibrosis: 1.2 vs 0.6%, p = 0.06 Cardiac disease: 6.5 vs 5.6%, p = 0.25	10-year OS: 82.3 vs 80.7%, p = 0.06 10-year DFS: 72.1 vs 69.1%, p = 0.04 10-year distant DFS: 78.0 vs 75.0%, p = 0.02 10-year breast-ca mortality: 12.5 vs 14.4%, p = 0.02 10-year breast ca. relapse: 19.4 vs 22.9%, p = 0.02
MA 20, 2015 [25]	WBRT + nodal RT (MI, supra, axilla) vs WBRT	– N (+), – N (−) high-risk[a], – SN (+): level I or II dissection, – BCS with adjuvant CT – T4, N2–3 excluded	916 vs 916	9.5	Number of positive LN 0: 9.6 vs 9.7% 1: 50.2 vs 48.8% 2: 22.8 vs 25.4% 3: 11.9 vs 10.9% Acute pneumonitis: 1.2 vs 0.2%, p = 0.01 Lymphedema: 8.4 vs 4.5%, p = 0.001	10-year OS: 82.8 vs 81.8%, p = 0.38 10-year DFS: 82.0 vs 77.0%, p = 0.01
French trial, 2013 [74]	CWRT + supra + IM RT vs CWRT + supra RT	pN (+), central/medial tumors ± pN (+) Age <75, Karnofsky index ≥7	1334	11.3		10-year OS: 62.6 vs 59.3%, p = 0.8 No OS benefit in all subgroups (medial/central or lateral tumor, pN0 [only for medial/central] or pN+, and chemotherapy or not)

Abbreviation: *ALN* axillary lymph node, *ALND* axillary lymph node dissection, *BCS* breast-conserving surgery, *CWRT* chest wall radiotherapy, *DFS* disease-free survival, *LN* lymph node, *MI* mammaria interna lymph node, *OS* overall survival, *SN* sentinel node, *SLND* sentinel lymph node dissection, *supra* supraclavicular lymph node, *WBRT* whole-breast radiotherapy

[a]High risk: ≥5 cm or ≥2 cm with <10 axillary nodes removed and at least one of the following: grade 3, estrogen-receptor negativity, or lymphovascular invasion

humeral head, including some part of the axillary LN) were used in 50% of patients in the ALND group and 52.6% in the SLND group. Among the 228 patients, 18.9% received directed regional nodal RT using three fields: 22 in the ALND arm and 21 in the SLND arm [70].

2. *International Breast Cancer Study Group Trial (IBCSG) 23-01:* Patients with cT1–2, cN0, and ≥1 sentinel LN micrometastasis were randomized to SLND + ALND + whole-breast RT (n = 464) versus SLND + whole-breast RT without ALND (n = 467). Five-year DFS was similar between groups (84.4 vs. 87.8%, p = 0.16), whereas side effects including sensory neuropathy (18 vs. 12%, p = 0.012), lymphoedema (13 vs. 3%, p < 0.0001) and motor neuropathy (8 vs. 3%, p = 0.0004) were significantly increased in the ALND arm [71].
3. *EORTC 10981-22023 AMAROS:* Patients with cT1–2, cN0, positive sentinel LN metastases were randomized to SLND + ALND (n = 744) versus SLND + axillary RT without ALND (n = 681). Nonsentinel LN metastases were detected in 33% of patients assigned to the ALND group. Sentinel LN macrometastases were found in 59% and 62% of patients in the ALND and axillary RT groups, respectively. There was no difference between groups in terms of 5-year axillary relapse (0.43 vs. 1.19%), DFS (86.9 vs. 82.7%, p = 0.18) and OS (93.3 vs. 92.5%, p = 0.34) whereas the incidences of lymphedema at 1 year (28 vs. 15%, p < 0.0001), 3 years (23 vs. 14%, p = 0.003) and 5 years (23 vs. 11%, p < 0.0001) were increased in the ALND arm [72].
4. *EORTC 22922/10925:* Patients with stage I, II, or III disease (centrally medially located tumor irrespective of axillar LN involvement) or axillary LN involvement (externally located tumor) were randomized to whole-breast RT/chest-wall RT + nodal RT (including medial supraclavicular and mammaria interna) (n = 2002) versus whole-breast RT/chest-wall RT without nodal RT (n = 2002). Patients underwent BCS or mastectomy and ALND (in case of sentinel LN involvement during the final years of the study). Most tumors were ≤5 cm (96 vs. 95.8%), and the pN0 ratios were similar (44.4 vs. 45.4%). pN1a was present in 42.9% and 43.3%, respectively. Ten-year DFS (72.1 vs. 69.1%, p = 0.04) and distant DFS (78.0 vs. 75.0%, p = 0.02) were significantly longer in the nodal RT arm, whereas there was a trend in 10-year OS benefit (82.3 vs. 80.7%, p = 0.06) in favor of nodal RT. In addition, nodal irradiation significantly decreased the 10-year breast cancer mortality (12.5 vs. 14.4%, p = 0.02) and breast cancer relapse (19.4 vs. 22.9%, p = 0.02). The study showed that some patients with no axillary LN involvement may benefit from nodal RT including the medial supraclavicular and medial mammaria interna. By contrast, pulmonary fibrosis was increased in the nodal RT arm (4.4 vs. 1.7%, p < 0.001), whereas there was no difference between groups in terms of cardiac disease (6.5 vs 5.6%, p = 0.25) [73].
5. *MA 20:* Patients with axillary LN involvement or high-risk (≥5 cm or ≥2 cm with <10 axillary nodes removed and at least one of the following: grade 3, estrogen-receptor negativity, or lymphovascular invasion) without axillary LN involvement were randomized to whole-breast RT + nodal RT (including axillary, supraclavicular and mammaria interna) (n = 916) versus whole-breast RT

without nodal RT (n = 916). Patients with T4 or N2 disease were excluded from the study. If the sentinel LN was positive, level 1–2 dissection was performed in addition to BCS. The distribution of positive LNs was as follows: 0 (9.6 vs. 9.7%), 1 (50.2 vs. 48.8%), 2 (22.8 vs. 25.4%), and 3 (11.9 vs. 10.9%). Ten-year DFS (82.0 vs. 77.0%, p = 0.01) was significantly better in the nodal RT arm, whereas OS (82.8 vs. 81.8%, p = 0.38) was similar between arms. The incidences of acute pneumonitis (1.2 vs. 0.2%, p = 0.01) and lymphedema (8.4 vs 4.5%, p = 0.001) were higher in the nodal RT group. The most obvious DFS benefit with nodal RT was observed in pN0 patients, with a hazard ratio of 0.55 (0.28–1.09) and 10-year DFS of 83.7 vs. 72.4% [25].

6. *French Trial:* A total of 1334 patients with axillary LN involvement or central/medial located tumors, regardless of axillary LN involvement, were randomized to chest-wall RT+supraclavicular + mammaria interna RT versus chest-wall RT + supraclavicular RT without mammaria interna RT. No benefit in 10-year OS was detected with the addition of mammaria interna LN RT (62.6 vs 59.3%, p = 0.8) [74].

Conclusion

Radiotherapy is part of breast cancer treatment. The addition of RT to BCS decreases the risk of local recurrence by half in "insitu disease". In invasive disease, PMRT in patients with 4 or more lymph nodes with metastatic involvement is the standard of care. After lumpectomy, whole-breast RT is still considered the standard of care. In addition, boost RT to the tumor bed after breast-conserving surgery was shown to decrease local failure. The results of APBI in patients with low local recurrence risk are controversial. Hypofractionation is also an appropriate therapeutic option for most patients with early breast cancer with comparable long-term toxicity profiles. A disease-free survival benefit of regional lymphatic irradiation has been demonstrated in patients with high-risk features with no axillary nodal involvement.

References

1. Holmberg L, Garmo H, Granstrand B, Ringberg A, Arnesson LG, Sandelin K, et al. Absolute risk reductions for local recurrence after postoperative radiotherapy after sector resection for ductal carcinoma in situ of the breast. J Clin Oncol. 2008;26(8):1247–52.
2. Stuart KE, Houssami N, Taylor R, Hayen A, Boyages J. Long-term outcomes of ductal carcinoma in situ of the breast: a systematic review, meta-analysis and meta-regression analysis. BMC Cancer. 2015;15:890.
3. EORTC Breast Cancer Cooperative Group, EORTC Radiotherapy Group, Bijker N, Meijnen P, Peterse JL, Bogaerts J, Van Hoorebeeck I, Julien JP, et al. Breast-conserving treatment with or without radiotherapy in ductal carcinoma-in situ: ten-year results of European Organisation

for Research and Treatment of Cancer randomized phase III trial 10853—a study by the EORTC Breast Cancer Cooperative Group and EORTC Radiotherapy Group. J Clin Oncol. 2006;24(21):3381–7.
4. Fisher B, Dignam J, Wolmark N, Mamounas E, Costantino J, Poller W, et al. Lumpectomy and radiation therapy for the treatment of intraductal breast cancer: findings from National Surgical Adjuvant Breast and Bowel Project B-17. J Clin Oncol. 1998;16(2):441–52.
5. Vargas C, Kestin L, Go N, Krauss D, Chen P, Goldstein N, et al. Factors associated with local recurrence and cause-specific survival in patients with ductal carcinoma in situ of the breast treated with breast-conserving therapy or mastectomy. Int J Radiat Oncol Biol Phys. 2005;63(5):1514–21.
6. A randomized phase III study of conventional whole breast irradiation (WBI) versus partial breast irradiation (PBI) for women with stage 0, I or II breast cancer. NCT00103181. https://clinicaltrials.gov/ct2/show/NCT00103181.
7. Smith BD, Arthur DW, Buchholz TA, Haffty BG, Hahn CA, Hardenbergh PH, et al. Accelerated partial breast irradiation consensus statement from the American Society for Radiation Oncology (ASTRO). Int J Radiat Oncol Biol Phys. 2009;74(4):987–01.
8. ASBS: http://www.breastsurgeons.org/statements/APBI_statement_revised_100708.pdf.
9. Keisch M, Arthur D, Patel R, Rivard M, Vicini F. American brachytherapy society breast brachytherapy task group. http://www.americanbrachytherapy.org/recources/abs_breast_brachytherapy_taskgroup.pdf.
10. Hughes LL, Wang M, Page DL, Gray R, Solin LJ, Davidson NE, et al. Local excision alone without irradiation for ductal carcinoma in situ of the breast: a trial of the Eastern Cooperative Oncology Group. J Clin Oncol. 2009;27(32):5319–24.
11. McCormick B, Winter K, Hudis C, Kuerer HM, Rakovitch E, Smith BL, et al. RTOG 9804: a prospective randomized trial for good-risk ductal carcinoma in situ comparing radiotherapy with observation. J Clin Oncol. 2015;33(7):709–15.
12. Smith BD. When is good enough really good enough? Defining the role of radiation in low-risk ductal carcinoma in situ. J Clin Oncol. 2015;33(7):686–91.
13. Julien JP, Bijker N, Fentiman IS, Peterse JL, Dellodonne V, Rouanat P, et al. Radiotherapy in breast-conserving treatment for ductal carcinoma in situ: first results of the EORTC randomised phase III trial 10853. EORTC Breast Cancer Cooperative Group and EORTC Radiotherapy Group. Lancet. 2000;355(9203):528–33.
14. Houghton J, George WD, Cuzick J, Duggan C, Fentim IS, Spittle M. Radiotherapy and tamoxifen in women with completely excised ductal carcinoma in situ of the breast in the UK, Australia, and New Zealand: randomised controlled trial. Lancet. 2003;362(9378):95–02.
15. Fisher B, Land S, Mamounas E, Dignam J, Fisher ER, Wolmark N. Prevention of invasive breast cancer in women with ductal carcinoma in situ: an update of the National Surgical Adjuvant Breast and Bowel Project experience. Semin Oncol. 2001;28(4):400–18.
16. Morrow M, Van Zee KJ, Solin LJ, Houssami N, Chavez-MacGregor M, Harris JR, et al. Society of Surgical Oncology-American Society for Radiation Oncology-American Society of Clinical Oncology consensus guideline on margins for breast-conserving surgery with whole-breast irradiation in ductal carcinoma in situ. Pract Radiat Oncol. 2016;6(5):287–95.
17. National Comprehensive Cancer Network. Breast cancer guidelines. http://nccn.org/professionals/physicians_gls/PDF/breast.pdf. Accessed April 27.
18. Nilsson C, Valachis A. The role of boost and hypofractionation as adjuvant radiotherapy in patients with DCIS: a meta-analysis of observational studies. Radiother Oncol. 2015;114(1):50–5.
19. Moran MS, Zhao Y, Ma S, Kirova YM, Fourquet A, Chen PY, et al. Radiation boost for ductal carcinoma in situ after whole-breast radiation therapy (WBRT) improves local control: analysis from 10 pooled academic institutions. Int J Radiat Oncol Biol Phys. 2016;96(2):144.
20. Harris JR, Halpin-Murphy P, McNeese M, Mendenhall NP, Morrow M, Robert NJ. Consensus Statement on postmastectomy radiation therapy. Int J Radiat Oncol Biol Phys. 1999;44(5):989–90.

21. Overgaard M, Hansen PS, Overgaard J, Rose C, Andersson M, Bach F, et al. Postoperative radiotherapy in high-risk premenopausal women with breast cancer who receive adjuvant chemotherapy. Danish Breast Cancer Cooperative Group 82b Trial. N Engl J Med. 1997;337(14):949–55.
22. Overgaard M, Jensen MB, Overgaard J, Hansen PS, Rose C, Andersson M, et al. Postoperative radiotherapy in high-risk postmenopausal breast-cancer patients given adjuvant tamoxifen: Danish Breast Cancer Cooperative Group DBCG 82c randomised trial. Lancet. 1999;353(9165):1641–8.
23. Ragaz J, Jackson SM, Le N, Plenderleith IH, Spinelli JJ, Basco VE. Adjuvant radiotherapy and chemotherapy in node-positive premenopausal women with breast cancer. N Engl J Med. 1997;337(14):956–62.
24. McGale P, Taylor C, Correa C, Cutter D, Duane F, Ewertz M, et al. Effect of radiotherapy after mastectomy and axillary surgery on 10-year recurrence and 20-year breast cancer mortality: meta-analysis of individual patient data for 8135 women in 22 randomised trials. Lancet. 2014;383(9935):2127–35.
25. Whelan TJ, Olivotto IA, Parulekar WR, Ackerman I, Chua BH, Nabid A, et al. Regional nodal irradiation in early-stage breast cancer. N Engl J Med. 2015;373(4):307–16.
26. Taghian AG, Jeong JH, Mamounas EP, Parda DS, Deutsch M, Costantino JP, et al. Low locoregional recurrence rate among node-negative breast cancer patients with tumors 5 cm or larger treated by mastectomy, with or without adjuvant systemic therapy and without radiotherapy: results from five national surgical adjuvant breast and bowel project randomized clinical trials. J Clin Oncol. 2006;24(24):3927–32.
27. NCI: http://www.cancer.gov/cancertopics/pdq/treatment/breast/healthprofessional/page5#section_5.71.
28. Recht A, Comen EA, Fine RE, Fleming GF, Hardenbergh PH, Ho AY, et al. Postmastectomy radiotherapy: an American Society of Clinical Oncology, American Society for Radiation Oncology, and Society of Surgical Oncology focused guideline update. Ann Surg Oncol. 2017;24(1):38–51.
29. Fisher B, Anderson S, Bryant J, Margolese RG, Deutsch M, Fisher ER, et al. Twenty-year follow-up of a randomized trial comparing total mastectomy, lumpectomy, and lumpectomy plus irradiation for the treatment of invasive breast cancer. N Engl J Med. 2002;347(16):1233–41.
30. van Dongen JA, Voogd AC, Fentiman IS, Legrand C, Sylvester RJ, Tong D, et al. Long-term results of a randomized trial comparing breast-conserving therapy with mastectomy: European Organization for Research and Treatment of Cancer 10801 trial. J Natl Cancer Inst. 2000;92(14):1143–50.
31. Veronesi U, Marubini E, Mariani L, Galimberti V, Luini A, Veronesi P, et al. Radiotherapy after breast-conserving surgery in small breast carcinoma: long-term results of a randomized trial. Ann Oncol. 2001;12(7):997–1003.
32. Veronesi U, Saccozzi R, Del Vecchio M, Banfi A, Clemente C, De Lena M, et al. Comparing radical mastectomy with quadrantectomy, axillary dissection, and radiotherapy in patients with small cancers of the breast. N Engl J Med. 1981;305(1):6–11.
33. Darby S, McGale P, Correa C, Taylor C, Arriagada R, Clarke M, et al. Effect of radiotherapy after breast-conserving surgery on 10-year recurrence and 15-year breast cancer death: meta-analysis of individual patient data for 10,801 women in 17 randomised trials. Lancet. 2011;378(9804):1707–16.
34. Valdaya JS, Joseph DJ, Tobias JS, Bulsara M, Wenz F, Saunders C, et al. Targeted intraoperative radiotherapy versus whole breast radiotherapy for breast cancer (TARGIT-A trial): an international, prospective, randomised, non-inferiority phase 3 trial. Lancet. 2010;376(9735):91–102.
35. Veronesi U, Orecchia R, Maisonneuve P, Viale G, Rotmensz N, Sangalli C, et al. Intraoperative radiotherapy versus external radiotherapy for early breast cancer (ELIOT): a randomised controlled equivalence trial. Lancet Oncol. 2013;14(13):1269–77.
36. Strnad V, Ott OJ, Hildebrandt G, Kauer-Dorner D, Knauerhase H, Major T, et al. 5-year results of accelerated partial breast irradiation using sole interstitial multicatheter brachytherapy

versus whole-breast irradiation with boost after breast-conserving surgery for low-risk invasive and in-situ carcinoma of the female breast: a randomised, phase 3, non-inferiority trial. Lancet. 2016;387(10015):229–38.

37. Smith GL, Xu Y, Buchholz TA, Smith BD, Giordano SH, Haffty BG, et al. Brachytherapy for accelerated partial-breast irradiation: a rapidly emerging technology in breast cancer care. J Clin Oncol. 2011;29(2):157–65.
38. Olivotto IA, Whelan TJ, Parpia S, Kim DH, Berrang T, Truong PT, et al. Interim cosmetic and toxicity results from RAPID: a randomized trial of accelerated partial breast irradiation using three-dimensional conformal external beam radiation therapy. J Clin Oncol. 2013;31(32):4038–45.
39. Julian TB, Costantino JP, Vicini FA, White JR, Cecchini RS, Winter KA, et al. A randomized phase III study of conventional whole breast irradiation (WBI) versus partial breast irradiation (PBI) for women with stage 0, 1, or 2 breast cancer: NSABP B-30/RTOG 0413. Cancer Res. 2012;71(24 Suppl.):Abstract nr OT2-06-02.
40. Kunkler IH, Williams LJ, Jack WJ, Cameron DA, Dixon JM, Bissett D, et al. Breast-conserving surgery with or without irradiation in women aged 65 years or older with early breast cancer (PRIME II): a randomised controlled trial. Lancet Oncol. 2015;16(3):266–73.
41. Hughes KS, Schnaper LA, Bellon JR, Cirrincione CT, Berry DA, McCormick B, et al. Lumpectomy plus tamoxifen with or without irradiation in women age 70 years or older with early breast cancer: long-term follow-up of CALGB 9343. J Clin Oncol. 2013;31(19):2382–7.
42. Romestaing P, Lehingue Y, Carrie C, Couquard R, Montbarbon X, Ardiet JM, et al. Role of a 10-Gy boost in the conservative treatment of early breast cancer: results of a randomized clinical trial in Lyon, France. J Clin Oncol. 1997;15(3):963–8.
43. Bartelink H, Horiot JC, Poortmans P, Struikmans H, Van den Bogaert W, Barillot I, et al. Recurrence rates after treatment of breast cancer with standard radiotherapy with or without additional radiation. N Engl J Med. 2001;345(19):1378–87.
44. Bartelink H, Maingon P, Poortmans P, Weltens C, Fourquet A, Jager J, et al. Whole-breast irradiation with or without a boost for patients treated with breast-conserving surgery for early breast cancer: 20-year follow-up of a randomised phase 3 trial. Lancet Oncol. 2015;16(1):47–56.
45. Poortmans P, Bartelink H, Horiot JC, Struikmans H, Van den Bogaert W, Fourquet A, et al. The influence of the boost technique on local control in breast conserving treatment in the EORTC 'boost versus no boost' randomised trial. Radiother Oncol. 2004;72(1):25–33.
46. Holland R, Veling SH, Mravunac M, Hendriks JH. Histologic multifocality of Tis, T1-2 breast carcinomas. Implications for clinical trials of breast-conserving surgery. Cancer. 1985;56(5):979–90.
47. Vaidya JS, Vyas JJ, Chinoy RF, Merchant N, Sharma OP, Mittra I. Multicentricity of breast cancer: whole-organ analysis and clinical implications. Br J Cancer. 1996;74(5):820–4.
48. Faverly DR, Hendriks JH, Holland R. Breast carcinomas of limited extent: frequency, radiologic-pathologic characteristics, and surgical margin requirements. Cancer. 2001;91(4):647–59.
49. Frazier TG, Wong RW, Rose D. Implications of accurate pathologic margins in the treatment of primary breast cancer. Arch Surg. 1989;124(1):37–8.
50. Rosen PP, Fracchia AA, Urban JA, Schottenfeld D, Robbins GF. "Residual" mammary carcinoma following simulated partial mastectomy. Cancer. 1975;35(3):739–47.
51. Khan AJ, Arthur DW, Dale RG, Haffty BG, Vicini FA. Ultra-short courses of adjuvant breast radiotherapy: promised land or primrose path? Int J Radiat Oncol Biol Phys. 2012;82(2):499–501.
52. Khan AJ, Arthur DW, Vicini FA. On the road to intraoperative radiotherapy: more 'proceed with caution' signs. Oncology (Williston Park). 2013;27(2):113–4.
53. Yarnold J, Ashton A, Bliss J, Homewood J, Harper C, Hanson J, et al. Fractionation sensitivity and dose response of late adverse effects in the breast after radiotherapy for early breast cancer: long-term results of a randomised trial. Radiother Oncol. 2005;75(1):9–17.
54. Whelan TJ, Pignol JP, Levine MN, Julian JA, MacKenzie R, Parpia S, et al. Long-term results of hypofractionated radiation therapy for breast cancer. N Engl J Med. 2010;362(6):513–20.

55. Bentzen SM, Agrawal RK, Aird EG, Barrett JM, Barrett-Lee PJ, Bliss JM, et al. The UK Standardisation of Breast Radiotherapy (START) Trial A of radiotherapy hypofractionation for treatment of early breast cancer: a randomised trial. Lancet Oncol. 2008;9(4):331–41.
56. Bentzen SM, Agrawal RK, Aird EG, Barrett JM, Barrett-Lee PJ, Bentzen SM, et al. The UK Standardisation of Breast Radiotherapy (START) Trial B of radiotherapy hypofractionation for treatment of early breast cancer: a randomised trial. Lancet. 2008;371(9618):1098–107.
57. Agrawal RK, Alhasso A, Barrett-Lee PJ, Bliss JM, Bliss P, Bloomfield D, et al. First results of the randomised UK FAST Trial of radiotherapy hypofractionation for treatment of early breast cancer (CRUKE/04/015). Radiother Oncol. 2011;100(1):93–100.
58. Hickey BE, James ML, Lehman M, Hider PN, Jeffery M, Francis DP, et al. Fraction size in radiation therapy for breast conservation in early breast cancer. Cochrane Database Syst Rev. 2016;7:CD003860.
59. Zhou ZR, Mei X, Chen XX, Yang ZZ, Hou J, Zhang L, et al. Systematic review and meta-analysis comparing hypofractionated with conventional fraction radiotherapy in treatment of early breast cancer. Surg Oncol. 2015;24(3):200–11.
60. Smith BD, Bentzen SM, Correa CR, Hahn CA, Handenberg PH, Ibbott GS, et al. Fractionation for whole breast irradiation: an American Society for Radiation Oncology (ASTRO) evidence-based guideline. Int J Radiat Oncol Biol Phys. 2011;81(1):59–68.
61. Fisher B, Jeong JH, Anderson S, Bryant J, Fisher ER, Wolmark N. Twenty-five-year follow-up of a randomized trial comparing radical mastectomy, total mastectomy, and total mastectomy followed by irradiation. N Engl J Med. 2002;347(8):567–75.
62. Motwani SB, Strom EA, McNeese MD, Buchholz TA. Breast cancer. In: Brady LW, Heliman PH, Molls M, editors. Technical basis of radiation therapy. 4th ed. Berlin: Springer; 2014. p. 485–510.
63. Galper S, Recht A, Silver B, Manola J, Gelman R, Schnitt SJ, et al. Factors associated with regional nodal failure in patients with early stage breast cancer with 0-3 positive axillary nodes following tangential irradiation alone. Int J Radiat Oncol Biol Phys. 1999;45(5):1157–66.
64. Reddy SG, Kiel KD. Supraclavicular nodal failure in patients with one to three positive axillary lymph nodes treated with breast conserving surgery and breast irradiation, without supraclavicular node radiation. Breast J. 2007;13(1):12–8.
65. Yates L, Kirby A, Crichton S, Gillett C, Cane P, Fentiman I, et al. Risk factors for regional nodal relapse in breast cancer patients with one to three positive axillary nodes. Int J Radiat Oncol Biol Phys. 2012;82(5):2093–103.
66. Strom EA, Woodward WA, Katz A, Buchholz TA, Perkins GH, Jhingran A, et al. Clinical investigation: regional nodal failure patterns in breast cancer patients treated with mastectomy without radiotherapy. Int J Radiat Oncol Biol Phys. 2005;63(5):1508–13.
67. Truong PT, Jones SO, Kader HA, Wai ES, Speers CH, Alexander AS, et al. Patients with t1 to t2 breast cancer with one to three positive nodes have higher local and regional recurrence risks compared with node-negative patients after breast-conserving surgery and whole-breast radiotherapy. Int J Radiat Oncol Biol Phys. 2009;73(2):357–64.
68. Veronesi U, Amone P, Veronesi P, Galimberti V, Luini A, Rotmensz N, et al. The value of radiotherapy on metastatic internal mammary nodes in breast cancer. Results on a large series. Ann Oncol. 2008;19(9):1553–60.
69. Giuliano AE, McCall L, Beitsch P, Whitworth PW, Blumencranz P, Leitch AM, et al. Locoregional recurrence after sentinel lymph node dissection with or without axillary dissection in patients with sentinel lymph node metastases: the American College of Surgeons Oncology Group Z0011 randomized trial. Ann Surg. 2010;252(3):426–32.
70. Jagsi R, Chadha M, Moni J, Ballman K, Laurie F, Buchholz TA, et al. Radiation field design in the ACOSOG Z0011 (Alliance) Trial. J Clin Oncol. 2014;32(32):3600–6.
71. Galimberti V, Cole BF, Zurrida S, Viale G, Luini A, Veronesi P, et al. Axillary dissection versus no axillary dissection in patients with sentinel-node micrometastases (IBCSG 23-01): a phase 3 randomised controlled trial. Lancet Oncol. 2013;14(4):297–305.
72. Donker M, van Tienhoven G, Straver ME, Meijnen P, van de Velde CJ, Mansl RE. Radiotherapy or surgery of axilla after a positive sentinel node in breast cancer (EORTC 10981-22023

AMAROS): a randomised, multicenter, open-label, phase 3 non-inferiority trial. Lancet Oncol. 2014;15(12):1303–10.
73. Poortmans PM, Collette S, Kirkove C, Van Limbergen E, Budach V, Struikmans H, et al. Internal mammary and medial supraclavicular irradiation in breast cancer. N Engl J Med. 2015;373(4):317–27.
74. Hennequin C, Bossard N, Servagi-Vernat S, Maingon P, Dubois JB, Datchary J, et al. Ten-year survival results of a randomized trial of irradiation of internal mammary nodes after mastectomy. Int J Radiat Oncol Biol Phys. 2013;86(5):860–6.

Chapter 20
Adjuvant Radiotherapy After Preoperative Chemotherapy

Makbule Tambas, Kamuran Arslan Ibis, and Merdan Fayda

Introduction

- Neoadjuvant systemic chemotherapy has been widely employed for the treatment of locally advanced operable breast cancer, and its use during the early stages of breast cancer has increased [1]. Randomized trials have not observed differences in survival or locoregional control between preoperative and postoperative chemotherapy, with hazard ratios (HRs) of 0.98 (95% CI, 0.87–1.09; $p = 0.67$) and 1.12 (95% CI, 0.92–1.37; $p = 0.25$), respectively [2].
- pCR to neoadjuvant chemotherapy is associated with better survival rates compared to non-complete responders [2]. The pathological complete nodal response of the axilla was 41% (95% CI, 36.7–45.3%) in a modern neoadjuvant study [3]. This research also indicates that preoperative treatment supports breast-conserving surgery (BCS) due to tumor shrinkage before surgical intervention (HR 0.82; 95% CI, 0.76–0.89) [2].
- However, many women who receive neoadjuvant chemotherapy still undergo mastectomy, due to either patient preference or a lack of feasibility of BCS [1]. Herein, we attempt to determine whether postmastectomy radiotherapy (PMRT) and regional irradiation in the breast-conserving setting are necessary for all patients undergoing systemic neoadjuvant treatment.

M. Tambas
Department of Radiation Oncology, University of Health Sciences, Okmeydanı Training and Research Hospital, Istanbul, Turkey

K. Arslan Ibis
Istanbul Medical Faculty, Department of Radiation Oncology, Istanbul University, Institute of Oncology, Istanbul, Turkey

M. Fayda (✉)
Istinye University, Faculty of Medicine, Department of Radiation Oncology, Istanbul, Turkey

A. Aydiner et al. (eds.), *Breast Cancer*, https://doi.org/10.1007/978-3-319-96947-3_20

Radiotherapy Considerations After Preoperative Chemotherapy

- The decision to prescribe radiotherapy after preoperative chemotherapy is still largely based on the initial clinical staging of the patients. Therefore, the initial clinical staging information should be available prior to systemic treatment.
- History and physical examination, complete blood count, liver function tests, alkaline phosphatase, diagnostic bilateral mammogram (ultrasound as necessary), determination of tumor estrogen (ER)/progesterone receptor (PR), and human epidermal growth factor receptor 2 *neu* (HER2) status should be routinely performed before the start of neoadjuvant chemotherapy in patients at clinical stages IIA–IIB [4].
- Chest computed tomography (CT), abdominal CT, and bone scan can be considered for early-stage patients with symptoms (i.e., pulmonary symptoms, abnormal liver function tests, bone pain, or elevated alkaline phosphatase) or clinical stage IIIA or higher disease. Positron emission tomography and magnetic resonance imaging (MRI) of the breast are not considered part of the standard staging procedure. However, MRI could be helpful in patients with mammographically occult tumors [4]. MRI is also more accurate than mammography in detecting residual tumors after neoadjuvant chemotherapy but requires standardization [5]. Before systemic therapy, a pathological confirmation of the axilla via fine needle aspiration biopsy is also strongly suggested [4, 6]. Radiopaque marker insertion before systemic therapy may be helpful for clarifying the lumpectomy area after systemic treatment, particularly in patients with a complete tumor response [4, 7].
- There is a lack of randomized data to guide decision-making for PMRT after preoperative chemotherapy. Lymphatic irradiation in patients treated with breast-conserving protocols after preoperative chemotherapy and who are staged ypN0 is another area of controversy for which higher-level evidence is urgently needed.
- Our current source of information in these controversial areas are the retrospective series, the prospective dataset from a pooled analysis of the National Surgical Adjuvant Breast and Bowel Project (NSABP) B18 and B27 trials, and the results of adjuvant randomized trials. A pooled analysis of the NSABP B18 and B27 trials has been published. This analysis included cT1–3 cN0–1 patients who underwent preoperative systemic treatment. The median follow-up time was 11.75 years. PMRT and lymphatic irradiation in a breast-conserving setting were not allowed in this trial [8].
- In a recent meta meta-analysis of 4756 patient individual data from ten randomized trials which compared the long-term outcomes for neoadjuvant versus adjuvant chemotherapy in early breast cancer, found that patients who received neoadjuvant chemotherapy had increased rate of breast-conserving therapy at an expense of increased 15-year local recurrence risk (21.4% vs. 15.9%, $p = 0.0001$) while there was no significant difference in terms of distant

recurrence or mortality. It should be noted that none of patients received trastuzumab while most of the patients did not chemotherapy regimen containing taxane [9].

Prognostic Factors for Locoregional Control After Preoperative Neoadjuvant Systemic Treatment

- The literature suggests that the most important factors impacting the risk of LRR are the initial clinical stage, the younger age at the diagnosis, the extent of residual disease after preoperative chemotherapy, and adverse risk factors such as lymphovascular space invasion (LVSI), extracapsular extension (ECE), and a triple-negative (TN) phenotype [10].

PMRT After Preoperative Systemic Treatment for Initial Clinical Stage I (T1 N0) Disease

There are insufficient data to conclude whether PMRT is necessary for cT1N0 disease treated with neoadjuvant chemotherapy and mastectomy.

PMRT After Preoperative Systemic Treatment for Initial Clinical Stage IIA (T0–1 N1 or T2 N0) Disease

- In two retrospective studies, no locoregional failure was observed in cT2N0 patients with complete pathological remission (pCR, no invasive disease in the pathological specimen) [11, 12]. The rates of LRR were 0–7% in patients with cT1N1 that finally staged ypN0 after neoadjuvant chemotherapy, even with the TN phenotype [10, 13, 14].
- In studies from MDACC, the LRR was 4–5% in older (>35 to 40) patients with an initial cT1N1 that finally staged ypN(1–3+) after systemic chemotherapy, unless there were adverse risk factors (LVSI, ECE, TN) [13, 15].
- In another study from MDACC, patients with cT1–2 N0–1 disease were evaluated. In the total cohort of patients who did not receive RT ($n = 181$), those with ypN(≥4+) had the worst 5-year LRR (ypN0 1%, ypN(1–3+) 5.4%, yp(≥4+) 20%, $p = 0.034$). The presence of LVSI was also associated with worse 5-year LRR (no LVSI 2% vs. LVSI(+) 15.4%, $p = 0.006$) [15].
- The 10-year incidences of LRR were 6.5%, 11.2%, and 11.1% without PMRT in patients with cT1–2 N0 disease that finally staged ypN0, ypN(1–3+), or ypN(≥4+), respectively, in the NSABP trial [8].

PMRT After Preoperative Systemic Treatment for Initial Clinical Stage IIB (T2 N1 or T3 N0) Disease

- Retrospective data from younger patients (<35) with stage IIB or worse disease treated with preoperative chemotherapy and mastectomy indicate that these patients should also be treated with PMRT [16]. In a study from MDACC, 0% LRR was observed in patients with cT2N1 disease that finally staged pCR after neoadjuvant chemotherapy [11].
- Two retrospective studies have investigated whether PMRT is necessary for patients with clinical stage II–III disease that finally staged ypN0. In a French single-center study, PMRT had no effect on LRR-free survival (HR, 0.37; 95% CI, 0.09–1.61; $p = 0.18$) or OS (HR, 2.06; 95% CI, 0.71–6; $p = 0.18$) for clinical stage II or III disease staged ypN0. A trend was observed toward poorer OS among patients without a pathologically complete in-breast tumor response after neoadjuvant chemotherapy (HR, 6.65; 95% CI, 0.82–54.12; $p = 0.076$) [14].
- In a Korean multicenter retrospective study, the addition of PMRT was not correlated with a difference in DFS, LRR-free survival, or OS by multivariate analysis for clinical stage II or III disease that finally staged ypN0. In multivariate analysis, age (≤40 vs. >40 years) and pathological T-stage (0-is vs. 1 vs. 2–4) were significant prognostic factors affecting DFS (HR, 0.35, 95% CI, 0.135–0.928; $p = 0.035$ and HR 2.22, 95% CI 1.074–4.604; $p = 0.031$, respectively) [17].
- The 10-year incidences of LRR were 0%, 10.8%, 14.4%, and 19.5% without PMRT in patients with cT1–2 N1 disease that finally staged pCR, ypN0 (no breast pCR), ypN(1–3+), or ypN(>4+), respectively, in the NSABP trial [8].
- Another study from MDACC evaluated patients with cT3N0 disease treated with neoadjuvant chemotherapy (NAC) and mastectomy. Although all patients were clinically determined to have no nodal disease prior to NAC, 45% had pathologically confirmed disease in the lymph node. The 5-year LRR rate differed significantly between patients who received PMRT and those who did not: 4% (95% CI, 1–9%) with PMRT vs. 24% (95% CI, 10–39%) without PMRT ($p < 0.001$) [18]. Although the LRR rate was 0% in patients with cT3N0 disease that finally staged pCR after preoperative chemotherapy, MDACC suggests PMRT for all patients with cT3N0 disease [1, 11, 13, 18].
- The 10-year incidences of LRR were 6.2%, 11.8%, 10.6%, and 17.6% without PMRT in patients with cT3N0 disease that finally staged pCR, ypN0 (no breast pCR), ypN(1–3+), or ypN(>4+), respectively, in the NSABP trial [8].

PMRT After Preoperative Systemic Treatment for Initial Clinical Stage IIIA (T3 N1 or T0–3 N2) Disease

- The role of PMRT in cases of pCR in patients with clinical stage III disease was evaluated at MDACC. The 10-year LRR rate for patients with stage III disease was significantly improved with radiation therapy (7.3% ± 3.5% with vs. 33.3% ± 15.7% without; $p = 0.04$). In this cohort, the 10-year distant metastasis-free survival (DMFS) rate was 87.9% ± 4.6% for irradiated patients and 40.7% ± 15.5% for non-irradiated patients ($p = 0.0006$). The 10-year OS rate was 77.3% ± 6% for irradiated patients and 33.3% ± 14% for non-irradiated patients [11].

- The 10-year incidences of LRR were 0%, 9.2%, 14.7%, and 27.2% without PMRT in patients with cT3N1 disease that finally staged pCR, ypN0 (no breast pCR), ypN(1–3+), or ypN(>4+), respectively, in the NSABP trial [8].
- The indications for PMRT in stage III patients achieving pCR varies between institutions. MDACC suggests PMRT for all clinical stage III patients [11]. If pCR is achieved in patients with cT3N1 disease, aged >40 years, and with no TN histology, PMRT is not necessary, according to NSABP data [8]. Clearly, validation is needed for this controversial topic [10].

PMRT After Preoperative Systemic Treatment for Initial Clinical Stage IIIB (T4 N0–2) Disease

- The 5-year LRR risk in clinical stage IIIB patients treated with neoadjuvant chemotherapy and without PMRT was 42% in a retrospective study from MDACC [18].

Lymphatic Irradiation After Preoperative Systemic Treatment and Breast-Conserving Surgery

- The complete nodal pathological response rate in the axilla was 41% (95%CI, 36.7–45.3) in a modern neoadjuvant study [3]. This encouraging result questions the necessity of axillary lymph node dissection for cN1 patients with good clinical response to neoadjuvant chemotherapy. However, the false-negative rate of sentinel lymph node biopsy after neoadjuvant chemotherapy remains high (12.6%), and studies are needed to decrease axillary surgical interventions, particularly in patients with cN1 disease and a good clinical response to neoadjuvant chemotherapy [19].
- The contribution of lymphatic irradiation to DFS and possibly to survival improvement has been demonstrated in modern adjuvant studies such as NCI-C MA20 and EORTC 22922/10925 [20, 21]. How this information will or should be applied in the neoadjuvant setting is not clear. There is no consensus on the optimal management of regional radiotherapy in patients receiving neoadjuvant chemotherapy and axillary dissection.
- The role of lymphatic irradiation in clinical stage II–III disease was investigated in a French retrospective study. These researchers compared the outcomes of patients with pN0 status after neoadjuvant chemotherapy and BCS according to whether they received lymphatic irradiation. No improvement in the rates of LRR or survival was observed for nodal irradiation. All patients with initially

positive axillary cytology received lymphatic radiotherapy, and 83% of patients in the no-lymphatic-RT arm had cN0 disease in that study [14].

- The risk of regional recurrence was less than 10% in the NSABP trial after BCS and breast-only RT. Age and the residual disease burden in the axilla had an impact on the 10-year incidence of LRR in the NSABP trial [8]. The 10-year incidences of LRR (<50 years vs. ≥50 years) were 12% vs. 5.9% and 15.6% vs. 11.3% with breast-only RT in patients with cN0 disease that finally staged ypN(1–3+) and ypN(>4+), respectively. The 10-year incidences of LRR (<50 years vs. ≥50 years) were 21.1% vs. 11.4% and 24% vs. 19.6% with breast-only RT in patients with cN+ disease that finally staged ypN(1–3+) and ypN(>4+), respectively [8].
- There are no conclusive data as to whether lymphatic irradiation can be omitted in patients with clinical stage N2 disease that finally staged pCR after neoadjuvant chemotherapy.

Radiotherapy Fields After Preoperative Systemic Chemotherapy

- Whole-breast radiotherapy is the standard of practice in patients treated with neoadjuvant chemotherapy and BCS. If radiotherapy is indicated in the postmastectomy setting, the chest wall should be treated. In most studies from MDACC, full lymphatic irradiation (mammaria interna, supra, level 3, and axillary apex) was also performed [13, 16].
- In general, there is no controversy about whether patients with initial clinical stage cN0–1 disease that finally staged ypN(4+) should receive lymphatic radiotherapy including the undissected portion of the axilla (i.e., supraclavicular and level 3). Lymphatic radiotherapy fields may vary between institutions in patients with clinical stage II disease that finally staged ypN(1–3+) [22].
- PMRT could be omitted for stage II patients with pCR who are not TN and who are >40 years. All patients with stage II disease but who have had residual disease in the axilla should receive PMRT. One institution is using a supra-level 3 field for stage II patients with no residual axillary cancer but no pCR at the tumor, particularly for younger patients who have no reasonable options for adjuvant systemic therapy (i.e., estrogen receptor (−) and Her-2 Neu(−)).
- All patients with stage III disease should receive PMRT [22]. The decision to use lymphatic radiotherapy in patients with stage III disease should be based on the pathological status of the axilla, but in a retrospective study from Florida, the omission of the supraclavicular field was significantly associated with LRR by multivariate analysis (HR 3.39; $p = 0.024$) [23].
- There are insufficient data examining the omission of radiotherapy in patients with cT4 or cN2 disease. Thus, PMRT with whole lymphatics should be advised for these patients.

Future Directions

- Clearly, there is a need for randomized studies to assess the safe omission of PMRT and regional radiotherapy in women with a good response to chemotherapy without compromising breast cancer outcomes. In the NSABP B51/Radiotherapy Oncology Group (RTOG) 1304 study, patients with involved axillary nodes (histologically confirmed) are treated with neoadjuvant chemotherapy. Those who are node negative at subsequent mastectomy are randomly assigned to ± postmastectomy RT (PMRT) to the chest wall and regional nodes. Similarly, patients who undergo subsequent breast conservation surgery and whose nodes have become negative after preoperative chemotherapy will be randomly assigned to breast RT ± regional nodal RT [24].
- An analysis of sentinel lymph node biopsy (SLNB) after systemic chemotherapy in patients with cN1 disease has been published (Z1071 study) [19]. The false-negative rate after the SLNB procedures was 12.6% (90% Bayesian credible interval, 9.85–16.05%) in the entire group. Both the use of dual-agent mapping (blue dye and radiolabeled colloid) and the recovery of more than 2 SLNs were associated with a lower likelihood of false-negative SLN findings (9.1% for ≥3 SLNs). According to the results of the AMAROS trial, both axillary dissection and lymphatic radiotherapy had the same rates of disease control but fewer side effects with RT in patients with positive SLNB cT1–2 N0 disease [25]. For women who receive neoadjuvant chemotherapy and whose lymph nodes remain pathologically positive after surgery, regional radiotherapy is indicated.
- However, the ALLIANCE (Alliance for Clinical Trials in Oncology) A011202 phase III clinical trial (NCT01901094) has been designed to answer whether axillary node dissection improves the rate of breast cancer recurrence over that observed with SLNB alone when regional radiotherapy is delivered. If SLNB becomes a standard approach in the neoadjuvant setting, some cN1 patients could be treated with SLNB and axillary radiotherapy without axillary dissection. Clearly, more studies are also needed in this area [26].

References

1. Hoffman KE, Mittendorf EA, Buchholz TA. Optimizing radiation treatment decisions for patients who receive neoadjuvant chemotherapy and mastectomy. Lancet Oncol. 2012;13(6):e270–6.
2. Mieog JS, van der Hage JA, van de Velde CJ. Preoperative chemotherapy for women with operable breast cancer. Cochrane Database Syst Rev. 2007;2:CD005002.
3. Boughey JC, Suman VJ, Mittendorf EA, Ahrendt GM, Wilke LG, Taback B, et al. Sentinel lymph node surgery after neoadjuvant chemotherapy in patients with node-positive breast cancer: the ACOSOG Z1071 (Alliance) clinical trial. JAMA. 2013;310(14):1455–61.
4. National Comprehensive Cancer Network Clinical Practice Guidelines in Oncology. Breast Cancer, Version 1; 2018.

5. Marinovich ML, Houssami N, Macaskill P, Sardanelli F, Minckwitz G, Mamounas E, et al. Meta-analysis of magnetic resonance imaging in detecting residual breast cancer after neoadjuvant therapy. J Natl Cancer Inst. 2013;105(5):321–33.
6. Park SH, Kim MJ, Park BW, Moon HJ, Kwak JY, Kim EK. Impact of preoperative ultrasonography and fine-needle aspiration of axillary lymph nodes on surgical management of primary breast cancer. Ann Surg Oncol. 2011;18(3):738–44.
7. Oh JL, Nguyen G, Whitman GJ, Hunt KK, Yu TK, Woodward WA, et al. Placement of radiopaque clips for tumor localization in patients undergoing neoadjuvant chemotherapy and breast conservation therapy. Cancer. 2007;110(11):2420–7.
8. Mamounas EP, Anderson SJ, Dignam JJ, James JD, Harry DB, Thomas BJ, et al. Predictors of locoregional recurrence after neoadjuvant chemotherapy: results from combined analysis of national surgical adjuvant breast and bowel project B-18 and B-27. J Clin Oncol. 2012;30:3960–6.
9. Early Breast Cancer Trialists' Collaborative Group (EBCTCG), Asselain B, Barlow W, Bartlett J, Bergh J, Bergsten-Nordström E, Bliss J, et al. Long-term outcomes for neoadjuvant versus adjuvant chemotherapy in early breast cancer: meta-analysis of individual patient data from ten randomized trials. Lancet Oncol. 2018;19(1):27–39.
10. Fowble BL, Einck JP, Kim DN, McCloskey S, Mayadev J, Yashar C, et al. Role of postmastectomy radiation after neoadjuvant chemotherapy in stage II–III breast cancer. Int J Radiat Oncol Biol Phys. 2012;83(2):494–503.
11. McGuire SE, Gonzalez-Angulo AM, Huang EH, Tucker SL, Kau SW, Yu TK, et al. Postmastectomy radiation improves the outcome of patients with locally advanced breast cancer who achieve a pathologic complete response to neoadjuvant chemotherapy. Int J Radiat Oncol Biol Phys. 2007;68:1004–9.
12. Settle S, Gonzalez-Angulo AM, Buchholz TA, Woodward WA, Yu TK, Oh JL, et al. Locoregional outcomes and radiotherapy response in patients with triple negative breast cancer (abstract). Int J Radiat Oncol Biol Phys. 2009;75:S9–10.
13. Garg AK, Strom EA, McNeese MD, Buzdar AU, Hortobagyi GN, Kuerer HM, et al. T3 disease at presentation or pathologic involvement of four or more lymph nodes predict for locoregional recurrence in stage II breast cancer treated with neoadjuvant chemotherapy and mastectomy without radiotherapy. Int J Radiat Oncol Biol Phys. 2004;59(1):138–45.
14. Le Scodan R, Selz J, Stevens D, Bollet MA, de la Lande B, Daveau C, et al. Radiotherapy for stage II and stage III breast cancer patients with negative lymph nodes after preoperative chemotherapy and mastectomy. Int J Radiat Oncol Biol Phys. 2012;82(1):e1–7.
15. Buchholz TA, Katz A, Strom EA. Pathologic tumor size and lymph node status predict for different rates of locoregional recurrence after mastectomy for breast cancer patients treated with neoadjuvant versus adjuvant chemotherapy. Int J Radiat Oncol Biol Phys. 2002;53:880–8.
16. Garg AK, Oh JL, Oswald MJ, Huang E, Strom EA, Perkins GH, et al. Effect of postmastectomy radiotherapy in patients <35 years old with stage II–III breast cancer treated with doxorubicin-based neoadjuvant chemotherapy and mastectomy. Int J Radiat Oncol Biol Phys. 2007;69(5):1478–83.
17. Shim SJ, Park W, Huh SJ, Choi SJ, Shin DH, Lee KH, et al. The role of postmastectomy radiation therapy after neoadjuvant chemotherapy in clinical stage II-III breast cancer patients with pN0: a multicenter, retrospective study (KROG 12-05). Int J Radiat Oncol Biol Phys. 2014;88(1):65–72.
18. Buchholz TA, Tucker SL, Masullo L, Kuerer HM, Erwin J, Salas J, et al. Predictors of local-regional recurrence after neoadjuvant chemotherapy and mastectomy without radiation. J Clin Oncol. 2002;20(1):17–23.
19. Daveau C, Stevens D, Brain E, Berges O, Villette S, Moisson P, et al. Is regional lymph node irradiation necessary in stage II to III breast cancer patients with negative pathologic node status after neoadjuvant chemotherapy? Int J Radiat Oncol Biol Phys. 2010;78(2):337–42.
20. Whelan T, Olivotto IA, Ackerman I. NCICCTG MA.20: an intergroup trial of regional nodal irradiation in early breast cancer. J Clin Oncol. 2011;29:779s. abstr LBA1003.
21. Poortmans P, Struikmans H, Kirkove C, Budach V, Matuschek C. Irradiation of the internal mammary and medial supraclavicular lymph nodes in stage I to III breast cancer: 10 years

results of the EORTC radiation oncology and breast cancer groups phase III trial 22922/10925. Eur J Cancer. 2013;49(Suppl 3):S1.

22. Bellon JR, Wong JS, Burstein HJ. Should response to preoperative chemotherapy affect radiotherapy recommendations after mastectomy for stage II breast cancer? J Clin Oncol. 2012;30(32):3916–20.
23. Wright JL, Takita C, Reis IM, Zhao W, Saigal K, Wolfson A, et al. Predictors of locoregional outcome in patients receiving neoadjuvant therapy and postmastectomy radiation. Cancer. 2013;119(1):16–25.
24. White J, Mamounas E. Locoregional radiotherapy in patients with breast cancer responding to neoadjuvant chemotherapy: a paradigm for treatment individualization. J Clin Oncol. 2014;32(6):494–5.
25. Rutgers EJ, Donker M, Straver ME, Meijnen, P, Van De Velde CJH, Mansel RE, et al. Radiotherapy or surgery of the axilla after a positive sentinel node in breast cancer patients: final analysis of the EORTC AMAROS trial (10981/22023). J Clin Oncol. 2013;31(15)suppl: abstract LBA1001.
26. Marks LB, Prosnitz LR. Reducing local therapy in patients responding to preoperative systemic therapy: are we outsmarting ourselves? J Clin Oncol. 2014;32(6):491–3.

Chapter 21
Advanced-Stage Breast Cancer Radiotherapy

Kamuran Arslan Ibis and Seden Kucucuk

Introduction

Advanced breast cancer represent a heterogeneous collection of diseases. Radiotherapy (RT) is an effective treatment modality in patients with locally advanced, local recurrent or metastatic disease. In this chapter, RT after neoadjuvant chemotherapy (NACT) and RT in unresectable disease, locally recurrent disease, and metastatic disease are discussed.

Radiotherapy After Neoadjuvant Chemotherapy

No randomized trial data exist to define which women will benefit from postmastectomy radiotherapy (PMRT) after NACT. Retrospective data suggest that both clinical stage at presentation and response to NACT could be used to indicate RT for these patients [1].

Patients with clinical stage III disease and lymph node involvement at the time of surgery are routinely given PMRT. In clinical stage II disease, PMRT is considered for those with lymph node involvement at the time of surgery or with features suggesting high-risk disease, such as triple-negative disease, partial response to chemotherapy, low hormone receptor levels, T3 tumor, close surgical margin, diffuse lymphovascular space involvement, or very young age. PMRT can be omitted in

K. Arslan Ibis (✉) · S. Kucucuk
Istanbul Medical Faculty, Department of Radiation Oncology, Istanbul University, Institute of Oncology, Istanbul, Turkey

A. Aydiner et al. (eds.), *Breast Cancer*, https://doi.org/10.1007/978-3-319-96947-3_21

patients with low locoregional relapse risk (<10%), defined as older than 40 years with estrogen-receptor positivity and pCR after NACT [2].

The results of the ongoing NSABP B-51/ RTOG 1304 trial will reveal any benefit of PMRT for clinical T1-3N1 disease that became node negative after NACT [3]. In another ongoing trial, Alliance 011202, patients with positive sentinel lymph node after NACT are randomly assigned to receive either level 1–2 axillary lymph node dissection (ALND) and nodal irradiation, including undissected axilla, supraclavicular and internal mammary nodes, or full axilla, supraclavicular and internal mammary node irradiation without ALND. This trial will establish if ALND may be omitted or not in this group of patients [4]. Until then, RT should be applied according to pre-chemotherapy clinical disease stage.

Patients with Unresectable Disease

In non-metastatic patients whose tumors remain unresectable after chemotherapy, RT may be administered to all pre-chemotherapy tumor extensions followed by boost to the residual sites. The initial RT dose of 50 Gy with an additional boost dose of 10–26 Gy for the organ at risk may be an appropriate approach. However, patients should be monitored at 45–50 Gy to assess suitability for surgery [5–7].

Radiotherapy in Locally Recurrent Disease

Approximately one third of recurrences occur as local relapse in breast cancer. The local recurrence rate is reported to be 3–14% after BCS+RT but 8–13% following mastectomy plus RT [8, 9]. When breast cancer recurs only on the chest wall after mastectomy or as in-breast recurrence after breast conserving surgery (BCS), intense local–regional therapies including surgical resection alone, surgical resection followed by RT, RT alone (when surgery is not applicable), concurrent chemoradiotherapy or RT combined with hyperthermia should be administered.

Surgical excision with negative margins not only reduces the necessary total RT dose but also increases disease control rates. While complete excision alone results in a 5-year disease free survival (DFS) rate of 35% [10], RT addition to surgery increases local control rates up to 60–77% [11, 12]. If not previously administered, chest wall and regional lymphatic irradiation should be administered in case of local recurrence after mastectomy [13]. In previously irradiated patients, superficial recurrences can be irradiated with interstitial brachytherapy or using a mold. Photons or electron RT may be used according to the dose to organs at risk from previous irradiation. Although the reported case series are inhomogeneous, the local control rates are in the range of 62–89%, at the expense of skin reactions, rib fracture and radiation pneumonitis [14, 15].

Following local recurrence after primary BCS + RT, second BCS alone results in local recurrence rates of 7–19% [16, 17]. Thus, partial breast irradiation with tumor bed boost has been applied at several centers. The reported local control rates are in the range of 77–93% [18, 19]. Re-irradiation after second BCS has been reported to have similar effectiveness as electrons, conventional external RT, interstitial brachytherapy, MammoSite and IORT [17, 19–21]. Attention should be paid to possible skin ulceration, brachial plexus injury, osteonecrosis, rib fractures and cardiomyopathy in chest wall re-irradiation at doses above 100 Gy [22].

In patients with prior irradiation who are considered to tolerate additional RT, combination therapies with chemotherapy or hyperthermia may be feasible options since recurrent tumors are generally radioresistant. A meta-analysis of hyperthermia and RT combination studies showed improved complete response rates (59% vs. 41%) compared with RT alone, with no survival benefit (both 18 months) [23]. Similar results were reported in a prospective randomized trial by Jones et al. (complete response 68.2% vs. 23.5%, $p = 0.02$), with no OS advantage [24]. In a more recent meta-analysis by Datta et al., the complete response was higher in the combination arm compared with RT alone ($n = 627$, 60.2% vs 38.1%, $p < 0.0001$) with a mean RT dose of 38.2 Gy (range 26–60 Gy); mean acute and late grade 3–4 toxicities for combination therapy were 14.4% and 5.2%, respectively [25]. Furthermore, a complete response rate as high as 80% was reported with the combination of thermo-chemoradiotherapy [26].

Radiotherapy in Metastatic Disease

Although there are no prospective randomized trials showing that local RT provides a survival benefit in patients with metastatic breast cancer (MBC), a recently published literature review analyzed 27 retrospective studies with more than 33,000 MBC patients. The role of RT was mentioned in 14 (52%) of the studies, and 5 of 6 that examined RT effects separately demonstrated a benefit of local RT [27]. Patients who are expected to have good survival prognosis may be candidates for local RT combined with surgery. Still, the role of RT in these patients remains to be clarified in further randomized prospective studies.

The percentage of patients with *oligometastatic disease* among breast cancer patients is not fully known. However, when prospective trials of first-line chemotherapy regimens were analyzed in terms of oligometastasis prevalence, approximately 50% of patients who were candidates for first-line MBC trials had ≤2 metastatic sites, and 75% had ≤4 [28–33]. When early-stage patients progressed to metastatic disease, approximately 17% presented with 1–5 metastatic sites; among these patients, oligometastasis was more common than in asymptomatic patients (26.7 vs. 14.5%, $p = 0.022$) [34]. Most of these patients may be more suitable for ablative RT than surgery due to their medical comorbidities; the lack of required interval time for postsurgical recovery, which causes systemic treatment interruptions; patient preference; or unresectable metastases. In addition, the determination of the subgroup that will benefit most from stereotactic ablative RT (SART) is a challenging issue, although patients with only bone metastasis seem to have improved outcomes [35].

The biological effects of SART can be summarized as follows: (1) suspension of progression of the irradiated metastatic focus, (2) prevention of new seeding of metastases from the irradiated site to other regions, and (3) inhibition of the progression of unirradiated sites via the abscopal effect [36, 37]. The control rates of SART are promising and reported to be 67–95% [38–40]. In addition, breast cancer patients have been shown to benefit from SART much more than patients with other types of cancer, as evidenced by 2-year PFS and 6-year OS rates of 36 vs. 13% and 47 vs. 9%, respectively. Furthermore, local control outcomes were also higher in breast cancer patients (87 vs. 74%) [41].

The reported 2-year local control rates and toxicities of SART according to metastatic sites irradiated are as follows: 80% for lung metastasis (5% rate of grade ≥3 side effects), with a 2-year survival rate of 50%; 57–92% for liver metastases (uncommon liver toxicities) [38, 39]. Available data are derived from retrospective studies, and ongoing phase II and randomized studies will provide more evidence about the role of SART in MBC patients [40].

One of the most common metastatic sites in SART is the *brain*, since 10–15% of MBC develops symptomatic brain metastasis [42, 43]. No obvious benefit has been shown for early detection, and screening for brain metastasis during the routine follow-up program of breast cancer patients is not recommended [44]. The prognostic factors for OS following SART for brain metastasis are triple-negative histology and progressive extracranial metastasis [45]. Since the ratio of breast cancer among phase III randomized trials of SART for brain metastasis is 6.8–11.7%, further studies including only breast cancer patients are warranted [46]. However, a systematic review of the literature comparing surgery, whole-brain RT (WBRT), single-dose stereotactic radiosurgery (SRS), and their combination [47–50] indicated the following:

1. SRS + WBRT is superior to WBRT in terms of local control in patients with ≤4 brain metastases and good performance status.
2. SRS + WBRT is superior to WBRT in term of survival in patients with single brain metastases [51].
3. SRS is equal to SRS + WBRT in terms of survival (one randomized trial showed superior survival with SRS alone) [52].
4. SRS alone is superior to WBRT alone in terms of survival benefit in patients with ≤3 brain metastases.
5. Further studies are warranted to determine the optimal dose for SRS alone and WBRT + SRS.
6. SRS + WBRT is equal to surgery + WBRT in terms of survival.
7. SRS may be used instead of surgery + WBRT.
8. Surgery + WBRT is superior to both WBRT alone and surgery alone in patients with good performance status and limited extracranial metastases.

9. Surgery is superior to SRS alone in patients with tumors that are larger (>3 cm) or cause a 1-cm midline shift.

In addition, retrospective and prospective data support increased local control and survival for the application of SRS to the surgical bed compared to WBRT. SRS of the surgical cavity in patients who have had complete resection of one, two, or three brain metastases significantly lowers local recurrence compared with that noted for observation alone [12-month freedom from local recurrence was 43% (95% CI 31–59) in the observation group and 72% (60–87) in the SRS group (hazard ratio 0.46; p = 0.015)] [53]. Thus, the use of SRS after brain metastasis resection could be an alternative to WBRT.

Regarding *bone metastases*, radiological assessment is needed to define whether a pathological fracture has occurred or is likely to happen. In this case, RT may be administered following surgical stabilization. If surgical intervention is not feasible, RT should be performed. In case of spinal cord compression, surgical decompression is recommended. If decompression/stabilization is not applicable, immediate RT should be planned [54].

References

1. Mamounas EP, Anderson SJ, Dignam JJ, Bear HD, Julian TB, Geyer CE Jr, et al. Predictors of locoregional recurrence after neoadjuvant chemotherapy: results from combined analysis of National Surgical Adjuvant Breast and Bowel Project B-18 and B-27. J Clin Oncol. 2012;30(32):3960–6.
2. De Felice F, Osti MF, De Sanctis V, Musio D, Tombolini V. Critical decision-making in radiotherapy for early stage breast cancer in a neo-adjuvant treatment era. Expert Rev Anticancer Ther. 2017;17(5):481–5.
3. Garg AK, Buchholz TA. Influence of neoadjuvant chemotherapy on radiotherapy for breast cancer. Ann Surg Oncol. 2015;22(5):1434–40.
4. National Cancer Institute Trial. Standard or comprehensive radiation therapy in treating patients with early-stage breast cancer previously treated with chemotherapy and surgery. www.clinicaltrials.gov.
5. Kao J, Conzen SD, Jaskowiak NT, Song DH, Recant W, Singh R, et al. Concomitant radiation therapy and paclitaxel for unresectable locally advanced breast cancer: results from two consecutive phase I/II trials. Int J Radiat Oncol Biol Phys. 2005;61(4):1045–53.
6. Karasawa K, Saito M, Hirowatari H, Izawa H, Furuya T, Ozawa S, et al. The role of chemoradiotherapy in patients with unresectable T4 breast tumors. Breast Cancer. 2013;20(3):254–61.
7. Shaughnessy JN, Meena RA, Dunlap NE, Jain D, Riley EC, Quillo AR, et al. Efficacy of concurrent chemoradiotherapy for patients with locally recurrent or advanced inoperable breast cancer. Clin Breast Cancer. 2015;15(2):135–42.
8. Fisher B, Jeong JH, Anderson S, Bryant J, Fisher ER, Wolmark N. Twenty-five-year follow-up of a randomized trial comparing radical mastectomy, total mastectomy, and total mastectomy followed by irradiation. N Engl J Med. 2002;347(8):567–75.
9. Ragaz J, Olivotto IA, Spinelli JJ, Philips N, Jackson SM, Wilson KS, et al. Locoregional radiation therapy in patients with high-risk breast cancer receiving adjuvant chemotherapy: 20-year results of the British Columbia randomized trial. J Natl Cancer Inst. 2005;97(2):116–26.
10. Faneyte IF, Rutgers EJ, Zoetmulder FA. Chest wall resection in the treatment of locally recurrent breast carcinoma: indications and outcome for 44 patients. Cancer. 1997;80(5):886–91.

11. Schwaibold F, Fowble BL, Solin LJ, Schultz DJ, Goodman RL. The results of radiation therapy for isolated local regional recurrence after mastectomy. Int J Radiat Oncol Biol Phys. 1991;21(2):299–310.
12. Skinner HD, Strom EA, Motwani SB, Woodward WA, Green MC, Babiera G, et al. Radiation dose escalation for loco-regional recurrence of breast cancer after mastectomy. Radiat Oncol. 2013;8:13.
13. Halverson KJ, Perez CA, Kuske RR, Garcia DM, Simpson JR, Fineberg B. Locoregional recurrence of breast cancer: a retrospective comparison of irradiation alone versus irradiation and systemic therapy. Am J Clin Oncol. 1992;15(2):93–101.
14. Delanian S, Housset M, Brunel P, Rozec C, Maulard C, Huart J, et al. Iridium 192 plesiocurietherapy using silicone elastomer plates for extensive locally recurrent breast cancer following chest wall irradiation. Int J Radiat Oncol Biol Phys. 1992;22(5):1099–104.
15. Harms W, Krepien R, Hensley FW, Berns C, Wannenmacher M, Fritz P. Results of chest wall reirradiation using pulsed-dose-rate (PDR) brachytherapy molds for breast cancer local recurrences. Int J Radiat Oncol Biol Phys. 2001;49(1):205–10.
16. Chadha M, Feldman S, Boolbol S, Wang L, Harrison LB. The feasibility of a second lumpectomy and breast brachytherapy for localized cancer in a breast previously treated with lumpectomy and radiation therapy for breast cancer. Brachytherapy. 2008;7(1):22–8.
17. Guix B, Lejarcegui JA, Tello JI, Zanon G, Henriquez I, Finestres F, et al. Exeresis and brachytherapy as salvage treatment for local recurrence after conservative treatment for breast cancer: results of a ten-year pilot study. Int J Radiat Oncol Biol Phys. 2010;78(3):804–10.
18. Deutsch M. Repeat high-dose external beam irradiation for in-breast tumor recurrence after previous lumpectomy and whole breast irradiation. Int J Radiat Oncol Biol Phys. 2002; 53(3):687–91.
19. Wadasadawala T, Vadgaonkar R, Bajpai J. Management of isolated locoregional recurrences in breast cancer: a review of local and systemic modalities. Clin Breast Cancer. 2017;17(7):493–502.
20. Chadha M, Mehta P, Feldman S, Boolbol SK, Harrison LB. Intraoperative high-dose-rate brachytherapy—a novel technique in the surgical management of axillary recurrence. Breast J. 2009;15(2):140–5.
21. Hannoun-Levi JM, Houvenaeghel G, Ellis S, Teissier E, Alzieu C, Lallement M, et al. Partial breast irradiation as second conservative treatment for local breast cancer recurrence. Int J Radiat Oncol Biol Phys. 2004;60(5):1385–92.
22. Siglin J, Champ CE, Vakhnenko Y, Anne PR, Simone NL. Radiation therapy for locally recurrent breast cancer. Int J Breast Cancer. 2012;2012:571946.
23. Vernon CC, Hand JW, Field SB, Machin D, Whaley JB, van der Zee J, et al. Radiotherapy with or without hyperthermia in the treatment of superficial localized breast cancer: results from five randomized controlled trials. International Collaborative Hyperthermia Group. Int J Radiat Oncol Biol Phys. 1996;35(4):731–44.
24. Jones EL, Oleson JR, Prosnitz LR, Samulski TV, Vujaskovic Z, Yu D, et al. Randomized trial of hyperthermia and radiation for superficial tumors. J Clin Oncol. 2005;23(13):3079–85.
25. Datta NR, Puric E, Klingbiel D, Gömez S, Bodis S. Hyperthermia and radiation therapy in locoregional recurrent breast cancers: a systematic review and meta-analysis. Int J Radiat Oncol Biol Phys. 2016;94(5):1073–87.
26. Zagar TM, Higgins KA, Miles EF, Vujaskovic Z, Dewhirst MW, Clough RW, et al. Durable palliation of breast cancer chest wall recurrence with radiation therapy, hyperthermia, and chemotherapy. Radiother Oncol. 2010;97(3):535–40.
27. Janssen S, Rades D. Primary breast cancer with synchronous metastatic disease - indications for local radiotherapy to the breast and chest wall. Anticancer Res. 2015;35(11):5807–12.
28. Albain KS, Nag SM, Calderillo-Ruiz G, Jordaan JP, Llombart AC, Pluzanska A, et al. Gemcitabine plus paclitaxel versus paclitaxel monotherapy in patients with metastatic breast cancer and prior anthracycline treatment. J Clin Oncol. 2008;26(24):3950–7.

29. Bergh J, Bondarenko IM, Lichinitser MR, Liljegren A, Greil R, Voytko NL, et al. First-line treatment of advanced breast cancer with sunitinib in combination with docetaxel versus docetaxel alone: results of a prospective, randomized phase III study. J Clin Oncol. 2012;30(9):921–9.
30. Tawfik H, Rostom Y, Elghazaly H. All-oral combination of vinorelbine and capecitabine as first-line treatment in HER2/Neu-negative metastatic breast cancer. Cancer Chemother Pharmacol. 2013;71(4):913–9.
31. Hurvitz SA, Dirix L, Kocsis J, Bianchi GV, Lu J, Vinholes J, et al. Phase II randomized study of trastuzumab emtansine versus trastuzumab plus docetaxel in patients with human epidermal growth factor receptor 2-positive metastatic breast cancer. J Clin Oncol. 2013;31(9):1157–63.
32. Gianni L, Romieu GH, Lichinitser M, Serrano SV, Mansutti M, Pivot X, et al. AVEREL: a randomized phase III Trial evaluating bevacizumab in combination with docetaxel and trastuzumab as first-line therapy for HER2-positive locally recurrent/metastatic breast cancer. J Clin Oncol. 2013;31(14):1719–25.
33. Sledge GW, Neuberg D, Bernardo P, Ingle JN, Martino S, Rowinsky EK, et al. Phase III trial of doxorubicin, paclitaxel, and the combination of doxorubicin and paclitaxel as front-line chemotherapy for metastatic breast cancer: an intergroup trial (E1193). J Clin Oncol. 2003;21(4):588–92.
34. Dorn PL, Meriwether A, LeMieux M, Weichsel baum RR, Chmura SJ, Hasan Y. Patterns of distant failure and progression in breast cancer: implications for the treatment of oligometastatic disease. Int J Radiat Oncol Biol Phys. 2011;81:S643.
35. Milano MT, Zhang H, Metcalfe SK, Muhs AG, Okunieff P. Oligometastatic breast cancer treated with curative-intent stereotactic body radiation therapy. Breast Cancer Res Treat. 2009;115(3):601–8.
36. Formenti SC, Friedman K, Chao K, Adams S, Fenton-Kerimian M, Donach ME, et al. Abscopal response in irradiated patients: results of a proof of priniciple trial. Int J Radiat Oncol Biol Phys. 2008;72:6–7.
37. Postow MA, Callahan MK, Barker CA, Yamada Y, Yuan J, Kitano S, et al. Immunologic correlates of the abscopal effect in a patient with melanoma. N Engl J Med. 2012;366(10):925–31.
38. Dellas K. Does radiotherapy have curative potential in metastatic patients? The concept of local therapy in oligometastatic breast cancer. Breast Care. 2011;6(5):363–8.
39. Tree AC, Khoo VS, Eeles RA, Ahmed M, Dearnaley DP, Hawkins MA, et al. Stereotactic body radiotherapy for oligometastases. Lancet Oncol. 2013;14(1):e28–37.
40. Corbin KS, Hellman S, Weichselbaum RR. Extracranial oligometastases: a subset of metastases curable with stereotactic radiotherapy. J Clin Oncol. 2013;31(11):1384–90.
41. Milano MT, Katz AW, Zhang H, Okunieff P. Oligometastases treated with stereotactic body radiotherapy: long-term follow-up of prospective study. Int J Radiat Oncol Biol Phys. 2012;83(3):878–86.
42. Dawood S, Gonzalez-Angulo AM. Progress in the biological understanding and management of breast cancer-associated central nervous system metastases. Oncologist. 2013;18(6):675–84.
43. Karaman Ş, Kücücük S. Neurological metastases. In: Aydiner A, İgci A, Soran A, editors. Breast disease. Cham: Springer; 2016.
44. Cardoso F, Costa A, Norton L, Cameron D, Cufer T, Fallowfield L, et al. 1st International consensus guidelines for advanced breast cancer (ABC 1). Breast. 2012;21(3):242–52.
45. Dyer MA, Kelly PJ, Chen YH, Pinnell NE, Claus EB, Lee EQ, et al. Importance of extracranial disease status and tumor subtype for patients undergoing radiosurgery for breast cancer brain metastases. Int J Radiat Oncol Biol Phys. 2012;83(4):e479–86.
46. Anders CK, Deal AM, Miller CR, Khorram C, Meng H, Burrows E, et al. The prognostic contribution of clinical breast cancer subtype, age, and race among patients with breast cancer brain metastases. Cancer. 2011;117(8):1602–11.
47. Linskey ME, Andrews DW, Asher AL, Burri SH, Kondziolka D, Robinson PD, et al. The role of stereotactic radiosurgery in the management of patients with newly diagnosed brain

metastases: a systematic review and evidence-based clinical practice guideline. J Neuro-Oncol. 2010;96(1):45–68.
48. Gaspar LE, Mehta MP, Patchell RA, Burri SH, Robinson PD, Morris RE, et al. The role of whole brain radiation therapy in the management of newly diagnosed brain metastases: a systematic review and evidence-based clinical practice guideline. J Neuro-Oncol. 2010;96(1):17–32.
49. Kalkanis SN, Kondziolka D, Gaspar LE, Burri SH, Asher AL, et al. The role of surgical resection in the management of newly diagnosed brain metastases: a systematic review and evidence-based clinical practice guideline. J Neuro-Oncol. 2010;96(1):33–43.
50. Patil CG, Pricola K, Sarmiento JM, Garg SK, Bryant A, Black KL. Whole brain radiation therapy (WBRT) alone versus WBRT and radiosurgery for the treatment of brain metastases. Cochrane Database Syst Rev. 2012;9:CD006121.
51. Andrews DW, Scott CB, Sperduto PW, Flanders AE, Gaspar LE, Schell MC, et al. Whole brain radiation therapy with or without stereotactic radiosurgery boost for patients with one to three brain metastases: phase III results of the RTOG 9508 randomised trial. Lancet. 2004;363(9422):1665–72.
52. Combs SE, Schulz-Ertner D, Thilmann C, Edler L, Debus J. Treatment of cerebral metastases from breast cancer with stereotactic radiosurgery. Strahlenther Onkol. 2004;180(9):590–6.
53. Mahajan A, Ahmed S, McAleer MF, Weinberg JS, Li J, Brown P, et al. Post-operative stereotactic radiosurgery versus observation for completely resected brain metastases: a single-centre, randomised, controlled, phase 3 trial. Lancet Oncol. 2017;18(8):1040–8.
54. Cardoso F, Costa A, Norton L, Senkus E, Aapro M, Andre F, et al. ESO-ESMO 2nd international consensus guidelines for advanced breast cancer (ABC2) dagger. Ann Oncol. 2014;25(10):1871–88.

Part VIII
Treatment of Metastatic Breast Cancer

Chapter 22
Systemic Treatment of HER2-Negative Metastatic Breast Cancer

Soley Bayraktar and Adnan Aydiner

Introduction

Breast cancer is the most common cancer in women, with more than 200,000 new cases in 2014, and it is the second leading cause of cancer death in women [1]. Although often curable when localized to the breast and local lymph nodes, if the disease becomes metastatic, it is usually not curable. Breast cancer is a heterogeneous disease comprising several molecular subtypes, which are commonly extrapolated into clinical subtypes based on receptor status [2]. The specific receptors that are assessed in standard clinical practice are the estrogen receptor (ER), progesterone receptor (PR), and human epidermal growth factor 2-neu (HER2) receptor. These receptors are both prognostic but also predictive of response to targeted therapy; thus, when metastasis is suspected, it is crucial to perform a biopsy not only to confirm recurrent disease but also to confirm receptor status [3]. In addition, tissue availability may increase clinical trial access because many studies now assess targetable molecular aberrancies. Figure 22.1 outlines the therapeutic approach to women with ER/PR+ and HER2-negative or 'triple-negative' metastatic breast cancer (MBC); the evidence supporting these treatment strategies is discussed below.

S. Bayraktar
Department of Medical Oncology, Memorial Hospital, Istanbul, Turkey

A. Aydiner (✉)
Internal Medicine, Medical Oncology, Istanbul Medical Faculty, Department of Medical Oncology, Institute of Oncology, Istanbul University, Istanbul, Turkey

A. Aydiner et al. (eds.), *Breast Cancer*, https://doi.org/10.1007/978-3-319-96947-3_22

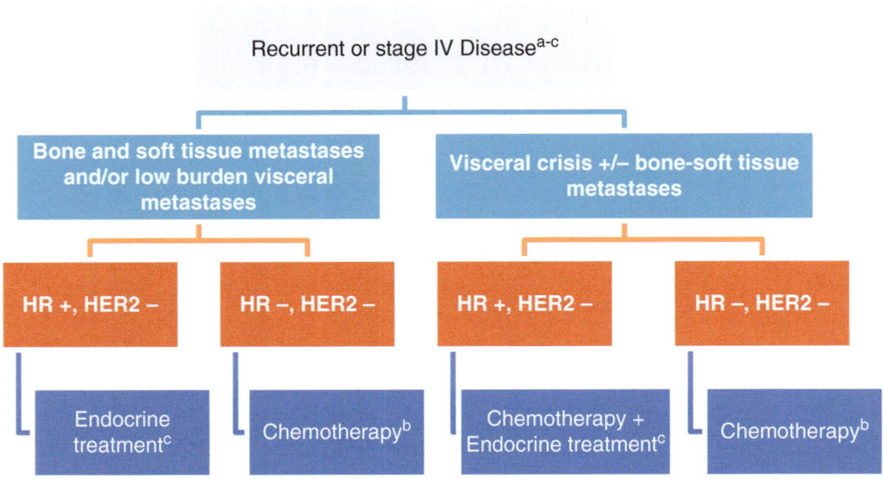

Fig. 22.1 Systemic treatment for recurrent or stage IV and HER2-negative disease. [a]If possible, a biopsy should be performed for pretreatment receptor assessment in relapse tumors. The benefit of palliative local breast surgery to women presenting with stage IV disease remains unclear. This local therapy should be considered only after a response to initial systemic therapy. Notably, some studies suggest that surgery is only valuable if performed with the same attention to detail (e.g., attaining clear margins and addressing disease in the axilla) as in patients with early-stage disease. If bone disease is present, add denosumab, zoledronic acid, ibandronic acid, or pamidronate. [b]"Anti-programmed death-1" (PD-1)/"Programmed death ligand" (PDL-1) antibodies were found to be effective alone or with taxanes in patients with triple-negative tumors. [c]The major determinants of the treatment plan include the number of lesions, extent of visceral involvement, receptor status of the primary lesion, sites of recurrence and metastasis, and previous response to endocrine treatment. The addition of CD4/6 inhibitors to the first- or second-choice endocrine treatment was found to be effective in randomized clinical trials. The combination of exemestane, tamoxifen or fulvestrant with everolimus can be considered for patients who progressed within 12 months on a non-steroidal AI or on tamoxifen at any time. Fulvestrant can be used as the first choice in de novo metastatic disease not previously treated with any endocrine treatment

Systemic Chemotherapy of HER2-Negative Metastatic Breast Cancer

Considerable advances have been made in the treatment of certain subtypes of breast cancer, such as HER2-positive disease. In this subtype, targeted therapies against HER2 have changed the clinical outcome for patients with metastatic disease by providing them with several effective therapies that can extend survival by many years [4]. The ER- and PR-positive subtypes also have several targeted therapies available that use endocrine therapies; however, when the disease becomes metastatic, all patients eventually develop endocrine resistance and eventually require cytotoxic chemotherapy [5]. Patients with ER-, PR-, and HER2-negative tumors, so-called triple-negative breast cancers (TNBCs), biologically tend to display an aggressive phenotype, currently do not have targeted therapy options as a standard of care, and have only a limited number of cytotoxic agents available to treat their disease [6]. This chapter narrates and expands on some of the recent efforts in drug development for HER2-negative MBC, and the current standard of care of these different subtypes of breast cancer is summarized.

Treatment of ER/PR-Positive HER2-Negative Metastatic Breast Cancer

Two-thirds of all women diagnosed with breast cancer have a disease that is ER/PR+. These tumors are highly responsive to anti-estrogen therapeutic strategies. However, despite widespread use of hormonal adjuvant therapy, a quarter of women with ER+ disease will relapse. In this situation, a determination regarding further hormonal therapy versus chemotherapy as the next step must be made. Patients whose disease is viscerally relatively 'low'-volume, bone/soft tissue-predominant, and asymptomatic are reasonable candidates for upfront endocrine therapy. Table 22.1 outlines the treatment strategies for women with ER+ MBC. The current standart practice for these patients will be discussed in Chap. 24.

Tamoxifen, Fulvestrant, and Ovarian Suppression

The current practice for premenopausal women with MBC previously unexposed to hormone blockade is treatment in the first-line setting with tamoxifen as initial endocrine therapy or with aromatase inhibitor (AI) therapy in combination with ovarian suppression (via oophorectomy, radiation, or a GnRH agonist). Ovarian radiation is a less optimal mode of ablation as the success rate and time to ablation vary, in contrast to the irreversible and immediate ablation afforded by oophorectomy. An Eastern Cooperative Oncology Group study examining adjuvant estrogen blockade in premenopausal patients randomly assigned patients to tamoxifen monotherapy versus tamoxifen plus ovarian ablation via radiotherapy, oophorectomy, or GnRH agonists [7]. The trial was closed early for inadequate accrual; however, 75% of those undergoing radiotherapy achieved estradiol or follicle-stimulating hormone (FSH) levels consistent with those of ovarian ablation at 6 months after completing 20 Gy in 10 fractions. Further evidence supporting the need for ovarian suppression in addition to tamoxifen is lacking; data pertaining to premenopausal women in the adjuvant setting suggest that the combination of goserelin and tamoxifen is not superior to tamoxifen alone [8].

Fulvestrant (Faslodex; AstraZeneca, London, UK) is a synthetic ER antagonist that downregulates and degrades ERs by competitively binding them without tamoxifen's partial agonist effect. Intramuscular injections of fulvestrant were compared with those of tamoxifen in a large randomized trial to determine whether the absence of the partial agonist properties of fulvestrant improved outcomes among

Table 22.1 Selected phase III clinical trials of endocrine therapy in MBC

Regimen	Line of endocrine therapy	Number of patients included	Findings
Tamoxifen [103]	1st Line	156	RR: 16%, TTP: 6.7 mo, 5-year PFS: 8%, OS: 27.2 mo
Tamoxifen vs. BSO [10]	1st line	53	CR: 0% vs. 15% PR: 31% vs. 20% TTP: 160 vs. 144 days OS: 749 vs. 722 days
BSO/RT vs. goserelin vs. BSO/RT + tamoxifen vs. Tamoxifen + goserelin [104]	1st line	85	RR: 47% vs. 27% vs. 11% vs. 45% OS: 37(ovarian) vs. 36 mo (goserelin)
Buserelin vs. tamoxifen vs. Buserelin + tamoxifen [105]	1st line	161	RR: 34% vs. 28% vs. 48% PFS: 6.3 vs. 5.6 vs. 9.7 mo[a] OS: 2.5 vs. 2.9 vs. 3.7 years[a]
Fulvestrant 500 mg vs. 250 mg every 30 days [9]	1st/2nd line	736	RR: 9% vs. 10% PFS HR: 0.8[a] OS HR: 0.78
Fulvestrant 250 mg vs. tamoxifen 20 mg [106]	1st line	587	RR: 33% vs. 31% TTP: 8.2 vs. 8.3 OS: 39.3 vs. 40.7 mo
Fulvestrant vs. anastrozole [11]	1st line	205	CBR: 73% vs. 67% TTP: not reached vs. 12.5 mo[a]
Anastrozole → tamoxifen vs. Tamoxifen → anastrozole [107]	1st line	60	TTP: 28.2 vs.19.5 mo OS: 69.7 vs. 59.3 mo
Letrozole vs. tamoxifen [14]	1st line	977	TTP: 42 vs. 21 weeks[a]
Exemestane vs. megestrol [16]	1st line	769	TTP: 20 vs. 17 weeks[a] OS: not reached vs. 123.4 weeks[a]
Exemestane vs. tamoxifen [15]	1st line	371	RR: 46% vs. 31%[a] PFS: 9.9 vs. 5.8 mo[a] but NS after 47 mo follow-up OS HR: 1.13
Anastrozole vs. exemestane [17]	1st line	130	Insufficient accrual RR: 16% vs. 16% TTP: 3.71 vs. 4.24 mo OS: 33.3 vs 30.5 mo
Tamoxifen vs. megestrol [108]	1st line	182	RR: 17% vs. 34%[a] TTF: 5.5 vs. 6.3 mo OS: 23.8 vs. 33 mo
Vorozole vs. megestrol [12]	1st/2nd line	452	RR: 10% vs. 7% Duration response: 18.2 vs. 12.5 mo TTP: 2.6 vs. 3.3 mo OS: 26.3 vs. 28.8 mo

[a]Statistically significant, *Mo* months, *BSO* bilateral salpingo-oophorectomy, *CBR* clinical benefit rate, *CR* complete response, *NS* not significant, *OS* overall survival, *PFS* progression-free survival, *PR* partial response, *RR* response rate, *RT* radiotherapy, *TTF* time-to treatment failure, *TTP* time-to treatment progression, *HR* hazard ratio

postmenopausal women with MBC. Despite the lack of first-line superiority over tamoxifen, the NCCTG (North Central Cancer Treatment Group) N0032 and CONFIRM (Comparison of Faslodex in Recurrent or Metastatic Breast Cancer) trials demonstrated that fulvestrant has efficacy as sequential endocrine therapy in postmenopausal women in the second- and even third-line settings [9, 10]. The latter study also established the current standard dose of fulvestrant at 500 mg monthly due to its superior efficacy compared with 250 mg monthly [9]. Subsequently, the FALCON trial, a phase III study that randomly assigned women who were endocrine therapy naïve to fulvestrant (500 mg monthly) versus anastrozole (1 mg daily), showed a comparable clinical benefit rate (CBR) and a longer PFS for fulvestrant, suggesting its potential as an alternative to AIs as a first-line endocrine agent in postmenopausal women [11].

Aromatase Inhibitors (AI): Exemestane, Anastrozole, and Letrozole

Estrogen production in postmenopausal women is derived from the peripheral aromatization of androgens. Inhibition of aromatase is consequently a cornerstone of hormonal blockade in the management of postmenopausal breast cancer [12]. These drugs cannot be used alone safely in premenopausal women without concomitant ovarian suppression or ablation since aromatase inhibition in the setting of functional ovaries will lead to ovarian hyperstimulation. AIs currently in use include anastrozole (AstraZeneca, London, UK), letrozole (Novartis, East Hanover, NJ, USA), and exemestane (Pfizer Inc, New York, NY, USA). An analysis of two large randomized trials showed that anastrozole was at least equivalent to tamoxifen in the first-line setting in postmenopausal women who were endocrine therapy-naïve in the metastatic setting; unplanned subgroup analysis restricted to patients with known hormone receptor positivity demonstrated a superior TTP for anastrozole [13]. Letrozole has also been directly compared with tamoxifen in the first-line setting among women with MBC, revealing a similar increase in TTP [14]. Consequently, anastrozole and letrozole, non-steroidal AIs, are first-line endocrine options in postmenopausal MBC.

Exemestane, in contrast to the non-steroidals in this class, is a steroidal AI that irreversibly inhibits aromatase. In women who progressed on tamoxifen, exemestane resulted in prolonged TTP and OS compared with megestrol [15, 16]. In addition to utility in the second-line setting, exemestane yielded a significant early improvement in TTP compared with tamoxifen in the first-line setting, although after a longer follow-up, the two drugs were found to have comparable efficacy [15]. There is a paucity of data comparing AIs directly to each other in the metastatic setting; however, extrapolation from a small trial showed that exemestane and anastrozole produced similar RRs among postmenopausal women who had MBC and who were tamoxifen refractory [17].

Progestins: Megestrol

Progestins such as megestrol acetate (MA) are some of the oldest compounds used in the treatment of MBC and indirectly reduce serum estrogen levels by reducing androgen levels. Although the use of these agents has dropped dramatically since the introduction of AIs and GNRH agonists, there are data demonstrating efficacy of these agents in the MBC setting. Although randomized trials comparing MA and tamoxifen show comparable RRs and TTP, ultimately tamoxifen remains preferable to MA because of its toxicity profile. Analyses comparing AI and MA have shown that anastrozole confers a survival advantage over MA, whereas letrozole confers an improved RR and time to treatment failure [12]. After failure on first- and second-line therapies, data suggest that the use of MA as a second- or third-line therapy is reasonable for 'durable' disease stabilization but not with the goal of response [18].

Treatment of ER/PR-Positive HER2-Negative Endocrine-Refractory Metastatic Breast Cancer

Mechanisms of Endocrine Therapy Resistance in ER+ Breast Cancer

Acquired resistance (defined as recurrence at least 6–12 months after completion of adjuvant therapy or disease progression more than 6 months after endocrine therapy initiated in the metastatic setting) and occasionally primary resistance (recurrence either during adjuvant therapy or within 6–12 months of completion of adjuvant therapy or disease progression less than 6 months after treatment in the metastatic setting) to antiestrogen therapy is inevitable in patients with ER+ metastatic breast cancer (MBC).

A variety of mechanisms have been implicated in primary and acquired resistance to endocrine agents (Sidebar 22.1). Below we review some strategies for overcoming endocrine therapy resistance.

Sidebar 22.1 Mechanisms of resistance to endocrine agents
Primary resistance

- Receptor tyrosine kinase/growth factor signaling pathway
- *FGFR* amplification
- *EGFR*/*ERBB2* mutations
- Cell cycle control signaling pathway
- Cyclin D1 amplification or expression
- *MYC* amplification and overexpression
- Hormone signaling pathway
- Loss of ERα
- Post-translational modification of ERα
- Expression of ER coactivation/corepression factors

Acquired resistance

- PI3K/AKT1/MTOR signaling pathway
- PI3K/AKT/mTOR pathway activation
- Mitogen-activated protein (MAP) kinase pathway
- MAPK/ERK pathway activation
- Hormone signaling pathway
- *ESR1* mutations
- Changes in the tumor microenvironment

mTOR Inhibitors

The PI3K–Akt–mTOR signaling pathway is a major intracellular signaling pathway that plays a significant role in cell growth and proliferation and has been implicated in resistance to endocrine therapy [19]. The Breast Cancer Trials of Oral Everolimus-2 (BOLERO-2) study [20] demonstrated that inhibiting mTOR with everolimus in combination with exemestane improved progression-free survival (PFS) compared with exemestane alone in patients with ER-positive MBC previously treated with a nonsteroidal AI (NSAI). However, the phase III HORIZON trial [21] found no survival benefit of combining temsirolimus with letrozole in the first-line setting, suggesting that mTOR signaling may have a specific role in acquired resistance to endocrine therapy. Although the BOLERO-2 study combination has become a standard of care in patients whose disease has progressed after treatment with a NSAI, it is unknown if everolimus has meaningful single-agent activity that could explain the results [22, 23]. Several ongoing trials will better define the role of everolimus in advanced disease: BOLERO-6 (NCT01783444), a phase II trial comparing exemestane/everolimus to capecitabine in ER+/HER2-negative disease refractory to AI, and BOLERO-4 (NCT01698918), a phase II single-arm study evaluating the role of everolimus as a first-line treatment. Everolimus is also being evaluated in the adjuvant setting in two studies using two different approaches: (1) SWOG1207 (NCT01674140), which will randomly assign high-risk premenopausal and postmenopausal patients to add everolimus or placebo to their standard adjuvant endocrine therapy; and (2) NCT01805271, which will evaluate the addition of everolimus to adjuvant endocrine therapy in high-risk ER+/HER2-negative patients with breast cancer who remain disease free after at least 1 year of treatment.

PI3K Inhibitors

PI3K inhibitors consist of pan-PI3K targeting all class I isoforms, isoform-specific PI3K inhibitors, and dual PI3K/mTOR inhibitors. Compounds may also display differential activity for wild-type and mutant PI3K proteins. The response rates for single-agent PI3K inhibitors are far below those for other kinase inhibitors in other cancer types (such as EGFR, ALK, or BRAF inhibitors).

Buparlisib (BKM120) is a pan-PI3K inhibitor with potent activity against mutant PI3Kα [24]. Early-phase trials of buparlisib plus endocrine therapy reported activity and a manageable safety profile characterized by transaminitis, hyperglycemia, diarrhea, and mood disorders (anxiety, depression, irritability) [25]. The randomized phase III BELLE-2 trial studied fulvestrant 500 mg plus buparlisib 100 mg daily or placebo in postmenopausal MBC progressing on AIs [26]. Buparlisib increased the median PFS by 1.9 months (6.9 months vs. 5.0 months, $p < 0.001$). For patients with PI3K/AKT pathway activation (defined as PIK3CA mutation or PTEN loss, assayed in the archival primary tumor for the majority of patients), there was no difference in the benefit of buparlisib. However, in the subset of patients in whom PIK3CA mutation was assessed by circulating tumor DNA at trial entry, buparlisib plus fulvestrant increased PFS in PIK3CA mutant cases compared with fulvestrant alone (7 months vs. 3.2 months; HR, 0.56; $p < 0.001$).

Using the same treatment arms as BELLE-2, the phase III BELLE-3 trial enrolled AI-experienced patients with disease progression in the past 30 days on an mTOR inhibitor plus endocrine therapy [27]. The median PFS for patients in the buparlisib arm was 3.9 months versus 1.8 months for fulvestrant/placebo, and the 6-month PFS rates were 30.6% and 20.1%, respectively. Of the 349 patients for whom PIK3CA mutation status from circulating tumor DNA was available, 147 had mutations in the gene. Among those with PIK3CA mutations, PFS was 4.7 months in the buparlisib arm versus 1.6 months in the placebo arm. A similar result was obtained for PIK3CA status in tumor tissue.

Fulvestrant

Another strategy used to overcome resistance to single-agent endocrine therapy is to target the ER. Fulvestrant binds to the ER, causing its downregulation; thus, estradiol may compete for receptor site occupancy. Preclinical studies [28] have suggested that the antitumor effects of fulvestrant can be increased in a low-estrogen environment, and studies in breast cancer xenografts have found the combination of an AI with fulvestrant to have synergistic antitumor effects. Combination endocrine therapy using AIs and fulvestrant in the metastatic setting has been studied in large randomized clinical trials with discordant results [29, 30]. The Southwest Oncology Group (SWOG) 0226 study demonstrated a median PFS of 13.5 months (95% CI, 12.1–15.1 months) for the anastrozole arm compared with 15 months (95% CI, 13.2–18.4 months) for the combination arm (HR, 0.8; $p = 0.007$), with overall survival (OS) favoring the combination arm as well (HR, 0.81; $p = 0.049$). However, subgroup analysis demonstrated that the benefit was restricted to patients who had not received prior tamoxifen (HR, 0.74; $p = 0.006$) rather than those previously treated with tamoxifen (HR, 0.89; $p = 0.39$) [30]. The Fulvestrant and Anastrozole Combination Therapy (FACT) study [29] and the Study of Faslodex with or without concomitant Arimidex vs Exemestane following progression on NSAIs (SoFEA) [28], on the other hand, showed no difference in median PFS. These results therefore have had limited applicability in clinical practice. However, neither the SWOG

0226 study nor the FACT study investigated fulvestrant alone as a control arm, although data from SoFEA suggest that fulvestrant and exemestane are equivalent in patients whose disease progressed during treatment with a NSAI (HR, 0.95; p = 0.56). Notably, these studies used the 250-mg dose of fulvestrant, which was subsequently shown to be inferior to the 500-mg dose in the Comparison of Faslodex in Recurrent or Metastatic Breast Cancer (CONFIRM) study. The 500-mg dose is now the standard of care dose [9]. In addition, in the front-line setting, the Fulvestrant FIRST-line Study comparing endocrine Treatments (FIRST) suggested that 500 mg of fulvestrant compared with anastrozole may improve median time to progression (HR, 0.63; p = 0.049), and an update at the 2014 SABCS suggested a similar benefit in median OS (HR, 0.7; p = 0.04). The FALCON trial, a phase III study that randomly assigned women who were endocrine therapy naïve to fulvestrant (500 mg monthly) versus anastrozole (1 mg daily), showed a comparable clinical benefit rate (CBR) and a longer PFS for fulvestrant, suggesting its potential as an alternative to AIs as a first-line endocrine agent in postmenopausal women [11].

Cyclin-Dependent Kinases 4 and 6 Inhibitors

A new strategy in treating patients with ER-positive breast cancer is to target cyclin-dependent kinases 4 and 6 (CDK4/6), a key pathway involved in regulating the G1/S transition of the cell cycle. Preclinical studies combining tamoxifen with the CDK4/6 inhibitor palbociclib demonstrated synergistic antitumor effects, which led to a phase 2 study randomizing 165 women with ER-positive MBC to front-line letrozole alone or in combination with palbociclib. This study showed a significant difference in PFS between the letrozole arm (10.2 months; 95% CI, 5.7–12.6 months) and the combination arm (20.2 months; 95% CI, 13.8–27.5 months) (HR, 0.488; 95% CI, 0.139–0.748; p < 0.001) [31]. The confirmatory phase III PALOMA-2 study randomized a total of 666 postmenopausal patients with ER+ MBC and no prior systemic therapy to receive letrozole with palbociclib or letrozole with placebo. Median PFS (the primary endpoint) was 24.8 months versus 14.5 months in favor of the palbociclib arm (hazard ratio [HR], 0.58; 95% CI, 0.46–0.72; p < 0.000001) [32]. The response rate was also improved in the palbociclib arm (42.1% vs. 34.7%, p = 0.031), and the clinical benefit rate was 84.9% versus 70.3% (p < 0.0001). Similar evidence of efficacy was observed in the phase III PALOMA-3 trial for the combination of fulvestrant plus palbociclib, in which PFS was 9.2 months versus 3.8 months with fulvestrant plus placebo (HR, 0.42; p < 0.000001) in patients with disease progression after at least one line of hormonal therapy and at most one line of chemotherapy but naive to CDK4/6 inhibitors [33, 34]. In both phase III trials, the most common grade 3 or 4 adverse event in the palbociclib arms was neutropenia (incidence 62–65%), but treatment was otherwise well-tolerated. Both palbociclib (or other CDK4/6 inhibitors) with letrozole for first-line treatment and palbociclib (or other CDK4/6 inhibitors) with fulvestrant for second-line treatment of patients with ER+/HER2-negative MBC are approved by the U.S. Food and Drug Administration (FDA). The current standart practice for these patients will be discussed in Chap. 24.

Treatment of Endocrine-Refractory or Triple-Negative Metastatic Breast Cancer that Presents with Visceral Threat

Admittedly, using receptor status and sensitivity to guide management of therapy in MBC oversimplifies the discrete molecular subtypes identified through advances in genomic analysis. For example, the biological behavior and drivers of an ER+ luminal breast cancer that becomes hormone-insensitive are presumably distinct from those of triple-negative basal-like subtypes, as evidenced by different patterns of relapse and response to treatment [35].

A guiding principle of treatment of metastatic disease is to respect the palliative goal of this therapy given the absence of data demonstrating superior survival benefit with combination cytotoxics rather than sequential strategies. Sequential administration of single agents has been considered a viable and acceptable standard of care, and this is due, in part, to Intergroup trial E1193, in which, despite increased RR and time to treatment failure with combination paclitaxel and doxorubicin in metastatic disease, sequential doxorubicin followed by paclitaxel and vice versa showed similar efficacy and no difference in survival benefit [36]. Many patients will require multiple lines of therapy for advanced disease, and consequently, use of combination chemotherapy regimens rather than sequential use of single-agent cytotoxics should be limited to specific circumstances in which performance status permits it and rapid response is critical, as with impending organ failure. Cytotoxics that have FDA-approved indications in MBC and activity as single agents include anthracyclines, taxanes, non-taxane microtubule inhibitors, and antimetabolites (Table 22.2).

Anthracycline Single-Agent Cytotoxic Therapy: Doxorubicin, Epirubicin, and Pegylated Liposomal Doxorubicin

Many patients will have been exposed to anthracyclines in the adjuvant setting; however, with the advent of docetaxel/cyclophosphamide as a standard adjuvant doublet, more patients may present with recurrent disease without having been exposed to these agents. Women with metastatic disease (receptor status not reported) exposed to alkylators in the adjuvant setting or to, at most, one line of therapy in the advanced setting or to both were randomly assigned to doxorubicin 75 mg/m^2 versus docetaxel 100 mg/m^2 every 3 weeks. Although docetaxel resulted in a higher objective RR in this pretreated population with visceral disease, there was no statistically significant difference in median TTP or OS. Neutropenic fever, infection, cardiac toxicity, nausea, and vomiting were more likely with anthracycline therapy, whereas the primary toxicities caused by docetaxel consisted of diarrhea, neuropathy, fluid retention, and skin and nail changes [37]. In a trial designed to establish the optimal dose of first-line epirubicin in MBC, women who had mostly positive/unknown hormone receptor status and whose adjuvant regimens

Table 22.2 Selected phase III clinical trials of single-agent and synergistic combination therapies in ER-positive, endocrine-refractory or triple-negative MBC

Drug/regimen	Line of therapy	Number of patients included	Findings
Doxorubicin 60 mg/m^2 every 3 weeks vs. liposomal doxorubicin 50 mg/m^2 every 3 weeks [39]	± adjuvant anthracycline or endocrine	509	PFS: 7.8 vs. 6.9 mo OS: 22 vs. 21 mo
Doxorubicin 75 mg/m^2 every 3 weeks vs. docetaxel 100 mg/m^2 every 3 weeks [37]	Prior alkylator	326	RR: 33% vs 48%[a] TTP: 21 vs. 26 weeks OS: 14 vs 15 mo
Docetaxel 100 mg/m^2 every 3 weeks vs. paclitaxel 175 mg/m^2 every 3 weeks [40]	1st and 2nd line	449	TTP: 5.7 vs. 3.6 mo[a] OS: 15.4 vs.12.7 mo[a]
Nab-paclitaxel 260 mg/m^2 every 3 weeks vs. paclitaxel 175 mg/m^2 every 3 weeks [44]	Unlimited, no prior taxane in metastatic setting	225	RR: 33% vs. 19%[a] TTP: 23 vs. 16.9 weeks[a] OS: 60.5 vs. 55.7 weeks
Docetaxel 100 mg/m^2 every 3 weeks vs. capecitabine 1250 mg/m^2 twice a day × 14 days every 3 weeks + docetaxel 75 mg/m^2 every 3 weeks [78]	1st/2nd line	511	RR: 30% vs. 42%[a] TTP: 6.1 vs. 4.2 mo[a] OS: 14.5 vs. 11.5 mo[a]
Paclitaxel 175 mg/m^2 every 3 weeks vs. paclitaxel 175 mg/m^2 every 3 weeks + gemcitabine 1250 mg/m^2 day 1 and day 8 every 3 weeks [79]	1st line	529	RR: 41% vs. 26%[a] TTP: 6.14 vs. 3.98 mo[a] OS: 18.6 vs. 15.8 mo[a]
Eribulin 1.4 mg/m^2 every week × 2 weeks every 3 weeks vs. physicians' choice [53]	Median 4 prior	762	PFS: 3.7 vs. 2.2 mo OS: 13.1 vs. 10.6 mo[a]
Capecitabine 1250 mg/m^2 twice a day × 14 days every 3 weeks vs. ixabepilone 40 mg/m^2 every 3 weeks + capecitabine 1000 mg/m^2 twice a day × 14 days every 3 weeks [109]	3rd line	1221	RR: 29% vs. 43%[a] PFS: 4.2 vs. 6.2 mo[a] OS: 15.6 vs. 16.4 mo

[a]Statistically significant, *Mo* months, *CBR* clinical benefit rate, *OS* overall survival, *PFS* progression-free survival, *RR* response rate, *TTP* time to progression

were nonanthracycline-based were randomly assigned to four dose levels of epirubicin, including 90 mg/m^2, which is hematologically equivalent to the maximum tolerated dose of 75 mg/m^2 of doxorubicin. This dose was found to afford the greatest TTP with the least toxicity and is further evidence of the efficacy of single-agent anthracyclines [38]. Pegylated liposomal doxorubicin (PLD) has also been examined in the hope that preferential accumulation in tumor tissue would limit cardiotoxicity. In a noninferiority trial designed to assess efficacy and cardiac safety, women who could have received prior adjuvant anthracycline were randomly assigned to either PLD or doxorubicin. Non-inferiority was achieved; however, not surprisingly, significantly more doxorubicin-treated patients met the protocol-defined criteria for cardiotoxicity [39].

Taxane Single-Agent Cytotoxic Therapy: Paclitaxel and Docetaxel

Single-agent taxanes are an effective option in metastatic patients, particularly in those who were treated with only anthracycline-based adjuvant therapy. Taxanes induce mitotic arrest by inhibiting depolymerization of the microtubules. Although the mechanisms of binding to tubulin and cell cycle arrest through stabilization of microtubules of paclitaxel and docetaxel are similar, preclinical studies have shown that docetaxel has greater affinity, longer retention time, and higher intracellular concentration in target cells [40]. The side-effect profiles are also different because fluid retention and fatigue are more characteristic of docetaxel toxicity, whereas hyper sensitivity and neurotoxicity are more common with paclitaxel. This difference is thought to be related to the solvents requirı́ng for stabilization of these hydrophobic compounds. Several studies have examined optimal dosing regimens of taxanes. Weekly paclitaxel appears to be as effective as or more effective than every-21-day dosing [41, 42]. Docetaxel administered every 3 weeks has better efficacy compared with either weekly or every-3-week paclitaxel but at the expense of greater toxicity [40]. Docetaxel on a weekly schedule still results in some fatigue, fluid retention, and excess lacrimation but less myelosuppression and neuropathy [43]. Nab-paclitaxel appears to be more effective and convenient than paclitaxel and docetaxel and affords the benefit of taxane therapy without steroid premedication [44].

Non-Taxane Microtubule Inhibitor Single-Agent Cytotoxic Therapy: Vinorelbine, Ixabepilone, and Eribulin

Other microtubule inhibitors efficacious in the treatment of metastatic disease in those exposed/resistant to anthracyclines and taxanes include vinorelbine, ixabepilone, and eribulin. Nearly a quarter of patients who progressed through anthracyclines and taxanes treated with weekly *vinorelbine* (dose modified to 25 mg/m^2 because of hematological toxicity and neurotoxicity) had an objective response [45]. Vinorelbine binds to tubulin, inhibiting tubulin polymerization, and this may explain why sensitivity to vinorelbine is retained among patients pretreated with taxanes because excess depolymerized tubulin has been noted in vitro.

Ixabepilone is an epothilone B analog that increases polymerization but, unlike taxanes, has the capacity to bind to multiple isomers of tubulin. Ixabepilone has been evaluated in the setting of patients pretreated with anthracyclines, taxanes, and capecitabine as well as in first-line metastatic treatment of patients treated with adjuvant anthracyclines. In the first-line setting, women with MBC achieved an overall RR of 41.5% and a median survival of 22 months [46, 47]. Modifications in the administration schedule of ixabepilone in a group of women who had not had prior taxane exposure did reduce neurotoxicity while maintaining RRs comparable to those of historical controls of docetaxel or paclitaxel in the first- or second-line metastatic setting [48]. Women with taxane-resistant MBC or those pretreated with taxanes and capecitabine had RRs ranging from 11% to 12% and a durable response of nearly 6 months [49, 50]. In this heavily pretreated population with prior exposure to taxane therapy, half experienced reversible sensory neuropathy.

Eribulin is the latest non-taxane microtubule inhibitor with a mechanism distinct from that of taxanes, epothilones, and vinca alkaloids in that it affects centromere dynamics and sequesters tubulin into nonfunctional aggregates. Like vinorelbine, eribulin decreases polymerization of microtubules [51]. Phase II studies have shown efficacy in populations pretreated with anthracyclines and taxane as well as capecitabine. Despite a median of four prior regimens, women still achieved RRs ranging from 9% to 14% and a PFS of approximately 2.6 months [52]. A phase III trial randomly assigning heavily pretreated patients to eribulin showed an improvement in OS of 13.1 months compared with 10.6 months in women treated according to physician's choice. Neutropenia (52%), fatigue (54%), and neuropathy (35%) were common toxicities [53].

Antimetabolite Single-Agent Cytotoxic Therapy: Capecitabine and Gemcitabine

Antimetabolite therapy should be considered in women with prior exposure to anthracycline and taxane therapy. Capecitabine is an orally administered precursor of 5-deoxy-5-fluorouridine monotherapy that is preferentially converted to 5-fluorouracil in tumor tissue by exploiting the high intratumoral concentrations of thymidine phosphorylase. A group of women who had received over three prior cytotoxic regimens, including prior anthracycline and taxane therapy, achieved an objective RR of 26% and a median survival of 12.2 months with capecitabine monotherapy, even though nearly half required dose reduction. Retrospective analysis suggested that dose reduction for palmar-plantar erythrodysesthesia, diarrhea, and nausea did not affect efficacy [54]. Capecitabine monotherapy was also tested in the first-line setting against cyclophosphamide/methotrexate/fluorouracil with comparable RRs, although palmar-plantar erythrodysesthesia induced by capecitabine required treatment interruptions and dose reductions in a third of patients [54]. Capecitabine at a lower dose of 1000 mg/m^2 daily for 14 days of a 21-day cycle was compared with previously tested regimens of 1250 mg/m^2 to assess safety in women at least 65 years of age, half of whom had received prior systemic treatments. The lower dose afforded similar rates of tumor response with better tolerability in the lower-dose group [55].

Gemcitabine has also been evaluated as a single-agent therapy in multiple trials in both the first-line and refractory/resistant settings at doses ranging from 800 to 1200 mg/m^2 weekly for 3 weeks on a 28-day cycle. RRs varied from 14.5% to 37% with an OS of 21 months in the first-line setting to RRs of 20–37.1% with an OS of 11 months in a pretreated setting [56, 57].

Platinum Agents

The efficacy of platinum agents in TNBC documented in the neoadjuvant setting has made them attractive agents for consideration in the metastatic setting [58]. A retrospective study [59] has shown that in patients with metastatic TNBC, platinum-based chemotherapy is associated with improved survival. The Triple-Negative Breast Cancer Trial (TNT), recently presented at the 2014 SABCS, randomized 376 unselected patients with metastatic TNBC to carboplatin vs docetaxel. In the overall analysis, median PFS was not statistically significant (P = 0.29; 3.1 vs 4.5 months for the carboplatin and docetaxel arms, respectively). However, for patients with breast cancer susceptibility gene (BRCA) germline mutations, the ORR for the carboplatin arm was more than double that of the docetaxel arm (ORR, 68.0 vs 33.3%; P = 0.03); homologous recombination deficiency (HRD) scores did not predict a benefit [60]. Moving forward, it will also be important to delineate which patients are most likely to derive benefit from platinum-based therapy and whether BRCA germline mutations or HRD biomarkers can predict who is most likely to benefit.

New Approaches for Triple-Negative Breast Cancer (TNBC): PARP Inhibitors and Beyond

Subtypes of TNBC have been described on the basis of histopathological features and gene expression profiling, highlighting the heterogeneity and complexity of these tumors [61]. Four distinct breast cancer subtypes (luminal A, luminal B, HER2 enriched, and basal-like) of prognostic and predictive significance were first described by Perou et al. [2] in 2000 using microarray analysis. Of the four subtypes, basal-like tumors are typically of the triple-negative phenotype, and the vast majority (approximately 80%) of TNBCs are of the basal-like subtype [62]. In analyzing gene expression profiles of TNBC, Lehmann et al. [63] identified six distinct molecular subtypes (basal-like 1, basal-like 2, immunomodulatory, mesenchymal, mesenchymal stem-like, and luminal androgen receptor). These molecular subtypes were refined into four tumor-specific subtypes (basal-like 1, basal-like 2, mesenchymal, and luminal androgen receptor) following histopathology and laser capture microdissection, which identified infiltrating lymphocytes and tumor-associated stromal cells contributing to the immunomodulatory and mesenchymal stem-like subtypes, respectively [62]. In addition to microarray-based studies, the genomic landscape of this disease has been extensively interrogated, resulting in the identification of alterations that add to our burgeoning knowledge of TNBC [64]. The features and alterations unique to these various subtypes have been incorporated into many ongoing, rationally designed trials to refine treatment strategies. In this section, we discuss notable novel approaches in the treatment of TNBC.

PARP Inhibitors

The effectiveness of poly(adenosine diphosphate-ribose) polymerase (PARP) inhibitors has been of great interest in TNBC, especially in women with BRCA germline mutations. Iniparib, initially thought to be a PARP inhibitor, was studied in a phase 2 study in an unselected population of patients with metastatic TNBC and showed improved PFS (3.6–5.9 months) and OS (7.7–12.3 months), prompting a larger phase 3 study that did not show improved PFS or OS [65, 66]. Subsequent definitive preclinical studies, however, demonstrated that in fact iniparib has weak, if any PARP, inhibitory effects [67]. Although these studies nearly put an end to the development of PARP inhibitors in breast cancer, several agents, including olaparib and veliparib among many others, are now actively being developed [68]. An ongoing phase III trial evaluating PARP inhibition in BRCA-mutant MBCs including olaparib, OlympiAD (NCT02000622), has reached its primary endpoint. In this trial, 302 patients with inherited BRCA mutations who had MBC that was either ER-positive or triple-negative were randomly assigned to receive olaparib tablets or standard chemotherapy (capecitabine, vinorelbine, or eribulin) until the cancer worsened or the patient developed severe side effects [69]. Tumors shrank in approximately 60% of patients who received olaparib, compared with 29% of those who received chemotherapy. At a median follow-up of approximately 14 months, patients who received olaparib had a 42% lower chance of cancer progression than those who received chemotherapy. The median time to progression was 7 months with olaparib and 4.2 months with chemotherapy. For women who have a BRCA germline mutation with metastatic ovarian cancer, the first PARP inhibitor, olaparib, has already been approved based on a phase 2 study and compelling ORR [70]. Ongoing efforts are focused on molecular diagnostics beyond BRCA testing to predict benefit from PARP inhibition as well as the application of PARP inhibitors in a broader population through combination strategies.

Androgen Receptor Blockers

The androgen receptor (AR) has been identified as a possible predictive biomarker for antiandrogen therapy in breast cancer. The Translational Breast Cancer Research Consortium (TBCRC) 011 study [71], a phase 2 study investigating bicalutamide in AR-positive, ER-negative breast cancer, found a clinical benefit rate (defined as complete or partial response or stable disease for >6 months) of 19% (95% CI, 7–39%), suggesting an antitumor effect even though only 12% of the 424 patients tested had AR positivity. Similarly, in a phase II trial of enzalutamide, a potent AR inhibitor, clinical benefit rate at 16 weeks was 25% (95% CI, 17% to 33%) in the intent-to-treat (ITT) population (all enrolled patients) and 33% (95% CI, 23% to 45%) in the evaluable subgroup. Median progression-free survival was 2.9 months (95% CI, 1.9 to 3.7 months) in the ITT population and 3.3 months (95% CI, 1.9 to 4.1 months) in the evaluable (whose tumor expressed ≥10% nuclear AR) subgroup. Median overall survival was 12.7 months (95% CI, 8.5 months to not yet reached) in the ITT population and 17.6 months (95% CI, 11.6 months to not yet reached) in the evaluable subgroup [72]. In this study, an androgen-driven diagnostic gene signature was associated with greater clinical benefit, and the phase III ENDEAR trial of paclitaxel plus enzalutamide/placebo and enzalutamide monotherapy has been initiated in diagnostic signature-positive TNBC (NCT02929576) [73].

Antibody-Drug Conjugates

Antibody-drug conjugates (ADCs) are a novel class of cancer therapeutics that combine the selectivity of a targeted treatment with the cytotoxicity of chemotherapy, resulting in an improved therapeutic index. Sacituzumab govitecan (IMMU-132) is an anti-Trop-2 ADC consisting of humanized IgG antibody against Trop-2 linked to SN-38, an active metabolite of irinotecan. The Trop-2 protein is an epithelial cancer antigen that is highly expressed in a majority of TNBC compared with normal tissues and is associated with a poor prognosis and aggressive disease [74]. In the first-in-human phase I trial, sacituzumab govitecan had an acceptable safety profile and evidence of efficacy, including one confirmed response and two minor responses in three of four patients with TNBC [75].

In the ongoing multicenter phase II trial, promising PFS of 5.6 months (95% CI, 3.6–7.1 months), OS of 14.3 months (95% CI, 10.5–18.8 months), and a response rate of 29% were observed in a heavily pretreated (median of five prior therapies) population of TNBC [76]. Sacituzumab govitecan has been given breakthrough therapy and fast-track designation from the FDA, and a phase III international multicenter randomized trial versus treatment of physician's choice in refractory mTNBC is planned for initiation in 2017 (NCT02574455).

Glembatumumab vedotin (CDX-011) is a fully human IgG2 monoclonal antibody with high affinity for the extracellular domain of glycoprotein nonmetastatic B linked to the microtubule inhibitor monomethyl auristatin E (MMAE). Glycoprotein nonmetastatic B is highly expressed in TNBC compared to normal tissue, predicts breast cancer recurrence, and is associated with reduced overall survival [77]. Early activity was observed in mTNBC and high-gpNMB-expressing tumors in the phase II EMERGE study [65]. The METRIC trial, a randomized phase III study evaluating glembatumumab vedotin versus capecitabine, is ongoing in gpNMB overexpressing TNBC (NCT01997333).

Combination Cytotoxic Therapy

Combination therapies generally increase RR and TTP but with a concomitant increase in toxicity. Moreover, a critical shortcoming of studies in this area is the use of study designs in which the combination is compared with one or the other of the agents alone. The lack of comparison between sequential use of both agents and the combination biases these studies in favor of the combination. Many cytotoxic combinations have been assessed in the metastatic setting; however, only a few have shown synergy in phase III studies to prolong OS over single-agent cytotoxics with manageable toxicities, and these regimens will be reviewed here.

The low myelotoxicity of capecitabine makes it an attractive agent for combination with other cytotoxics, and preclinical work showing tumor overexpression of thymidine phosphorylase by taxanes suggested that this was an opportunity for synergy. Patients pretreated with anthracycline (prior paclitaxel was permitted) were randomly assigned to capecitabine/docetaxel or docetaxel monotherapy, and the combination resulted in an increased RR, TTP, and OS. However, the improvement in efficacy was at the cost of more grade 3 adverse events (71% versus 49%) in the combination arm. The 1250 mg/m^2 twice-daily dose of capecitabine may have been too high to use in combination with docetaxel given evidence that 1000 mg/m^2 twice daily of capecitabine monotherapy is equivalent to higher doses in women at least 65 years old. Treatment interruption was required in 34% of capecitabine cycles and 27% of docetaxel cycles compared with 20% in the single-agent arm [78]. This trial did not answer the question of whether sequential administration would have had equivalent benefit with less toxicity.

Another study compared the combination of gemcitabine plus paclitaxel to gemcitabine alone in the first-line treatment of metastatic disease. Median survival was 18.6 versus 15.8 months (P = 0.0489) with a longer TTP (6.14 versus 3.98 months; P = 0.0002) and a higher RR (41.4% versus 26.2%; P = 0.0002). However, the 22% improvement in OS and 43% improvement in TTP were at the expense of more neutropenia, fatigue, and neuropathy. Again, the trial did not answer the question of whether sequential single-agent therapy would have yielded equivalent results [79]. The study design also precluded comparison with a weekly paclitaxel schedule, which appears preferential to a three-weekly schedule in the advanced setting [79, 80].

Given the proposed deficiency of DNA-repair mechanisms in triple-negative and basal-like tumors, platinum-based chemotherapy combinations have been presented as a strategy to treat these subtypes of MBC. Although phase II studies of carboplatin- or cisplatin-based combination regimens have demonstrated overall RRs ranging from 29% to 41% in triple-negative MBC, these responses are often at the expense of significant hematological and non-hematological side effects, including peripheral neuropathy, nephrotoxicity, and nausea [81, 82]. In light of the high rates of grade 3/4 toxicities for a palliative regimen and absence of prospective phase III data showing improvement in PFS and OS, the use of combination platinum-based therapy in triple-negative MBC warrants further study [83].

In summary, women whose MBC requires cytotoxic therapy have multiple alternatives. Monotherapy is preferable to minimize side effects given the paucity of data comparing combination regimens to sequential use of single agents. Presuming adequate performance status, women with prior exposure to anthracyclines should only receive paclitaxel, albumin-bound paclitaxel, or docetaxel as first-line treatment for their triple-negative or endocrine-refractory metastatic disease. Women who have progressed through taxane therapy can be treated with alternative microtubule inhibitors such as vinorelbine or eribulin if they do not have prohibitive residual neuropathy. A reasonable alternative is to treat these women with either capecitabine or gemcitabine. Combination cytotoxic regimens should be reserved for women who have good performance status and whose organ function is threatened by rapidly progressive disease.

New Directions in Targeting Angiogenesis

Although numerous studies investigating [84] anti–vascular endothelial growth factor (VEGF) therapy in the neoadjuvant setting have suggested improved pathologic complete response rates, especially in TNBC, studies to date have not demonstrated a survival benefit in the adjuvant setting or metastatic setting. Multiple studies have now been conducted in unselected patients with MBC. The Eastern Cooperative Oncology Group (ECOG) 2100 study [85] found that adding bevacizumab to paclitaxel in unselected patients with MBC improved PFS (11.8 vs 5.9 months; HR, 0.60; $p < 0.001$) but not OS (26.7 vs 25.2 months; HR, 0.88; $p = 0.16$). The Regimens in Bevacizumab for Breast Oncology-1 (RIBBON-1) trial [86, 87] showed that adding bevacizumab to chemotherapy in HER2-negative MBC also improved PFS but not OS in the first-line setting; the RIBBON-2 study had similar results in the second-line setting. Subgroup analysis, however, suggested that in patients with TNBC, there may be a trend toward OS benefit (HR, 0.624; $p = 0.05$) [88].

The phase 3 IMELDA study randomized patients with HER2-negative MBC to bevacizumab with or without capecitabine after induction with docetaxel and bevacizumab and found that the addition of capecitabine improved PFS (11.9 vs 4.3 months; $p < 0.001$) and OS (39.0 vs 23.7 months; $P = 0.003$) despite premature termination of the study [89]. An update at the 2014 SABCS meeting revealed no differences among different subgroups in terms of OS and no significant changes in quality of life measures. These results are difficult to apply in clinical practice because there was no control arm investigating capecitabine without bevacizumab. The TANIA phase 3 study, an investigation of bevacizumab continuation through second-line therapy in patients with HER2-negative MBC, reported that PFS was improved in those continuing bevacizumab (6.3 vs 4.2 months; $p = 0.007$); however, OS has not been reported to date [90]. A subgroup analysis of the TANIA study presented at the 2014 SABCS meeting suggested a slight benefit in the TNBC populations (median PFS, 4.9 vs 2.1 months) and that plasma-based VEGF biomarkers did not predict efficacy [91, 92]. The fact there are no data suggesting an improvement in OS in patients receiving bevacizumab compared to those who do not and the failure to identify patients who are more likely to benefit from anti-VEGF therapy have hindered the development of these drugs for MBC.

A key growth factor in angiogenesis is the fibroblast growth factor receptor gene (FGFR), and this may be an important mechanism of resistance to anti-VEGF therapy. Many genetic aberrations in FGFR have been identified in breast cancer. Approximately 10% of breast cancers will have FGFR aberrations, which are associated with inferior prognosis, especially in luminal-type breast cancers [93]. Several targeted drugs are currently under development to target tumors that have FGFR amplification [94].

Promises of Immune Therapies

The immune system can identify tumor antigens through immune surveillance, a process in which antigen-presenting cells present non–self-antigens to T cells, allowing them to recognize and destroy cells expressing such antigens. A hallmark of oncogenesis is that tumor cells can develop mechanisms to evade such immune recognition [95]. The success of immune checkpoint blockade in certain cancers has served as proof-of-concept that immune therapy is a viable therapeutic strategy. Cytotoxic T-lymphocyte antigen (CTLA) inhibitors have shown significant and sustained antitumor activity in melanoma [96]. Blockade of programmed cell death 1 (PD-1) and PD-L1 has also been found to have antitumor activity in certain cancers, with 6–17% overall response rates [97]. The effects of single-agent checkpoint blockade are modest, with only a small fraction of patients having clinically significant responses; however, combination checkpoint blockade with CTLA and PD-1 inhibitors has recently demonstrated synergistic activity, with an ORR of 40% and 31% of patients achieving greater than 80% reduction in their tumors by 12 weeks [98]. These results suggest that combination immune therapy may improve antitumor responses.

Approximately 20% of TNBCs express PD-L1, and the expression of PD-L1 is associated with poor prognosis in patients with breast cancer, particularly those with luminal B and basal-like subtypes, thus making the aggressive phenotype ER-positive and TNBC attractive subtypes in which to investigate PD-L1 blockade [99]. An early-phase study [100] presented at the 2014 SABCS meeting demonstrated clinical activity of the anti-PD-L1 monoclonal antibody pembrolizumab in patients with heavily treated TNBC. In this phase IB study of monotherapy with pembrolizumab, the ORR was 18.5% in evaluable patients with TNBC displaying PD-L1 expression (positive staining in stroma or on at least 1% of tumor cells by immunohistochemistry). The median duration of response was not reached, and three responders remained on the study for at least 1 year. These promising results led to the initiation of KEYNOTE-086 (NCT02447003), a larger single-arm phase II study to evaluate the role of pembrolizumab in advanced TNBC and identify biomarkers of efficacy. The preliminary results of this study were reported at the 2017 ASCO Annual Meeting. Of 170 patients enrolled, 44% had ≥3 prior lines of therapy, 74% had visceral metastases, and 62% had PD-L1+ tumors. ORR was 5% regardless of PD-L1 expression: 0.6% CR, 4% PR, 21% SD. The disease control rate was 8% (95% CI: 4–13). Median PFS and OS were 2.0 months (95% CI: 1.9–2.0) and 8.9 months (95% CI: 7.2–11.2), with 6 months rates of 12% and 69%, respectively. ORR was numerically lower in patients with poor prognostic factors (e.g., high LDH and liver/visceral metastases) [101]. In addition, KEYNOTE-119 (NCT02555657), a randomized phase III study of pembrolizumab versus physician's choice single-agent chemotherapy in pretreated advanced TNBC, is estimated to complete recruitment in late 2017. Finally, atezolizumab has also shown efficacy as a single agent in PD-L1–positive tumors in a phase IA trial in which a cohort of 12 patients with mTNBC were treated, with an ORR of 33% [102].

Conclusions

An understanding of the biology of breast cancer has led to important advances in the development of targeted therapies; however, MBC remains an incurable disease for most patients. As we learn to use genomic medicine and harness the immune system to guide drug development, it is important to start combining drugs using biologically informed translational science to optimize patient outcomes.

References

1. American Cancer Society. *Cancer facts & figures 2014*. Atlanta: American Cancer Society; 2014.
2. Perou CM, Sorlie T, Eisen MB, van de Rijn M, Jeffrey SS, Rees CA, et al. Molecular portraits of human breast tumours. Nature. 2000;406(6797):747–52.
3. Niikura N, Odisio BC, Tokuda Y, Symmans FW, Hortobagyi GN, Ueno NT. Latest biopsy approach for suspected metastases in patients with breast cancer. Nat Rev Clin Oncol. 2013;10(12):711–9.
4. Figueroa-Magalhaes MC, Jelovac D, Connolly RM, Wolff AC. Treatment of HER2-positive breast cancer. Breast. 2014;23(2):128–36.
5. Dalmau E, Armengol-Alonso A, Munoz M, Segui-Palmer MA. Current status of hormone therapy in patients with hormone receptor positive (HR+) advanced breast cancer. Breast. 2014;23(6):710–20.
6. Foulkes WD, Smith IE, Reis-Filho JS. Triple-negative breast cancer. N Engl J Med. 2010;363(20):1938–48.
7. Hughes LL, Gray RJ, Solin LJ, Robert NJ, Martino S, Tripathy D, et al. Efficacy of radiotherapy for ovarian ablation: results of a breast intergroup study. Cancer. 2004;101(5):969–72.
8. Sverrisdottir A, Johansson H, Johansson U, Bergh J, Rotstein S, Rutqvist L, et al. Interaction between goserelin and tamoxifen in a prospective randomised clinical trial of adjuvant endocrine therapy in premenopausal breast cancer. Breast Cancer Res Treat. 2011;128(3):755–63.
9. Di Leo A, Jerusalem G, Petruzelka L, Torres R, Bondarenko IN, Khasanov R, et al. Results of the CONFIRM phase III trial comparing fulvestrant 250 mg with fulvestrant 500 mg in postmenopausal women with estrogen receptor-positive advanced breast cancer. J Clin Oncol. 2010;28(30):4594–600.
10. Ingle JN, Krook JE, Green SJ, Kubista TP, Everson LK, Ahmann DL, et al. Randomized trial of bilateral oophorectomy versus tamoxifen in premenopausal women with metastatic breast cancer. J Clin Oncol. 1986;4(2):178–85.
11. Robertson JFR, Bondarenko IM, Trishkina E, Dvorkin M, Panasci L, Manikhas A, et al. Fulvestrant 500 mg versus anastrozole 1 mg for hormone receptor-positive advanced breast cancer (FALCON): an international, randomized, double-blind, phase 3 trial. Lancet. 2016;388(10063):2997–3005.
12. Goss PE, Winer EP, Tannock IF, Schwartz LH. Randomized phase III trial comparing the new potent and selective third-generation aromatase inhibitor vorozole with megestrol acetate in postmenopausal advanced breast cancer patients. North American Vorozole Study Group. J Clin Oncol. 1999;17(1):52–63.
13. Bonneterre J, Buzdar A, Nabholtz JM, Robertson JF, Thurlimann B, von Euler M, et al. Anastrozole is superior to tamoxifen as first-line therapy in hormone receptor positive advanced breast carcinoma. Cancer. 2001;92(9):2247–58.

14. Mouridsen H, Gershanovich M, Sun Y, Perez-Carrion R, Boni C, Monnier A, et al. Superior efficacy of letrozole versus tamoxifen as first-line therapy for postmenopausal women with advanced breast cancer: results of a phase III study of the International Letrozole Breast Cancer Group. J Clin Oncol. 2001;19(10):2596–606.
15. Paridaens RJ, Dirix LY, Beex LV, Nooij M, Cameron DA, Cufer T, et al. Phase III study comparing exemestane with tamoxifen as first-line hormonal treatment of metastatic breast cancer in postmenopausal women: the European Organisation for Research and Treatment of Cancer Breast Cancer Cooperative Group. J Clin Oncol. 2008;26(30):4883–90.
16. Kaufmann M, Bajetta E, Dirix LY, Fein LE, Jones SE, Zilembo N, et al. Exemestane improves survival in metastatic breast cancer: results of a phase III randomized study. Clin Breast Cancer. 2000;1(Suppl 1):S15–8.
17. Campos SM, Guastalla JP, Subar M, Abreu P, Winer EP, Cameron DA. A comparative study of exemestane versus anastrozole in patients with postmenopausal breast cancer with visceral metastases. Clin Breast Cancer. 2009;9(1):39–44.
18. Brufman G, Isacson R, Haim N, Gez E, Sulkes A. Megestrol acetate in advanced breast carcinoma after failure to tamoxifen and/or aminoglutethimide. Oncology. 1994;51(3):258–61.
19. Paplomata E, O'Regan R. The PI3K/AKT/mTOR pathway in breast cancer: targets, trials and biomarkers. Ther Adv Med Oncol. 2014;6(4):154–66.
20. Baselga J, Campone M, Piccart M, Burris HA, Rugo HS, Sahmoud T, et al. Everolimus in postmenopausal hormone-receptor-positive advanced breast cancer. N Engl J Med. 2012;366(6):520–9.
21. Wolff AC, Lazar AA, Bondarenko I, Garin AM, Brincat S, Chow L, et al. Randomized phase III placebo-controlled trial of letrozole plus oral temsirolimus as first-line endocrine therapy in postmenopausal women with locally advanced or metastatic breast cancer. J Clin Oncol. 2013;31(2):195–202.
22. Maass N, Harbeck N, Mundhenke C, Lerchenmuller C, Barinoff J, Luck HJ, et al. Everolimus as treatment for breast cancer patients with bone metastases only: results of the phase II RADAR study. J Cancer Res Clin Oncol. 2013;139(12):2047–56.
23. Fleming GF, Ma CX, Huo D, Sattar H, Tretiakova M, Lin L, et al. Phase II trial of temsirolimus in patients with metastatic breast cancer. Breast Cancer Res Treat. 2012;136(2):355–63.
24. Ma CX, Luo J, Naughton M, Ademuyiwa F, Suresh R, Griffith M, et al. A phase I trial of BKM120 (Buparlisib) in combination with fulvestrant in postmenopausal women with estrogen receptor-positive metastatic breast cancer. Clin Cancer Res. 2016;22(7):1583–91.
25. Mayer IA, Abramson VG, Isakoff SJ, Forero A, Balko JM, Kuba MG, et al. Stand up to cancer phase Ib study of pan-phosphoinositide-3-kinase inhibitor buparlisib with letrozole in estrogen receptor-positive/human epidermal growth factor receptor 2-negative metastatic breast cancer. J Clin Oncol. 2014;32(12):1202–9.
26. Baselga J, Im SA, Iwata H, editors. PIK3CA status in circulating tumor DNA (ctDNA) predicts efficacy of buparlisib (BUP) plus fulvestrant (FULV) in postmenopausal women with endocrine-resistant HR+/HER2– advanced breast cancer (BC): first results from the randomized, phase III BELLE-2 trial. In: San Antonio breast cancer symposium, San Antonio, TX; 2015.
27. Di Leo A, Seok Lee K, Ciruelos E, editors. BELLE-3: a phase III study of buparlisib + fulvestrant in postmenopausal women with HR+, HER2-, aromatase inhibitor-treated, locally advanced or metastatic breast cancer, who progressed on or after mTOR inhibitor-based treatment. In: San Antonio breast cancer symposium, San Antonio, TX; 2016.
28. Johnston SR, Kilburn LS, Ellis P, Dodwell D, Cameron D, Hayward L, et al. Fulvestrant plus anastrozole or placebo versus exemestane alone after progression on non-steroidal aromatase inhibitors in postmenopausal patients with hormone-receptor-positive locally advanced or metastatic breast cancer (SoFEA): a composite, multicentre, phase 3 randomised trial. Lancet Oncol. 2013;14(10):989–98.
29. Bergh J, Jonsson PE, Lidbrink EK, Trudeau M, Eiermann W, Brattstrom D, et al. FACT: an open-label randomized phase III study of fulvestrant and anastrozole in combination com-

pared with anastrozole alone as first-line therapy for patients with receptor-positive postmenopausal breast cancer. J Clin Oncol. 2012;30(16):1919–25.
30. Mehta RS, Barlow WE, Albain KS, Vandenberg TA, Dakhil SR, Tirumali NR, et al. Combination anastrozole and fulvestrant in metastatic breast cancer. N Engl J Med. 2012;367(5):435–44.
31. Finn RS, Crown JP, Lang I, Boer K, Bondarenko IM, Kulyk SO, et al. The cyclin-dependent kinase 4/6 inhibitor palbociclib in combination with letrozole versus letrozole alone as first-line treatment of oestrogen receptor-positive, HER2-negative, advanced breast cancer (PALOMA-1/TRIO-18): a randomised phase 2 study. Lancet Oncol. 2015;16(1):25–35.
32. Finn RS, Martin M, Rugo HS, Jones S, Im SA, Gelmon K, et al. Palbociclib and Letrozole in Advanced Breast Cancer. N Engl J Med. 2016;375(20):1925–36.
33. Turner NC, Ro J, Andre F, Loi S, Verma S, Iwata H, et al. Palbociclib in hormone-receptor-positive advanced breast cancer. N Engl J Med. 2015;373(3):209–19.
34. Cristofanilli M, Turner NC, Bondarenko I, Ro J, Im SA, Masuda N, et al. Fulvestrant plus palbociclib versus fulvestrant plus placebo for treatment of hormone-receptor-positive, HER2-negative metastatic breast cancer that progressed on previous endocrine therapy (PALOMA-3): final analysis of the multicentre, double-blind, phase 3 randomised controlled trial. Lancet Oncol. 2016;17(4):425–39.
35. Kennecke H, Yerushalmi R, Woods R, Cheang MC, Voduc D, Speers CH, et al. Metastatic behavior of breast cancer subtypes. J Clin Oncol. 2010;28(20):3271–7.
36. Early Breast Cancer Trialists' Collaborative Group. Effects of chemotherapy and hormonal therapy for early breast cancer on recurrence and 15-year survival: an overview of the randomised trials. Lancet. 2005;365(9472):1687–717.
37. Chan S, Friedrichs K, Noel D, Pinter T, Van Belle S, Vorobiof D, et al. Prospective randomized trial of docetaxel versus doxorubicin in patients with metastatic breast cancer. J Clin Oncol. 1999;17(8):2341–54.
38. Bastholt L, Dalmark M, Gjedde SB, Pfeiffer P, Pedersen D, Sandberg E, et al. Dose-response relationship of epirubicin in the treatment of postmenopausal patients with metastatic breast cancer: a randomized study of epirubicin at four different dose levels performed by the Danish Breast Cancer Cooperative Group. J Clin Oncol. 1996;14(4):1146–55.
39. O'Brien ME, Wigler N, Inbar M, Rosso R, Grischke E, Santoro A, et al. Reduced cardiotoxicity and comparable efficacy in a phase III trial of pegylated liposomal doxorubicin HCl (CAELYX/Doxil) versus conventional doxorubicin for first-line treatment of metastatic breast cancer. Ann Oncol. 2004;15(3):440–9.
40. Jones SE, Erban J, Overmoyer B, Budd GT, Hutchins L, Lower E, et al. Randomized phase III study of docetaxel compared with paclitaxel in metastatic breast cancer. J Clin Oncol. 2005;23(24):5542–51.
41. Seidman AD, Berry D, Cirrincione C, Harris L, Muss H, Marcom PK, et al. Randomized phase III trial of weekly compared with every-3-weeks paclitaxel for metastatic breast cancer, with trastuzumab for all HER-2 overexpressors and random assignment to trastuzumab or not in HER-2 nonoverexpressors: final results of Cancer and Leukemia Group B protocol 9840. J Clin Oncol. 2008;26(10):1642–9.
42. Perez EA, Vogel CL, Irwin DH, Kirshner JJ, Patel R. Multicenter phase II trial of weekly paclitaxel in women with metastatic breast cancer. J Clin Oncol. 2001;19(22):4216–23.
43. Burstein HJ, Manola J, Younger J, Parker LM, Bunnell CA, Scheib R, et al. Docetaxel administered on a weekly basis for metastatic breast cancer. J Clin Oncol. 2000;18(6):1212–9.
44. Gradishar WJ, Tjulandin S, Davidson N, Shaw H, Desai N, Bhar P, et al. Phase III trial of nanoparticle albumin-bound paclitaxel compared with polyethylated castor oil-based paclitaxel in women with breast cancer. J Clin Oncol. 2005;23(31):7794–803.
45. Zelek L, Barthier S, Riofrio M, Fizazi K, Rixe O, Delord JP, et al. Weekly vinorelbine is an effective palliative regimen after failure with anthracyclines and taxanes in metastatic breast carcinoma. Cancer. 2001;92(9):2267–72.

46. Roche H, Yelle L, Cognetti F, Mauriac L, Bunnell C, Sparano J, et al. Phase II clinical trial of ixabepilone (BMS-247550), an epothilone B analog, as first-line therapy in patients with metastatic breast cancer previously treated with anthracycline chemotherapy. J Clin Oncol. 2007;25(23):3415–20.
47. Rivera E, Gomez H. Chemotherapy resistance in metastatic breast cancer: the evolving role of ixabepilone. Breast Cancer Res. 2010;12(Suppl 2):S2.
48. Denduluri N, Low JA, Lee JJ, Berman AW, Walshe JM, Vatas U, et al. Phase II trial of ixabepilone, an epothilone B analog, in patients with metastatic breast cancer previously untreated with taxanes. J Clin Oncol. 2007;25(23):3421–7.
49. Perez EA, Lerzo G, Pivot X, Thomas E, Vahdat L, Bosserman L, et al. Efficacy and safety of ixabepilone (BMS-247550) in a phase II study of patients with advanced breast cancer resistant to an anthracycline, a taxane, and capecitabine. J Clin Oncol. 2007;25(23):3407–14.
50. Thomas E, Tabernero J, Fornier M, Conte P, Fumoleau P, Lluch A, et al. Phase II clinical trial of ixabepilone (BMS-247550), an epothilone B analog, in patients with taxane-resistant metastatic breast cancer. J Clin Oncol. 2007;25(23):3399–406.
51. Cortes J, Vahdat L, Blum JL, Twelves C, Campone M, Roche H, et al. Phase II study of the halichondrin B analog eribulin mesylate in patients with locally advanced or metastatic breast cancer previously treated with an anthracycline, a taxane, and capecitabine. J Clin Oncol. 2010;28(25):3922–8.
52. Vahdat LT, Pruitt B, Fabian CJ, Rivera RR, Smith DA, Tan-Chiu E, et al. Phase II study of eribulin mesylate, a halichondrin B analog, in patients with metastatic breast cancer previously treated with an anthracycline and a taxane. J Clin Oncol. 2009;27(18):2954–61.
53. Cortes J, O'Shaughnessy J, Loesch D, Blum JL, Vahdat LT, Petrakova K, et al. Eribulin monotherapy versus treatment of physician's choice in patients with metastatic breast cancer (EMBRACE): a phase 3 open-label randomised study. Lancet. 2011;377(9769):914–23.
54. Blum JL, Dieras V, Lo Russo PM, Horton J, Rutman O, Buzdar A, et al. Multicenter, phase II study of capecitabine in taxane-pretreated metastatic breast carcinoma patients. Cancer. 2001;92(7):1759–68.
55. Bajetta E, Procopio G, Celio L, Gattinoni L, Della Torre S, Mariani L, et al. Safety and efficacy of two different doses of capecitabine in the treatment of advanced breast cancer in older women. J Clin Oncol. 2005;23(10):2155–61.
56. Blackstein M, Vogel CL, Ambinder R, Cowan J, Iglesias J, Melemed A. Gemcitabine as first-line therapy in patients with metastatic breast cancer: a phase II trial. Oncology. 2002;62(1):2–8.
57. Rha SY, Moon YH, Jeung HC, Kim YT, Sohn JH, Yang WI, et al. Gemcitabine monotherapy as salvage chemotherapy in heavily pretreated metastatic breast cancer. Breast Cancer Res Treat. 2005;90(3):215–21.
58. von Minckwitz G, Schneeweiss A, Loibl S, Salat C, Denkert C, Rezai M, et al. Neoadjuvant carboplatin in patients with triple-negative and HER2-positive early breast cancer (GeparSixto; GBG 66): a randomised phase 2 trial. Lancet Oncol. 2014;15(7):747–56.
59. Villarreal-Garza C, Khalaf D, Bouganim N, Clemons M, Pena-Curiel O, Baez-Revueltas B, et al. Platinum-based chemotherapy in triple-negative advanced breast cancer. Breast Cancer Res Treat. 2014;146(3):567–72.
60. Tutt A, Tovey H, Cheang MCU, Kernaghan S, Kilburn L, Gazinska P, et al. Carboplatin in BRCA1/2-mutated and triple-negative breast cancer BRCAness subgroups: the TNT Trial. Nat Med. 2018;24(5):628–37.
61. Penault-Llorca F, Viale G. Pathological and molecular diagnosis of triple-negative breast cancer: a clinical perspective. Ann Oncol. 2012;23(Suppl 6):vi19–22.
62. Lehmann BD, Jovanovic B, Chen X, Estrada MV, Johnson KN, Shyr Y, et al. Refinement of triple-negative breast cancer molecular subtypes: implications for neoadjuvant chemotherapy selection. PLoS One. 2016;11(6):e0157368.

63. Lehmann BD, Bauer JA, Chen X, Sanders ME, Chakravarthy AB, Shyr Y, et al. Identification of human triple-negative breast cancer subtypes and preclinical models for selection of targeted therapies. J Clin Invest. 2011;121(7):2750–67.
64. Nik-Zainal S, Davies H, Staaf J, Ramakrishna M, Glodzik D, Zou X, et al. Landscape of somatic mutations in 560 breast cancer whole-genome sequences. Nature. 2016;534(7605):47–54.
65. O'Shaughnessy J, Osborne C, Pippen JE, Yoffe M, Patt D, Rocha C, et al. Iniparib plus chemotherapy in metastatic triple-negative breast cancer. N Engl J Med. 2011;364(3):205–14.
66. O'Shaughnessy J, Schwartzberg L, Danso MA, Miller KD, Rugo HS, Neubauer M, et al. Phase III study of iniparib plus gemcitabine and carboplatin versus gemcitabine and carboplatin in patients with metastatic triple-negative breast cancer. J Clin Oncol. 2014;32(34):3840–7.
67. Patel AG, De Lorenzo SB, Flatten KS, Poirier GG, Kaufmann SH. Failure of iniparib to inhibit poly(ADP-Ribose) polymerase in vitro. Clin Cancer Res. 2012;18(6):1655–62.
68. Audeh MW. Novel treatment strategies in triple-negative breast cancer: specific role of poly(adenosine diphosphate-ribose) polymerase inhibition. Pharmacogenomics Pers Med. 2014;7:307–16.
69. Robson M, Im SA, Senkus E, Xu B, Domchek SM, Masuda N, et al. Olaparib for metastatic breast cancer in patients with a germline BRCA mutation. N Engl J Med. 2017;377(6):523–33.
70. Kaufman B, Shapira-Frommer R, Schmutzler RK, Audeh MW, Friedlander M, Balmana J, et al. Olaparib monotherapy in patients with advanced cancer and a germline BRCA1/2 mutation. J Clin Oncol. 2015;33(3):244–50.
71. Gucalp A, Tolaney S, Isakoff SJ, Ingle JN, Liu MC, Carey JA, Consortium TBCR, et al. Phase II trial of bicalutamide in patients with androgen receptor-positive, estrogen receptor-negative metastatic breast cancer. Clin Cancer Res. 2013;19(19):5505–12.
72. Traina TA, Miller K, Yardley DA, Eakle J, Schwartzberg LS, O'Shaughnessy J, et al. Enzalutamide for the treatment of androgen receptor—expressing triple-negative breast cancer. J Clin Oncol. 2018;36(9):884–90.
73. Dent R, Schmid P, Cortes J, editors. ENDEAR: a randomized international phase 3 study comparing the efficacy and safety of enzalutamide in combination with paclitaxel chemotherapy or as monotherapy vs placebo with paclitaxel in patients with advanced diagnostic-positive triple-negative breast cancer. In: San Antonio breast cancer symposium, San Antonio, TX; 2016.
74. Goldenberg DM, Cardillo TM, Govindan SV, Rossi EA, Sharkey RM. Trop-2 is a novel target for solid cancer therapy with sacituzumab govitecan (IMMU-132), an antibody-drug conjugate (ADC). Oncotarget. 2015;6(26):22496–512.
75. Starodub AN, Ocean AJ, Shah MA, Guarino MJ, Picozzi VJ Jr, Vahdat LT, et al. First-in-human trial of a novel anti-Trop-2 antibody-SN-38 conjugate, sacituzumab govitecan, for the treatment of diverse metastatic solid tumors. Clin Cancer Res. 2015;21(17):3870–8.
76. Bardia A, Diamond J, Mayer IA, editors. Safety and efficacy of anti-Trop-2 antibody drug conjugate, sacituzumab govitecan (IMMU-132), in heavily pretreated patients with TNBC. In: San Antonia breast cancer symposium, San Antonio, TX; 2016.
77. Rose AA, Grosset AA, Dong Z, Russo C, Macdonald PA, Bertos NR, et al. Glycoprotein nonmetastatic B is an independent prognostic indicator of recurrence and a novel therapeutic target in breast cancer. Clin Cancer Res. 2010;16(7):2147–56.
78. O'Shaughnessy J, Miles D, Vukelja S, Moiseyenko V, Ayoub JP, Cervantes G, et al. Superior survival with capecitabine plus docetaxel combination therapy in anthracycline-pretreated patients with advanced breast cancer: phase III trial results. J Clin Oncol. 2002;20(12):2812–23.
79. Albain KS, Nag SM, Calderillo-Ruiz G, Jordaan JP, Llombart AC, Pluzanska A, et al. Gemcitabine plus Paclitaxel versus Paclitaxel monotherapy in patients with metastatic breast cancer and prior anthracycline treatment. J Clin Oncol. 2008;26(24):3950–7.
80. Mauri D, Kamposioras K, Tsali L, Bristianou M, Valachis A, Karathanasi I, Georgiou C, Polyzos NP. Overall survival benefi t for weekly vs. three-weekly, taxanes regimens in advanced breast cancer: a meta-analysis. Cancer Treat Rev. 2010;36:69.

81. Sirohi B, Arnedos M, Popat S, Ashley S, Nerurkar A, Walsh G, et al. Platinum-based chemotherapy in triple-negative breast cancer. Ann Oncol. 2008;19(11):1847–52.
82. Chew HK, Doroshow JH, Frankel P, Margolin KA, Somlo G, Lenz HJ, et al. Phase II studies of gemcitabine and cisplatin in heavily and minimally pretreated metastatic breast cancer. J Clin Oncol. 2009;27(13):2163–9.
83. Staudacher L, Cottu PH, Dieras V, Vincent-Salomon A, Guilhaume MN, Escalup L, et al. Platinum-based chemotherapy in metastatic triple-negative breast cancer: the Institut Curie experience. Ann Oncol. 2011;22(4):848–56.
84. Kumler I, Christiansen OG, Nielsen DL. A systematic review of bevacizumab efficacy in breast cancer. Cancer Treat Rev. 2014;40(8):960–73.
85. Miller K, Wang M, Gralow J, Dickler M, Cobleigh M, Perez EA, et al. Paclitaxel plus bevacizumab versus paclitaxel alone for metastatic breast cancer. N Engl J Med. 2007;357(26):2666–76.
86. Robert NJ, Dieras V, Glaspy J, Brufsky AM, Bondarenko I, Lipatov ON, et al. RIBBON-1: randomized, double-blind, placebo-controlled, phase III trial of chemotherapy with or without bevacizumab for first-line treatment of human epidermal growth factor receptor 2-negative, locally recurrent or metastatic breast cancer. J Clin Oncol. 2011;29(10):1252–60.
87. Brufsky AM, Hurvitz S, Perez E, Swamy R, Valero V, O'Neill V, et al. RIBBON-2: a randomized, double-blind, placebo-controlled, phase III trial evaluating the efficacy and safety of bevacizumab in combination with chemotherapy for second-line treatment of human epidermal growth factor receptor 2-negative metastatic breast cancer. J Clin Oncol. 2011;29(32):4286–93.
88. Brufsky A, Valero V, Tiangco B, Dakhil S, Brize A, Rugo HS, et al. Second-line bevacizumab-containing therapy in patients with triple-negative breast cancer: subgroup analysis of the RIBBON-2 trial. Breast Cancer Res Treat. 2012;133(3):1067–75.
89. Gligorov J, Doval D, Bines J, Alba E, Cortes P, Pierga JY, et al. Maintenance capecitabine and bevacizumab versus bevacizumab alone after initial first-line bevacizumab and docetaxel for patients with HER2-negative metastatic breast cancer (IMELDA): a randomised, open-label, phase 3 trial. Lancet Oncol. 2014;15(12):1351–60.
90. Vrdoljak E, Marschner N, Zielinski C, Gligorov J, Cortes J, Puglisi F, et al. Final results of the TANIA randomized phase III trial of bevacizumab after progression on first-line bevacizumab therapy for HER2-negative locally recurrent/metastatic breast cancer. Ann Oncol. 2016;27(11):2046–52.
91. Puglisi F, Cortes J, Vrdoljak E, Gligorov J, Marschner N, Zielinski C, et al. Subgroup efficacy analyses of the randomized phase III TANIA trial evaluating continued or reintroduced bevacizumab (BEV) after 1st-line BEV for HER2-negative locally recurrent/metastatic breast cancer (LR/mBC). SABCS; 2014, PD2-4.
92. Cortes J, Vrdoljak E, Puglisi F, Marschner N, Gligorov J, Zielinski C, et al. Plasma (p) biomarker results from the TANIA trial evaluating continued or reintroduced bevacizumab (BEV) after 1st-line BEV for HER2-negative metastatic breast cancer (mBC). SABCS; 2014, PD2-4.
93. Turner N, Pearson A, Sharpe R, Lambros M, Geyer F, Lopez-Garcia MA, et al. FGFR1 amplification drives endocrine therapy resistance and is a therapeutic target in breast cancer. Cancer Res. 2010;70(5):2085–94.
94. Soria JC, DeBraud F, Bahleda R, Adamo B, Andre F, Dienstmann R, et al. Phase I/IIa study evaluating the safety, efficacy, pharmacokinetics, and pharmacodynamics of lucitanib in advanced solid tumors. Ann Oncol. 2014;25(11):2244–51.
95. de la Cruz-Merino L, Palazón-Carrión N, Henao-Carrasco F, Nogales-Fernández E, Álamo-de la Gala M, Vallejo-Benítez A, et al. New horizons in breast cancer: the promise of immunotherapy. Clin Transl Oncol. 2018. https://doi.org/10.1007/s12094-018-1907-3.
96. Hodi FS, O'Day SJ, McDermott DF, Weber RW, Sosman JA, Haanen JB, et al. Improved survival with ipilimumab in patients with metastatic melanoma. N Engl J Med. 2010;363(8):711–23.

97. Brahmer JR, Tykodi SS, Chow LQ, Hwu WJ, Topalian SL, Hwu P, et al. Safety and activity of anti-PD-L1 antibody in patients with advanced cancer. N Engl J Med. 2012;366(26):2455–65.
98. Wolchok JD, Kluger H, Callahan MK, Postow MA, Rizvi NA, Lesokhin AM, et al. Nivolumab plus ipilimumab in advanced melanoma. N Engl J Med. 2013;369(2):122–33.
99. Muenst S, Soysal SD, Gao F, Obermann EC, Oertli D, Gillanders WE. The presence of programmed death 1 (PD-1)-positive tumor-infiltrating lymphocytes is associated with poor prognosis in human breast cancer. Breast Cancer Res Treat. 2013;139(3):667–76.
100. Nanda R, Chow LQ, Dees EC, Berger R, Gupta S, Geva R, et al. Pembrolizumab in patients with advanced triple-negative breast cancer: phase Ib KEYNOTE-012 study. J Clin Oncol. 2016;34(21):2460–7.
101. Adams S, Schmid P, Hope S, editors. Phase 2 study of pembrolizumab (pembro) monotherapy for previously treated metastatic triple-negative breast cancer (mTNBC): KEYNOTE-086 cohort A. In: 2017 ASCO annual meeting, Chicago, IL; 2017.
102. Emens LA, Braiteh FS, Cassier P, editors. Inhibition of PDL1 by MPDL3280A leads to clinical activity in patients with metastatic triple-negative breast cancer (TNBC). In: San Antonio breast symposium, San Antonio, TX; 2015.
103. Kuss JT, Muss HB, Hoen H, Case LD. Tamoxifen as initial endocrine therapy for metastatic breast cancer: long term follow-up of two Piedmont Oncology Association (POA) trials. Breast Cancer Res Treat. 1997;42(3):265–74.
104. Boccardo F, Rubagotti A, Perrotta A, Amoroso D, Balestrero M, De Matteis A, et al. Ovarian ablation versus goserelin with or without tamoxifen in pre-perimenopausal patients with advanced breast cancer: results of a multicentric Italian study. Ann Oncol. 1994;5(4):337–42.
105. Klijn JG, Beex LV, Mauriac L, van Zijl JA, Veyret C, Wildiers J, et al. Combined treatment with buserelin and tamoxifen in premenopausal metastatic breast cancer: a randomized study. J Natl Cancer Inst. 2000;92(11):903–11.
106. Howell A, Robertson JF, Abram P, Lichinitser MR, Elledge R, Bajetta E, et al. Comparison of fulvestrant versus tamoxifen for the treatment of advanced breast cancer in postmenopausal women previously untreated with endocrine therapy: a multinational, double-blind, randomized trial. J Clin Oncol. 2004;22(9):1605–13.
107. Thurlimann B, Hess D, Koberle D, Senn I, Ballabeni P, Pagani O, et al. Anastrozole ('Arimidex') versus tamoxifen as first-line therapy in postmenopausal women with advanced breast cancer: results of the double-blind cross-over SAKK trial 21/95—a sub-study of the TARGET (Tamoxifen or 'Arimidex' Randomized Group Efficacy and Tolerability) trial. Breast Cancer Res Treat. 2004;85(3):247–54.
108. Muss HB, Case LD, Atkins JN, Bearden JD, Cooper MR, Cruz JM, et al. Tamoxifen versus high-dose oral medroxyprogesterone acetate as initial endocrine therapy for patients with metastatic breast cancer: a Piedmont Oncology Association study. J Clin Oncol. 1994;12(8):1630–8.
109. Sparano JA, Vrdoljak E, Rixe O, Xu B, Manikhas A, Medina C, et al. Randomized phase III trial of ixabepilone plus capecitabine versus capecitabine in patients with metastatic breast cancer previously treated with an anthracycline and a taxane. J Clin Oncol. 2010;28(20):3256–63.

Chapter 23
Systemic Treatment of HER2-Overexpressing Metastatic Breast Cancer

Adnan Aydiner

Introduction

HER2 is a transmembrane tyrosine kinase receptor that belongs to the EGFR (epidermal growth factor receptor) family and is overexpressed in 25–30% of human breast cancers [1]. HER2 has several features of an ideal target for breast cancer treatment, and HER2 overexpression is an adverse prognostic factor in women with breast cancer [2]. The level of HER2 in human cancer cells with membrane overexpression is much higher than that in normal adult tissues, and HER2 overexpression is found in both the primary tumor and in metastatic sites, indicating that anti-HER2 therapy may be effective at all disease sites. Trastuzumab was the first of such agents registered for use in patients with HER2-overexpressing breast cancer. A key first step in appropriately deciding on the use of HER2-targeted therapy is the accurate determination of HER2 overexpression by either immunohistochemistry (IHC) or fluorescence in situ hybridization (FISH). The current American Society of Clinical Oncology (ASCO)/ College of American Pathologists (CAP) guidelines, updated in 2018, define HER2 positivity as 3+ on IHC (circumferential membrane staining in >10% of invasive tumor cells that is complete and intense) or amplified on FISH (single-probe average HER2 copy number ≥6.0 signals/cell, or dual-probe HER2/CEP17 ratio ≥2.0 with an average HER2 copy number ≥4.0 signals per cell) [1]. The 2018 update on recommendations for HER2 testing with ISH method cancelled an equivocal result. Instead, forced pathologists to make a judgement as positive or negative using combination of repeated IHC and dual-probe ISH method. According to final update, if the HER2/ CEP 17 ratio ≥2.0 and average HER2 copy number is <4.0 the result should be

A. Aydiner (✉)
Internal Medicine, Medical Oncology, Istanbul Medical Faculty, Department of Medical Oncology, Institute of Oncology, Istanbul University, Istanbul, Turkey

A. Aydiner et al. (eds.), *Breast Cancer*, https://doi.org/10.1007/978-3-319-96947-3_23

negative after completion of a work-up. If the average HER2 copy number is ≥6.0 and the ratio is <2.0 the result should be positive after completion of a work-up.

Clinicians should recommend HER2-targeted combinations for first-line treatment. When the best treatment response has been obtained (usually after 6–12 months of combined therapy), cytotoxic chemotherapy is stopped, and anti-HER2 therapy is continued, although the optimal duration of treatment is unknown. Following discontinuation of chemotherapy, endocrine therapy must be added to

Box 23.1 Summary of the Optimal HER2-Targeted Therapy for Advanced Human Epidermal Growth Factor Receptor 2 (HER2)–Positive Breast Cancer

- Clinicians should recommend HER2-targeted therapy–based combinations for first-line treatment. If HER2-positive advanced breast cancer progresses during or after first-line HER2-targeted therapy, clinicians should recommend second-line HER2-targeted therapy–based treatment.
- If HER2-positive advanced breast cancer progresses during or after second-line or greater HER2-targeted treatment, clinicians should recommend third-line or greater HER2-targeted therapy–based treatment.
- If available, the clinicians should recommend the combination of trastuzumab, pertuzumab, and a taxane for first-line and trastuzumab emtansine (T-DM1) as second-line treatment. If HER2-positive advanced breast cancer progresses during or after second-line or greater HER2-targeted treatment but the patient has not received pertuzumab, clinicians may offer pertuzumab.
- If the patient has already received trastuzumab, pertuzumab, and T-DM1, clinicians should recommend third-line or greater HER2-targeted therapy–based treatment (lapatinib plus chemotherapy, trastuzumab plus lapatinib, trastuzumab plus chemotherapy, trastuzumab or lapatinib plus hormonal therapy in patients with hormone receptor–positive disease).
- If a patient is receiving HER2-targeted therapy and chemotherapy combinations, chemotherapy should continue to the time of maximal response, depending on toxicity and in the absence of progression. When chemotherapy ends, clinicians should continue the HER2-targeted therapy, and no further change in the regimen is needed until time of progression or unacceptable toxicities.
- If a patient finished trastuzumab-based adjuvant treatment >12 months before recurrence, clinicians should follow the first-line HER2-targeted therapy–based treatment recommendations.
- If a patient's cancer is hormone receptor positive and HER2 positive, clinicians may recommend either HER2-targeted therapy plus chemotherapy or

in select cases endocrine therapy plus trastuzumab/pertuzumab or lapatinib/trastuzumab. Clinicians may add endocrine therapy to the HER2-targeted therapy when chemotherapy ends and/or when the cancer progresses.

- Management of hormone receptor-positive and HER2-positive metastatic disease without chemotherapy could conceivably include combinations of available endocrine therapies, with one or more of the currently approved HER2-targeted agents including trastuzumab, pertuzumab, or lapatinib.

the HER2-directed therapy of patients whose tumors are also hormone receptor positive. Further treatment of patients with MBC who progress on HER2-directed therapy must be based on individual considerations (Box 23.1).

First-Line Treatment

The trial by Slamon et al. and other randomized controlled trials of trastuzumab reported a benefit for HER2-targeted therapy combinations [2]. Other agents that improve survival include lapatinib and the combination of trastuzumab plus pertuzumab.

There are a number of effective options for single-agent chemotherapy and anti-HER2 agents. Taxanes [2], vinorelbine [3], and capecitabine [4, 5] are generally preferred regimens with anti-HER2 partners. Double-agent chemotherapy with HER2-targeted agents is generally avoided because PFS is improved at the cost of significantly increased toxicity [6].

Many clinically important randomized trials of first-line treatments for HER2 MBC, including trastuzumab, lapatinib, pertuzumab, trastuzumab emtansine (T-DM1) and mammalian target of rapamycin (mTOR) inhibitor (everolimus), have affected medical practice (Table 23.1).

Trastuzumab

Single-agent trastuzumab treatment may be reasonable when avoiding the cytotoxic side effects of chemotherapy is desirable but may result in poorer outcomes compared with trastuzumab administered in combination with chemotherapy [7]. If a patient progresses on single-agent trastuzumab therapy, adding single-agent chemotherapy to trastuzumab is an option.

Table 23.1 First-line randomized phase III studies in HER2-positive metastatic breast cancer patients

		ORR		PFS		OS	
Trial	Study arms	%	P	Months		Months	
Slamon [2]	Trastuzumab + chemotherapy	50	p < 0.001	7.4	RR = 0.51 P < 0.001	25.1	RR = 0.80 p = 0.046
	Chemotherapy	32		4.6		20.3	
HERNATA (Andersson [3])	Trastuzumab + docetaxel	59.3	NS	15.3	HR = 0.94 P = 0.67	35.7	HR 1.01 p = 0.98
	Trastuzumab + vinorelbine	59.3		12.4		38.8	
NCIC CTG MA-31 (Gelmon [12])	Lapatinib + taxane	54	NS	9.0	HR 1.37 p = 0.001	NR	HR 1.28 p = 0.11
	Trastuzumab + taxane	55		11.3		NR	
CLEOPATRA (Swain [13])	Pertuzumab + trastuzumab + docetaxel	80.2	p = 0.0001	18.7	HR 0.69 p < 0.0001	56.5	HR 0.66 p = 0.0001
	Placebo + trastuzumab + docetaxel	69.3		12.4		40.8	
MARIANNE (Perez [14])	Trastuzumab + taxane	67.9	NR	13.7	HR 0.91 P = 0.31 HR 0.87 P = 0.14	NR	HR 0.86 p = NR HR: 0.82 p = NR
	T-DM1 + placebo	59.7		14.1		NR	
	T-DM1 + pertuzumab	64.2		15.2		NR	
BOLERO-1 (Hurvitz [15])	Everolimus + trastuzumab + paclitaxel	NR	NS	15 ER(−) 20.3	HR 0.89 p = 0.11 ER (−) HR: 0.66 p = 0.049	NR	NR
	Placebo + trastuzumab + paclitaxel	NR		14.5 ER (−) 13.1		NR	

ORR objective response rate, *PFS* progression-free survival, *OS* overall survival, *HR* hazard ratio, *RR* relative risk, *ER* estrogen receptor, *NR* not reported, *NS* non-significant, *T-DM1* T-DM1

Table 23.2 Dosage dose modification of trastuzumab based on asymptomatic left ventricular ejection fraction decrease from baseline

Relationship of left ventricular ejection fraction (LVEF) to the lower limit of normal (LLN)	Trastuzumab dose modification based on asymptomatic LVEF decrease from baseline		
	≤10% points	10–15% points	≥15% points
Within a facility's normal limits	Continue	Continue	Hold and repeat MUGA/ECHO after 4 weeks[a]
<6% below LLN	Continue[a]	Hold and repeat MUGA/ECHO after 4 weeks[a,b]	Hold and repeat MUGA/ECHO after 4 weeks[b,c]
≥6% below LLN	Continue and repeat MUGA/ECHO after 4 weeks[c]	Hold and repeat MUGA/ECHO after 4 weeks[b,c]	Hold and repeat MUGA/ECHO after 4 weeks[b,c]

[a]Consider cardiac assessment. Cardiotoxicity associated with trastuzumab typically responds to appropriate medical therapy but may be severe and lead to cardiac failure
[b]After 2 holds, consider permanent trastuzumab discontinuation
[c]Refer to cardiologist

Table 23.3 Dosage dose modification of trastuzumab and pertuzumab combination based on asymptomatic left ventricular ejection fraction decrease from baseline

Left ventricular ejection fraction	Trastuzumab and pertuzumab		
	Action	LVEF at reassessment	Dose
<40% AND asymptomatic	Pause and repeat MUGA in 3 weeks	>45% OR 40–45% AND <10% ↓ from baseline	Restart
40–50%[a] AND ≥10% points below baseline AND asymptomatic		<40% OR 40–50%[a] AND ≥ 10% points below baseline OR symptomatic	Discontinue
Symptomatic	Consider discontinuing	Not applicable	Not applicable

[a]In the CLEOPATRA trial, trastuzumab and pertuzumab treatments were paused if LVEF was 40–45% and ≥10% below baseline and asymptomatic. At LVEF reassessment, pertuzumab and trastuzumab may be restarted if LVEF "≥46%" or "40–45% and <10% ↓ from baseline"; otherwise, discontinue

Trastuzumab Plus Chemotherapy

Trastuzumab is more active when used in combination with various chemotherapeutic agents, resulting in significantly improved ORR and OS [3] (Table 23.1). The combination of an anthracycline and trastuzumab is not recommended because of the risk of significant cardiotoxicity [2].

The cardiotoxicity of trastuzumab is reversible in the majority of patients. Additional treatment with trastuzumab can be considered after recovery of cardiac function among patients who experience a cardiac event (Tables 23.2 and 23.3).

Trastuzumab is generally not given in combination with multi-agent chemotherapy because of the excess risk of toxicity [8, 9]. No trials have demonstrated that this approach improves OS.

Lapatinib

As a second-line combination therapy, lapatinib and capecitabine improve TTP compared with capecitabine monotherapy for the treatment of HER2-positive MBC refractory to anthracycline-, taxane-, and trastuzumab-containing regimens [10]. The use of lapatinib in the first-line setting has been explored in two phase III trials, one of which compared lapatinib against placebo [11, 12]. The evidence suggests that trastuzumab-based regimens should still be considered the standard of care in this setting (Table 23.1).

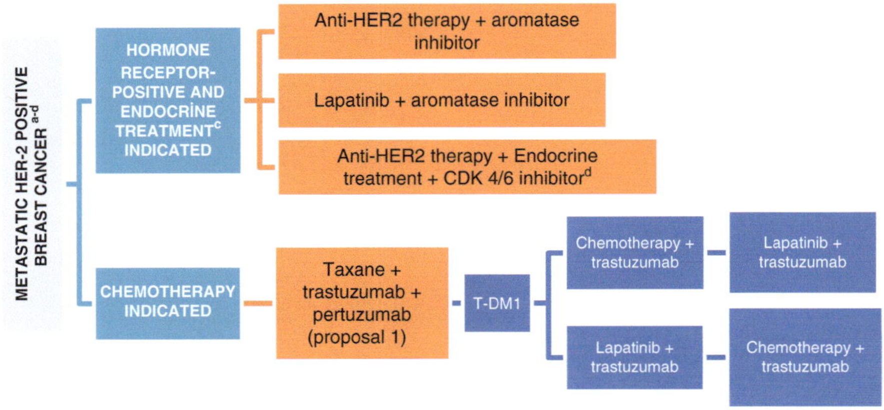

Fig. 23.1 Systemic treatment of recurrent or metastatic HER2-overexpressing breast cancer. [a]Administration of ado-trastuzumab emtansine and pertuzumab was not superior to treatment with chemotherapy + trastuzumab or ado-trastuzumab alone as the first choice treatment in HER2-positive disease. According to the PERTAIN trial (Rimawi, J Clin Oncol, 2018), addition of pertuzumab to trastuzumab and endocrine treatment in the first choice prolonged progression-free survival. The addition of pertuzumab in the second choice in patients who did not receive pertuzumab in the first choice provided a minor clinical benefit. [b]T-DM1 may be used as the front line if the patient develops metastasis within 6 months of finishing adjuvant therapy with anti-HER2 treatment. [c]In premenopausal patients, medical or surgical oophorectomy must be performed. [d]Clinical trials are ongoing for anti-HER2 therapy + endocrine treatment + CDK 4/6 inhibitor, or anti-HER2 therapy + immunotherapy

Pertuzumab

In the CLEOPATRA trial, the survival of patients with HER2 positive MBC was significantly improved after first-line therapy with pertuzumab, trastuzumab and docetaxel compared with placebo, trastuzumab, and docetaxel [13]. Compared with the addition of placebo, the addition of pertuzumab to trastuzumab and docetaxel significantly improved the median OS of patients with HER2-positive MBC. The median overall survival was 56.5 months in the group receiving the pertuzumab combination, compared to 40.8 months (95% CI, 35.8–48.3) in those receiving the placebo combination (hazard ratio favoring the pertuzumab group, 0.68; $P < 0.001$). Median PFS, as assessed by the investigators, improved by 6.3 months in the pertuzumab group (hazard ratio, 0.68; 95% CI, 0.58–0.80). Pertuzumab extended the median duration of response by 7.7 months, as independently assessed. Dual HER2 blockade did not increase the risk of cardiac toxicity. Febrile neutropenia was more common with pertuzumab (13.8% vs.7.6%), driven mostly by a high incidence in Asian patients (26% vs. 10%), for reasons not currently clearly understood. The rate of grade 3 and 4 diarrhea (7.9% vs. 5.0%) was increased in the pertuzumab arm.

In conclusion, compared with the addition of placebo, the addition of pertuzumab to trastuzumab and docetaxel significantly improved median OS of patients with HER2-positive MBC (Table 23.1, Fig. 23.1).

T-DM1 (Trastuzumab-Emtansine)

The MARIANNE (NCT01120184) trial recruited more than 1000 patients with HER2-positive MBC who had not received any chemotherapy in the metastatic setting [14]. According to the primary results from the phase III MARIANNE study, patients with HER2-positive, advanced breast cancer and no prior therapy for advanced disease were randomly assigned to control (trastuzumab plus taxane), T-DM1 plus placebo, hereafter T-DM1, or T-DM1 plus pertuzumab at standard doses. Neither experimental arm showed PFS superiority to trastuzumab plus taxane. The response rate was 67.9% in patients who were treated with trastuzumab plus taxane, 59.7% with T-DM1, and 64.2% with T-DM1 plus pertuzumab; the median response duration was 12.5 months, 20.7 months, and 21.2 months, respectively. The incidence of grade ≥3 adverse events was numerically higher in the control arm (54.1%) versus the T-DM1 arm (45.4%) and T-DM1 plus pertuzumab arm (46.2%). In conclusion, T-DM1 showed noninferior but not superior efficacy and better tolerability compared to taxane plus trastuzumab for first-line treatment of HER2-positive, advanced breast cancer [14].

These results suggest that T-DM1 may be an alternative to trastuzumab plus taxane in previously untreated HER2-positive MBC.

Everolimus (M-TOR Inhibitor)

The BOLERO-1 trial evaluated the combination of everolimus with trastuzumab plus paclitaxel as a first-line treatment for women with HER2-positive, locally advanced breast cancer or MBC [15]. In this phase 3 trial, patients who had not received previous trastuzumab or chemotherapy for advanced breast cancer within 12 months of randomization and without previous systemic treatment for advanced disease except endocrine therapy were enrolled. Patients were randomly assigned to receive either 10 mg of everolimus once daily orally or placebo plus weekly trastuzumab intravenously at 4 mg/kg loading dose on day 1 with subsequent weekly doses of 2 mg/kg of each 4-week cycle plus paclitaxel intravenously at a dose of 80 mg/m^2 on days 1, 8, and 15 of each 4-week cycle. First-line therapy with everolimus plus trastuzumab plus paclitaxel did not show a PFS benefit in patients with HER2-positive advanced breast cancer; the hormone receptor-negative subpopulation derived a clinically robust benefit to a median PFS of 7.2 months, suggesting that everolimus may have a role in this patient subpopulation. The most frequently reported grade 3 or 4 adverse events in the everolimus group versus the placebo group were neutropenia (25% vs 15%), stomatitis (13% vs 1%), anemia (10% vs 3%) and diarrhea (9% vs 4%). The authors concluded that proactive monitoring and early management of adverse events in patients given everolimus and chemotherapy are crucial [15] (Table 23.1).

To identify biomarkers to predict the clinical efficacy of everolimus treatment, BOLERO-1 and BOLERO-3 data were retrospectively analyzed. In both studies, differential progression-free survival (PFS) benefits of everolimus were consistently observed in patient subgroups defined by their PI3K pathway status. When analyzing the combined data sets from both studies, everolimus was associated with a decreased hazard of progression in patients with PIK3CA mutations (HR 0.67), PTEN loss (HR 0.54), or hyperactive PI3K pathway (HR 0.67).This analysis, although exploratory, suggests that patients with human epidermal growth factor receptor 2-positive advanced breast cancer and tumors with PIK3CA mutations, PTEN loss, or a hyperactive PI3K pathway could derive PFS benefit from everolimus [16].

Anti-HER2 Treatment Plus Endocrine Treatment

The data justify addition of endocrine treatment whenever possible for ER-positive breast cancer, leading to the current NCCN, ASCO and ESMO recommendations to add endocrine agents to treatment for most triple-positive breast cancer patients in the metastatic setting. Addition of hormonal agents to HER2-targeted treatment is recommended after the completion of cytotoxic chemotherapy. Importantly, the guidelines emphasize that addition of endocrine therapy is not based on direct evidence. In addition, they provide no reason why endocrine therapy should be delayed until completion of cytotoxic treatment.

Anti-HER2 treatment is less effective in Luminal B, hormone receptor-positive breast cancer. Loibl et al. combined individual patient data from five clinical trials evaluating PIK3CA mutations. Patients received either trastuzumab (T), lapatinib (L) or combination T/L in addition to taxane-based chemotherapy. Within the hormone-receptor positive (HR+) subgroup, the PIK3CA mutant group had a lower pCR rate. HR+/PIK3CA mutant patients appeared to have significantly worse DFS (HR 1.56 P = 0.050) [17].

For select patients with HER2-positive and hormone receptor–positive (ER-positive/PgR- positive or negative) breast cancer, endocrine treatment with either trastuzumab/pertuzumab or lapatinib/trastuzumab may be an acceptable first-line treatment [18, 19]. We do not typically recommend endocrine therapy alone for hormone receptor-positive, HER2-positive disease. Management could conceivably include combinations of available endocrine therapies such as aromatase inhibitors (AIs), selective estrogen receptor down-regulators or tamoxifen, with one or more of the currently approved HER2-targeted agents including trastuzumab, pertuzumab, or lapatinib. Several trials have examined the addition of HER2-targeted agents to AIs in postmenopausal women [18, 20, 21]. In ALTERNATIVE and PERTAIN trials, dual HER2 blockade + AI showed superior PFS benefit versus trastuzumab + AI in patients with HER2-positive/HR-positive metastatic breast cancer. These combinations offer an effective and safe chemotherapy-sparing alternative treatment regimen for this patient population. Patients with low-volume disease, a long disease-free interval, indolent disease or significant comorbidities would be the most appropriate candidates for endocrine therapy with anti-HER2 therapy (Fig. 23.1). A number of studies combining HER2-targeting with fulvestrant, AIs, or CDK4/6 inhibitors are ongoing.

Table 23.4 Second-line randomized phase III studies in HER2-positive metastatic breast cancer patients

Trial	Study arms	ORR (CR/PR) %	ORR (CR/PR) P	PFS Months	PFS Hazard ratio (95% CI), p	OS Months	OS Hazard ratio (95% CI), p
GBG26/BIG03-05 (von Minckwitz [5])	Capecitabine + trastuzumab	48.1	OR = 2.5 P = 0.0115	8.2	HR = 0.69 P = 0.0338	25.5	HR = 0.76 P = 0.257
	Capecitabine	27		5.6		20.4	
EGF100151 (Cameron [56])[a]	Lapatinib + capecitabine	NR	NR	31.3 (weeks)	HR 0.5 P < 0.001	71.4 (weeks)	HR = 0.79 P = 0.077
	Capecitabine	NR		18.6 (weeks)		56.6 (weeks)	
EMILIA (Diéras [23])	T-DM1	43.6	<0.001	9.6	HR 0.65 P < 0.001	29.9	HR 0.75 p < 0.001
	Lapatinib + capecitabine	30.8		6.4		25.9	
BOLERO-3 (André [57])	Everolimus + trastuzumab + vinorelbine	41	=0.210	7	HR 0.78 (0.65–0.95) P < 0.001	NR	
	Trastuzumab + vinorelbine	37		5.8		NR	
TH3RESA (Krop [30])	T-DM1	31	=0.0001	6.2	HR 0.53 P < 0.0001	22·7	HR = 0·68; p = 0·0007
	Physician's choice[b]	9		3.3		15·8	
EGF 104900 (Blackwell [58])	Lapatinib + trastuzumab	NR		11.1	HR 0.74 (0.58–0.94)	14	HR 0.74 (0.57–0.97)
	Lapatinib[c]	NR		8.1		9.5	
LUX Breast I (Harbeck [59])	Afatinib + vinorelbine	46.1	=0.851	5.5	P = 0.4272	20.5	p = 0.0048
	Trastuzumab + vinorelbine	47		5.6		28.6	

MBC metastatic breast cancer, *ORR* objective response rare, *CR* complete response, *PR* partial response, *PFS* progression-free survival, *OS* overall survival, *HR* hazard ratio, *T-DM1* T-DM1, *NE* not evaluable, *NS* non-significant

[a]The lapatinib plus trastuzumab study did include a heavily pretreated population. The results for patients receiving only one prior trastuzumab-based regimen are included in the table.

[b]Physician's choice included single-agent chemotherapy, hormonal therapy, HER2-directed therapy or a combination of HER2-directed therapy with chemotherapy, hormonal therapy, or other HER2-directed therapy: 68% chemotherapy + trastuzumab, 10.3% trastuzumab + lapatinib, and 2.7% chemotherapy + lapatinib.

[c]Lapatinib is not approved as a single agent.

Second-Line Therapy

Multiple phase III clinical trials have demonstrated that continuation of anti-HER2 therapy in the second-line setting improves the clinical outcome of patients whose disease has recurred or progressed on first-line trastuzumab-based therapy (Table 23.4).

The efficacy and safety of trastuzumab plus capecitabine with or without pertuzumab in patients with human epidermal growth factor receptor 2-positive metastatic breast cancer who experienced disease progression during or after trastuzumab-based therapy and received a prior taxane were assessed in a randomized trial [22]. Patients were randomly assigned to arm A: trastuzumab plus capecitabine 1250 mg/m^2 twice a day (2 weeks on, 1 week off, every 3 weeks); or arm B: pertuzumab plus trastuzumab at the same dose and schedule as arm A plus capecitabine 1000 mg/m^2 on the same schedule as arm A. Median PFS at 28.6 and 25.3 months' median follow-up was 9.0 v 11.1 months (HR, 0.82; P = 0.0731), and interim OS was 28.1 v 36.1 months (HR, 0.68). In conclusion, the addition of pertuzumab to trastuzumab and capecitabine did not significantly improve PFS. Statistical significance for OS cannot be claimed because of the hierarchical testing of OS after the primary PFS end point [22].

The evaluated therapeutic options included continuing trastuzumab with a different chemotherapy partner, switching to T-DM1, adding the mTOR pathway inhibitor everolimus, or switching to a regimen of capecitabine plus lapatinib.

T-DM1

The superiority of T-DM1 to capecitabine plus lapatinib in the second-line setting was established in the EMILIA trial [23]. EMILIA was a randomized phase 3 study of patients with HER2-positive unresectable, locally advanced or metastatic breast cancer previously treated with trastuzumab and a taxane. Enrolled patients were randomly assigned (1:1) to trastuzumab emtansine (3.6 mg/kg intravenously every 3 weeks) or the control (capecitabine 1000 mg/m^2 self-administered orally twice daily on days 1–14 on each 21-day cycle, plus lapatinib 1250 mg orally once daily on days 1–21). A total of 991 eligible patients were enrolled and randomly assigned to either trastuzumab emtansine (n = 495) or capecitabine and lapatinib (control; n = 496). In this final descriptive analysis, median overall survival was longer with trastuzumab emtansine than with the control (29.9 months vs. 25.9 months; HR 0.75). In the safety population, fewer grade 3 or worse adverse events occurred with trastuzumab emtansine [48%] than with the capecitabine plus lapatinib control treatment [60%]. In the control group, the most frequently reported grade 3 or worse adverse events were diarrhea [21%], followed by palmar-plantar erythrodysesthesia syndrome [18%] and vomiting [5%]. The safety profile of trastuzumab emtansine was similar to that reported previously; the most frequently reported grade 3 or worse adverse events in the trastuzumab emtansine group were thrombocytopenia [14%], increased aspartate aminotransferase levels [5%], and anemia [4%]. This descriptive analysis of final overall survival in the EMILIA trial shows that trastuzumab emtansine improved

Table 23.5 Dosage dose modification of T-DM1 based on asymptomatic left ventricular ejection fraction decrease from baseline

<table>
<tr><th>Criteria</th><th>Left ventricular ejection fraction (LVEF)</th><th>Action</th><th>Action at LVEF reassessment</th></tr>
<tr><td>1</td><td>>45%</td><td>Continue and follow routine monitoring guidelines</td><td>Follow actions based on criteria</td></tr>
<tr><td>2</td><td>40–45% AND < 10% below baseline and asymptomatic</td><td>Continue and repeat LVEF in 3 weeks</td><td rowspan="3">Discontinue permanently if no recovery. If improved to criterion #1 (for #2, 3 or 4) or #2 (for #3 or 4), treatment may be restarted; monitor closely</td></tr>
<tr><td>3</td><td>40–45% AND ≥10% below baseline, and asymptomatic</td><td rowspan="2">Pause and repeat LVEF in 3 weeks</td></tr>
<tr><td>4</td><td><40% and asymptomatic</td></tr>
<tr><td>5</td><td>Symptomatic or confirmed CHF</td><td>Discontinue</td><td>Not applicable</td></tr>
</table>

overall survival in patients with previously treated HER2-positive metastatic breast cancer even in the presence of crossover treatment. The safety profile was similar to that reported in previous analyses, reaffirming trastuzumab emtansine as an efficacious and tolerable treatment in this patient population [23] (Table 23.5).

Afatinib

Afatinib is an oral small molecule that irreversibly inhibits HER1, 2 and 4 [24]. In a phase II study, 4 of 35 patients with trastuzumab-resistant metastatic breast cancer showed partial responses [24]. Adverse events included diarrhea and rash. However, the recently published LUX-Breast 1 [25] trial was a negative trial for afatinib. This was a phase III study comparing vinorelbine plus trastuzumab or afatinib plus vinorelbine for metastatic patients who progressed to one chemotherapy regimen containing trastuzumab. Recruitment was stopped on April 26, 2013, after a benefit-risk assessment by the independent data monitoring committee was unfavorable for the afatinib group. Patients on afatinib plus vinorelbine were required to switch to trastuzumab plus vinorelbine.

Neratinib

Neratinib is also an oral, irreversible inhibitor of HER1,-2 and -4. On the basis of the ExteNET study, neratinib was recently approved by the FDA for extended post-trastuzumab adjuvant treatment [26]. However, neratinib failed to show superiority over comparators in metastatic settings. Neratinib was compared with trastuzumab (both in combination with taxanes) as first-line treatment by the NEfERT trial, which reported identical PFS in both arms (12.9 months) and much higher toxicity in the neratinib arm (grade 3 diarrhea developed in up to 30% of patients) [27]. In a second-line trial that compared neratinib monotherapy with the combination of lapatinib + capecitabine, the neratinib arm showed shorter PFS and OS than the combination [28]. In addition, a subanalysis of NEfERT-T trial showed that neratinib was more effective against brain metastases (relative risk of central nervous system [CNS] recurrences 0.48, $p = 0.002$). New trials of neratinib may be expected in patients with brain metastases.

MM-111

MM-11 is a bi-specific monoclonal antibody that reversibly targets the HER2 and HER3 heterodimer. A phase I–II study is currently evaluating the efficacy of MM-111 as a single agent in HER2 positive advanced breast cancer patients who have received prior trastuzumab or lapatinib therapy (clinicaltrials.gov, NCT00911898). Another phase I trial is studying MM-111 plus trastuzumab in HER2-positive, heregulin-positive, advanced and refractory breast cancer (clinicaltrials.gov, NCT01097460).

MM-302 (HER2-Targeted Antibody-Liposomal Doxorubicin Conjugate)

MM-302 is a novel, HER2-targeted antibody-liposomal doxorubicin conjugate that specifically targets HER2-overexpressing cells. HERMIONE is an open-label, multicenter, randomized Phase 2 trial of MM-302 plus trastuzumab versus chemotherapy of physician's choice (gemcitabine, capecitabine, or vinorelbine) plus trastuzumab planned to enroll 250 anthracycline-naïve patients with locally advanced/metastatic HER2-positive breast cancer. The HERMIONE study will evaluate the efficacy and safety of MM-302 plus trastuzumab in patients with refractory HER2-positive advanced/metastatic breast cancer for whom there are no standard of care therapies with a proven survival advantage [29].

Third-Line Therapy and Beyond

The lapatinib plus trastuzumab study did include a heavily pretreated population and showed a benefit for continuing trastuzumab in combination with lapatinib after progression during previous trastuzumab-containing regimens [5]. These data support the continuation of HER2-targeted therapy in the third-line setting and beyond.

Patients with progressive disease after two or more HER2-directed regimens for recurrent or MBC have few effective therapeutic options. TH3RESA is a phase III trial to specifically address the efficacy of anti-HER2 therapy in this third-line setting [30]. Results from the final overall survival analysis of the TH3RESA trial have been reported. Eligible patients for the TH3RESA trial were those with centrally confirmed HER2-positive advanced breast cancer previously treated with both trastuzumab and lapatinib (advanced setting) and a taxane (any setting) and with progression on two or more HER2-directed regimens in the advanced setting (n = 602). Overall survival was significantly longer with trastuzumab emtansine versus treatment of physician's choice (median 22.7 months vs. 15.8 months; HR = 0.68; p = 0.0007). In conclusion, in patients who had progressed on two or more HER2-directed regimens, trastuzumab emtansine treatment resulted in a significant improvement in overall survival versus treatment of physician's choice [30].

T-DM1 should be considered as a new standard for patients with HER2-positive advanced breast cancer who have previously received trastuzumab and lapatinib.

Trastuzumab Deruxtecan

Trastuzumab deruxtecan (ds-8201a), a HER2-targeting antibody-drug conjugate, demonstrated significant clinical activity in heavily pretreated patients with HER2-expressing metastatic breast cancers who previously received T-DM1. Whereas T-DM1 is a tubulin-targeting chemotherapy, trastuzumab deruxtecan is a topoisomerase 1 inhibitor. It is highly potent, with a drug-to-antibody ratio of 7.8, compared with 3.5 for T-DM1.

In an ongoing 2-part phase I study, the ORR to trastuzumab deruxtecan in 57 evaluable patients with HER2-positive tumors was 61.4%. In the HER2-positive cohort, the ORR was 56.4% (22 of 39) among those with ER-positive disease and 75.0% (12 of 16) among those with ER-negative disease. Notably, the ORR was 62.5% among the 50 patients in this cohort with prior pertuzumab treatment. The disease control rate was 94.7% overall in the HER2-positive subset: 92.3% in the ER-positive group, 100.0% in the ER-negative group, and 94.0% among those who had received prior pertuzumab. Median PFS was not yet reached in the ER-positive group and was 10.3 months in the ER-negative group. Median PFS was 10.3 months in the HER2-positive cohort who had received prior pertuzumab, as reported by Shanu Modi, MD, at the 2017 San Antonio Breast Cancer Symposium [31]. The main toxicity was grade 1/2 gastrointestinal toxicity. Grade 1/2 nausea was reported by 67.9%. Grade 3 and 4 events were hematological in nature. The rates of grade 3/4 anemia were 8.7% in the HER2-positive group and 0.9% in the HER2-low group. The rates of grade 3 decreases in neutrophil count and white blood cell count were each 10.4%. Across the study, 5 patients (4.3%) had a grade 4 decrease in neutrophil count.

In August 2017, trastuzumab deruxtecan received an FDA breakthrough therapy designation for the treatment of patients with HER2-positive, locally advanced, or metastatic breast cancer who have been treated with trastuzumab and pertuzumab and have disease progression after T-DM1. An ongoing pivotal phase II trial called DESTINY-Breast 01 is examining the efficacy and safety of trastuzumab

Table 23.6 Combined usage of cytotoxic drugs with dual anti-HER2 inhibition for HER2-positive advanced breast cancer

Regimen	Drug	Dosage	Route of administration	Frequency of cycles
Trastuzumab plus pertuzumab with docetaxel	Trastuzumab	8 mg/kg IV day 1 followed by 6 mg/kg	Intravenous	Cycled every 21 days
	Pertuzumab	840 mg IV day 1 followed by 420 mg	Intravenous	Cycled every 21 days
	Docetaxel	75–100 mg/m²	Intravenous	Cycled every 21 days
Trastuzumab plus pertuzumab with paclitaxel	Trastuzumab	8 mg/kg IV day 1 followed by 6 mg/kg	Intravenous	Cycled every 21 days OR
		4 mg/kg day 1 followed by 2 mg/kg	Intravenous	Weekly
	Pertuzumab	840 mg IV day 1 followed by 420 mg	Intravenous	Cycled every 21 days
	Paclitaxel	175 mg/m²	Intravenous	Cycled every 21 days OR
	Paclitaxel	80–90 mg/m²	Intravenous	Cycled every 7 days

Table 23.7 Combined usage of cytotoxic drugs with trastuzumab for HER2-positive advanced breast cancer

Regimen	Drug	Dosage	Route of administration	Frequency of cycles
Trastuzumab plus the following cytotoxic(s)	Trastuzumab	4 mg/kg day 1 followed by 2 mg/kg	Intravenous	Weekly
		8 mg/kg IV day 1 followed by 6 mg/kg	Intravenous	Cycled every 21 days
Paclitaxel/carboplatin	Carboplatin	AUC 6	Intravenous	Day 1 Cycled every 21 days
	Paclitaxel	175 mg/m²	Intravenous	Day 1 Cycled every 21 days
Weekly paclitaxel/carboplatin	Carboplatin	AUC 2	Intravenous	Days 1, 8, and 15 Cycled every 28 days
	Paclitaxel	80 mg/m²	Intravenous	Days 1, 8, and 15 Cycled every 28 days
Paclitaxel	Paclitaxel	175 mg/m²	Intravenous	Day 1 Cycled every 21 days
	Paclitaxel	80–90 mg/m²	Intravenous	Days 1 Cycled every 7 days
Docetaxel	Docetaxel	80–100 mg/m²	Intravenous	Day 1 Cycled every 21 days
	Docetaxel	35 mg/m²	Intravenous	Day 1 Cycled every week
Vinorelbine	Vinorelbine	25 mg/m²	Intravenous	Day 1 weekly Cycled every 21 days
	Vinorelbine	30–35 mg/m²	Intravenous	Days 1 and 8 Cycled every 21 days
Capecitabine	Capecitabine	1000–1250 mg/m²	Peroral	Twice daily days 1–14 Cycled every 21 days

Table 23.8 Systemic therapy for previously trastuzumab–treated HER2-positive advanced breast cancer patients

Regimen	Drug	Dosage	Route of administration	Frequency of cycles
T-DM1	Ado-trastuzumab emtansine	3.6 mg/kg	Intravenous	Day 1 Cycled every 21 days
Lapatinib + capecitabine	Lapatinib PO daily	1250 mg	Peroral	Days 1–21 Cycled every 21 days
	Capecitabine	1000 mg/m^2	Peroral	Twice daily days 1–14 Cycled every 21 days
Trastuzumab + capecitabine	Capecitabine	1000–1250 mg/m^2	Peroral	Twice daily days 1–14 Cycled every 21 days
	Trastuzumab	4 mg/kg day 1 followed by 2 mg/kg	Intravenous	Weekly
		8 mg/kg IV day 1 followed by 6 mg/kg	Intravenous	Cycled every 21 days
Trastuzumab + lapatinib (without cytotoxic therapy)	Lapatinib	1000 mg	Peroral	Days 1–21 Cycled every 21 days
	Trastuzumab	4 mg/kg day 1 followed by 2 mg/kg	Intravenous	Weekly
		8 mg/kg IV day 1 followed by 6 mg/kg	Intravenous	Cycled every 21 days

deruxtecan in patients with HER2-positive unresectable and/or metastatic breast cancer who are resistant or refractory to T-DM1.

Treatment Influence of Previous HER2 Therapy

First-Line Treatment

1. For patients with recurrence ≤12 months after adjuvant treatment:
   If the patient finished trastuzumab-based adjuvant treatment ≤12 months before recurrence, clinicians should follow the second-line HER2-targeted therapy–based treatment recommendations. For patients who progress 6 months or longer after the completion of adjuvant trastuzumab (without pertuzumab), trastuzumab plus pertuzumab in combination with a taxane can also be suggested [32] (Tables 23.6, 23.7, and 23.8).
2. For patients with recurrence >12 months after adjuvant treatment:
   If the patient finished trastuzumab-based adjuvant treatment >12 months before recurrence, clinicians should follow the first-line HER2-targeted therapy–based treatment recommendations [32].

Patients Who Require Second- or Later-Line Treatment

For patients with HER2-positive MBC who experience disease progression on a regimen that includes an HER2-directed agent, available options are shown in Fig. 23.1. Ongoing studies are evaluating novel therapeutic approaches to overcome primary and secondary drug resistance in tumors.

Duration of Chemotherapy or HER2-Targeted Therapy

There are insufficient data to make a single statement on when to stop administering HER2-targeted therapy. In most trials, HER2-targeted therapy was administered until disease progression or until toxic adverse events caused the clinician and patient to decide to discontinue therapy. For patients who have an optimal treatment response and for whom cytotoxic chemotherapy has been discontinued, the decision to discontinue HER2-directed therapy should be individualized because there are no prospective data to provide guidance. Anti-HER2-directed therapy can be continued for many years in such patients without disease progression. However, the same can be said for patients who discontinue treatment. While continuation of HER2-directed treatment can increase the risk of cumulative toxicity (particularly cardiotoxicity), increase healthcare costs, and may be inconvenient, these considerations

Box 23.2 Summary of Recommendations on Disease Management for Patients with Advanced HER2-Positive Breast Cancer and Brain Metastases

- For patients with a favorable prognosis for survival and limited (one to four) metastases, treatment options include ± surgery and radiation therapy (RT) (whole-brain radiation therapy (WBRT) or stereotactic radiosurgery (SRS) or both).
- For other patients with diffuse disease/extensive metastases, options include WBRT and, in select cases, only best supportive care and/or palliative care.
- For patients with leptomeningeal metastases options include involved field RT to bulky disease or symptomatic sites and intratechal treatment for select cases with normal cerebrospinal fluid flow (consider placing ventricular catheter and subcutaneous reservoir).
- For patients whose systemic disease is not progressive at the time of brain metastasis diagnosis, the same systemic therapy should be continued, and for patients whose systemic disease is progressive at the time of brain metastasis diagnosis, clinicians should use the algorithms for treatment of HER2-positive metastatic breast cancer.

- If a patient does not have a known history or symptoms of brain metastases, routine surveillance with brain magnetic resonance imaging (MRI) should not be performed. Clinicians should have a low threshold for performing diagnostic brain MRI testing in the setting of any neurological symptoms suggestive of brain involvement.

must be balanced by the potential benefit of treatment in delaying (or preventing) disease progression [32].

Targeting HER2 in Breast Cancer Brain Metastases

Patients with brain metastases should receive appropriate local therapy and systemic therapy. Local therapies include surgery, whole-brain radiotherapy (WBRT), and stereotactic radiosurgery (SRS). Treatments depend on factors such as patient prognosis, presence of symptoms, resectability, number and size of metastases, prior therapy, and whether metastases are diffuse [33]. Other options include systemic therapy, best supportive care, enrollment in a clinical trial, and/or palliative care (Box 23.2).

The data strongly support the hypothesis that the best overall treatment also improves survival in cases of brain metastases [13, 34–39]. Other conventional cytotoxic agents that can cross the blood-brain barrier may act with anti-HER2 therapy on CNS metastases, and further research is needed.

Neratinib is an irreversible pan-ERBB tyrosine kinase inhibitor. In a randomized trial, in first-line HER2-positive metastatic breast cancer, neratinib-paclitaxel was not superior to trastuzumab-paclitaxel in terms of progression-free survival. With neratinib-paclitaxel, the incidence of central nervous system recurrences was lower (relative risk, 0.48; P = 0.002) and time to central nervous system metastases was delayed (HR, 0.45; P = 0.004). In spite of its similar overall efficacy, neratinib-paclitaxel may delay the onset and reduce the frequency of central nervous system progression, but this finding requires a larger study for confirmation [26].

Breast cancer is one of the most common tumors involving the leptomeninges. Leptomeningeal carcinomatosis (LCM) of HER2-overexpressing breast carcinoma remains potentially sensitive to HER2-type receptor inhibition if the meningeal blood brain barrier is bypassed. Importantly, the receptor status of a metastasis can change [40]. Several studies and case reports of intrathecal (IT) trastuzumab to treat LCM have been published. Extremely low levels of the antibody are detected in the CSF after intravenous trastuzumab; much higher levels could be reached after intra-ventricular or IT administration, potentially reaching therapeutic concentrations.

Seventeen patients were evaluable for the efficacy and safety of IT trastuzumab for the treatment of metastatic cancer in HER2-positive breast cancer patients [41]. The mean age at IT trastuzumab administration was 48 years, and the mean total dose was 400 mg. IT trastuzumab alone or as part of combination therapies appeared to be safe; no serious adverse events were reported in 88% of cases. In 69% of cases, there was a significant clinical improvement, whereas 31% exhibited stabilization or progression of the disease. A CSF response was observed in 67% of cases. The median OS was 13.5 months, whereas the median CNS-PFS was 7.5 months. In 24% of cases, IT trastuzumab was administered after CNS progression, with a response observed in 75% of cases and a CNS-PFS of 9.4 months. The cumulative dose of IT trastuzumab given was 1040 mg (median 1215; range 55–1675). Clinical improvement (hazard ratio 0.14, 95% CI 0.02–0.91) and cerebrospinal fluid response (hazard ratio 0.09, 95% CI 0.01–0.89) were associated with longer CNS-PFS [41].

IT trastuzumab thus might be a promising treatment for leptomeningeal involvement in HER2-positive breast cancer patients, and further studies are warranted to optimize the dose, interval, duration, and combination of drugs for treatment.

New Exploratory Strategies

Anti-HER-2 Blocking Strategies

Ongoing trials combining anti-HER-2 agents with drugs blocking other signaling pathways hold the promise of further improvement. An auspicious approach appears to be the combination of anti-HER-2 therapy with insulin growth factor receptor (IGFR-1) blocking agents. IGFR-1 inhibition has been shown to restore sensitivity to trastuzumab in animal models [42]. Another potential combination is the dual blockade of HER-2 and SRC, which was recently shown to work as a central node downstream of multiple trastuzumab-resistance mechanisms [43]. Finally, HER-3 is a strong activator of the PI3K/Akt signaling pathway and has been demonstrated to be up-regulated after HER-2 blockade [44]. Although still in the early phases of development, Rb disruption strategies and the use of CDK-4/6 inhibitors may be clinically useful [45]. At present, CDK4/6 inhibition is perceived as one of the most promising new directions in the treatment of HER2-positive MBC and may soon be used in clinical practice. A series of trials showed that the addition of CDK4/6-inhibitors to endocrine treatment significantly improves PFS in the metastatic setting [46]. None of these trials have included HER2-positive patients. The success of these trials led to regulatory approvals and supported a wave of interest in CDK4/6 inhibitors for the treatment of HER2-positive disease. A number of studies combining HER2 targeting with fulvestrant, AIs, or CDK4/6 inhibitors are already ongoing (PATINA, PATRICIA, and monarcHER trials: NCT02947685, NCT02448420, NCT02675231).

Future studies of HER2-positive patients will be challenging because of the small window to improve the outcome beyond what is achievable today.

Imvmunotherapy

Cancer vaccines designed to induce specific anti-HER-2 immunity are being investigated. Different strategies include protein-based vaccines, plasmid DNA-based vaccines, and vaccines that deliver HER-2 in a viral vector. HER-2 peptide-based vaccines have been tested in patients with metastatic HER-2-positive breast cancer [47]. Immunized patients developed delayed-type hypersensitivity reactions and strong CD8+ cell responses specific for HER-2 [48]. A dendritic cell-based vaccine was also tested in a small group of patients with stage IV breast cancer [49]. One patient showed a partial response, and three had stable disease for ≥12 months. Using a different strategy, cell-based GM-CSF secreting vaccines were tested in combination with trastuzumab [50].

There is a broad array of ongoing breast cancer immunotherapy clinical trials. Immune-therapeutics that augment CD8 T-cell anti-tumor activity—such as anti-PD1, anti-PDL1 and anti-CTLA4 mAbs—given in combination with trastuzumab in patients with HER2-positive breast cancer may improve outcome by involving and enhancing critical host immunity [51–55]. A search for trials of immunotherapies yielded more than 90 clinical trials that are currently enrolling breast cancer patients. The application of immunotherapeutic strategies to the treatment of breast cancer holds promise.

Conclusion

Many clinically important randomized trials of first- and second-line treatments for HER2 metastatic breast cancer, including trastuzumab, lapatinib, pertuzumab, trastuzumab emtansine (T-DM1) and mammalian target of rapamycin (mTOR) inhibitor (everolimus), have affected medical practice. New studies are evaluating novel therapeutic approaches to overcome primary and secondary drug resistance in tumors. Ongoing trials combining anti-HER-2 agents with drugs blocking other signaling pathways hold the promise of further improvement.

References

1. Wolff AC, Hammond MEH, Allison KH, Harvey BE, Mangu PB, Bartlett JMS, et al. Human epidermal growth factor receptor 2 testing in breast cancer: American Society of Clinical Oncology/College of American Pathologists clinical practice guideline focused update. J Clin Oncol. 2018. https://doi.org/10.1200/JCO.2018.77.8738.

2. Slamon DJ, Leyland-Jones B, Shak S, Fuchs H, Paton V, Bajamonde A, et al. Use of chemotherapy plus a monoclonal antibody against HER2 for metastatic breast cancer that overexpresses HER2. N Engl J Med. 2001;344:783–92.
3. Andersson M, Lidbrink E, Bjerre K, Wist E, Enevoldsen K, Jensen AB, et al. Phase III randomized study comparing docetaxel plus trastuzumab with vinorelbine plus trastuzumab as first-line therapy of metastatic or locally advanced human epidermal growth factor receptor 2-positive breast cancer: the HERNATA study. J Clin Oncol. 2011;29(3):264–71.
4. Geyer CE, Forster J, Lindquist D, Chan S, Romieu CG, Pienkowski T, et al. Lapatinib plus capecitabine for HER2-positive advanced breast cancer. N Engl J Med. 2006;355(26):2733–43.
5. von Minckwitz G, du Bois A, Schmidt M, Maass N, Cufer T, de Jongh FE, et al. Trastuzumab beyond progression in human epidermal growth factor receptor 2-positive advanced breast cancer: a German Breast Group 26/Breast International Group 03-05 study. J Clin Oncol. 2009;27(12):1999–2006.
6. Wardley AM, Pivot X, Morales-Vasquez F, Zetina LM, de Fátima Dias Gaui M, Reyes DO, et al. Randomized phase II trial of first-line trastuzumab plus docetaxel and capecitabine compared with trastuzumab plus docetaxel in HER2-positive metastatic breast cancer. J Clin Oncol. 2010;28(6):976–83.
7. Hamberg P, Bos MM, Braun HJ, Stouthard JM, van Deijk GA, Erdkamp FL, et al. Randomized phase II study comparing efficacy and safety of combination-therapy trastuzumab and docetaxel vs. sequential therapy of trastuzumab followed by docetaxel alone at progression as first-line chemotherapy in patients with HER2+ metastatic breast cancer: HERTAX trial. Clin Breast Cancer. 2011;11:103.
8. Valero V, Forbes J, Pegram MD, Pienkowski T, Eiermann W, von Minckwitz G, et al. Multicenter phase III randomized trial comparing docetaxel and trastuzumab with docetaxel, carboplatin, and trastuzumab as first-line che- motherapy for patients with her2-gene-amplified metastatic breast cancer (BCIRG 007 Study): two highly active therapeutic regimens. J Clin Oncol. 2011;29:149–56.
9. Robert N, Leyland-Jones B, Asmar L, Belt R, Ilegbodu D, Loesch D, et al. Randomized phase III study of trastuzumab, paclitaxel, and carboplatin compared with trastuzumab and paclitaxel in women with her-2–overexpressing metastatic breast cancer. J Clin Oncol. 2006;24:2786–92.
10. Paul B, Trovato JA, Thompson J. Lapatinib: a dual tyrosine kinase inhibitor for metastatic breast cancer. Am J Health Syst Pharm. 2008;65(18):1703–10.
11. Guan Z, Xu B, DeSilvio ML, Shen Z, Arpornwirat W, Tong Z, et al. Randomized trial of lapatinib versus placebo added to paclitaxel in the treatment of human epidermal growth factor receptor 2–overexpressing metastatic breast cancer. J Clin Oncol. 2013;31:1947–53.
12. Gelmon KA, Boyle FM, Kaufman B, Huntsman DG, Manikhas A, Di Leo A, et al. Lapatinib or trastuzumab plus taxane therapy for human epidermal growth factor receptor 2-positive advanced breast cancer: final results of NCIC CTG MA.31. J Clin Oncol. 2015;33(14):1574–83.
13. Swain SM, Baselga J, Kim SB, Ro J, Semiglazov V, Campone M, CLEOPATRA Study Group, et al. Pertuzumab, trastuzumab, and docetaxel in HER2-positive metastatic breast cancer. N Engl J Med. 2015;372(8):724–34.
14. Perez EA, Barrios C, Eiermann W, Toi M, Im YH, Conte P, et al. Trastuzumab emtansine with or without pertuzumab versus trastuzumab plus taxane for human epidermal growth factor receptor 2-positive, advanced breast cancer: primary results from the phase III MARIANNE study. J Clin Oncol. 2017;35(2):141–8.
15. Hurvitz SA, Andre F, Jiang Z, Shao Z, Mano MS, Neciosup SP, et al. Combination of everolimus with trastuzumab plus paclitaxel as first-line treatment for patients with HER2-positive advanced breast cancer (BOLERO-1): a phase 3, randomised, double-blind, multicentre trial. Lancet Oncol. 2015;16(7):816–29.
16. André F, Hurvitz S, Fasolo A, Tseng LM, Jerusalem G, Wilks S, et al. Molecular alterations and everolimus efficacy in human epidermal growth factor receptor 2-overexpressing metastatic breast cancers: combined exploratory biomarker analysis from BOLERO-1 and BOLERO-3. J Clin Oncol. 2016;34:2115–24.

17. Loibl S, Majewski I, Guarneri V, Nekljudova V, Holmes E, Bria E, et al. PIK3CA mutations are associated with reduced pathological complete response rates in primary HER2-positive breast cancer: pooled analysis of 967 patients from five prospective trials investigating lapatinib and trastuzumab. Ann Oncol. 2016;27:1519–25.
18. Kaufman B, Mackey JR, Clemens MR, Bapsy PP, Vaid A, Wardley A, et al. Trastuzumab plus anastrozole versus anastrozole alone for the treatment of postmenopausal women with human epidermal growth factor receptor 2-positive, hormone receptor-positive metastatic breast cancer: results from the randomized phase III TAnDEM study. J Clin Oncol. 2009;27(33):5529–37.
19. Johnston S, Pippen J Jr, Pivot X, Lichinitser M, Sadeghi S, Dieras V, et al. Lapatinib combined with letrozole versus letrozole and placebo as first-line therapy for postmenopausal hormone receptor-positive metastatic breast cancer. J Clin Oncol. 2009;27(33):5538–46.
20. Huober J, Fasching PA, Barsoum M, Petruzelka L, Wallwiener D, Thomssen C, et al. Higher efficacy of letrozole in combination with trastuzumab compared to letrozole monotherapy as first-line treatment in patients with HER2-positive, hormone-receptor-positive metastatic breast cancer: results of the eLEcTRA trial. Breast. 2012;21:27–33.
21. Johnston SRD, Hegg R, Im SA, Park IH, Burdaeva O, Kurteva G, et al. Phase III, randomized study of dual human epidermal growth factor receptor 2 (HER2) blockade with lapatinib plus trastuzumab in combination with an aromatase inhibitor in postmenopausal women with HER2-positive, hormone receptor-positive metastatic breast cancer: ALTERNATIVE. J Clin Oncol. 2018;36(8):741–8.
22. Urruticoechea A, Rizwanullah M, Im SA, Ruiz ACS, Láng I, Tomasello G, et al. Randomized phase III trial of trastuzumab plus capecitabine with or without pertuzumab in patients with human epidermal growth factor receptor 2-positive metastatic breast cancer who experienced disease progression during or after trastuzumab-based therapy. J Clin Oncol. 2017;35(26):3030–8.
23. Diéras V, Miles D, Verma S, Pegram M, Welslau M, Baselga J, et al. Trastuzumab emtansine versus capecitabine plus lapatinib in patients with previously treated HER2-positive advanced breast cancer (EMILIA): a descriptive analysis of final overall survival results from a randomised, open-label, phase 3 trial. Lancet Oncol. 2017;18(6):732–42.
24. Lin NU, Winer EP, Wheatley D, Carey LA, Houston S, Mendelson D, et al. A phase II study of afatinib (BIBW 2992), an irreversible ErbB family blocker, in patients with HER2-positive metastatic breast cancer progressing after trastuzumab. Breast Cancer Res Treat. 2012;133(3):1057–65.
25. Harbeck N, Huang CS, Hurvitz S, Yeh DC, Shao Z, Im SA, et al. Afatinib plus vinorelbine versus trastuzumab plus vinorelbine in patients with HER2-overexpressing metastatic breast cancer who had progressed on one previous trastuzumab treatment (LUX-Breast 1): an open-label, randomised, phase 3 trial. Lancet Oncol. 2016;17(3):357–66.
26. Chan A, Delaloge S, Holmes FA, Moy B, Iwata H, Harvey VJ, et al. Neratinib after trastuzumab-based adjuvant therapy in patients with HER2-positive breast cancer (ExteNET): a multicentre, randomised, double-blind, placebo-controlled, phase 3 trial. Lancet Oncol. 2016;17(3):367–77.
27. Awada A, Colomer R, Inoue K, Bondarenko I, Badwe RA, Demetriou G, et al. Neratinib plus paclitaxel vs trastuzumab plus paclitaxel in previously untreated metastatic ERBB2-positive breast cancer: the NEfERT-T randomized clinical trial. JAMA Oncol. 2016;2(12):1557–64.
28. Martin M, Bonneterre J, Geyer CE Jr, Ito Y, Ro J, Lang I, et al. A phase two randomised trial of neratinib monotherapy versus lapatinib plus capecitabine combination therapy in patients with HER2+ advanced breast cancer. Eur J Cancer. 2013;49(18):3763–72.
29. Miller K, Cortes J, Hurvitz SA, Krop IE, Tripathy D, Verma S, et al. HERMIONE: a randomized phase 2 trial of MM-302 plus trastuzumab versus chemotherapy of physician's choice plus trastuzumab in patients with previously treated, anthracycline-naïve, HER2-positive, locally advanced/metastatic breast cancer. BMC Cancer. 2016;16:352.

30. Krop IE, Kim SB, Martin AG, LoRusso PM, Ferrero JM, Badovinac-Crnjevic T, et al. Trastuzumab emtansine versus treatment of physician's choice in patients with previously treated HER2-positive metastatic breast cancer (TH3RESA): final overall survival results from a randomised open-label phase 3 trial. Lancet Oncol. 2017;18(6):743–54.
31. Modi S, Tsurutani J, Takahashi S. Safety and efficacy results from a phase 1 study of DS-8201a in patients with HER2 expressing breast cancers. In: Presented at 2017 San Antonio breast cancer symposium, 5–9 Dec 2017, San Antonio, TX. Abstract PD3-07.
32. Giordano SH, Temin S, Chandarlapaty S, Crews JR, Esteva FJ, Kirshner JJ, et al. Systemic therapy for patients with advanced human epidermal growth factor receptor 2-positive breast cancer: ASCO clinical practice guideline update. J Clin Oncol. 2018:JCO2018792697. https://doi.org/10.1200/JCO.2018.79.2697.
33. Ramakrishna N, Temin S, Chandarlapaty S, Crews JR, Davidson NE, Esteva FJ, et al. Recommendations on disease management for patients with advanced human epidermal growth factor receptor 2-positive breast cancer and brain metastases: ASCO clinical practice guideline update. J Clin Oncol. 2018:JCO2018792713. https://doi.org/10.1200/JCO.2018.79.2713.
34. Brufsky AM, Mayer M, Rugo HS, Kaufman PA, Tan-Chiu E, Tripathy D, et al. Central nervous system metastases in patients with HER2-positive metastatic breast cancer: incidence, treatment, and survival in patients from registHER. Clin Cancer Res. 2011;17(14):4834–43.
35. Lin NU, Diéras V, Paul D, Lossignol D, Christodoulou C, Stemmler HJ, et al. Multicenter phase II study of lapatinib in patients with brain metastases from HER2-positive breast cancer. Clin Cancer Res. 2009;15:1452–9.
36. Bachelot T, Romieu G, Campone M, Diéras V, Cropet C, Dalenc F, et al. Lapatinib plus capecitabine in patients with previously untreated brain metastases from HER2-positive metastatic breast cancer (LANDSCAPE): a single-group phase 2 study. Lancet Oncol. 2013;14:64–71.
37. Pivot X, Manikhas A, Żurawski B, Chmielowska E, Karaszewska B, Allerton R, et al. CEREBEL (EGF111438): a phase III, randomized, open-label study of lapatinib plus capecitabine versus trastuzumab plus capecitabine in patients with human epidermal growth factor receptor 2-positive metastatic breast cancer. J Clin Oncol. 2015;33:1564–73.
38. Krop IE, Lin NU, Blackwell K, Guardino E, Huober J, Lu M, et al. T-DM1 (T-DM1) versus lapatinib plus capecitabine in patients with HER2-positive metastatic breast cancer and central nervous system metastases: a retrospective, exploratory analysis in EMILIA. Ann Oncol. 2015;26:113–9.
39. Yuan P, Gao SL. Management of breast cancer brain metastases: focus on human epidermal growth factor receptor 2-positive breast cancer. Chronic Dis Transl Med. 2017;3(1):21–32.
40. Curigliano G, Bagnardi V, Viale G, Fumagalli L, Rotmensz N, Aurilio G, et al. Should liver metastases of breast cancer be biopsied to improve treatment choice? Ann Oncol. 2011;22:2227–33.
41. Zagouri F, Sergentanis TN, Bartsch R, Berghoff AS, Chrysikos D, de Azambuja E, et al. Intrathecal administration of trastuzumab for the treatment of meningeal carcinomatosis in HER2-positive metastatic breast cancer: a systematic review and pooled analysis. Breast Cancer Res Treat. 2013;139(1):13–22.
42. Nahta R, Yuan LX, Zhang B, Kobayashi R, Esteva FJ. Insulin-like growth factor-I receptor/human epidermal growth factor receptor 2 heterodimerization contributes to trastuzumab resistance of breast cancer cells. Cancer Res. 2005;65(23):11118–28.
43. Zhang S, Huang WC, Li P, Guo H, Poh SB, Brady SW, et al. Combating trastuzumab resistance by targeting SRC, a common node downstream of multiple resistance pathways. Nat Med. 2011;17(4):461–9.
44. Garrett JT, Olivares MG, Rinehart C, Granja-Ingram ND, Sanchez V, Chakrabarty A, et al. Transcriptional and posttranslational up-regulation of HER3 (ErbB3) compensates for inhibition of the HER2 tyrosine kinase. Proc Natl Acad Sci U S A. 2011;108(12):5021–6.
45. Witkiewicz AK, Ertel A, McFalls J, Valsecchi ME, Schwartz G, Knudsen ES. RB-pathway disruption is associated with improved response to neoadjuvant chemotherapy in breast cancer. Clin Cancer Res. 2012;18(18):5110–22.

46. Messina C, Cattrini C, Buzzatti G, Cerbone L, Zanardi E, Messina M, et al. CDK4/6 inhibitors in advanced hormone receptor-positive/HER2-negative breast cancer: a systematic review and meta-analysis of randomized trials. Breast Cancer Res Treat. 2018 Jul 27. https://doi.org/10.1007/s10549-018-4901-0.
47. Disis ML, Gooley TA, Rinn K, Davis D, Piepkorn M, Cheever MA, et al. Generation of T-cell immunity to the HER-2/neu protein after active immunization with HER-2/neu peptide-based vaccines. J Clin Oncol. 2002;20(11):2624–32.
48. Knutson KL, Schiffman K, Cheever MA, Disis ML. Immunization of cancer patients with a HER-2/neu, HLA-A2 peptide, p369–377, results in short-lived peptide-specific immunity. Clin Cancer Res. 2002;8(5):1014–8.
49. Park JW, Melisko ME, Esserman LJ, Jones LA, Wollan JB, Sims R. Treatment with autologous antigen-presenting cells activated with the HER-2 based antigen Lapuleucel-T: results of a phase I study in immunologic and clinical activity in HER-2 overexpressing breast cancer. J Clin Oncol. 2007;25(24):3680–7.
50. Hamilton E, Blackwell K, Hobeika AC, Clay TM, Broadwater G, Ren XR, et al. Phase 1 clinical trial of HER2-specific immunotherapy with concomitant HER2 kinase inhibition [corrected]. J Transl Med. 2012;10:28.
51. Stagg J, Loi S, Divisekera U, Ngiow SF, Duret H, Yagita H, et al. Anti-ErbB-2 mAb therapy requires type I and II interferons and synergizes with anti-PD-1 or anti-CD137 mAb therapy. Proc Natl Acad Sci U S A. 2011;108(17):7142–7.
52. Park S, Jiang Z, Mortenson ED, Deng L, Radkevich-Brown O, Yang X, et al. The therapeutic effect of anti-HER2/neu antibody depends on both innate and adaptive immunity. Cancer Cell. 2010;18(2):160–70.
53. Pondé N, Brandão M, El-Hachem G, Werbrouck E, Piccart M. Treatment of advanced HER2-positive breast cancer: 2018 and beyond. Cancer Treat Rev. 2018;67:10–20.
54. Al-Awadhi A, Lee Murray J, Ibrahim NK. Developing anti-HER2 vaccines: breast cancer experience. Int J Cancer. 2018. https://doi.org/10.1002/ijc.31551.
55. Nicolini A, Barak V, Biava P, Ferrari P, Rossi G, Carpi A. Use of immunotherapy to treat metastatic breast cancer. Curr Med Chem. 2018. https://doi.org/10.2174/09298673256661802091 24052.
56. Cameron D, Casey M, Oliva C, Newstat B, Imwalle B, Geyer CE. Lapatinib plus capecitabine in women with her-2–positive advanced breast cancer: final survival analysis of a phase III randomized trial. Oncologist. 2010;15:924–34.
57. André F, O'Regan R, Ozguroglu M, Toi M, Xu B, Jerusalem G, et al. Everolimus for women with trastuzumab-resistant, HER2-positive, advanced breast cancer (BOLERO-3): a randomised, double-blind, placebo-controlled phase 3 trial. Lancet Oncol. 2014;15(6):580–91.
58. Blackwell KL, Burstein HJ, Storniolo AM, Rugo HS, Sledge G, Aktan G, et al. Overall survival benefit with lapatinib in combination with trastuzumab for patients with human epidermal growth factor receptor 2–positive metastatic breast cancer: final results from the EGF104900 study. J Clin Oncol. 2012;30:2585–92.
59. Harbeck N, Huang CS, Hurvitz S, Harbeck N, Huang CS, Hurvitz S, et al. Randomized phase III trial of afatinib plus vinorelbine versus trastuzumab plus vinorelbine in patients with HER2-overexpressing metastatic breast cancer who had progressed on one prior trastuzumab treatment: LUX-Breast 1. In: Poster P5-19-01 presented at the San Antonio breast cancer symposium (SABCS) 2014 congress, San Antonio, TX, 9–13 Dec 2014.

Chapter 24
Endocrine Therapy of Metastatic Breast Cancer

Fatma Sen and Adnan Aydiner

Introduction

Breast cancer is one of the most commonly diagnosed malignant neoplasms worldwide, and breast cancer remains the second leading cause of cancer death in females according to the 2018 WHO Cancer Statistics. The 5-year survival rate of females with metastatic disease is approximately 22% [1]. Early diagnosis via mammographic screening and implementation of post-surgical [1]. Early diagnosis via mammographic screening and implementation of post-surgical systemic adjuvant therapy have provided a significant decrease in breast cancer mortalities in developed countries. However, breast cancer remains the leading cause of cancer death, with ~90% of these mortalities due to metastasis of tumor cells to other organs. The median survival rate of females with metastatic disease is only 2–3 years [2]. Approximately two-thirds of breast cancers are hormone receptor positive (HR+) based on the immunohistochemical expression of estrogen receptor (ER), progesterone receptor (PgR), or both receptors [3]. Recent data suggest that if the current trends continue, the incidence of HR+ breast cancers will increase, whereas the incidence of HR-negative breast cancers will continue to decrease, and the overall incidence of breast cancer will remain similar to its current level [4]. In general, HR positivity is considered both a favorable prognostic factor and a predictor of the efficacy of endocrine therapy (ET) [5]. However, one-third of patients with early-stage HR+ breast cancer who are treated with adjuvant ET with curative intent will experience disease recurrence with local or distant metastasis. Additionally, approximately 5–10% of patients have distant metastasis at initial presentation [6]. The

F. Sen
Department of Medical Oncology, Avrasya Hospital, Istanbul, Turkey

A. Aydiner (✉)
Internal Medicine, Medical Oncology, Istanbul Medical Faculty, Department of Medical Oncology, Institute of Oncology, Istanbul University, Istanbul, Turkey

A. Aydiner et al. (eds.), *Breast Cancer*, https://doi.org/10.1007/978-3-319-96947-3_24

goal of treatment in metastatic breast cancer is to improve quality of life and prolong survival [7].

The role of hormones in the growth of some tumors was first discovered more than a century ago when the tumor of a patient with metastatic breast carcinoma regressed following ovariectomy [8]. Later, estradiol was shown to be the most powerful hormone stimulator of breast cancer [9]. Thus, ET including medical or surgical deprivation and/or antagonism of estradiol is the mainstay of systemic treatment of patients with HR+ breast cancer [10].

Cytotoxic drugs or targeted therapies are other systemic treatment options for HR+ advanced breast cancer. Several systematic reviews or meta-analyses have revealed that in patients with HR+ advanced breast cancer, ET should be chosen as the first-line treatment option instead of chemotherapy unless a life-threatening disease that requires sudden improvement with cytotoxics exists [11]. Overall survival is similar between chemotherapy and ET. Unfortunately, chemotherapy leads to greater toxicity, particularly emesis and alopecia. Thus, ET is recommended as the first-line treatment option in the absence of severe symptomatic disease in which an immediate tumor response is necessary [12]. However, the definition of the exact number or volume or symptom level as the cutoff to start chemotherapy rather than endocrine therapy remains a topic of debate. There is no uniform consensus among international breast cancer guidelines on the optimal chemotherapeutic agent as the first line and subsequent lines, and the number of agents and types of agents are decided based on the characteristics of the patient and the tumor, including previous types of therapy, severity of adverse reactions, performance status, medical comorbidities, and patient choices. When an indication of chemotherapy exists in patients with HR+ breast cancer, a single-agent approach should be preferred over combination chemotherapy [11].

During the selection of the ET option, the history of previous or ongoing ET, including the type of endocrine agent and response to that agent, the setting in which ET has been given, and the time of progression are important features. If the tumor progresses one year after adjuvant ET completion, patients should be accepted and treated as endocrine treatment–naive patients. By contrast, if disease metastasis or recurrence occurs under adjuvant ET, under first-line ET in the metastatic setting or within 1 year after adjuvant ET ended, eligible patients should be evaluated for subsequent ET. The mechanism of action, possible side effects, pharmacological interactions, cost, availability and route of administration are factors to be considered in selecting the type of endocrine agent.

Although sequencing of ET was the recommended approach until recently, few randomized trials had directly compared the effects of the order in which different agents are used. Thus, definitive recommendations regarding the optimal ET sequencing in patients with HR+ metastatic breast cancer were difficult to provide due to lack of sufficient scientific data on ET sequencing [13]. However, based on data about ET plus other targeted agents from recently published phase II/III randomized trials, some ET options can be used sequentially or preferentially as the first line or second line (Figs. 24.1 and 24.2).

The main sources of estrogens that should be suppressed and the choices of ET differ between premenopausal and postmenopausal women. The ovaries are the

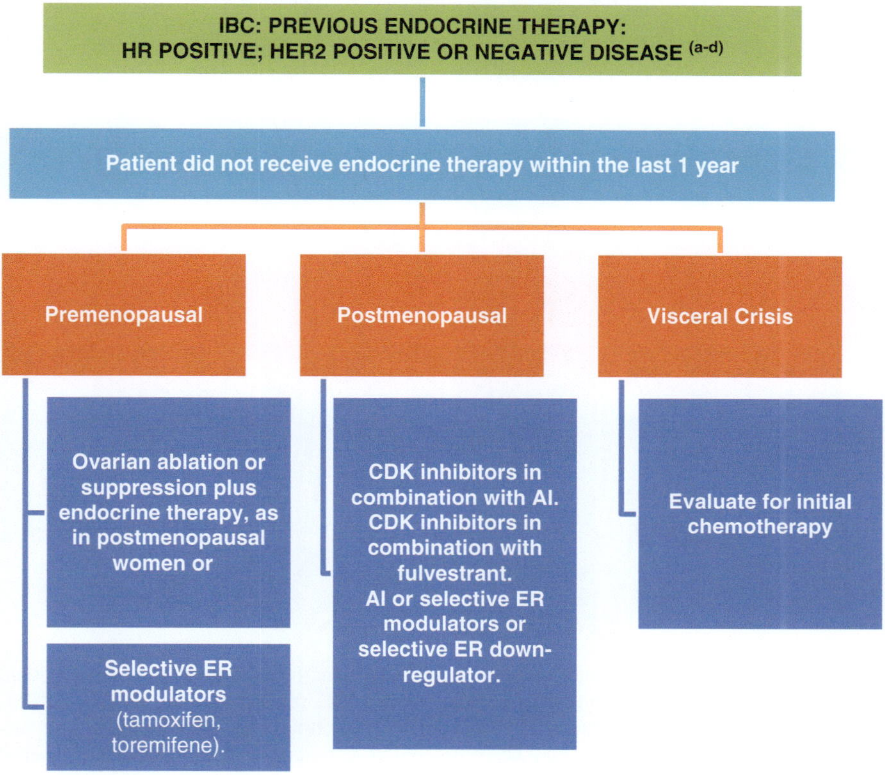

Fig. 24.1 Systemic treatment of recurrent stage IV hormone receptor-positive disease (patient did not received endocrine therapy during the last year). [a]If bone disease is present, add denosumab, zoledronic acid, ibandronic acid or pamidronate. [b]AI ± CDK 4/6 inhibitor may be considered as a treatment option for first-line therapy for postmenopausal patients with ER-positive, HER2-negative breast cancer. [c]Fulvestrant (selective ER downregulator) can be used in the first choice in de novo metastatic disease that has never received any endocrine treatment. Fulvestrant was found to be superior to anastrozole in patients with bone metastases. [d]Anti-HER2 therapy must be added to HER2-positive patients

main source of estrogen in premenopausal women, whereas estrogen synthesis occurs mainly in peripheral tissues, particularly fat tissues, in postmenopausal women, whose ovaries fail to produce estrogen. Aromatase, also called estrogen synthetase or estrogen synthase, is a member of the cytochrome P450 superfamily and is the main enzyme in estrogen biosynthesis in postmenopausal women. In particular, aromatase is responsible for the aromatization of androgens into estrogens. Aromatase inhibitors (AI) cannot inhibit the ovaries from making estrogen. In premenopausal women, AIs reduce hypothalamic–pituitary estrogen feedback, leading to increased gonadotropin-releasing hormone (GnRH) secretion that could, in turn, stimulate the ovarian production of estrogen. Due to the potential for ovary stimulation and the probability of resumption of menses, AIs should not be offered alone in premenopausal women. Thus, the definition of menopause is an important issue in

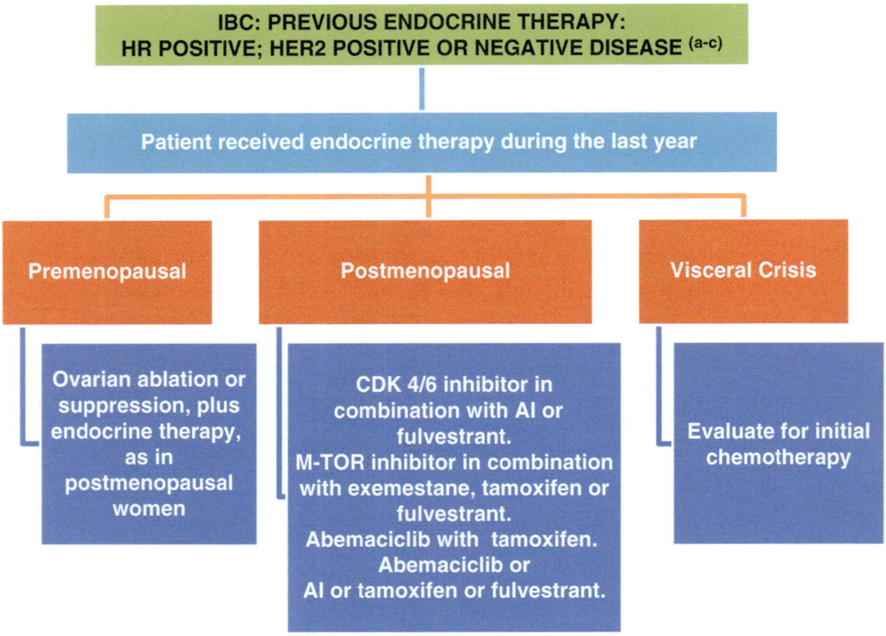

Fig. 24.2 Systemic treatment of recurrent stage IV hormone receptor-positive disease (patient received endocrine therapy during the last year). [a]Anti-HER2 therapy must be added to HER2-positive patients. [b]AI or fulvestrant ± CDK 4/6 inhibitor, everolimus (M-TOR inhibitor) + exemestane or tamoxifen or fulvestrant, may be considered as a treatment option for postmenopausal patients with ER-positive, HER2-negative breast cancer.[c] If bone disease is present, add denosumab, zoledronic acid, ibandronic acid or pamidronate

women with breast cancer. Women who become amenorrhoeic after chemotherapy should not be considered postmenopausal. The cessation of menses is not synonymous with true ovarian failure because estrogen levels can remain in the premenopausal range despite one year or chemotherapy-induced amenorrhea or longer, and the AIs might induce the resumption of ovarian function. Patients with a history of bilateral oophorectomy or older than 60 years are accepted as postmenopausal without further requirement for any laboratory testing. For young women (<60 years) without a history of chemotherapy, ovarian function suppression, tamoxifen and toremifene, amenorrhea for at least for 1 year and plasma estradiol and FSH levels in the postmenopausal range are required to classify patients as postmenopausal [14]. Monitoring of estradiol, FSH and LH values should be performed before prescribing an AI. Patients who are receiving a luteinizing hormone-releasing hormone (LHRH) agonist or LHRH antagonist should not be evaluated based on plasma FSH or estradiol levels or menstrual status to determine menopausal status (Box 24.1).

Selective ER modulators (SERMs), AIs (with ovarian function suppression in premenopausal women), and ER downregulators (SERDs) are the main ET options in HR+ metastatic breast cancer. Recently, targeted agents in combination with ET have become an alternative treatment approach in this patient population.

Approximately 20% of HR+ breast cancers are also HER2-positive (HER2+). HER2-directed targeted therapy should be considered in patients with both HR+ and HER2+ breast cancer.

Endocrine Therapy in HER2-Negative and Hormone Receptor-Positive Breast Cancer

First-Line Treatment

Ovarian ablation/suppression: In premenopausal women, pulses of LHRH induce the pituitary gland to release pulses of gonadotrophins and provide the menstrual cycles. Treatment with a long-term depot formulation of an LHRH agonist initially stimulates gonadotrophin release and later leads to a reduction in gonadotrophin secretion and circulating estrogen to postmenopausal ranges [15]. In a randomized trial, premenopausal women with HR+ MBC were treated with either goserelin 3.6 mg repeated monthly or surgical oophorectomy. Goserelin achieved a reduction of serum estradiol levels to postmenopausal levels. Failure-free survival and OS were not different between the treatment arms [16].

Tamoxifen, a nonsteroidal antiestrogenic compound synthesized in 1966, is an estrogen receptor modifier (SERMs). Tamoxifen and its derivatives have both partial agonist activity on ERs located in certain tissues and antagonistic activity on ERs located in other tissues. The well-defined agonistic effects that limit their clinical efficacy are endometrial stimulation and induction of tumor growth after previous response to tamoxifen [17]. After the clinical efficacy of tamoxifen for metastatic breast cancer was proven in several studies, Food and Drug Administration approved it for the treatment of MBC in postmenopausal women in 1977. Tamoxifen is currently the most widely prescribed agent for the treatment of both postmenopausal and premenopausal women with breast cancer. Tamoxifen is considered a chemosuppressive agent based on in vitro studies. Tamoxifen has been shown to prevent the transition of cells from early-*G1* phase to mid-*G1* phase, induce the accumulation of cells in early-*G1* phase of the cell cycle, and reduce the number of cells in *S* and G2 plus M phases [18]. These shifts have cytostatic effects.

Tamoxifen has similar effects as ovarian ablation in terms of the overall response rate, progression-free survival and overall survival in premenopausal, HR+ metastatic breast cancer as first-line therapy and is unlikely to be substantially inferior. However, combined use of tamoxifen with an LHRH agonist was found to be superior to single-agent therapy in several clinical trials [19]. A meta-analysis of randomized trials comparing combination therapy with an LHRH agonist alone in premenopausal women with HR+ metastatic breast cancer with respect to overall survival, progression-free survival, and objective response supported the combination therapy [20].

Tamoxifen has several adverse effects including nausea, menstrual irregularity, vaginal bleeding or discharge; fluid retention, hot flashes, reduction of antithrombin III activity, and central nervous system symptoms (e.g., depression, irritability, headache, dizziness, nervousness, inability to concentrate, sleep disturbance, lethargy, and fatigue) [21, 22]. Bone mineral density is not reduced by tamoxifen [23].

Toremifene, another SERM, has efficacy against HR+ breast cancer [24]. However, toremifene is cross-resistant with tamoxifen and is ineffective as sequential therapy in patients who are refractory to tamoxifen.

Aromatase inhibitors reduce circulating estrogen levels in both pre- and postmenopausal women without partial agonist effects. Aromatase, a member of the cytochrome P450 enzyme system, catalyzes the final enzymatic step of estrogen biosynthesis and converts androstenedione to estrone and testosterone to estradiol, thereby increasing estrogen levels. Aromatase inhibition alone is not recommended in premenopausal women because inhibition of the hypothalamus pituitary aromatase increases gonadotropin, which in turn stimulates ovarian follicular growth, producing high levels of circulating estrogen that can induce mammary tumor proliferation [25]. The clinical efficacies of combination therapy with AIs (letrozole, anastrozole, exemestane) and ovarian suppression (e.g., goserelin) in premenopausal patients with HR+ breast cancer were shown to be comparable to those of single-agent aromatase inhibitors in postmenopausal women [26, 27].

In postmenopausal women, third-generation AIs have well-established efficacy in HR+ breast cancer as single-agent ET. Steroidal (exemestane) and nonsteroidal (anastrozole and letrozole) are the 2 main classes of available third-generation AIs. NSAIs inhibit aromatase reversibly by binding to the heme moiety of the enzyme and preventing androgens from binding to the catalytic site [28]. Steroidal AIs, analogs of androstenedione, which is the substrate of natural aromatase, bind covalently to the substrate-binding site of aromatase and irreversibly inactivate the enzyme [28]. Therefore, steroidal nonreversible AIs are also known as aromatase inactivators, whereas NSAIs are reversible inhibitors of aromatase. The major side effects of AIs are osteoporosis and abnormalities of serum lipid levels. However, AIs cause vaginal bleeding and thromboembolic events less frequently than tamoxifen. Overall survival was found to be similar to that of tamoxifen in the different individual trials of the three third-generation AIs, but a meta-analysis showed an OS benefit of using AIs compared with tamoxifen as first-line therapy for HR+ breast cancer [29]. Currently, both steroidal and NSAIs are one of the standard first-line treatment options for postmenopausal women with HR+ breast cancer [30, 31].

Fulvestrant is a novel, steroidal estrogen antagonist with 100 times greater affinity for the ER than that of tamoxifen. Fulvestrant lacks the uterotrophic activity-blocking estrogen agonist effects found in ER agonists and partial agonists such as tamoxifen and raloxifene. Fulvestrant functionally blocks and decreases the cellular ER levels so the ERs become unavailable or unresponsive to estrogen or estrogen agonists in breast cancer. Therefore, fulvestrant is now known as a selective ER downregulator (SERD) and has neither cross-resistance with tamoxifen nor the ER-agonist activity associated with tamoxifen. Since fulvestrant has an attractive mode of action, it has been studied in several phase II and III trials that included postmenopausal and/or premenopausal women. However, until recently, the dosage, line of therapy and comparison groups were not uniform [32].

The Fulvestrant First-Line Study Comparing Endocrine Treatments (FIRST trial), a phase II, randomized, open-label, multicenter trial conducted by Robertson et al. [33], compared fulvestrant 500 mg (days 0, 14, 28, and every 28 days thereafter) with anastrozole 1 mg (daily) in postmenopausal women (fulvestrant 500 mg, n = 102; anastrozole, n = 103) with ER+ advanced breast cancer in the first-line setting. The primary endpoint (clinical benefit rate [72.5% and 67.0%]) and a follow-up analysis (median time to progression [23.4 months and 13.1 months]) have been reported for fulvestrant 500 mg and anastrozole, respectively [33]. Later, OS data were published, and the hazard ratio (95% CI) for OS with fulvestrant 500 mg versus anastrozole was 0.70 (0.50–0.98; P = 0.04; median OS, 54.1 months v 48.4 months) [34]. The treatment effects were generally consistent across the subgroups analyzed.

Prospective confirmation has been demonstrated in the larger phase III FALCON (Fulvestrant and Anastrozole Compared in Hormonal Therapy Naïve Advanced Breast Cancer) trial, which showed that intramuscular fulvestrant 500 mg/month (plus an additional dose at 2 weeks) was significantly more effective in terms of PFS than was anastrozole 1 mg/day (particularly in the non-visceral disease subgroup, PFS: 22.3 months in the non-visceral subgroup vs 13.8 months in the visceral group, HR: 0.80) [35]. The objective response rate was similar between the arms, but the median OS was not yet calculable. Fulvestrant was well-tolerated in this trial. Thus, monotherapy with intramuscular fulvestrant is well-tolerated and a more effective treatment option than standard-of-care anastrozole for ER+ or HR+/HER2- advanced breast cancer in postmenopausal women not previously treated with endocrine therapy [35, 36].

The combined use of multiple endocrine agents has been studied in several studies in the first-line setting. The Fulvestrant and Anastrozole Combination Trial (FACT) was an open-label randomized phase III clinical trial designed to compare the efficacy of anastrozole (1 mg daily, n = 256) alone with that of combined fulvestrant (initiated with a loading dose of 500 mg, 250 mg on days 14, 28 then 250 mg every month) and anastrozole therapy (1 mg daily and n = 258) in women who had experienced the first relapse of breast cancer after primary treatment of early disease [37]. Postmenopausal women or premenopausal women receiving an LHRH agonist were included. The median time to progression was similar between the experimental and standard arms (10.8 and 10.2 months, respectively, P = 0.91). The median OS was also similar between the 2 treatment groups (37.8 and 38.2 months, respectively, P = 1.00) [37].

The Southwest Oncology Group (SWOG) conducted a similarly designed randomized phase III trial [38]. Treatment-naïve postmenopausal women with advanced breast cancer were randomized into 2 groups to receive either anastrozole (1 mg orally every day with permission to crossover to fulvestrant (500 mg on day 1 and 250 mg on days 14 and 28 and monthly) alone as the disease progressed or anastrozole in combination with fulvestrant. The combination therapy resulted in improvement in PFS (15 vs 14 months; HR 0.80) and OS (48 months versus 41 months; HR 0.81).

In subgroup analyses, among women without prior tamoxifen, OS was significantly different between groups, with HR for death with combination therapy of 0.74 (95% CI; p = 0.04), whereas OS was similar among women with prior tamoxifen history (HR, 0.91; p = 0.59). The combination therapy resulted in a benefit in both groups [38].

A meta-analysis of these prospective randomized clinical trials was performed to compare the effectiveness of fulvestrant plus anastrozole with anastrozole alone as first-line treatment in postmenopausal women with HR+, HER2-negative advanced breast cancer. For endpoints including PFS, OS, and response rates, a non-significant trend of only marginal improvement was observed for anastrozole plus fulvestrant compared to anastrozole. The current evidence is not sufficient to recommend the combination of monthly fulvestrant with anastrozole instead of anastrozole or fulvestrant alone to all women with postmenopausal HR+ breast cancer as first-line therapy.

A systematic review of 8 randomized trials was performed by Al-Mubarak et al. to compare fulvestrant with other endocrine therapies [39]. The meta-regression analysis demonstrated that fulvestrant, when used in the first-line setting, reduced hazards for time to progression compared with AIs in studies where fewer patients were administered adjuvant endocrine therapy and at higher doses. Rates of serious adverse events and treatment discontinuation were reported to be similar between the fulvestrant and other groups, but fulvestrant monotherapy was associated with less frequent arthralgia (OR: 0.73, p = 0.02). Combining fulvestrant with AI did not improve time to progression but increased toxicity. High-dose fulvestrant monotherapy, when used as the first line or in patients with limited prior exposure to adjuvant endocrine therapy, may delay progression compared with AI [39].

Combined Use of Endocrine Agents with Other Targeted Agents in the First-Line Setting: Despite the efficacy of several endocrine agents, response rates for first-line metastatic patients of up to 40% have been described, with all initial responders eventually developing resistance over time [40]. Due to its clinical significance, extensive research has focused on determining the potential mechanisms of endocrine resistance. Initially, ER expression loss and polymorphisms of CYP2D6 and CYP19A1 were suggested as the main mechanisms of primary resistance to tamoxifen and AIs [41, 42]. However, further studies did not support these data. Preclinical evidence indicated that targeting the phosphatidylinositol-3-kinase (PI3K)/protein kinase B (AKT)/mammalian target of rapamycin (mTOR) pathway, the cell machinery and growth receptor signaling may improve endocrine responsiveness. More recently, studies of HR+ metastatic breast cancer designed with high-throughput technologies revealed a large number of molecular aberrations in potential driver genes, including PI3K3CA mutations, FGFR1 and CCND1 amplifications and ESR1 mutations [43, 44]. These findings led to the development of several therapies targeting these pathways to circumvent or delay the occurrence of endocrine resistance. The combination of endocrine agents with targeted agents is becoming a promising approach in HR+ metastatic breast cancer (Table 24.1).

Table 24.1 Endocrine therapy in hormone receptor positive HER2-negative advanced breast cancer

Ovarian suppression (GnRH agonist) or ablation to all premenopausal patients			
Endocrine treatment naïve		Previous endocrine treatment	
No contraindication to CDK inhibitors	*Contraindication to CDK inhibitors*	*Under endocrine treatment or within 12 months after the end of adjuvant endocrine treatment*	*Disease recurrence at least one year after the end of adjuvant endocrine treatment*
CDK inhibitor[a] and aromatase inhibitors	Fulvestrant	CDK inhibitor and fulvestrant	Treat as patients who are endocrine treatment naïve
CDK inhibitor[b] and Fulvestrant	Aromatase inhibitors	CDK inhibitor and aromatase inhibitors	
Fulvestrant	Tamoxifen	Everolimus and exemestane OR tamoxifen OR fulvestrant	
		Abemeciclib and tamoxifen if not used previously	
		Abemaciclib	
		Fulvestrant if not used previously	
		If an aromatase inhibitor used previously, switch to other (steroidal to nonsteroidal or vice versa)	
		Tamoxifen	
		Progestins	
		Estrogens or androgens	

[a]Pablociclib, ribociclib, abemaciclib
[b]Ribociclib

CDK4/6 Inhibitors: Analysis of the Cancer Genome Atlas revealed associations of deregulated cyclin D, CDK4/6 and retinoblastoma (Rb) interaction with luminal B cancer [45]. Cyclin D activates CDK4/6 and induces Rb phosphorylation and progression of the cell cycle into S phase, eventually resulting in endocrine resistance [46]. CDK4/6 inhibitors have been demonstrated to improve the efficacy of ET. Palbociclib, ribociclib and abemaciclib are oral small-molecule inhibitors of CDK4/6 with preclinical and clinical evidence of growth-inhibitory activity in HR+ breast cancer cells and synergy with anti-estrogens [47–54].

Palbociclib: *Palbociclib in combination with letrozole* received US Food and Drug Administration (FDA) accelerated approval as a first-line treatment option for HR+ advanced breast cancer in February 2015 [48]. The approval was based on a randomized, multicenter, open-label phase I/II trial (PALOMA-1) in which 165 patients were randomized to receive palbociclib (125 mg orally daily for 21 consecutive days, followed by 7 days off treatment) plus letrozole (2.5 mg orally daily) or letrozole alone [49]. A significant improvement in PFS was observed in patients receiving palbociclib plus letrozole (median 20 months) compared with patients receiving letrozole alone (median 10 months) (HR, 0.49; 95% confidence interval, 0.32–0.75). An improvement in OS was observed in the combination arm versus the letrozole-alone arm (median 37.5 versus 33 months, respectively, p = 0.819), although this improvement did not reach statistical significance. The most common adverse reaction in patients receiving palbociclib plus letrozole was neutropenia (grade ¾ toxicity 54% in the combination arm vs 15% in the letrozole-alone arm) [48].

The results from the phase III trial, PALOMA-2, which compared letrozole with letrozole plus palbociclib in the first-line setting for HR+ HER2- metastatic breast cancer, supported the findings of previous trials [50, 51]. At a median follow up of 23 months, the median PFS of the combination arm was longer than that of the letrozole-alone arm (HR: 0.58, 24.8 months vs 14.5 months, respectively). A consistent benefit of palbociclib–letrozole was demonstrated across all subgroups. The subgroups were visceral disease (HR, 0.63; 95% CI, 0.47–0.85), nonvisceral disease (HR, 0.50; 95% CI, 0.36–0.70), presence of previous hormonal therapy (HR, 0.53; 95% CI, 0.40–0.70), no history of prior hormonal therapy (HR, 0.63; 95% CI, 0.44–0.90), a disease-free interval of 12 months or less (HR, 0.50; 95% CI, 0.33–0.76), a disease-free interval of more than 12 months (HR, 0.52; 95% CI, 0.36–0.73), and newly metastatic disease (HR, 0.67; 95% CI, 0.46–0.99). The rate of clinical benefit response was 84.9% in the palbociclib–letrozole group and 70.3% in the placebo–letrozole group [51]. However, overall survival data are immature.

Ribociclib: LEE011 is another CDK4/6 inhibitor that has been tested in a phase III clinical trial in association with letrozole as a first-line treatment in postmenopausal women with HR+ advanced breast cancer (MONALEESA-2) [52]. Patients were randomized to ribociclib (600 mg/day; 3 weeks-on/1 week-off) plus letrozole (2.5 mg/day; continuous) or placebo plus letrozole until disease progression, unacceptable toxicity, death, or treatment discontinuation. Median PFS was not reached in the combination arm versus 16.4 months in the letrozole arm in patients with de novo advanced breast cancer (HR 0.45). The overall response rate was 41% in the ribociclib and letrozole combination arm versus 28% in the placebo and letrozole arm.

In MONALEESA-7, a phase 2 trial, ribociclib was studied in association with NSAI/tamoxifen plus goserelin for premenopausal patients [53]. Adding the CDK4/6 inhibitor ribociclib to standard first-line endocrine therapy significantly prolonged survival in premenopausal and perimenopausal women with advanced HR-positive, HER2-negative breast cancer. This is the first definitive evidence that CDK4/6 inhibitor–based therapy is effective for first-line treatment of premenopausal and perimenopausal women.

Abemaciclib: Abemaciclib (Verzenio™) is an orally administered inhibitor of cyclin-dependent kinases 4 and 6 that is being developed by Eli Lilly and Company. In the MONARCH-3 trial, abemaciclib in combination with an aromatase inhibitor (letrozole or anastrozole) was compared with aromatase inhibitor monotherapy in endocrine treatment naïve first-line HR+ advanced breast cancer patients [54].

Median PFS was found to be significantly prolonged in the abemaciclib arm (HR, 0.54; p = 0.000021; median: not reached in the abemaciclib arm, 14.7 months in the placebo arm). In patients with measurable disease, the objective response rate was 59% in the abemaciclib arm and 44% in the placebo arm (p = 0.004). Comparing abemaciclib and placebo, the most frequent grade 3 or 4 adverse events were neutropenia (21.1% v 1.2%), diarrhea (9.5% v 1.2%), and leukopenia (7.6% v 0.6%).

Although increased expression of cyclin D1 and pRb and decreased expression of p16 (a natural CDK4/6 inhibitor) were found to be associated with response in in vitro preclinical studies, patient selection on the basis of cyclin D1 amplification or p16 loss was not associated with an improved outcome from palbociclib treatment in the PALOMA-1/TRIO-18 trial [49, 55].

Anti-VEGF Monoclonal Antibody, Bevacizumab: Preclinical findings have indicated that estradiol regulates angiogenesis under both physiological and pathological conditions. High VEGF levels in breast tumors have been shown to be related to a decreased response to endocrine agents [10]. Bevacizumab has been extensively evaluated in the treatment of HR+ and negative breast cancer in several trials. In 2014, Kümler et al. performed a meta-analysis of 14 phase III trials in which bevacizumab was investigated [56]. More than 4400 patients with advanced breast cancer had benefits in relapse rate and PFS; however, no trial demonstrated an OS advantage. Recently, the results of 2 phase III trials have been published [57, 58]. In the LEA trial, the addition of bevacizumab to letrozole or fulvestrant in the first-line setting was studied for postmenopausal women with HR+ HER2-negative advanced breast cancer [57]. The time to treatment failure and OS were comparable in the treatment arms, although ORR was improved with the bevacizumab combination. In the CALGB 40503 trial, bevacizumab plus letrozole was compared with letrozole monotherapy. PFS was improved with the combination (20 months versus 16 months, HR:0.74; p = 0.016) [58]. Unfortunately, OS was similar between the 2 treatment arms at the cost of a higher frequency of grade 3 or 4 toxicities with bevacizumab-based treatment regimens. Thus, bevacizumab is not currently recommended in combination with ET in HR+ advanced breast cancer patients.

Second-Line Treatment

Until recently, there were insufficient data to guide the optimal sequence of therapy in the second-line and subsequent settings. However, PFS and OS data from several clinical trials including endocrine agents and targeted drugs have been published recently. Ovarian ablation or ovarian function suppression should be recommended to all premenopausal women to facilitate treatment with endocrine agents approved only for postmenopausal women. For premenopausal patients who have been treated with an ovarian function-suppressing agent, serum estradiol levels should be measured to confirm that menopausal status is maintained. In the case of estradiol levels in the premenopausal range with ovarian suppression, ovarian ablation via surgery or radiation should be offered.

Tamoxifen: Limited data have demonstrated the clinical benefit of tamoxifen in the second-line setting. In a combined analysis of 2 randomized trials evaluating the sequence strategy, such as tamoxifen followed by anastrozole or vice versa, the overall response rate was 10%, and the clinical benefit rate (overall response rate and stable disease ≥6 months) was 49% in 137 patients who crossed over to tamoxifen [59].

Aromatase Inhibitors: As second-line ET, there is no specific AI that has shown superior activity in terms of PFS or OS compared to any other AI [60].

Switching AIs: Total cross-resistance is lacking between steroidal (exemestane) AIs and NSAIs as far as their anti-tumoral efficacy is concerned. Thus, upon progression of metastatic disease following treatment with NSAIs, exemestane may be effective as sequential hormone therapy or vice versa [61, 62]. The clinical benefit of exemestane after progression on a NSAI was supported by the findings of a systemic review published in 2011 [63]. On average, 25–30% of patients in the crossover studies experienced objective response or stable disease for 6 months or more.

Fulvestrant: In second-line setting trials, fulvestrant was used at a lower dose (250 mg monthly) than in current clinical practice and had no OS or overall response rate advantage compared to AIs [36, 64]. Furthermore, the combination of fulvestrant with steroidal or NSAIs as a second-line treatment option did not provide any PFS advantage over AI monotherapy or fulvestrant monotherapy [65]. Currently, fulvestrant in combination with other endocrine agents is not a recommended approach for second-line endocrine treatment.

The strategy of increasing the dose of fulvestrant has been explored in patients with prior exposure to ET. The phase III, multicenter CONFIRM trial randomized postmenopausal patients with HR+ advanced breast cancer who received tamoxifen or AI and experienced disease progression to receive 500 mg or 250 mg of fulvestrant on days 0, 14, 28 and every 28 days thereafter [66]. There were no clinically important differences in serious adverse effect profiles between the treatment groups, and no clustering of serious adverse effects was detected in either treatment group. The overall response rate and clinical benefit rate were similar between high and low doses of fulvestrant. Although the absolute benefit in PFS was only one month with the high dose, the PFS benefit reached statistical significance (HR:0.80; $p = 0.006$). A longer follow-up revealed a 4-month difference in favor of a higher dose of fulvestrant [67]. The median OS was 26.4 months for fulvestrant 500 mg and 22.3 months for 250 mg ($HR = 0.81$; $p = 0.02$). After this unique OS advantage, fulvestrant at a dose of 500 mg has become the standard schedule in clinical practice and clinical trials.

PI3K–Akt–mTOR Signaling Pathway: Accumulating evidence suggests that both the levels and activity of ER and PgR are dramatically influenced by growth-factor receptor (GFR) signaling pathways and that this crosstalk is a major determinant of both breast cancer progression and response to therapy [68]. The PI3K pathway, a key mediator of GFR signaling, is one of the most altered pathways in breast cancer [10, 45]. For example, breast tumors may have mutation or loss of PTEN or both, amplification and activating mutations in PIK3CA, amplification of Akt2 and p70S6kinase, and overexpression of Akt3 [69]. Consistent with the mutational spectrum of PI3K signaling intermediates in breast cancer, direct analysis of PI3K activation has shown an association with poor outcome [70]. Similarly, loss of PTEN is associated with low ER and PgR and poor outcome [71]. Recently, Generali et al. demonstrated the significance of downregulation of key molecules in the PI3K pathway in response to letrozole, further emphasizing the predictive and therapeutic role of this pathway in ET [72].

Inhibition of proliferation has been shown to be synergistically enhanced by the addition of an mTOR inhibitor to endocrine treatment [73]. The Breast Cancer Trials of Oral Everolimus-2 (BOLERO-2) study investigated the safety and efficacy of the mTOR inhibitor everolimus in combination with exemestane in breast cancer patients who had been previously treated with NSAIs [74]. The study showed that concomitant use prolonged PFS (median 7 versus 3 months; HR for mortality 0.43, 95% CI 0.35–0.54) and provided a higher overall response rate (9.5 versus 0.4%). The combination therapy resulted in a higher incidence of serious adverse events, including stomatitis (8%), dyspnea (4%), noninfectious pneumonitis (3%) and elevated liver enzymes (3%) compared with exemestane monotherapy and led to a higher percentage of treatment discontinuation [75]. There was no statistically significant improvement in OS [76]. Given the remarkable PFS benefit, everolimus was approved by the FDA for the treatment of HR+ advanced breast cancer in combination with exemestane after failure with NSAIs.

A phase III trial (HORIZON) was conducted in the first-line setting with temsirolimus, another mTOR inhibitor [77]. Unfortunately, adding temsirolimus to letrozole did not improve PFS (median, 9 months; HR, 0.90; 95% CI, 0.76–1.07; $P = 0.25$) as first-line therapy in patients with AI-naïve advanced breast cancer nor in the 40% patient subset with prior adjuvant endocrine therapy [77].

In a randomized phase II study of neoadjuvant everolimus and letrozole versus placebo and letrozole, the addition of everolimus marginally improved the sonographic response rate (68% versus 59%, respectively; $P = 0.062$) but markedly enhanced the antiproliferative response (defined as the natural logarithm of percentage positive for Ki67 <1 on day 15 versus baseline; 57% versus 30%, respectively; $P < 0.01$) [78]. In TAMRAD, which was conducted by Groupe d'Investigateurs Nationaux pour I'Etude des Cancers Ovariens et du sein (GINECO) as a randomized phase II trial of everolimus and tamoxifen versus tamoxifen alone in postmenopausal patients with advanced disease pre-exposed to AIs, the addition of everolimus was associated with a 4-month improvement in time to progression (median 9 versus 5 months, HR = 0.54, 95% CI 0.36–0.81) and reduced risk of death (HR 0.45,

95% CI 0.24–0.81) [79]. However, the overall response rates of the 2 arms were similar (14 versus 13%). Furthermore, grade 3–4 stomatitis (11 versus 0%), anorexia (7 versus 4%), and the incidence of pneumonitis were higher in combination therapy.

Drugs targeting other components of these pathways, including AKT inhibitors, PIK3CA inhibitors (e.g., pictilisib) and dual kinase inhibitors targeting both mTOR and PI3KCA, are currently in development.

Next-generation sequencing of BOLERO-2 did not show any relationship between somatic mutation patterns, particularly in the catalytic subunit of PI3K3CA, and clinical outcomes [80]. The progression-free survival benefit of everolimus was maintained regardless of the alteration status of PIK3CA, FGFR1, and CCND1 or the pathways of which they are components. However, quantitative differences in everolimus benefit were observed between patient subgroups defined by exon-specific mutations in PIK3CA (exon 20 v 9) or by different degrees of chromosomal instability in the tumor tissues [80]. The data from this exploratory analysis suggest that the efficacy of everolimus is largely independent of the most commonly altered genes or pathways in hormone receptor-positive, human epidermal growth factor receptor 2-negative breast cancer. The potential impact of chromosomal instabilities and low-frequency genetic alterations on everolimus efficacy warrants further investigation. Thus, the identification of predictive markers for PIK3CA/mTOR inhibition still needs to be addressed prospectively. Furthermore, PIK3CA mutational status has been shown to be discordant between the primary tumor and metastases [10]. In fact, mutational status is mainly analyzed in primary tumor samples. Thus, alterations in molecular pathways should be re-analyzed in the metastatic setting.

CDK4/6 Inhibitors in Second or Further Lines of Treatment

There is no evidence to recommend a CDK4/6 inhibitor as monotherapy or in combination with other drugs in patients who received another CDK4/6 inhibitor in previous lines. However, CDK4/6 inhibitors are one of the most effective treatment options in patients who are CDK4/6 inhibitor naïve and have progressive disease under prior antiestrogen treatment.

Palbociclib in Combination with Fulvestrant: PALOMA-3 trial is a phase III randomized trial that included patients with HR+ and HER2- advanced breast cancer to compare palbociclib plus fulvestrant with placebo plus fulvestrant [47]. Premenopausal women who were treated with goserelin were also included in the study. Patients were required to have progressive disease during or within 12 months after completion of adjuvant ET or on prior ET in the metastatic setting (with progression from prior AI required for postmenopausal women). The study was stopped early due to significant efficacy results reported at interim analysis favoring fulvestrant plus palbociclib (median PFS: 9.2 versus 3.8 months; HR:0.42, 95% CI 0.32–0.56; $p < 0.001$). Although higher rates of neutropenia and fatigue were reported in the combination arm, rates of discontinuation and febrile neutropenia were similar between the 2 arms. Although longer follow-up is required to determine the impact of combination therapy on OS, available PFS data support the use of palbociclib in combination with fulvestrant.

Abemaciclib with Fulvestrant: Abemaciclib at 150 mg twice daily plus fulvestrant has been approved in the USA for the treatment of HR+, HER2- advanced or metastatic breast cancer, in combination with fulvestrant in women with disease progression following endocrine therapy, and as monotherapy in adult patients with disease progression following endocrine therapy and prior chemotherapy in the metastatic setting based on the findings obtained in the phase 3 MONARCH 2 trial [81]. PFS was significantly longer with abemaciclib plus fulvestrant than with fulvestrant alone (median, 16.4 v 9.3 months; HR, 0.553; $p < 0.001$). In patients with measurable disease, abemaciclib plus fulvestrant achieved an ORR of 48.1% (95% CI, 42.6–53.6%) compared with 21.3% (95% CI, 15.1–27.6%) in the control arm. The most common adverse events were diarrhea (86.4% v 24.7%), neutropenia (46.0% v 4.0%), nausea (45.1% v 22.9%), and fatigue (39.9% v 26.9%) in the abemaciclib versus placebo arms.

Further Lines of Treatment

Until recently, there were no sufficient data to guide further lines of ET. In the MONARCH 1 trial, a phase II single-arm open-label study, patients with HR+/HER2- MBC who had progressed on or after prior endocrine therapy and had 1 or 2 chemotherapy regimens in the metastatic setting were treated with abemaciclib 200 mg 2 times daily on a continuous schedule until disease progression or unacceptable toxicity [82]. Patients had a median of 3 (range, 1–8) lines of prior systemic therapy in the metastatic setting, 90.2% had visceral disease, and 50.8% had ≥3 metastatic sites. At the 12-month final analysis, the objective response rate was 19.7%; the clinical benefit rate (CR + PR + SD ≥6 months) was 42.4%, median PFS was 6.0 months, and median OS was 17.7 months. Diarrhea, fatigue, and nausea were the most frequent side effects, but discontinuations due to AEs were infrequent (7.6%). In this poor-prognosis, heavily pretreated population with refractory HR+/HER2- metastatic breast cancer, continuous dosing of single-agent abemaciclib was well tolerated and approved by the FDA.

Patients who progressed on 2 prior lines of ET should receive treatment based on their individual clinical characteristics. Important factors affecting treatment decision include prior treatment response, duration of responses, tumor burden, risk of visceral crisis, and preferences of patients. In addition to tamoxifen, AIs and fulvestrant, progestins (e.g., megestrol acetate and medroxyprogesterone acetate), estrogens (e.g., diethylstilbestrol) and androgens (e.g., testosterone, fluoxymesterone and danazol) are other endocrine treatment options for patients with HR+ advanced breast cancer who previously received the standard 2 lines of ET.

Insulin-Like Growth Factors (IGF-1 and IGF-2): Ganitumab is a monoclonal IgG1 antibody that blocks IGF-1R. In a phase II double blind randomized controlled trial, the efficacy and safety of ganitumab in combination with endocrine therapy was investigated in postmenopausal patients with HR+ locally advanced breast cancer or MBC previously treated with endocrine agents [83]. Median PFS was similar between the ganitumab and placebo arms, and overall survival was shorter in the ganitumab arm than in the placebo arm. Because the addition of ganitumab to endocrine treatment in women with previously treated HR+ advanced breast cancer did not improve outcomes, further studies of ganitumab in this subgroup of patients have not been designed.

Class I Histone Deacetylases Inhibitors: Entinostat is a small-molecule inhibitor of class I histone deacetylases, which have a key function in the control of gene expression. Entinostat exerts antiproliferative effects and promotes apoptosis in breast cancer cell lines and has been evaluated as a second or later line of therapy in women with ER+ breast cancer. In the ENtinostat Combinations Overcoming REsistance (ENCORE 301) randomized phase II trial, women who had previously progressed on AI therapy and had multiple prior lines of therapy, including chemotherapy and endocrine agents, were randomly assigned to receive exemestane 25 mg daily with entinostat 5 mg daily or with placebo [84]. The preliminary findings showed that exemestane plus entinostat therapy improved PFS (median 4 versus 2 months) at the expense of greater fatigue (46 versus 26%) and uncomplicated neutropenia (25 versus 0%).

There are several other targeted agents, including CDK inhibitors, FGFR inhibitors (e.g., dovitinib), and heat shock protein 90 inhibitors, under evaluation in preclinical and clinical studies.

Endocrine Therapy in HER2-Positive and Hormone Receptor-Positive Breast Cancer

Mutual effects of ER and HER2 have been demonstrated in several studies. The overexpression of HER2 leads to resistance to established endocrine therapies. Thus, a combined therapeutic strategy might enhance endocrine effectiveness in patients with HR+, HER2+ breast cancer but delay disease progression for those with HR+, HER2-negative tumors at risk of early relapse. This treatment strategy has been evaluated in many clinical studies.

Trastuzumab in Combination with Endocrine Therapy

In an open-label, multicenter, 2-arm phase III trial, anastrozole monotherapy was compared with combination therapy of anastrozole with trastuzumab in HER2+, ER+ breast cancer patients [85]. Median PFS doubled in the anastrozole + trastuzumab arm compared to anastrozole alone (4.8 months vs 2.4 months, respectively, $P = 0.0016$). In the anastrozole-alone arm, 70% of patients were allowed to proceed to trastuzumab later in the course of disease. Overall survival, although not significantly different, was numerically superior in the combination arm (28.5 vs 23.9 months, $P = 0.325$).

Kaufman et al. investigated endocrine therapy in combination with anti-HER2 therapy in a randomized trial named "The Trastuzumab and Anastrozole Directed Against ER+ HER2+ Mammary Carcinoma (TAnDEM)" [86]. Postmenopausal women with HR+ and HER2+ MBC were randomized to receive anastrozole alone or combination therapy with anastrozole and trastuzumab. Approximately two thirds of patients on anastrozole alone received the combination treatment at progression. Treatment with trastuzumab plus anastrozole resulted in significantly longer PFS compared with treatment with anastrozole alone (4.8 versus 2.4 months, respectively; HR 0.63; log-rank P = 0.0016). However, the median OS was statistically similar between the treatment groups in both the overall and centrally confirmed HR+ subgroups, which may, in part, be explained by the high crossover rate [86].

The addition of an AI to HER2-targeted therapy may delay the use of chemotherapy in several patients and provides an important advantage. Based on these positive results, trastuzumab (±pertuzumab) used concurrently with an AI has been approved for treating postmenopausal patients with HR+ and HER2+ MBC who have not received prior trastuzumab. Based on conducted clinical trials, NSAIs have become one of the standard treatment options in this patient population, but there is no reason to believe that a different result would be obtained with a steroidal AI. Furthermore, there are no available data strongly supporting the use of tamoxifen in combination with trastuzumab. However, based on the clinical evidence of superiority of combination therapy in postmenopausal patients, tamoxifen in combination with trastuzumab can be offered to premenopausal women who have HR+ HER2+ advanced breast cancer.

Lapatinib in Combination with Endocrine Therapy

In the first-line setting, the combination of lapatinib with letrozole was compared with letrozole plus placebo in patients with HR+ advanced breast cancer. In HER2+ patients, lapatinib plus letrozole led to longer median PFS than letrozole plus placebo (8.2 versus 3 months; HR 0.71; p = 0.019) [87]. In patients with centrally confirmed HR+, HER2-negative disease (n = 952), lapatinib plus letrozole arm did not improve PFS.

The FDA approved lapatinib in combination with letrozole for the treatment of postmenopausal women with HR+ MBC overexpressing the HER2 receptor for whom hormonal therapy is indicated. However, lapatinib in combination with an AI has not been compared to a trastuzumab-containing chemotherapy regimen for the treatment of MBC.

Recently, the results of the CALGB 40302 trial were published. The authors investigated whether lapatinib would improve PFS among women with HR+ MBC treated with fulvestrant [88]. Adding lapatinib to fulvestrant did not improve PFS or OS in ER+ advanced breast cancer and led to greater toxicity [88].

In conclusion, the combination of an anti-HER2 agent with endocrine therapy is an active and safe method with favorable response rates and survival advantages in patients with HR+ and HER2+ advanced breast cancer. There are several other targeted agents, including CDK inhibitors with anti HER2 and endocrin agents, under evaluation in preclinical and clinical studies.

Conclusion

In conclusion, the major determinants of the treatment plan include the number of lesions, extent of visceral involvement, receptor status of the primary lesion, sites of recurrence and metastasis, and previous response to endocrine treatment. The combination of an anti-HER2 agent with endocrine therapy is an active and safe method with favorable response rates and survival advantages in patients with HR+ and HER2+ advanced breast cancer. The combination of exemestane with everolimus can be considered for patients who progressed within 12 months on a non-steroidal AI or on tamoxifen at any time. Fulvestrant can be used as the first choice in de novo metastatic disease not previously treated with any endocrine treatment. Cyclin inhibitors in combination with an aromatase inhibitor or fulvestrant may be considered a treatment option for first-line or second-line therapy for postmenopausal patients with ER-positive, HER2-negative breast cancer.

Box 24.1

The definition of menopause. Menopause can be defined as natural menopause (no menses for 12 months before starting chemotherapy or hormone therapy) or as menopause with ovarian ablation or suppression. Luteinizing hormone (LH), follicle-stimulating hormone (FSH), and serum estradiol (E2) levels should be at postmenopausal levels and should be measured before systemic treatment unless oophorectomy has been performed with hysterectomy in women aged 60 years or younger.

The definition of menopause: "Prior bilateral oophorectomy" OR "Age $\geq$ 60 years" OR "Age < 60 years" and amenorrheic for 12 or more months in the absence of chemotherapy, tamoxifen, toremifene, or ovarian suppression and follicle-stimulating hormone (FSH) and estradiol in the postmenopausal range OR "If taking tamoxifen or toremifene, and age <60 years, then FSH and plasma estradiol levels in postmenopausal ranges".

References

1. Siegel RL, Miller KD, Jemal A. Cancer statistics, 2018. CA Cancer J Clin. 2018;68:7–30.
2. Liotta LA, Kohn EC. The microenvironment of the tumour-host interface. Nature. 2001;411:375–9.
3. Li CI, Daling JR, Malone KE. Incidence of invasive breast cancer by hormone receptor status from 1992 to 1998. J Clin Oncol. 2003;21:28–34.
4. Anderson WF, Katki HA, Rosenberg PS. Incidence of breast cancer in the United States: current and future trends. J Natl Cancer Inst. 2011;103(18):1397–402.
5. Goldhirsch A, Ingle JN, Gelber RD, Coates AS, Thurlimann B, Senn HJ. Thresholds for therapies: highlights of the St Gallen International Expert Consensus on the primary therapy of early breast cancer 2009. Ann Oncol. 2009;20:1319–29.
6. Bayraktar S, Arun B. Epidemiology, risk factors, and prevention. In: Aydiner A, İğci A, Soran A, editors. Breast disease, vol. I. Cham: Springer; 2016. p. 57–89.
7. Chung CT, Carlson RW. Goals and objectives in the management of metastatic breast cancer. Oncologist. 2003;8(6):514–20.
8. Beatson GT. On the treatment of inoperable cases of carcinoma of the mamma: suggestion for a new method of treatment, with illustrative cases. Lancet. 1896;2:104–7.
9. Benz CC, Scott GK, Sarup JC, Johnson RM, Tripathy D, Coronado E, et al. Estrogen-dependent, tamoxifen-resistant tumorigenic growth of MCF-7 cells transfected with HER2/neu. Breast Cancer Res Treat. 1992;24(2):85–95.
10. Reinert T, Barrios CH. Optimal management of hormone receptor positive metastatic breast cancer in 2016. Ther Adv Med Oncol. 2015;7(6):304–20.
11. Partridge AH, Rumble RB, Carey LA, Come SE, Davidson NE, Di Leo A, et al. Chemotherapy and targeted therapy for women with human epidermal growth factor receptor 2-negative (or unknown) advanced breast cancer: American Society of Clinical Oncology clinical practice guideline. J Clin Oncol. 2014;32(29):3307–29.
12. Wilcken N, Hornbuckle J, Ghersi D. Chemotherapy alone versus endocrine therapy alone for metastatic breast cancer. Cochrane Database Syst Rev. 2003;2:CD002747.
13. Barrios C, Forbes JF, Jonat W, Conte P, Gradishar W, Buzdar A, et al. The sequential use of endocrine treatment for advanced breast cancer: where are we? Ann Oncol. 2012;23(6):1378–86.
14. National Comprehensive Cancer Network Clinical Practice Guidelines in Oncology. Breast cancer, version 1. 2018. http://www.nccn.org/professionals/physician_gls/pdf/breast.pdf.
15. Blamey RW, Jonat W, Kaufmann M, Bianco AR, Namer M. Goserelin depot in the treatment of premenopausal advanced breast cancer. Eur J Cancer. 1992;28:810–4.
16. Taylor CW, Green S, Dalton WS, Martino S, Rector D, Ingle JN. Multicenter randomized clinical trial of goserelin versus surgical oophorectomy in premenopausal patients with receptor-positive MBC: an intergroup study. J Clin Oncol. 1998;16(3):994–9.
17. Crump M, Sawka CA, DeBoer G, Buchanan RB, Ingle JN, Forbes J, et al. An individual patient-based meta-analysis of tamoxifen versus ovarian ablation as first line endocrine therapy for premenopausal women with MBC. Breast Cancer Res Treat. 1997;44(3):201–10.
18. Osborne CK, Boldt DH, Clark GM, Trent JM. Effects of tamoxifen on human breast cancer cell cycle kinetics: accumulation of cells in early G1 phase. Cancer Res. 1983;43(8):3583–5.
19. Jonat W, Kaufmann M, Blamey RW, Howell A, Collins JP, Coates A, et al. A randomised study to compare the effect of the luteinising hormone releasing hormone (LHRH) analogue goserelin with or without tamoxifen in pre- and perimenopausal patients with advanced breast cancer. Eur J Cancer. 1995;31(2):137–42.
20. Klijn JG, Blamey RW, Boccardo F, Tominaga T, Duchateau L, Sylvester R, Combined Hormone Agents Trialists' Group, European Organization for Research and Treatment of Cancer. Combined tamoxifen and luteinizing hormone-releasing hormone (LHRH) agonist versus LHRH agonist alone in premenopausal advanced breast cancer: a meta-analysis of four randomized trials. J Clin Oncol. 2001;19(2):343–53.

21. Sawka CA, Pritchard KI, Paterson AHG, Sutherland DJ, Thomson DB, Shelley WE, et al. Role and mechanism of action of tamoxifen in premenopausal women with metastatic breast carcinoma. Cancer Res. 1986;46:3152–6.
22. Margreiter R, Wiegle J. Tamoxifen (Nolvadex) for premenopausal patients with advanced breast cancer. Breast Cancer Res Treat. 1984;4:45–84.
23. Love RR, Mazess RB, Barden HS, Epstein S, Newcomb PA, Jordan VC, et al. Effects of tamoxifen on bone mineral density in postmenopausal women with breast cancer. N Engl J Med. 1992;326(13):852–6.
24. Mustonen MVJ, Pyrhönen S, Kellokumpu-Lehtinen P-L. Toremifene in the treatment of breast cancer. World J Clin Oncol. 2014;5(3):393–405.
25. Rao RD, Cobleigh MA. Adjuvant endocrine therapy for breast cancer. Oncology (Williston Park). 2012;26(6):541–7.
26. Carlson RW, Theriault R, Schurman CM, Rivera E, Chung CT, Phan SC, et al. Phase II trial of anastrozole plus goserelin in the treatment of HR+, metastatic carcinoma of the breast in premenopausal women. J Clin Oncol. 2010;28(25):3917–21.
27. Park IH, Ro J, Lee KS, Kim EA, Kwon Y, Nam BH, et al. Phase II parallel group study showing comparable efficacy between premenopausal MBC patients treated with letrozole plus goserelin and postmenopausal patients treated with letrozole alone as first-line hormone therapy. J Clin Oncol. 2010;28(16):2705–11.
28. Van Asten K, Neven P, Lintermans A, Wildiers H, Paridaens R. AIs in the breast cancer clinic: focus on exemestane. Endocr Relat Cancer. 2014;21(1):R31–49.
29. Mauri D, Pavlidis N, Polyzos NP, Ioannidis JP. Survival with aromatase inhibitors and inactivators versus standard hormonal therapy in advanced breast cancer: meta-analysis. J Natl Cancer Inst. 2006;98(18):1285–91.
30. Bonneterre J, Thurlimann B, Robertson JF, Krzakowski M, Mauriac L, Koralewski P, et al. Anastrozole versus tamoxifen as first-line therapy for advanced breast cancer in 668 postmenopausal women: results ofthe Tamoxifen or Arimidex Randomized Group Efficacy and Tolerability study. J Clin Oncol. 2000;18:3748–57.
31. Paridaens RJ, Dirix LY, Beex LV, Nooij M, Cameron DA, Cufer T, et al. Phase III study comparing exemestane with tamoxifen as first-line hormonal treatment of MBC inpostmenopausal women: the European Organisation for Research and Treatment of Cancer Breast Cancer Cooperative Group. J Clin Oncol. 2008;26:4883–90.
32. Ciruelos E, Pascual T, Arroyo Vozmediano ML, Blanco M, Manso L, Parrilla L, et al. The therapeutic role of fulvestrant in the management of patients with HR+ breast cancer. Breast. 2014;23(3):201–8.
33. Robertson JF, Lindemann JP, Llombart-Cussac A, Rolski J, Feltl D, Dewar J, et al. Fulvestrant 500 mg versus anastrozole 1 mg for the first-line treatment of advanced breast cancer: follow-up analysis from the randomized ‘FIRST’ study. Breast Cancer Res Treat. 2012;136(2):503–11.
34. Ellis MJ, Llombart-Cussac A, Feltl D, Dewar JA, Jasiówka M, Hewson N, et al. Fulvestrant 500 mg versus anastrozole 1 mg for the first-line treatment of advanced breast cancer: overall survival analysis from the phase II FIRST study. J Clin Oncol. 2015;33(32):3781–7.
35. Robertson JFR, Bondarenko IM, Trishkina E, Dvorkin M, Panasci L, Manikhas A, et al. Fulvestrant 500 mg versus anastrozole 1 mg for hormone receptor-positive advanced breast cancer (FALCON): an international, randomised, double-blind, phase 3 trial. Lancet. 2016;388(10063):2997–3005.
36. Robertson JF, Osborne CK, Howell A, Jones SE, Mauriac L, Ellis M, et al. Fulvestrant versus anastrozole for the treatment of advanced breast carcinoma in postmenopausal women: a prospective combined analysis of two multicenter trials. Cancer. 2003;98(2):229–38.
37. Bergh J, Jönsson PE, Lidbrink EK, Trudeau M, Eiermann W, Brattström D, et al. FACT: an open-label randomized phase III study of fulvestrant and anastrozole in combination compared with anastrozole alone as first-line therapy for patients with receptor-positive postmenopausal breast cancer. J Clin Oncol. 2012;30(16):1919–25.
38. Mehta RS, Barlow WE, Albain KS, Vandenberg TA, Dakhil SR, Tirumali NR, et al. Combination anastrozole and fulvestrant in MBC. N Engl J Med. 2012;367(5):435–44.

39. Al-Mubarak M, Sacher AG, Ocana A, Vera-Badillo F, Seruga B, Amir E. Fulvestrant for advanced breast cancer: a meta-analysis. Cancer Treat Rev. 2013;39(7):753–8.
40. Yamamoto-Ibusuki M, Arnedos M, André F. Targeted therapies for ER+/HER2- metastatic breast cancer. BMC Med. 2015;13:137.
41. Abraham JE, Maranian MJ, Driver KE, Platte R, Kalmyrzaev B, Baynes C, et al. CYP2D6 gene variants: association with breast cancer specific survival in a cohort of breast cancer patients from the United Kingdom treated with adjuvant tamoxifen. Breast Cancer Res. 2010;12(4):R64.
42. Ferraldeschi R, Arnedos M, Hadfield KD, A'Hern R, Drury S, Wardley A, et al. Polymorphisms of CYP19A1 and response to aromatase inhibitors in metastatic breast cancer patients. Breast Cancer Res Treat. 2012;133(3):1191–8.
43. Stephens PJ, Tarpey PS, Davies H, Van Loo P, Greenman C, Wedge DC, et al. The landscape of cancer genes and mutational processes in breast cancer. Nature. 2012;486(7403):400–4.
44. Curtis C, Shah SP, Chin SF, Turashvili G, Rueda OM, Dunning MJ, et al. The genomic and transcriptomic architecture of 2,000 breast tumours reveals novel subgroups. Nature. 2012;486(7403):346–52.
45. Ma CX, Ellis MJ. The Cancer Genome Atlas: clinical applications for breast cancer. Oncology (Williston Park). 2013;27(12):1263–9, 1274–9.
46. Thangavel C, Dean JL, Ertel A, Knudsen KE, Aldaz CM, Witkiewicz AK, et al. Therapeutically activating RB: reestablishing cell cycle control in endocrine therapy-resistant breast cancer. Endocr Relat Cancer. 2011;18(3):333–45.
47. Turner NC, Ro J, André F, Loi S, Verma S, Iwata H, PALOMA3 Study Group, et al. Palbociclib in hormone-receptor-positive advanced breast cancer. N Engl J Med. 2015;373(3):209–19.
48. Finn RS, Crown JP, Lang I, Boer K, Bondarenko IM, Kulyk SO, et al. The cyclin-dependent kinase 4/6 inhibitor palbociclib in combination with letrozole versus letrozole alone as first-line treatment of oestrogen receptor-positive, HER2-negative, advanced breast cancer (PALOMA-1/TRIO-18): a randomised phase 2 study. Lancet Oncol. 2015;16(1):25–35.
49. Beaver JA, Amiri-Kordestani L, Charlab R, Chen W, Palmby T, Tilley A, et al. FDA approval: palbociclib for the treatment of postmenopausal patients with estrogen receptor-positive, HER2-negative metastatic breast cancer. Clin Cancer Res. 2015;21(21):4760–6.
50. Kim ES, Scott LJ. Palbociclib: a review in HR-positive, HER2-negative, advanced or metastatic breast cancer. Target Oncol. 2017;12(3):373–83.
51. Finn RS, Martin M, Rugo HS, Jones S, Im SA, Gelmon K, et al. Palbociclib and letrozole in advanced breast cancer. N Engl J Med. 2016;375(20):1925–36.
52. Hortobagyi GN, Stemmer SM, Burris HA, Yap YS, Sonke GS, Paluch-Shimon S, et al. Updated results from MONALEESA-2, a phase III trial of first-line ribociclib plus letrozole versus placebo plus letrozole in hormone receptor-positive, HER2-negative advanced breast cancer. Ann Oncol. 2018;29(7):1541–7.
53. Tripathy D, Im SA, Colleoni M, Franke F, Bardia A, Harbeck N, et al. Ribociclib plus endocrine therapy for premenopausal women with hormonereceptor-positive, advanced breast cancer (MONALEESA-7): a randomised phase 3 trial. Lancet Oncol. 2018;19(7):904–15.
54. Goetz MP, Toi M, Campone M, Sohn J, Paluch-Shimon S, Huober J, et al. MONARCH 3: abemaciclib as initial therapy for advanced breast cancer. J Clin Oncol. 2017;35(32):3638–46.
55. Finn RS, Dering J, Conklin D, Kalous O, Cohen DJ, Desai AJ, et al. PD 0332991, a selective cyclin D kinase 4/6 inhibitor, preferentially inhibits proliferation of luminal estrogen receptor-positive human breast cancer cell lines in vitro. Breast Cancer Res. 2009;11(5):R77.
56. Kümler I, Christiansen OG, Nielsen DL. A systematic review of bevacizumab efficacy in breast cancer. Cancer Treat Rev. 2014;40(8):960–73.
57. Martín M, Loibl S, von Minckwitz G, Morales S, Martinez N, Guerrero A, et al. Phase III trial evaluating the addition of bevacizumab to endocrine therapy as first-line treatment for advanced breast cancer: the letrozole/fulvestrant and avastin (LEA) study. J Clin Oncol. 2015;33(9):1045–52.

58. Dickler MN, Barry WT, Cirrincione CT, Ellis MJ, Moynahan ME, Innocenti F, et al. Phase III trial evaluating letrozole as first-line endocrine therapy with or without bevacizumab for the treatment of postmenopausal women with hormone receptor-positive advanced-stage breast cancer: CALGB 40503 (alliance). J Clin Oncol. 2016;34(22):2602–9.
59. Thürlimann B, Robertson JF, Nabholtz JM, Buzdar A, Bonneterre J, Arimidex Study Group. Efficacy of tamoxifen following anastrozole ('Arimidex') compared with anastrozole following tamoxifen as first-line treatment for advanced breast cancer in postmenopausal women. Eur J Cancer. 2003;39(16):2310–7.
60. Rose C, Vtoraya O, Pluzanska A, Davidson N, Gershanovich M, Thomas R, et al. An open randomised trial of second-line endocrine therapy in advanced breast cancer: comparison of the aromatase inhibitors letrozole and anastrozole. Eur J Cancer. 2003;39(16):2318–27.
61. Bertelli G, Garrone O, Merlano M, Occelli M, Bertolotti L, Castiglione F, et al. Sequential treatment with exemestane and non-steroidal aromatase inhibitors in advanced breast cancer. Oncology. 2005;69(6):471–7.
62. Gennatas C, Michalaki V, Carvounis E, Psychogios J, Poulakaki N, Katsiamis G, et al. Third-line hormonal treatment with exemestane in postmenopausal patients with advanced breast cancer progressing on letrozole or anastrozole. A phase II trial conducted by the Hellenic Group of Oncology (HELGO). Tumori. 2006;92(1):13–7.
63. Beresford M, Tumur I, Chakrabarti J, Barden J, Rao N, Makris A, et al. A qualitative systematic review of the evidence base for non-cross-resistance between steroidal and non-steroidal aromatase inhibitors in metastatic breast cancer. Clin Oncol (R Coll Radiol). 2011;23(3):209–15.
64. Mauriac L, Romieu G, Bines J. Activity of fulvestrant versus exemestane in advanced breast cancer patients with or without visceral metastases: data from the EFECT trial. Breast Cancer Res Treat. 2009;117(1):69–75.
65. Johnston SR, Kilburn LS, Ellis P, Dodwell D, Cameron D, Hayward L, et al. Fulvestrant plus anastrozole or placebo versus exemestane alone after progression on non-steroidal aromatase inhibitors in postmenopausal patients with hormone-receptor-positive locally advanced or metastatic breast cancer (SoFEA): a composite, multicentre, phase 3 randomised trial. Lancet Oncol. 2013;14(10):989–98.
66. Di Leo A, Jerusalem G, Petruzelka L, Torres R, Bondarenko IN, Khasanov R, et al. Results of the CONFIRM phase III trial comparing fulvestrant 250 mg with fulvestrant 500 mg in postmenopausal women with estrogen receptor-positive advanced breast cancer. J Clin Oncol. 2010;28(30):4594–600.
67. Di Leo A, Jerusalem G, Petruzelka L, Torres R, Bondarenko IN, Khasanov R, et al. Final overall survival: fulvestrant 500 mg vs 250 mg in the randomized CONFIRM trial. J Natl Cancer Inst. 2014;106(1):djt337.
68. Creighton CJ, Fu X, Hennessy BT, Casa AJ, Zhang Y, Gonzalez-Angulo AM, et al. Proteomic and transcriptomic profiling reveals a link between the PI3K pathway and lower estrogen-receptor (ER) levels and activity in ER+ breast cancer. Breast Cancer Res. 2010;12(3):R40.
69. Hennessy BT, Smith DL, Ram PT, Lu Y, Mills GB. Exploiting the PI3K/AKT pathway for cancer drug discovery. Nat Rev Drug Discov. 2005;4(12):988–1004.
70. Creighton CJ. A gene transcription signature of the Akt/mTOR pathway in clinical breast tumors. Oncogene. 2007;26:4648–55.
71. Shi W, Zhang X, Pintilie M, Ma N, Miller N, Banerjee D, et al. Dysregulated PTEN-PKB and negative receptor status in human breast cancer. Int J Cancer. 2003;104:195–203.
72. Generali D, Fox S, Brizzi M, Allevi G, Bonardi S, Aguggini S, et al. Down-regulation of phosphatidylinositol 3'-kinase/AKT/molecular target of rapamycin metabolic pathway by primary letrozole-based therapy in human breast cancer. Clin Cancer Res. 2008;14:2673–80.
73. Boulay A, Rudloff J, Ye J, Zumstein-Mecker S, O'Reilly T, Evans DB, et al. Dual inhibition of mTOR and estrogen receptor signaling in vitro induces cell death in models of breast cancer. Clin Cancer Res. 2005;11(14):5319–28.
74. Baselga J, Campone M, Piccart M, Burris HA, Rugo HS, Sahmoud T, et al. Everolimus in postmenopausal hormone-receptor-positive advanced breast cancer. N Engl J Med. 2012;366(6):520–9.

75. Dhillon S. Everolimus in combination with exemestane: a review of its use in the treatment of patients with postmenopausal hormone receptor-positive, HER2-negative advanced breast cancer. Drugs. 2013;73(5):475–85.
76. Piccart M, Hortobagyi GN, Campone M, Pritchard KI, Lebrun F, Ito Y, et al. Everolimus plus exemestane for hormone-receptor-positive, human epidermal growth factor receptor-2-negative advanced breast cancer: overall survival results from BOLERO-2†. Ann Oncol. 2014;25(12):2357–62.
77. Wolff AC, Lazar AA, Bondarenko I, Garin AM, Brincat S, Chow L, et al. Randomized phase III placebo-controlled trial of letrozole plus oral temsirolimus as first-line endocrine therapy in postmenopausal women with locally advanced or metastatic breast cancer. J Clin Oncol. 2013;31(2):195–202.
78. Baselga J, Semiglazov V, van Dam P, Manikhas A, Bellet M, Mayordomo J, et al. Phase II randomized study of neoadjuvant everolimus plus letrozole compared with placebo plus letrozole in patients with estrogen receptor-positive breast cancer. J Clin Oncol. 2009;27:2630–7.
79. Bachelot T, Bourgier C, Cropet C, Ray-Coquard I, Ferrero JM, Freyer G, et al. Randomized phase II trial of everolimus in combination with tamoxifen in patients with hormone receptor-positive, human epidermal growth factor receptor 2-negative metastatic breast cancer with prior exposure to aromatase inhibitors: a GINECO study. J Clin Oncol. 2012;30:2718–24.
80. Hortobagyi GN, Chen D, Piccart M, Rugo HS, Burris HA 3rd, Pritchard KI, et al. Correlative analysis of genetic alterations and everolimus benefit in hormone receptor-positive, human epidermal growth factor receptor 2-negative advanced breast cancer: results from BOLERO-2. J Clin Oncol. 2016;34(5):419–26.
81. Sledge GW Jr, Toi M, Neven P, Sohn J, Inoue K, Pivot X, et al. MONARCH 2: abemaciclib in combination with fulvestrant in women with HR+/HER2- advanced breast cancer who had progressed while receiving endocrine therapy. J Clin Oncol. 2017;35(25):2875–84.
82. Dickler MN, Tolaney SM, Rugo HS, Cortés J, Diéras V, Patt D, et al. MONARCH 1, a phase II Study of abemaciclib, a CDK4 and CDK6 inhibitor, as a single agent, in patients with refractory HR+/HER2-metastatic breast cancer. Clin Cancer Res. 2017;23(17):5218–24.
83. Robertson JF, Ferrero JM, Bourgeois H, Kennecke H, de Boer RH, Jacot W, et al. Ganitumab with either exemestane or fulvestrant for postmenopausal women with advanced, hormone-receptor-positive breast cancer: a randomised, controlled, double-blind, phase 2 trial. Lancet Oncol. 2013;14(3):228–35.
84. Yardley DA, Ismail-Khan RR, Melichar B, Lichinitser M, Munster PN, Klein PM, et al. Randomized phase II, double-blind, placebo-controlled study of exemestane with or without entinostat in postmenopausal women with locally recurrent or metastatic estrogen receptor-positive breast cancer progressing on treatment with a nonsteroidal aromatase inhibitor. J Clin Oncol. 2013;31(17):2128–35.
85. Mackey JR, Kaufman B, Clemens M. Trastuzumab prolongs progression-free survival in hormone-dependent and HER2+ MBC. Breast Cancer Res Treat. 2006;100:5.
86. Kaufman B, Mackey JR, Clemens MR, Bapsy PP, Vaid A, Wardley A, et al. Trastuzumab plus anastrozole versus anastrozole alone for the treatment of postmenopausal women with human epidermal growth factor receptor 2- positive, HR+ MBC: results from the randomized phase III TAnDEM study. J Clin Oncol. 2009;27:5529–37.
87. Johnston S, Pippen J Jr, Pivot X, Lichinitser M, Sadeghi S, Dieras V, et al. Lapatinib combined with letrozole versus letrozole and placebo as first-line therapy for postmenopausal HR+ MBC. J Clin Oncol. 2009;27:5538–46.
88. Burstein HJ, Cirrincione CT, Barry WT, Chew HK, Tolaney SM, Lake DE, et al. Endocrine therapy with or without inhibition of epidermal growth factor receptor and human epidermal growth factor receptor 2: a randomized, double-blind, placebo-controlled phase III trial of fulvestrant with or without lapatinib for postmenopausal women with HR+ advanced breast cancer-CALGB 40302 (Alliance). J Clin Oncol. 2014;32(35):3959–66.

Chapter 25
Bone-Targeted Therapy in Advanced Breast Cancer

Ece Esin and Irfan Cicin

Introduction

In addition to the lungs and liver, bone is among the most common recurrence sites of breast cancer. In patients diagnosed with early breast cancer, the incidence of bone metastasis reaches 8% at 2 years and 27% at 10 years of follow-up. The risk of bone metastasis in early-diagnosed breast cancer is associated with early diagnosis age (<35 years), tumor size larger than 2 cm, and metastasis to greater than 4 axillary lymph nodes in pathology [1]. Historically, the reported incidence of bone metastasis is 70%, and skeletal event-related morbidity is estimated at 2.2–4% per year [2]. Although bone-only metastatic disease has a better prognosis than visceral metastatic disease does, the morbidity and decreases in quality of life due to symptomatic bone metastasis should not be underestimated.

Pain, pathologic fractures, hypercalcemia and spinal cord compression are named together as skeletal-related events (SRE) and contribute to the morbidity of bone metastasis of breast cancer. SRE creates a major symptom burden and decrease in quality of life by limiting daily instrumental activities, causing pain and requiring surgery or palliative radiotherapy.

This chapter focuses on the mechanism of bone metastasis, the impact of bone metastasis on the treatment and follow-up of breast cancer patients, bone-targeted treatment options and prevention in advanced metastatic breast cancer patients without bone metastasis.

E. Esin
Department of Medical Oncology, Dr. A. Y. Ankara Oncology Education and Research Hospital, Ankara, Turkey

I. Cicin (✉)
Department of Medical Oncology, Faculty of Medicine, Balkan Oncology Hospital, Trakya University of Medicine, Edirne, Turkey
e-mail: irfancicin@trakya.edu.tr

A. Aydiner et al. (eds.), *Breast Cancer*, https://doi.org/10.1007/978-3-319-96947-3_25

Pathophysiology of Bone Metastasis in Breast Cancer

Normally, bone health is a dynamic process that is internally coordinated by the equilibrium of osteoblasts and osteoclasts. A variety of local growth factors, chemokines and systemic proteins are responsible for this equilibrium. Osteoblasts are derived from mesenchymal cells and, under the influence of chemical factors, differentiate into mature osteocytes to create the bony matrix. By contrast, osteoclasts are derived from monocytes, are responsible for bone resorption and are coordinated by local factors in the bone microenvironment. The major influence on osteoclasts is receptor activator of nuclear factor (NF)-KB ligand (RANK-L). Under normal conditions, RANK-L binds to an extracellular receptor on osteoclasts and activates intracellular signaling, which is essential for survival. Osteoprotegerin is a negative regulator of RANK-L that is responsible for inhibiting the function and differentiation of osteoclasts. A study showed that tumor necrosis factor (TNF)-related apoptosis-inducing ligand secreted from tumor cells is associated with osteoprotogerin and enhances osteoclast survival [3]. Thus, the generation of osteoblasts and osteoclasts is strictly regulated, especially by local factors of the bone microenvironment.

As in any organ, the development of bone metastasis is not a random process but rather a cascade of events in which the expression of multiple genes and various proteins and aberrant intracellular signaling occur [4]. In an important pivotal study, chemokine receptor type 4 (CXCR4) and matrix metalloproteinase (MMP)-1 were shown to be crucial for homing of breast cancer cells to bone [5]. For many reasons, bone is an appropriate substrate for breast cancer cells. First, bone is a highly vascular organ, and bone marrow requires high blood flow. Second, intramedullary acidity, oxygen levels and extracellular calcium levels favor the maintenance of metastatic cells. Finally, the bone microenvironment includes various growth factors, chemokines and enzymes that create a suitable home for cancer cells, that is, a metastatic niche [6].

In bone metastasis, the delicate equilibrium between osteoblasts and osteoclasts is disturbed. Whether osteolytic or osteoblastic metastasis, the final cost is bone fragility and instability. Although breast cancer has a reputation for osteolytic bone metastasis, in reality, 48% of breast cancer bone metastases are reported to be purely lytic, 38% to be mixed and 13% to be purely osteoblastic. Therefore, both blastic and resorptive processes are involved in breast cancer bone metastasis [7].

Targeting Bone Metastasis in Metastatic Breast Cancer

Preventing Skeletal-Related Events Due to Bone Metastasis

Targeting with Bisphosphonates

Bisphosphonates are an important class of medications that inhibit bone resorption by inducing osteoclast apoptosis. First-generation, non-nitrogen bisphosphonates accumulate intracellularly, and an analogue of ATP is formed that results in apoptosis of osteoclasts [7]. Nitrogen-containing (N) bisphosphonates (pamidronate, ibandronate and zoledronic acid) target signaling proteins of osteoclasts that are important for cell survival [8]. In addition, experiments have shown that higher concentrations of N-bisphosphonates inhibit osteoblasts, epithelial and endothelial cells and breast cancer cells. Hence, the antitumoral properties of N-bisphosphonates may include multicellular pathways of inhibition [8]. Moreover, the integration and interaction of T cells, bone, osteoblasts and osteoclasts with N-bisphosphonates have been explained via immune mechanisms [9].

The effects of bisphosphonates have been extensively studied over the previous two decades due to the high burden of SREs in the course of advanced breast cancer (ABC). In a 2017 Cochrane meta-analysis, 44 randomized controlled studies involving more than 37,000 women were analyzed [10]. In bone metastatic breast cancer patients, SREs were reduced by 14% with bisphosphonates, and the first SRE was delayed by a median ratio of 1.43, with a moderate reduction of bone pain. Quality of life scores were slightly better with bisphosphonates, and overall survival was not affected by bisphosphonates.

Whether the effects of bisphosphonates are consistent with a class effect or whether there are any differences among bisphosphonates is an ongoing debate. One problem is that the methodology and expressions of SKE differ between studies. Rosen et al. published a head-to-head comparison study of zoledronic acid (ZA) [4–8 mg, intravenous (iv)] and pamidronate (90 mg, iv) every 3–4 weeks for up to 2 years in 1130 patients [11]. A protocol modification was needed due to concerns of renal toxicity for 8 mg ZA. After the dose was established, 4 mg ZA was shown to be noninferior to 90 mg pamidronate in terms of SRE excluding hypercalcemia. In the osteolytic metastasis subgroup, the skeletal morbidity rate and time to first SRE were lower when ZA was combined with radiotherapy or endocrine treatment, thus confirming the synergistic efficacy of N-bisphosphonates. More recently, oral ibandronic acid (IBA) was compared to ZA in the ZICE phase III trial, and oral IBA was found to be inferior with respect to the SRE rate endpoint [12].

The remaining questions are the duration of bisphosphonate treatment and the optimal time interval. For the optimal duration of bisphosphonates, there is a paucity of clinically relevant data. Two years, which is usually set as the duration in clinical trials, may be chosen, but continuation after 2 years is also an option. According to the American Society of Clinical Oncolgy (ASCO) 2017 updated guidelines, the use of bisphosphonates is reserved for patients with evident bone metastasis [13]. There is no advice regarding the choice of one bisphosphonate over another. If ZA is chosen, regimens of 4 mg every 3–4 weeks as well as every 12 weeks are suggested by the advisory board. The results of three randomized control trials were in favor of 12-week scheduling of iv ZA [14–16]. The advisory board addressed that bisphosphonates should not be used solely for bone pain since the effects are modest; instead, adjunct therapies such as radiotherapy, endocrine agents for hormone receptor-positive patients, and pain medications should be included.

Targeting RANK-L

The major signal of osteoclastic survival is receptor activator of nuclear factor (NF)-KB ligand (RANK-L). Denosumab is a fully human monoclonal antibody developed against RANK-L. Preclinical studies have proven that denosumab is effective against osteoclast-induced bone destruction [17, 18].

A set of trials of patients with breast cancer, prostate cancer and other cancers excluding breast and prostate cancer was conducted to demonstrate the importance of denosumab in bone metastasis [19–21]. In a landmark study by Stopeck et al., subcutaneous (sc) 120 mg denosumab was tested against iv 4 mg ZA every 4 weeks [21]. The primary endpoint was defined as delay of first SRE in the study. Denosumab met the criteria, as the median time to development of SRE with denosumab was 32.4 months vs. 26.4 months with ZA and it was shown to be noninferior to ZA (HR: 0.82, $p = 0.001$). In addition, bone metastasis-related pain, which was set as a secondary endpoint, developed later with denosumab than ZA (HR: 0.78, $p = 0.002$). Cochrane analyses showed that denosumab reduced the risk of developing SRE by 22% [10].

As a result, ASCO recommends denosumab as a first-line option at the first sign of metastasis to bone [22].

Preventing Bone Metastases in Advanced Breast Cancer Without Clinically Evident Skeletal Involvement

As far as the burden of bone metastasis is concerned, it is important to prevent skeletal involvement in advanced cancer patients without skeletal involvement. Three studies were included in Cochrane meta-analyses. Kanis et al. showed that clodronate use was associated with a decreased risk of bone metastases ($p < 0.005$); however, there was no survival benefit [23]. Pamidronate was tested, but there was no significant efficacy in skeletal morbidity, quality of life and survival [24]. In conclusion, the Cochrane meta-analyses reported that supportive bisphosphonates did not affect the primary endpoint of reducing SRE [10]. Given the available data regarding bisphosphonates in ABC without osseous involvement, ASCO does not support their use without any clinically evident bone metastases [22].

Toxicity Related to Bone-Targeted Therapy

Bisphosphonates and denosumab share common side effects. In general, they may result in acute-phase reactions, hypocalcemia, and osteonecrosis of the jaw (ONJ). Oral bisphosphonates may result in some degree of gastrointestinal irritation. Occasionally, subcutaneous local reactions may be seen with denosumab. In randomized studies, both medications resulted in serious side effects at the same rates, and the reported treatment discontinuation rates due to adverse events were similar for both agents [25]. Bisphosphonates are associated with renal toxicity. The renal toxicity of ZA may be reversible, but pamidronate is associated with nephrotic syndrome, which may not be reversible [26, 27]. By contrast, denosumab is relatively safe in renal aspects compared to bisphosphonates. In patients with normal function and in patients with a decreased glomerular filtration rate, denosumab can be safely administered without any dose change [13, 28–30]. To avoid bisphosphonate-induced nephrotoxicity, patients should be screened for glomerular filtration rate (GFR) before each bisphosphonate application, and bisphosphonates should not be given if the GFR is below 30 ml/min. Bisphosphonates have a relatively lower risk of developing hypocalcemia compared to denosumab [21] The risk of denosumab-associated hypocalcemia is higher if the GFR is less than 30 ml/min.

ONJ is one of the most debilitating complications of bone targeting in malignancies. The risk of ONJ increases continuously with repeated doses and shorter intervals of bone-targeted agent use [31]. No statistically significant difference was observed in ONJ rates between denosumab and bisphosphonates [31, 32]. In Cochrane analyses, the reported ONJ rate was increased by less than 0.5% compared to use in the adjuvant setting [10]. To avoid ONJ, preventive measures should be taken, such as oral hygiene, regular tooth control and avoiding dental procedures.

Conclusion

Bone metastatic disease has a favorable prognosis compared to visceral metastatic disease. However, the morbidity and decrease in quality of life due to possible skeletal events (pain, pathologic fractures, hypercalcemia and spinal cord compression) may have a large impact overall. Bisphosphonates inhibit bone resorption by inducing apoptosis of osteoclasts, and denosumab acts as a monoclonal antibody against receptor activator of nuclear factor (NF)-KB ligand, which is essential for osteoclast survival. Given the available data regarding bisphosphonates in ABC without osseous involvement, international guidelines do not support the preventive use of bone-targeted agents. Toxicities of bisphosphonates and denosumab include hypocalcemia, renal toxicity, gastrointestinal disturbance and osteonecrosis of the jaw and should be carefully reviewed when administering drugs and making decisions about dose, interval and duration.

References

1. Colleoni M, O'Neill A, Goldhirsch A, Gelber RD, Bonetti M, Thürlimann B, et al. Identifying breast cancer patients at high risk for bone metastases. J Clin Oncol. 2000;18:3925–35.
2. Body J. Biphosphonates in breast cancer and other solid tumors. In: Mundy RD, Rubens RD, editors. Cancer and the skeleton. London: Martin Dunitz; 2000.

3. Van Poznak C, Cross SS, Saggese M, Hudis C, Panageas KS, Norton L, et al. Expression of osteoprotegerin (OPG), TNF related apoptosis inducing ligand (TRAIL), and receptor activator of nuclear factor kappaB ligand (RANKL) in human breast tumours. J Clin Pathol. 2006;59:56–63.
4. Chambers AF, Groom AC, MacDonald IC. Dissemination and growth of cancer cells in metastatic sites. Nat Rev Cancer. 2002;2:563–72.
5. Kang Y, Siegel PM, Shu W, Drobnjak M, Kakonen SM, Cordón-Cardo C, et al. A multigenic program mediating breast cancer metastasis to bone. Cancer Cell. 2003;3:537–49.
6. Psaila B, Lyden D. The metastatic niche: adapting the foreign soil. Nat Rev Cancer. 2009;9:285–93.
7. Wong M, Pavlakis N. Optimal management of bone metastases in breast cancer patients. Breast Cancer. 2011;3:35–60.
8. Roelofs AJ, Thompson K, Gordon S, Rogers MJ. Molecular mechanisms of action of bisphosphonates: current status. Clin Cancer Res. 2006;12:6222s–30s.
9. Thompson K, Roelofs AJ, Jauhiainen M, Monkkonen H, Monkkonen J, Rogers MJ. Activation of gammadelta T cells by bisphosphonates. Adv Exp Med Biol. 2010;658:11–20.
10. O'Carrigan B, Wong MH, Willson ML, Stockler MR, Pavlakis N, Goodwin A. Bisphosphonates and other bone agents for breast cancer. Cochrane Database Syst Rev. 2017;10:CD003474.
11. Rosen LS, Gordon DH, Dugan W Jr, Major P, Eisenberg PD, Provencher L, et al. Zoledronic acid is superior to pamidronate for the treatment of bone metastases in breast carcinoma patients with at least one osteolytic lesion. Cancer. 2004;100:36–43.
12. Barrett-Lee P, Casbard A, Abraham J, Hood K, Coleman R, Simmonds P, et al. Oral ibandronic acid versus intravenous zoledronic acid in treatment of bone metastases from breast cancer: a randomised, open label, non-inferiority phase 3 trial. Lancet Oncol. 2014;15:114–22.
13. Dhesy-Thind S, Fletcher GG, Blanchette PS, Clemons MJ, Dillmon MS, Frank ES, et al. Use of adjuvant bisphosphonates and other bone-modifying agents in breast cancer: a Cancer Care Ontario and American Society of Clinical Oncology clinical practice guideline. J Clin Oncol. 2017;35:2062–81.
14. Amadori D, Aglietta M, Alessi B, Gianni L, Ibrahim T, Farina G, et al. Efficacy and safety of 12-weekly versus 4-weekly zoledronic acid for prolonged treatment of patients with bone metastases from breast cancer (ZOOM): a phase 3, open-label, randomised, non-inferiority trial. Lancet Oncol. 2013;14:663–70.
15. Hortobagyi GN, Van Poznak C, Harker WG, Gradishar WJ, Chew H, Dakhil SR, et al. Continued treatment effect of zoledronic acid dosing every 12 vs 4 weeks in women with breast cancer metastatic to bone: the OPTIMIZE-2 randomized clinical trial. JAMA Oncol. 2017;3:906–12.
16. Himelstein AL, Foster JC, Khatcheressian JL, Roberts JD, Seisler DK, Novotny PJ, et al. Effect of longer-interval vs standard dosing of zoledronic acid on skeletal events in patients with bone metastases: a randomized clinical trial. JAMA. 2017;317:48–58.
17. Bouganim N, Clemons MJ. Bone-targeted agents in the treatment of bone metastases: RANK outsider or new kid on the block? Future Oncol. 2011;7:381–3.
18. Lipton A, Jacobs I. Denosumab: benefits of RANK ligand inhibition in cancer patients. Curr Opin Support Palliat Care. 2011;5:258–64.
19. Fizazi K, Carducci M, Smith M, Damião R, Brown J, Karsh L, et al. Denosumab versus zoledronic acid for treatment of bone metastases in men with castration-resistant prostate cancer: a randomised, double-blind study. Lancet. 2011;377:813–22.
20. Henry DH, Costa L, Goldwasser F, Hirsh V, Hungria V, Prausova J, et al. Randomized, double-blind study of denosumab versus zoledronic acid in the treatment of bone metastases in patients with advanced cancer (excluding breast and prostate cancer) or multiple myeloma. J Clin Oncol. 2011;29:1125–32.
21. Stopeck AT, Lipton A, Body JJ, Steger GG, Tonkin K, de Boer RH, et al. Denosumab compared with zoledronic acid for the treatment of bone metastases in patients with advanced breast cancer: a randomized, double-blind study. J Clin Oncol. 2010;28:5132–9.

22. Van Poznak C, Somerfield MR, Barlow WE, Biermann JS, Bosserman LD, Clemons MJ, et al. Role of bone-modifying agents in metastatic breast cancer: an American Society of Clinical Oncology-Cancer Care Ontario focused guideline update. J Clin Oncol. 2017;35:3978–86.
23. Kanis JA, Powles T, Paterson AH, McCloskey EV, Ashley S. Clodronate decreases the frequency of skeletal metastases in women with breast cancer. Bone. 1996;19:663–7.
24. van Holten-Verzantvoort AT, Hermans J, Beex LV, Blijham G, Cleton FJ, van Eck-Smit BC, et al. Does supportive pamidronate treatment prevent or delay the first manifestation of bone metastases in breast cancer patients? Eur J Cancer. 1996;32A:450–4.
25. Sheedy KC, Camara MI, Camacho PM. Comparison of the efficacy, adverse effects, and cost of zoledronic acid and denosumab in the treatment of osteoporosis. Endocr Pract. 2015;21:275–9.
26. Markowitz GS, Fine PL, Stack JI, Kunis CL, Radhakrishnan J, Palecki W, et al. Toxic acute tubular necrosis following treatment with zoledronate (Zometa). Kidney Int. 2003;64:281–9.
27. Markowitz GS, Fine PL, D'Agati VD. Nephrotic syndrome after treatment with pamidronate. Am J Kidney Dis. 2002;39:1118–22.
28. Anghel R, Bachmann A, Beksac M, Brodowicz T, Finek J, Komadina R, American Society of Clinical Oncology, National Comprehensive Cancer Network, et al. Expert opinion 2011 on the use of new anti-resorptive agents in the prevention of skeletal-related events in metastatic bone disease. Wien Klin Wochenschr. 2013;125:439–47.
29. Prommer E. Palliative oncology: denosumab. Am J Hosp Palliat Care. 2015;32:568–72.
30. Domschke C, Schuetz F. Side effects of bone-targeted therapies in advanced breast cancer. Breast Care. 2014;9:332–6.
31. Campisi G, Fedele S, Fusco V, Pizzo G, Di Fede O, Bedogni A. Epidemiology, clinical manifestations, risk reduction and treatment strategies of jaw osteonecrosis in cancer patients exposed to antiresorptive agents. Future Oncol. 2014;10:257–75.
32. Wang X, Yang KH, Wanyan P, Tian JH. Comparison of the efficacy and safety of denosumab versus bisphosphonates in breast cancer and bone metastases treatment: a meta-analysis of randomized controlled trials. Oncol Lett. 2014;7:1997–2002.

Chapter 26
Biostatistical and Epidemiological Terms Frequently Used in Breast Cancer Research

Rian Disci

Introduction

Statistical methodology techniques are required in every stage of scientific research [1–3].

The phases of scientific research are as follows:

1. Definition of purpose (observation, choice of topic, establishment of hypotheses).
2. Planning (e.g., preparing a written protocol, defining the problem, the importance of the problem according to various sources, the hypotheses considered, defining dependent and independent variables, the obligatory and non-essential constraints, defining the concepts used, research management, determination of possibilities).
3. Application (collection of data).
4. Data analysis (descriptive statistics, testing hypotheses).
5. Interpreting the results and writing the report.

Statistics are regarded as a *common language of science* used in scientific research [2]. This section will summarize the biostatistical and epidemiological terms frequently used in medical research.

R. Disci (✉)
Istinye University, Medical Faculty, Department of Biostatistics and Medical Informatics, Istanbul, Turkey

A. Aydiner et al. (eds.), *Breast Cancer*, https://doi.org/10.1007/978-3-319-96947-3_26

Arithmetic Mean (Average)

The average is obtained by dividing the sum of the numerical values of the observations by the number of observations. The arithmetic mean of the sample is indicated by the $\overline{x}$ symbol, and that of the masterbatch (universe) is indicated by the μ symbol.

$$\overline{x} = \frac{\sum_{i=1}^{n} x_i}{n}$$

Median

The median is the value that divides the serial terms into two equal parts with regard to the number of terms when sorted in increasing or decreasing order. The median is indicated by the symbols Q_2 or Med. Values dividing serial terms into 4 equal parts are called *quartiles*, values dividing into 10 equal parts are called *decimals*, and values dividing into 100 equal parts are called *percentiles*. The 2nd quartile, 5th decimal and 50th percentile values correspond to the median value. Quartiles, decimals and percentiles are calculated in the same way as the median. The 1st quartile is indicated by Q_1, the 2nd by Q_2, and the 3rd by Q_3.

Peak Value (Mod)

The most frequently repeated value in a series is called the peak value (mod) and is indicated by $\hat{X}$.

Geometric Mean

The geometric mean is used instead of the arithmetic mean if the serial terms increase or decrease geometrically. The geometric mean is obtained by taking the root of the product of serial terms by the number of total observations. The geometric mean is indicated by the symbol G.M.

$$G.M. = \sqrt[n]{x_1 x_2 \cdots x_n}$$

Spreading Range

This is a measure of variability that does not depend on the whole units of the series. The spreading range is obtained by subtracting the smallest value from the largest value.

Variance

The variance is calculated as the arithmetic mean of the squares of the deviations of each term from the mean of the series. 'Variance' is used as a measure of variability in all statistical analyses due to its suitability for algebraic operations. Variance is indicated by σ^2 for the masterbatch and s^2 for the sample.

Standard Deviation

The standard deviation is the positive square root of the variance value. It is the most commonly used variability measure and is indicated by σ for the masterbatch and s for the sample.

Coefficient of Variance

The coefficient of variance refers to the percentage of the standard deviation relative to the arithmetic mean and is indicated by CV. The coefficient of variation is calculated by the following formula: $C.V. = \frac{S}{\overline{x}} \cdot 100$

Variable, Random Variable

We refer to properties that the units (subjects) carry that differ among the clumps (communities) we have studied with statistical methods as "variables". This variability may arise from biological differences between the subjects constituting the studied communities as well as from the measurement errors.

In a study consisting of randomly selected subjects, the variable is called the "*random variable*".

Probability Distribution

The values of the characteristics-variables (e.g., age, blood pressure, life span) can be presented as frequency distributions. The frequency distribution that summarizes the values for the random variable is called the "*probability distribution*". There are many theoretical probability distributions in statistics. The most commonly used probability distributions in Medicine are the "Binom", "Poisson" and "Normal (Gaussian)" distributions. The Binom and Poisson distributions are discrete, and the Normal distribution is in a continuous pattern.

Probability

Probability is the measure of the likelihood that an event will occur. It is obtained by dividing the number of cases of "success" recorded during the emergence of an event in different forms under the same conditions divided by the number of possible states; the successful cases or situations are called the "probability value".

Probability of Independent Events

This rule is valid for events independent of each other. If one of the two events does not affect the likelihood of the occurrence of the second event, it is said that these events are independent. The probability that A and B co-occur is calculated as follows:

$$P(\text{A and B}) = P(A) \cdot P(B)$$

Probability of Dependent Events

The probability that A and B co-occur is calculated as follows:

$$P(\text{A and B}) = P(A) \cdot PA(B)$$

Here, the PA (B) symbol indicates the probability of the occurrence of event B after event A has occurred.

Addition Rules for Probability

This is valid for events that are compatible and means that it is possible for the events to occur together. If A and B are two compatible events, the probability of the occurrence of A or B is calculated as follows:

$$P(\text{A or B}) = P(A) + P(B) - P(\text{A and B})$$

Here, P (A and B) indicates the probability of the co-occurrence of events A and B.

Theoretical Sampling Distribution

This is the distribution of the means of all samples in size (n), which can be taken from a masterbatch. Such a distribution indicates the likelihood of occurrence of certain mean values in a fixed-size sample that can be pulled from a masterbatch. For the mean, the theoretical sampling distributions can be established for parameters such as the standard deviation of the population or the rate of a particular property.

Standard Error

The standard deviation of the theoretical sampling distribution is called the "*standard error*".

"*Standard error*" and "*standard deviation*" should not be confused with each other. The standard deviation measures the variability between observation results for a population (σ) or for a sample in a given population, whereas the standard error is the measure of variability between the means of the (n) sized samples taken from the population. In other words, the standard error refers to how the determined mean values may vary from one sample to another.

The standard error is usually calculated by one of the following formulas:

$$\frac{\sigma}{\sqrt{n}}, \sqrt{\frac{(P \cdot Q)}{n}}$$

Sampling

Selection of a subgroup according to certain rules that can represent the whole masterbatch (universe) to conduct observations and examinations and generalizing the results to the universe is called "sampling". It is inevitable that there will be significant deviations and misstatements in a generalization based on a sample that does not have the power of representation of the universe. For this reason, care should be taken to comply with certain rules and to implement certain conditions during sampling.

Random Sampling (Probabilistic Sampling)

This is a type of sampling in which subjects are selected by the probability rules of the selection process. In random sampling, the probability of selecting each subject in the sample is equal.

Sample Size (n)

To make a correct prediction, it is necessary to calculate the minimum number of subjects that should be examined in the study group (sample). To calculate the sample size (n), the researcher first needs to determine the maximum value of the difference between the sample statistics and the parameters of the universe (acceptable sampling error). The acceptable sampling error must as low as possible to obtain sensitive and highly predictable results. In the study to be performed, the acceptable sampling error can be reduced by increasing the sample size. However, since increasing the sample size will increase the difficulty of the scientific study, the researcher must balance the working conditions and the accuracy and sensitivity of the results.

Estimate

Here, the value of particular parameters in the masterbatch is estimated by an approach moving from the tangential to the summit, with a mean or a rate of a selected sample.

Confidence Interval (CI)

Moving from the average value calculated in a sample while estimating the mean of the universe, the variability that exists from one sample to another is taken into account, and an estimation is made within a certain interval called the "*confidence interval*".

Hypothesis

A hypothesis is a proposition that is deemed to be valid and designed to relate or link events to specific causes. In the context of biostatistics, an assumption can be said to be a proposition designed between the parameters of the universe and the statistical values obtained for samples. In biostatistics, assumption tests are used to compare the statistical measures of different samples between themselves or to compare their parameters with the parameters of the universe.

Zero Assumption (Assumption of Indifference) (Null Hypothesis) H_o

This assumption proposes that the difference between the values we want to compare is actually (0); it differs from zero in practice, suggesting that this difference is only accidental.

(example: H_0: $\bar{x} = \mu$ or H_0: $|\bar{x} - \mu| = 0$)

Alternative Hypothesis (H_1)

The difference between the values that we want to compare is actually different than (0), which suggests that there is a reason for the difference other than coincidental causes [4–6].

(example: H_1: $\bar{x} \neq \mu$ or H_1: $|\bar{x} - \mu| \neq 0$)

As a result of hypothesis testing, the researcher will either agree that there is no real difference between the compared values and thus find correctness (accept H_o) or will reject it (reject H_o) and argue that the difference between the values examined is so great that it cannot be accidental.

Testing the Hypothesis, Type 1 Error, Type 2 Error and Power

Testing the H_o hypothesis will result in four ultimate situations rather than two. As can be clearly seen from the chart, the researcher will reach the correct conclusion in two cases and the wrong conclusion in the other two (Table 26.1).

The misconceptions that a researcher who tests a null hypothesis may encounter, which are referred to as "type 1 and 2 errors", may be different from each other in terms of scientific and practical consequences. The probability of type 1 error is indicated by the sign (α), and the probability of type 2 error is indicated

Table 26.1 Possible conclusions of hypothesis testing

	Real situation	
The results of the hypothesis test	Significant difference	No difference
Significant difference, H_0 reject	Correct result	Type I error
No difference, H_0 accept	Type II error	Correct result

by (β). Another important definition in hypothesis testing is the concept of "*power*". Power is the probability of rejecting an inaccurate null hypothesis (or accepting the correct alternative hypothesis). In another words, the power of a test indicates the ability to detect a difference that actually exists. The power is calculated as (1 − β).

P Value and Confidence Level

Prior to applying the statistical test, a selected and indeed valid null hypothesis is indicated by the level of confidence (α), which measures the probability of rejection by mistake. There is no doubt that (α) should be as small as possible for the results to be valid. In this respect, values of (0.05), (0.01), or (0.001) are used for (α) in accordance with common acceptance. As to the (p) value given in published scientific studies, this value should be equal to or greater than the observed difference if the null hypothesis is true; in other words, the probability that the observed difference will only be found incidentally. The (p) value is calculated after all tests have been completed. If $p < \alpha$, (H_o) is rejected [7, 8].

Correlation and Regression

These terms are used to show the relationship between two or more variables. The degree of the relationship is indicated by a number expressed as a correlation coefficient (relation coefficient). In addition, regression analysis is used to express the shape of the relationship between two or more variables.

The coefficient indicating the relationship between two continuous variables (analyzed at the interval or proportional measurement level) is called the "Pearson-Bravais moment product coefficient". In Medicine, this coefficient is referred to as the coefficient of association and represented by the symbol r.

The correlation coefficient (r) takes values between +1 and −1. If both variables are changing in the same direction, the sign of r is positive; if one of the variables is changing in the opposite direction of the other (that is, if one is decreasing while the other is increasing), the sign of r is negative. If there is no change in either the positive or negative direction between the variables, the correlation coefficient is zero. A correlation coefficient equal to zero indicates that there is no relationship between the variables. The absolute value of the correlation coefficient determines the power of the relationship, and the sign specifies the direction of the relationship. For example, correlation coefficients of +0.95 and −0.95 indicate strong relationships at the same level. The direction of the correlation is positive for the first and negative for the latter. In the two-way table, the shape of dots (Scatter Diagram) gets closer to a line as the *r* value approaches '+1' or '−1'. As the distribution of the dots in a scatter diagram takes the shape of a circle, the absolute value of *r* decreases and becomes zero when the dots are too messy.

If the variables studied are not normally distributed and the variables are examined only at the ranked measurement level, the Spearman ranking variation correlation coefficient is calculated instead of the Pearson-Bravais moment product correlation coefficient.

The technique used to determine the relationship between variables varies according to the form of the relationship, as well as the number of variables involved and the measurement results of these variables. Simple correlation techniques are used in the correlation analysis between two variables, multiple correlation techniques are used when the number of variables is three or more, and partial correlation techniques are used in cases where the effect of some variables is kept constant.

The relationship between variables can be in different forms. A relationship that can be expressed by a first-order mathematical equation (the line equation) is called a 'linear relation'. In contrast, if there is no possibility of expressing the relationship between variables with a first-order mathematical equation, then the relation is not linear, or there is a non-linear relationship. A non-linear relationship is expressed by a higher-order equation instead of a linear equation.

Coefficient of Determination

The determination coefficient ($d_{y \cdot x}$) indicates what percentage of the variance in 'y' depends on 'x' and is calculated by taking the square of the correlation coefficient.

Study Designs

We can classify scientific studies according to their purpose or style of conducting as follows:

Observational/Experimental
Descriptor/Analyzer
Retrospective/Prospective

The types of studies frequently used in health sciences are as follows:

Case Series Studies

Simple descriptive statistics for a group of patients are obtained. Regarding the disease being investigated, the answers to the questions "who", "where" and "when" are sought. Various hypotheses are established based on the results obtained in the study.

Cross-Sectional Studies

In such studies, an event is examined by a questionnaire or general screening within a very short time period. After collecting the necessary data, researchers attempt to determine the cause-result associations. Generally, the prevalence values of diseases (the incidence of the disease in the society) are obtained in such studies (Fig. 26.1).

Cohort Studies

The cohort formed by the individuals to be monitored will be randomly divided into two groups that will be exposed or not exposed to the factor. Both groups are monitored for a certain period of time, and data about disease development are collected (Fig. 26.2). In such studies, the incidence of the disease (the emergence of new cases with the particular disease during the time period examined), the relative risk ratio (relative risk, RR), and the attributable risk factor can be calculated. As the randomly formed groups are under monitoring, more accurate information about disease development can be obtained.

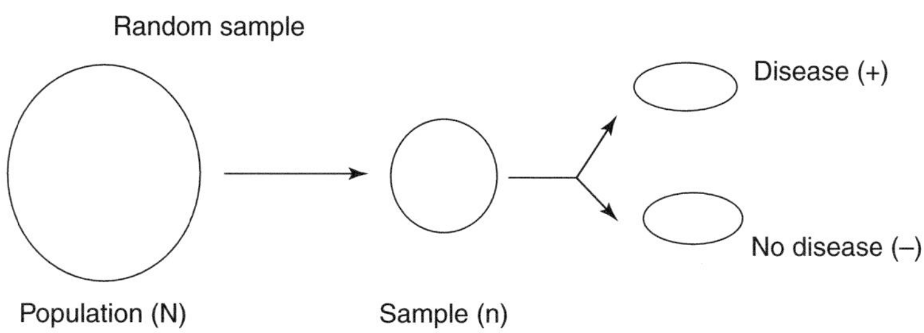

Fig. 26.1 Cross-sectional studies

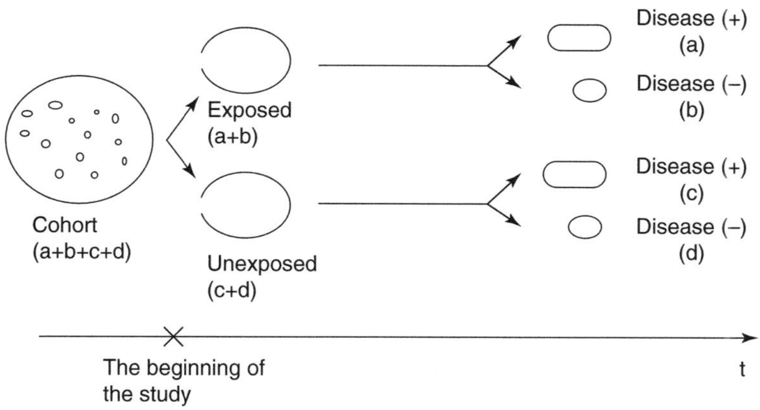

Fig. 26.2 Cohort study

Case-Control Studies

In Case-Control studies, the answer to the question "what happened in the past" is sought. In this type of study investigating causal relationships, the past histories of two groups of subjects, those who have a particular disease (study group) and those who do not (control group), are reviewed (Fig. 26.3). Usually, the patient files in the clinic constitute the research database. To conduct the research, the information about the disease and risk factors must be already recorded in the files. It is an appropriate type of research for investigating the causes of rare diseases. To ensure that the groups are comparable, both groups should be homogeneous (similar) with respect to variables other than the presence of the disease.

Parallel-Controlled Clinical Study

Patients presenting to the clinic who are eligible for the study (patients fulfilling the inclusion criteria specified in the study protocol) are randomly divided into two (or more) groups. One of these groups forms the experimental group, and the other forms the control group (Fig. 26.4). In the experimental group, a new drug or treatment method is used, whereas in the control group, placebo or traditional treatment is applied.

By comparing the treatment outcomes of the two groups, the results such as drug efficacy and side effects are evaluated. To ensure that the groups are comparable, the process of including patients in groups must be randomized. However, to reduce

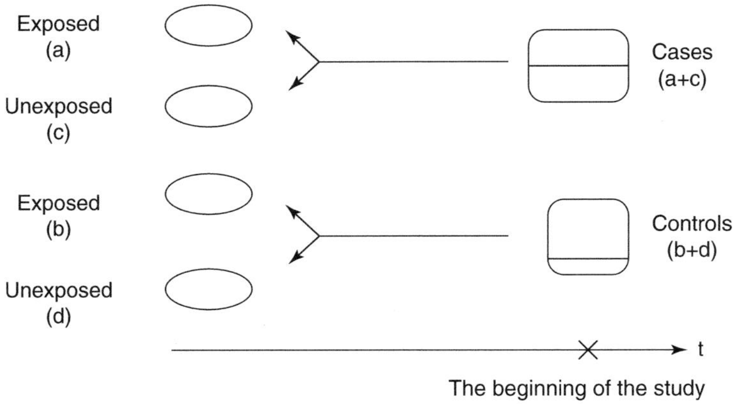

Fig. 26.3 Case-control study

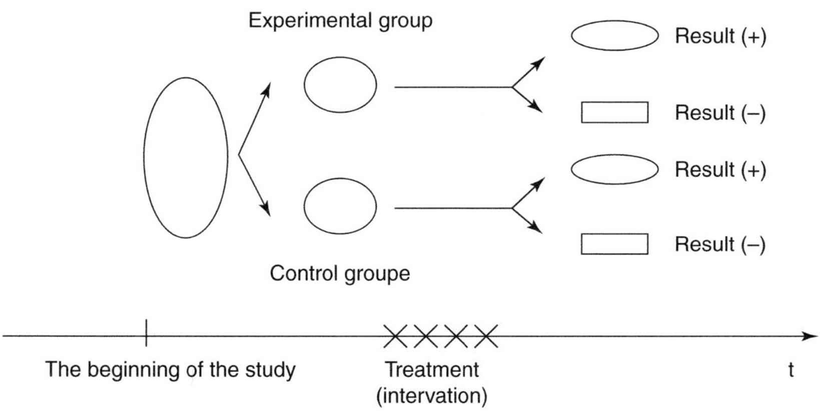

Fig. 26.4 Parallel-controlled clinical study

bias most likely to be caused by favoritism, the patients and practitioners (physicians, nurses, etc.) must not know which study arm the patients are located in (double blind).

Trials with External Controls

There is no control group in such studies. The results of previous studies are used for comparison (Fig. 26.5). Since randomization and blindness cannot be achieved, it is very difficult to make realistic comparisons.

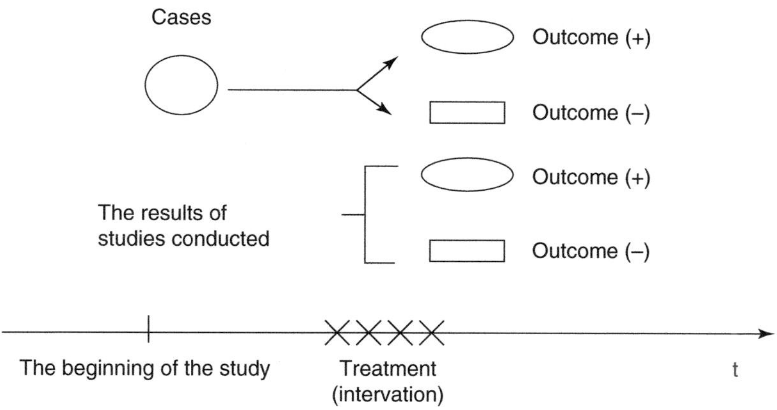

Fig. 26.5 Trials with external controls

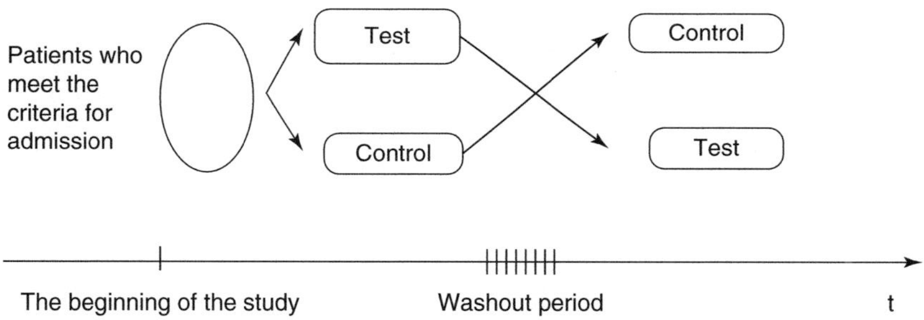

Fig. 26.6 Crossover study

Crossover Studies

Patients fulfilling the inclusion criteria are randomly assigned to experimental and control groups. In both groups, a suitable period of clearance (transition period) is implemented after application. The control group is then treated as the experimental group, and the experimental group is treated as the control group (Fig. 26.6). The involvement of individuals in both experimental and control groups ensures that individual differences are controlled.

Randomization

Randomization allows individuals fulfilling the inclusion criteria to be divided into groups with equal probability.

Table 26.2 Blinding types

	Single blind	Double blind	Triple blind
Subject	X	X	X
Practitioner, observer		X	X
Data analyzer, statistician			X

The most commonly used method for randomization is the "random numbers" method. Randomization ensures that the groups are homogeneous (similar) and therefore comparable.

Blinding

In blinding, the practitioners do not know what method is applied to which individual; similarly, the subjects do not know to which group they belong. Blinding (not being aware) is applied to prevent mistakes that may arise from bias (Table 26.2).

In single-blind studies, only the subjects are unaware of the group in which they participate. In double-blind studies, both practitioners and patients are unaware of which groups the patients are in. During the course of the statistical evaluation of the study results, if the data analyst does not know in which group the patients are involved, the study is called triple blind.

Evaluation Criteria for Diagnostic Tests

Sensitivity This shows the percentage of subjects known to have actually developed the disease that can be identified by the new method being tested.

Specificity This shows the percentage of those who do not have the disease (those who are healthy) that can be identified by the method being tested.

General Accuracy This shows the percentage of patients and healthy people who can be recognized by the method being tested.

Positive Predictive Value This demonstrates the percentage of positive results indicating disease presence with the method tested (compliance with the known method).

Negative Predictive Value This shows the percentage of the negative results indicating the absence of disease with the method tested.

We can also show the test results that are true positive (TP), false positive (FP), true negative (TN) and false negative (FN) (Table 26.3).

Table 26.3 Real situation and test results

	Real situation		
Test result	Disease (+)	Disease (−)	Total
(+)	TP	FP	TP + FP
(−)	FN	TN	FN + TN
Total	TP + FN	FP + TN	TP + FP + TN + FN

The definitions can be expressed as follows:

Sensitivity = TP/(TP + FN)
Specificity = TN/(TN + FP)
Total accuracy = (TP + TN)/(TP + FP + FN + TN)
Positive predictive value = TP/(TP + FP)
Positive predictive value = TN/(FN + TN)

Receiver Operating Characteristic (ROC) Curve

This analysis method aims to use a variable that receives continuous values in a given definition interval (continuous variable) as a diagnostic test. Sensitivity and (1-specificity) values are calculated for various "positive limit values" (cutoff values).

Sensitivity is represented on the (y) axis, and (1-specificity) values are represented on the (x) axis. We plot the ROC curve using the sensitivity and (1-selectivity) coordinate values obtained for various cutoff values. The power of the diagnostic value of the examined variable (the ability to distinguish between the patient and healthy subjects) is expressed by the area under the ROC curve (AUC). The diagnostic value increases as the area (AUC) approaches a value of 1. At a diagnostic power of 100%, the AUC value equals '1'. The 95% confidence intervals (CI) of the AUC are determined. If the value of 0.50 (theoretical discrepancy) is outside the confidence intervals, we may refer to a statistically significant diagnostic value.

Follow-Up Time and Result Endpoints in Survival Analysis

We can show the start time, the monitoring time and the end time of monitoring as follows (Fig. 26.7):

Two of the most common problems in prospective follow-up studies are an inability to fully monitor subjects during the research period and changes in treatment methods applied to patients in long follow-up durations. Patients who cannot be fully monitored for various reasons are taken into account for as long as they are followed-up in the survival analysis. We can consider death, recurrence (disease recurrence), metastasis and any event that shows the treatment result as endpoints.

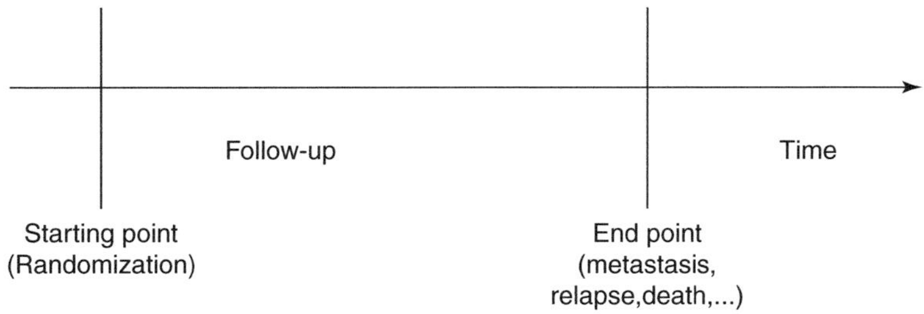

Fig. 26.7 Follow-up process

Table 26.4 Presentation of survival analysis results

Follow-up period	Median follow-up (min–max)
Event (result) frequency	Number of events/number of patients
Mean survival time	Mean survival time ± standard error (95% confidence interval)
Median survival time	Median survival time ± standard error (95% CI)
Cumulative survival rate for the year (n) (to calculate the cumulative survival rate for the year (n), at least 5 patients must be under follow-up at the end of the year (n))	(at the end of year n) R ± SE (95% CI:…)
Statistical comparison of survival curves	(Log rank = …; d.f. = …; p = …)

The length of time from the receipt of the patient for follow-up until reaching the outcome that is regarded as the "endpoint" is called the monitoring period.

Definitions Frequently Used in Survival Analysis

Overall Survival The time from start (randomization) to death.

Progression-Free Survival (PFS) or Disease-Free Survival (DFS) Duration from randomization to progression/recurrence or death.

Progression-Free Interval (PFI) or Disease-Free Interval (DFI) Duration from randomization to progression or recurrence.

Time to Event Duration from the initiation of the study (randomization) to any event that shows the treatment result.

Survival analysis results are presented as follows (Table 26.4):

Valid Statistical Procedures and Test Selection

In the evaluation of the hypothesis tests, first, the measurement level of the tested variable is defined. If the variable is classified or ranked, the statistical analyses that can be performed are very limited. It is possible to use only non-parametric tests (ranking statistical tests) at these measurement levels, whereas all parametric tests can be used at intermittent and proportional measurement levels. The most important prerequisites for the use of parametric tests are that the variable examined has to fit the normal distribution. If the normality condition is not fulfilled, it can be resumed by transforming the examined variable into another variable that shows a normal distribution.

If the number of subjects in the sample (sample size) is small, it is difficult to decide the distribution of the examined variable. Non-parametric tests are preferred in this case. In non-parametric tests, the distribution type of the examined variable has no significance.

Statistical analyses and hypothesis tests that are valid at various measurement levels are presented in the following table (Table 26.5):

Incidence of a Disease

This shows the frequency of new cases emerging within the particular period.

$$I = \frac{\text{New cases emerged during monitoring}}{\text{Populaion at risk}\left(\text{number of subjects monitored}\right)}$$

Relative Risk (RR)

In a cohort (prospective) study, we can show the results as follows (Table 26.6):

The incidence of disease is compared between the risk factor-exposed and risk factor-unexposed groups to determine whether there is a relationship between the risk factor and the disease.

The relationship between the risk factor and the disease is indicated by the "Relative Risk" (*RR*), which indicates the contribution of the exposure to the risk factor to disease development. The *RR* value is obtained by dividing the incidence of the disease in the exposed group by the incidence in the unexposed group.

$$RR = \frac{\text{Disease incidence in risk factor} - \text{exposed group}}{\text{Disease incidence in risk factor} - \text{unexposed group}}$$

Table 26.5 Measurement levels and appropriate statistical tests

Measurement levels	Valid descriptive statistics	Two independent groups	Three or more independent groups	Single group (before/after)	Multiple repeated measurements	The relationship between two variables
Nominal	– Frequency distribution – Mode	– Chi-square tests (chi-square, Yate's chi-square, Fisher exact chi-square) (or ε tests)	– Chi-square test	– McNemar test – Sign test	– Cochran Q test	– Contingency coefficient (in cohort studies) – RR, AR (in case-control studies), OR
Ordinal	(In addition to the above) – Median – Percentile	Mann-Whitney U	Kruskal-Wallis test	– Wilcoxon matched paired sign test	– Friedman test	– Spearman rank correlation coefficient rs
Interval or ratio (if it is normally distributed)	(In addition to the above) – Arithmetic mean – Variance – Standard deviation – Geometric mean (for ratio)	– Student's t test for independent groups	– Analysis of variance	– Paired Student's t test	– Analysis of variance in repeated measures	– Pearson-Bravais correlation coefficient r – Determination coefficient r^2 – Partial and multiple correlation – Regression equation

Table 26.6 Results of a cohort study

	Disease developed (D+)	Healthy survivors (D−)	Total
Exposed to risk factor (E+)	*a*	*b*	(*a* + *b*)
Unexposed to risk factor (E−)	*c*	*d*	(*c* + *d*)
Total	(*a* + *c*)	(*b* + *d*)	(*a* + *b* + *c* + *d*)

Table 26.7 Results of case-control studies

	Patients (D+)	Controls (D−)	Total
Risk factor present (E+)	*a*	*b*	(*a* + *b*)
Risk factor absent (E−)	*c*	*d*	(*c* + *d*)
Total	(*a* + *c*)	(*b* + *d*)	(*a* + *b* + *c* + *d*)

$$RR = \frac{I_{E+}}{I_{E-}} = \frac{P(D+/E+)}{P(D+/E-)} = \frac{\frac{a}{a+b}}{\frac{c}{c+d}}$$

Whereas *RR* scores close to 1 (the value of "1" is included between the confidence intervals of the *RR*) indicate that the relationship between the disease and the causal agent is not statistically significant, an *RR* value of less than 1 or greater than 1 indicates a statistically significant relationship between the disease and exposure to the causal agent.

RR can only be calculated in cohort studies or experimental studies. Since the incidence value cannot be calculated in case-control studies, *RR* cannot be calculated directly. In such studies, the odds ratio (OR) is calculated for the estimated *RR* value.

Odds Ratio (OR)

In case-control studies, we can show the study results as follows (Table 26.7):

The relationship between the disease and the agent is indicated by the "Relative Proportion" (Odds ratio, (OR)), which indicates the contribution of the causative agent to disease development. OR is calculated as follows:

$$OR = \frac{a \cdot d}{b \cdot c}$$

If an event has two outcomes denoted by (A) and (B), the Odds value of a given outcome is calculated as follows:

$$O = \frac{P(A)}{1-P(A)} = \frac{P(A)}{P(B)}$$

If *A* indicates presence of the disease (cases, *D*+) and *B* indicates subjects free of disease (controls, *D*−), the OR of a case-control study is calculated with the following formula:

$$OR = \frac{O_{E+/D+}}{O_{E+/D-}}$$

$$OR = \frac{\text{Odds value of the presence of the risk factor in patients (probability ratio)}}{\text{Odds value of the presence of the risk factor in controls (probability ratio)}}$$

$$OR = \frac{P(E+/D+)/P(E-/D+)}{P(E+/D-)/P(E-/D-)} = \frac{\dfrac{a/(a+c)}{c/(a+c)}}{\dfrac{b/(b+d)}{d/(b+d)}} = \frac{a \cdot d}{b \cdot c}$$

The calculated *OR* value indirectly shows the contribution of the risk factor to disease development. The odds value (probability ratio) of disease occurrence in the causative agent (+) group is *OR* times higher than that in the causative agent (−) group. The *OR* value is used as the estimated value of the *RR* calculated in the cohort studies.

Hazard Ratio (HR)

The relative risk (RR) calculated in prospective studies is shown as the hazard ratio (HR) in survival analysis. The interpretations of the relative risk and the hazard ratio are similar. When HR has a value close to 1 ("1" is included in between the confidence intervals of the calculated HR), there is no statistically significant relationship between the study group and the control group (reference group), whereas if HR is less than or greater than 1, there is a statistically significant relationship.

References

1. Dawson B, Trapp RG. Basic and clinical biostatistics. London: Prentice-Hill; 2004.
2. Disci R. Basic and clinical biostatistics. 3rd ed. Istanbul: Istanbul Tip Kitabevi; 2015.
3. Dupont WD. Statistical modeling for biomedical researchers. Cambridge: Cambridge University Press; 2002.

4. Glantz SA. Primer of biostatistics. 6th ed. New York: McGraw-Hill Medical; 2005.
5. Knapp RG, Miller MC. Clinical epidemiology and biostatistics. Baltimore: Williams & Wilkins; 1992.
6. Miettinen OS. Theoretical epidemiyology. New York: Delmar; 1988.
7. Motulsky H. Intuitive biostatistics. Oxford: Oxford University Press; 1995.
8. Riffenburgh RH. Statistics in medicine. San Diego: Academic Press; 2006.

Chapter 27
Systemic Treatment Drugs and Regimens

Naziye Ak and Adnan Aydiner

Preoperative/Adjuvant Therapy Regimens

Regimens for HER2 Negative Diseases

Dose dense AC (doxorubicin/cyclophosphamide) followed by weekly paclitaxel
Dose dense AC (doxorubicin/cyclophosphamide) followed by paclitaxel every 2 weeks
AC followed by weekly paclitaxel
AC followed by docetaxel every 3 weeks
TAC (docetaxel/doxorubicin/cyclophosphamide)
FEC (fluorouracil/epirubicin/cyclophosphamide)
TC (docetaxel and cyclophosphamide)
Dose dense AC (doxorubicin/cyclophosphamide)
AC (doxorubicin/cyclophsphamide) every 3 weeks
EC (epirubicin/cyclophosphamide)
CMF (cyclophosphamide/methotrexate/fluorouracil)

Dosing Schedules

Dose dense AC (doxorubicin/cyclophosphamide) followed by weekly paclitaxel
Cyclophosphamide 600 mg/m^2 IV day 1,
Doxorubicin 60 mg/m^2 IV day 1,

N. Ak · A. Aydiner (✉)
Internal Medicine, Medical Oncology, Istanbul Medical Faculty, Department of Medical Oncology, Institute of Oncology, Istanbul University, Istanbul, Turkey

A. Aydiner et al. (eds.), *Breast Cancer*, https://doi.org/10.1007/978-3-319-96947-3_27

Cycled every 14 days for 4 cycles, all cycles are with GCSF support.
Followed by:
Paclitaxel 80 mg/m^2 day 1, 1 h IV infusion weekly for 12 weeks.

Dose dense AC (doxorubicin/cyclophosphamide) followed by paclitaxel every 2 weeks
Doxorubicin 60 mg/m^2 IV day 1,
Cyclophosphamide 600 mg/m^2 IV day 1,
Cycled every 14 days for 4 cycles, all cycles are with GCSF support.
Followed by:
Paclitaxel 175 mg/m^2 IV day 1, 3 h IV infusion
Cycled every 14 days for 4 cycles, all cycles are with GCSF support.

AC (doxorubicin/cyclophosphamide) followed by weekly paclitaxel
Cyclophosphamide 600 mg/m^2 IV day 1,
Doxorubicin 60 mg/m^2 IV day 1,
Cycled every 21 days for 4 cycles.
Followed by:
Paclitaxel 80 mg/m^2 day 1, 1 h IV infusion weekly for 12 weeks.

AC (doxorubicin/cyclophosphamide) followed by docetaxel
Cyclophosphamide 600 mg/m^2 IV day 1,
Doxorubicin 60 mg/m^2 IV day 1,
Cycled every 21 days for 4 cycles.
Followed by:
Docetaxel 100 mg/m^2 IV day 1,
Cycled every 21 days for 4 cycles, with GCSF support.

TAC (docetaxel/doxorubicin/cyclophosphamide)
Docetaxel 75 mg/m^2 IV day 1,
Doxorubicin 50 mg/m^2 IV day 1,
Cyclophosphamide 500 mg/m^2 IV day 1,
Cycled every 21 days for 6 cycles, all cycles are with GCSF support.

FEC (fluorouracil/epirubicin/cyclophosphamide)
Fluorouracil 500 mg/m^2 IV day 1
Epirubicin 100 mg/m^2 IV day 1
Cyclophosphamide 500 mg/m^2 IV day 1,
Cycled every 21 days for 6 cycles, with GCSF support.

TC (docetaxel/cyclophosphamide)
Docetaxel 75 mg/m^2 IV day 1,
Cyclophosphamide 600 mg/m^2 IV day 1
Cycled every 21 days for 4 cycles, all cycles are with GCSF support.

Dose dense AC (doxorubicin/cyclophosphamide)
Doxorubicin 60 mg/m^2 IV day 1,
Cyclophosphamide 600 mg/m^2 IV day 1,

Cycled every 14 days for 4 cycles, with GCSF support.

AC (doxorubicin/cyclophosphamide)
Doxorubicin 60 mg/m^2 day 1,
Cyclophosphamide 600 mg/m^2 day 1,
Cycled every 21 days for 4 cycles.

CMF (cyclophosphamide/methotrexate/fluorouracil)
Cyclophosphamide 100 mg/m^2 PO, days 1–14
Methotrexate 40 mg/m^2 IV day 1, day 8
5-fluorouracil 600 mg/m^2 IV day 1, day 8
Cycled every 28 days for 6 cycles.

Regimens for HER2 Positive Disease

AC (doxorubicin/cyclophosphamide) followed by paclitaxel + trastuzumab
Dose dense AC followed by paclitaxel trastuzumab
AC followed by weekly paclitaxel + trastuzumab + pertuzumab
TCH (Docetaxel + carboplatin + trastuzumab)
TCHP (Docetaxel + carboplatin + trastuzumab) + pertuzumab
AC followed by docetaxel + trastuzumab
AC followed by docetaxel + trastuzumab + pertuzumab
Docetaxel + cyclophosphamid + trastuzumab
Paclitaxel + trastuzumab

Dosing Regimens

AC followed by paclitaxel + trastuzumab
Doxorubicin 60 mg/m^2 IV day 1,
Cyclophosphamide 600 mg/m^2 IV day 1,
Cycled every 21 days for 4 cycles.
Followed by:
Paclitaxel 80 mg/m^2 day 1, 1 h IV infusion weekly for 12 weeks.
With:
Trastuzumab 8 mg/kg IV with first dose of paclitaxel
Followed by:
Trastuzumab 6 mg/kg IV every 21 days to complete 1 year of treatment.
*Evaluate left ventricular ejection fraction prior to and every 3 months during treatment.

Dose dense AC (doxorubicin/cyclophosphamide) followed by paclitaxel trastuzumab
Doxorubicin 60 mg/m^2 IV day 1,
Cyclophosphamide 600 mg/m^2 IV day 1,

Cycled every 14 days for 4 cycles, all cycles are with GCSF support.
Followed by:
Paclitaxel 175 mg/m^2 day 1, 3 h IV infusion,
Cycled every 14 days for 4 cycles, all cycles are with GCSF support.
With:
Trastuzumab 4 mg/kg IV with first dose of paclitaxel
Followed by:
Trastuzumab 2 mg/kg IV weekly to complete 1 year of treatment.
As an alternative, trastuzumab 6 mg/kg IV every 21 days may be used following the completion of paclitaxel, and given to complete 1 year of trastuzumab treatment.
*Evaluate left ventricular ejection fraction prior to and every 3 months during treatment.

AC (doxorubicin/cyclophosphamide) followed by weekly paclitaxel + trastuzumab + pertuzumab
Doxorubicin 60 mg/m^2 IV day 1,
Cyclophosphamide 600 mg/m^2 IV day 1,
Cycled every 21 days for 4 cycles.
Followed by:
Pertuzumab 840 mg IV day 1 followed by 420 mg IV, every 21 days to complete 1 year of treatment,
Trastuzumab 8 mg/kg day 1 followed by 6 mg/kg IV, every 21 days to complete 1 year of treatment,
Paclitaxel 80 mg/m^2 day 1, 1 h IV infusion weekly for 12 weeks.
*Evaluate left ventricular ejection fraction prior to and every 3 months during treatment.

TCH (Docetaxel + carboplatin + trastuzumab)
Docetaxel 75 mg/m^2 IV day 1,
Carboplatin AUC 6 IV day 1,
Cycled every 21 days for 6 cycles.
Trastuzumab 4 mg/kg IV week 1
Followed by:
Trastuzumab 2 mg/kg IV weekly for 17 weeks.
Followed by:
Trastuzumab 6 mg/kg IV cycled every 21 days to complete 1 year of trastuzumab treatment.
OR
Trastuzumab 8 mg/kg IV week 1
Followed by:
Trastuzumab 6 mg/kg IV cycled every 21 days to complete 1 year of trastuzumab treatment.

*Evaluate left ventricular ejection fraction prior to and every 3 months during treatment.

TCH (Docetaxel + carboplatin + trastuzumab) + pertuzumab
Docetaxel 75 mg/m² IV day 1,
Carboplatin AUC 6 IV day 1,
Cycled every 21 days for 6 cycles.
AND
Pertuzumab 840 mg IV day 1
Trastuzumab 8 mg/kg IV day 1
Followed by:
Trastuzumab 6 mg/kg IV day 1
Pertuzumab 420 mg IV day 1
Cycled every 21 days to complete 1 year of therapy.
*Evaluate left ventricular ejection fraction prior to and every 3 months during treatment.

AC followed by docetaxel + trastuzumab
Cyclophosphamide 600 mg/m² IV day 1,
Doxorubicin 60 mg/m² IV day 1,
Cycled every 21 days for 4 cycles.
Followed by:
Docetaxel 100 mg/m² IV day 1, all cycles are with GCSF support.
Cycled every 21 days for 4 cycles.
With:
Trastuzumab 8 mg/kg IV week 1
Followed by:
Trastuzumab 6 mg/kg IV cycled every 21 days to complete 1 year of trastuzumab therapy.
*Evaluate left ventricular ejection fraction prior to and every 3 months during treatment.

AC followed by docetaxel + trastuzumab + pertuzumab
Cyclophosphamide 600 mg/m² IV day 1,
Doxorubicin 60 mg/m² IV day 1,
Cycled every 21 days for 4 cycles.
Followed by:
Pertuzumab 840 mg IV day 1 follewed by 420 mg IV
Trastuzumab 8 mg/kg IV day 1 followed by 6 mg/kg IV
Docetaxel 75–100 mg/m² IV day 1, with GCSF support.
Cycled every 21 days for 4 cycles.
Followed by:
Trastuzumab 6 mg/kg IV
Pertuzumab 420 mg IV day 1

Cycled every 21 days to complete 1 year of trastuzumab and pertuzumab therapy.
*Evaluate left ventricular ejection fraction prior to and every 3 months during treatment.

Docetaxel + cyclophosphamid + trastuzumab
Docetaxel 75 mg/m^2 IV day 1,
Cyclophosphamide 600 mg/m^2 IV day 1
Cycled every 21 days for 4 cycles, all cycles are with GCSF support.
With:
Trastuzumab 8 mg/kg IV week 1
Followed by:
Trastuzumab 6 mg/kg IV cycled every 21 days to complete 1 year of trastuzumab therapy.
*Evaluate left ventricular ejection fraction prior to and every 3 months during treatment.

Paclitaxel + trastuzumab
Paclitaxel 80 mg/m^2 day 1, 1 h IV infusion weekly for 12 weeks.
With:
Trastuzumab 4 mg/kg IV with first dose of paclitaxel
Followed by:
Trastuzumab 2 mg/kg IV weekly to complete 1 year of treatment.
As an alternative trastuzumab 6 mg/kg IV every 21 days may be used following the completion of paclitaxel, and given to complete 1 year of trastuzumab treatment.
*Evaluate left ventricular ejection fraction prior to and every 3 months during treatment.

Systemic Endocrine Therapy for Hormone-Positive Recurrent or Stage IV Disease

HER2 Negative Disease

Premenopausal:
Tamoxifen or,
Ovarian ablation or suppression plus endocrine therapy as for postmenopausal women

Postmenopausal:
Palbociclib + aromatase inhibitor (proposal 1)
Palbociclib + fulvestrant (proposal 1)
Ribociclib + aromatase inhibitor (proposal 1)
Ribociclib + fulvestrant (proposal 1)
Ribociclib + tamoxifen (proposal 1)

Abemaciclib + aromatase inhibitor (proposal 1)
Abemaciclib + fulvestrant (proposal 1)
Abemaciclib + tamoxifen
Fulvestrant (proposal 1)
Non-steroidal aromatase inhibitor (anastrozole, letrozole)
Steroidal aromatase inactivator (exemestane)
Tamoxifen or toremifene
Exemestane + everolimus
Everolimus + fulvestrant
Everolimus + tamoxifen
Megestrol acetate
Abemaciclib

HER2 Positive Disease

Premenopausal
Tamoxifen + trastuzumab (±pertuzumab) or
Ovarian ablation or suppression plus therapy as for post-menopausal women

Postmenopausal
Aromatase inhibitor + trastuzumab (±pertuzumab)
Aromatase inhibitor + lapatinib + trastuzumab
Aromatase inhibitor + lapatinib
Fulvestrant + trastuzumab (±pertuzumab)
Tamoxifen + trastuzumab (±pertuzumab)

Chemotherapy Regimens for Recurrent or Metastatic Breast Cancer

Regimens for HER2-Negative Disease

Single Agent

Doxorubicin
Liposomal doxorubicin
Paclitaxel
Vinorelbine
Capecitabine
Gemcitabine
Docetaxel
Eribulin

Albumin-bound paclitaxel
Carboplatin
Cisplatin
Epirubicin
Ixabepilone
Cyclophosphamide
Olaparib (option for HER2-negative, BRCA1/2-positive tumors)

Dosing Regimens

Doxorubicin 60–75 mg/m^2 IV day 1, cycled every 21 days or 20 mg/m^2 IV day 1, weekly.
Liposomal doxorubicin 50 mg/m^2 IV day 1, cycled every 28 days or 30 mg/m^2 IV day 1, cycled every 21 days.
Paclitaxel 80 mg/m^2 day 1, IV day 1 weekly or 175 mg/m^2 IV day 1, cycled every 21 days.
Vinorelbine 25 mg/m^2 IV day 1, weekly, or 30–35 mg/m^2 IV day 1, day 8 cycled every 3 weeks.
Capecitabine 850–1250 mg/m^2 PO twice daily days 1–14, cycled every 21 days.
Gemcitabine 800–1200 mg/m^2 IV days 1, 8, 15 cycled every 28 days.
Docetaxel 60–100 mg/m^2 day 1, cycled every 21 days or d*ocetaxel* 35 mg/m^2 day 1, weekly for 6 weeks followed by a 2-week rest, then repeat.
Eribulin 1.25–1.4 mg/m^2 IV day 1, day 8 cycled every 21 days.
Albumin-bound paclitaxel 100–125 mg/m^2 IV days 1, 8, 15 cycled every 28 days or 260 mg/m^2 IV day 1, cycled every 21 days.
Carboplatin AUC 5–6 on day 1, cycled every 21–28 days.
Cisplatin 75 mg/m^2 IV day 1, cycled every 21 days.
Epirubicin 60–90 mg/m^2 IV day 1, cycled every 21 days.
Ixabepilone 40 mg/m^2 IV day 1, cycled every 21 days.
Cyclophosphamide 50 mg PO daily on days 1–21, cycled every 28 days.
Olaparib tablet 300 mg PO twice daily cycled every 28 days.

Chemotherapy Combinations

AC (doxorubicin/cyclophosphamide)
EC (epirubicin/cyclophosphamide)
Docetaxel/capecitabine
Gemcitabine/paclitaxel
Paclitaxel/carboplatin (especially for triple negative tumors)
Gemcitabine/carboplatin (especially for triple negative tumors)
Gemcitabine/cisplatin (especially for triple negative tumors)
Paclitaxel/bevacizumab
CMF (cyclophosphamide/methotrexate/flurouracil)

Dosing Regimens

AC (doxorubicin/cyclophosphamide)
Doxorubicin 60 mg/m^2 IV day 1,
Cyclophosphamide 600 mg/m^2 IV day 1,
Cycled every 21 days.

EC (doxorubicin/cyclophosphamide)
Epirubicin 75 mg/m^2 IV day 1,
Cyclophosphamide 600 mg/m^2 IV day 1,
Cycled every 21 days.

Docetaxel/capecitabine
Docetaxel 75 mg/m^2 IV day 1
Capecitabine 950 mg/m^2 PO twice daily days 1–14,
Cycled every 21 days.

GT (gemcitabine/paclitaxel)
Paclitaxel 175 mg/m^2 IV day 1,
Gemcitabine 1250 mg/m^2 IV day 1, day 8 (following paclitaxel on day 1)
Cycled every 21 days.

Paclitaxel/carboplatin
Paclitaxel 80 mg/m^2 days 1, 8, 15
Carboplatin AUC 5–6 IV day 1
Cycled every 21–28 days.

Paclitaxel/carboplatin
Carboplatin AUC 5–6 IV day 1
Paklitaksel 175 mg/m^2 IV day 1,
Cycled every 21 days.

Gemcitabine/carboplatin
Gemcitabin 1000 mg/m^2 IV day 1, day 8
Carboplatin AUC 2 IV day 1, day 8
Cycled every 21 days.

Gemcitabine/cisplatin
Gemcitabin 1000 mg/m^2 IV day 1, day 8
Cisplatin 60–75 mg/m^2 IV day 1
Cycled every 21 days.

Paclitaxel/bevacizumab
Paclitaxel 90 mg/m^2 IV day 1, day 8, day 15.
Bevacizumab 10 mg/kg IV day 1, day 15.
Cycled every 28 days.

CMF (cyclophosphamide/methotrexate/fluorouracil)
Cyclophosphamide 100 mg/m^2 PO, days 1–14
Methotrexate 40 mg/m^2 day 1, day 8
5-fluorouracil 600 mg/m^2 IV day 1, day 8
Cycled every 28 days.

Regimens for HER2-Positive Disease

Pertuzumab + trastuzumab + docetaxel
Pertuzumab + trastuzumab + paclitaxel
Ado-trastuzumab emtansine (T-DM1)
Trastuzumab + paclitaxel ± carboplatin
Trastuzumab + docetaxel
Trastuzumab + vinorelbine
Trastuzumab + capecitabine
Trastuzumab + lapatinib
Trastuzumab + other agents
Lapatinib + capecitabine

Dosing Regimens

Pertuzumab + trastuzumab + docetaxel
Pertuzumab 840 mg IV day 1 followed by 420 mg IV
Trastuzumab 8 mg/kg IV day 1 followed by 6 mg/kg IV
Docetaxel 75–100 mg/m^2 IV day 1
Cycled every 21 days.

Pertuzumab + trastuzumab + paclitaxel
Pertuzumab 840 mg IV day 1 followed by 420 mg IV cycled every 21 days.
Trastuzumab 8 mg/kg IV day 1 followed by 6 mg/kg IV cycled every 21 days.
Paclitaxel 80 mg/m^2 IV day 1 weekly or 175 mg/m^2 IV day 1 cycled every 21 days.

Ado-trastuzumab emtansine (T-DM1)
3.6 mg/kg IV day 1, cycled every 21 days.

Trastuzumab + paclitaxel/carboplatin
Carboplatin AUC 5–6 IV day 1
Paklitaksel 175 mg/m^2 IV day 1,
Cycled every 21 days.
Trastuzumab 8 mg/kg IV day 1 followed by 6 mg/kg IV cycled every 21 days.

Weekly paclitaxel/carboplatin + trastuzumab
Paclitaxel 80 mg/m^2 IV days 1, 8, 15.
Carboplatin AUC 2 IV days 1, 8, 15 or AUC 5–6 day 1

Cycled every 28 days.
Trastuzumab 4 mg/kg IV day 1 followed by trastuzumab 2 mg/kg IV weekly or 8 mg/kg IV day 1 followed by 6 mg/kg IV cycled every 21 days.

Trastuzumab + paclitaxel
Paclitaxel 175 mg/m^2 IV day 1, cycled every 21 days or 80–90 mg/m^2 IV weekly.
Trastuzumab 8 mg/kg IV day 1 followed by 6 mg/kg IV cycled every 21 days or 4 mg/kg IV day 1 followed by trastuzumab 2 mg/kg IV weekly.

Trastuzumab + docetaxel
Docetaxel 75–100 mg/m^2 IV day 1 cycled every 21 days or 35 mg/m^2 IV weekly.
Trastuzumab 8 mg/kg IV day 1 followed by 6 mg/kg IV cycled every 21 days or 4 mg/kg IV day 1 followed by trastuzumab 2 mg/kg IV weekly.

Trastuzumab + vinorelbine
Vinorelbine 25 mg/m^2 IV day 1 weekly or 30–35 mg/m^2 IV days 1 and 8 cycled every 21 days.
Trastuzumab 4 mg/kg IV day 1 followed by trastuzumab 2 mg/kg IV weekly or 8 mg/kg IV day 1 followed by 6 mg/kg IV cycled every 21 days.

Trastuzumab + Capecitabine
Capecitabine 1000–1250 mg/m^2 PO twice daily, days 1–14 cycled every 21 days.
Trastuzumab 8 mg/kg IV day 1 followed by 6 mg/kg IV cycled every 21 days.

Trastuzumab + Lapatinib
Lapatinib 1000 mg PO daily,
Trastuzumab 8 mg/kg IV day 1 followed by 6 mg/kg IV cycled every 21 days.

Lapatinib + Capecitabine
Capecitabine 1000 mg/m^2 PO twice daily, days 1–14,
Lapatinib 1250 mg PO daily, days 1–21, cycled every 21 days.

Recommendations in Chemotherapy Dose Modification

Basic Recommendations for Dose Modification in Hematological Toxicity

New doses of chemotherapy according to the maximum toxicity in the previous chemotherapy:

Toxicity grade	Dose in the next cycle
ANC[a] < 0.5 (×10^9)/L for 5–7 days or febrile neutropenia	Reduce by 25%[b]
Thrombocyte < 25 (×10^9)/L or bleeding	Reduce by 25%

[a]ANC = Absolute neutrophil count = Neutrophils + number of rod cells
[b]Dosage may not be reduced by administering G-CSF in curative treatments

Chemotherapy is avoided until ANC $\geq 1.5 \times 10^9$/L, platelet $\geq 100 \times 10^9$/L and other toxicities are ≤grade 2. However, if it is necessary to administer chemotherapy despite lower blood laboratory results due to the patient's clinical condition, treatment may be given by reducing the doses by 25–50% and administering G-CSF, if necessary.

Basic Recommendations for Dose Modification in Non-Hematological Toxicity

New doses of chemotherapy according to the maximum toxicity in the previous chemotherapy:

Toxicity Grade 1: The treatment is continued, and the symptoms are treated. There is no change in dosage.

Toxicity Grade 2: The treatment is continued, and the symptoms are treated. No dose changes or modifications can be made according to the treatment regimen applied.

Toxicity Grade 3: Treatment is postponed, and the symptoms are treated; 75% of the previous dose is given.

Toxicity Grade 4: The treatment is postponed or completely discontinued. If continued, the doses are modified.

Everolimus

Dosage

10 mg once daily, in combination with exemestane, fulvestrant, tamoxifen (https://www.accessdata.fda.gov/scripts/cder/daf/index.cfm) [1, 2].

Dose Modifications at Toxicity

1. Thrombocytopenia
   - Thrombocyte count higher than 75,000/μL (Grade1 thrombocytopenia) does not require dose modification.
2. Neutropenia
   - Neutrophile count higher than 1,000/μL (Grade 1–2 neutropenia) does not require dose modification.
3. Non-infectious pneumonitis
   - If the patient has only radiological signs and no or few symptoms, no dose modification is required. Only observe and monitor the patient.

4. Stomatitis
   - Minimal symptoms do not need dose modification, only the standard approach to mucositis is recommended.
5. Metabolic events (e.g. hyperglycemia, hyperlipidemia)
   - Grade 1 and 2 hyperglycemia and hyperlipidemia do not need dose modification. Only observe and monitor the patient.

Hepatic Impairment

- Mild (Child-Pugh class A) (Table 27.1); 7.5 mg daily. (5 mg daily if 7.5 mg not tolerated)
- Moderate (Child-Pugh class B); 5 mg daily (2.5 mg daily if 5 mg not tolerated)
- Severe (Child-Pugh class C); Use only when benefits outweigh risks at 2.5 mg daily.

Renal Impairment

No dose adjustment is required.

Elderly

No dose adjustment is required.

Palbociclib

Dosage

125 mg once daily, 21 days for every 28 days in combination with either aromatase inhibitor or fulvestrant (https://www.accessdata.fda.gov/scripts/cder/daf/index.cfm) [1, 4].

Table 27.1 Child-Pugh classification [3]

Points	Albumin	Ascites	Bilirubin	Encephelopathy	INR
1	>3.5 g/dL	–	<2 mg/dL	–	<1.7
2	2.8–3.5 g/dL	Slight	2–3 mg/dL	Grade 1–2	1.7–2.3
3	<2.8 g/dL	Moderate	>3 mg/dL	Grade 3–4	>2.3

Score of 5–6 is considered Child-Pugh class A; 7–9 is class B; and 10–15 is class C
INR international normalized ratio

The recommended dose reduction is to 100 mg daily at the first level; if a second reduction is required, reduce the dose to 75 mg daily. If the 75 mg daily dose is not tolerated, discontinue treatment.

Dose Modifications at Toxicity

Hematologic Toxicities

1. Thrombocytopenia
   - A thrombocyte count higher than 50,000 (Grade1–2) does not need dose modification.
2. Neutropenia
   - A neutrophile count higher than 1,000/μL (Grade 1–2 neutropenia) does not need dose modification.

Nonhematologic Toxicities

- Grade 1 or 2 toxicities does not need dose modification.

Hepatic Impairment

No change is needed for mild hepatic impairment.

The drug has not been studied in patients with moderate and severe hepatic impairment.

Renal Impairment

No change is needed for patients with GFR >30 mL/dk.

The drug has not been studied in patients with severe renal impairment.

Dosage in the Elderly

No overall differences in efficacy and toxicity.

Ribociclib

Dosage

600 mg once daily for 21 days, with 28-day cycles in combination with either aromatase inhibitor or fulvestrant or tamoxifen (https://www.accessdata.fda.gov/scripts/cder/daf/index.cfm) [1, 5].

The recommended dose reduction is to 400 mg daily at the first level; if a second reduction is required, reduce the dose to 200 mg daily. If the 200 mg daily dose is not tolerated, discontinue treatment.

Dose Modifications at Toxicity

1. Neutropenia
   - Neutrophile count higher than 1,000/μL (Grade 1–2 neutropenia) does not require dose modification.
2. Hepatobiliary toxicity
   - Grade 1 ALT and/or AST elevation [1–3 times of upper limit of normal (ULN)] without total bilirubin increase >2 times the ULN, does not require dose modification.

Hepatic Impairment

No change is needed on mild hepatic impairment.

On moderate or severe impairment (Child-Pugh class B or C), the initial dose is 400 mg.

Renal Impairment

No change is needed on patients with GFR >30 mL/dk.

The drug has not been studied in patients with severe renal impairment.

Dosage in the Elderly

No dosing modification is needed.

Abemaciclib

Dosage

200 mg twice daily (400 mg/day) as a single-agent or 150 mg twice daily (300 mg/day) in combination with an aromatase inhibitor or fulvestrant or tamoxifen (https://www.accessdata.fda.gov/scripts/cder/daf/index.cfm) [1, 6].

The recommended dose reduction for monotherapy is to 150 mg twice daily at the first level; if a second reduction is required, reduce the dose to 100 mg twice daily and then 50 mg twice daily. If a 50-mg twice-daily dose is not tolerated, discontinue treatment.

The recommended dose reduction for aromatase inhibitor combined therapy is to 100 mg twice daily at the first level; if a second reduction is required, reduced the dose to 50 mg twice daily. If the 50-mg twice-daily dose is not tolerated, discontinue treatment.

Dose Modifications at Toxicity

1. Hematologic toxicities
   - No change is needed on Grade 1 and 2 hematologic toxicities.
2. Diarrhea
   - Less than 4 loose stools/day (Grade 1 diarrhea) does not require dose modification.
3. Hepatobiliary toxicity
   - Grade 1 (ALT, AST elevation up to 3 times ULN) and Grade 2 (ALT, AST elevation 3 to 5 times ULN) hepatocellular toxicities without increase in total bilirubin of more than 2 times of ULN, do not require dose adjustment.

Hepatic Impairment

No dose modification is needed for mild and moderate hepatic impairment (Child-Pugh class A or B).

At severe impairment (Child-Pugh class C), give drug once daily.

Renal Impairment

No dose modification is needed for patients with GFR >30 mL/dk.

The drug has not been studied in patients with severe renal impairment.

Dosage in the Elderly

No dose modification is needed.

Olaparib

Dosing

300 mg twice daily (600 mg/day), in tablet form for breast cancer (https://www.accessdata.fda.gov/scripts/cder/daf/index.cfm) [1, 7].

The recommended first dose reduction for tablet form is to 250 mg twice daily; if a second reduction is required, reduce the dose to 200 mg twice daily.

Dosing and bioavailability differ; do not substitute the capsules and the tablets on a mg-per-mg basis.

Hepatic Impairment

No change is needed for mild (Child-Pugh class A) hepatic impairment.

The drug has not been studied in patients with moderate and severe (Child-Pugh classes B and C) hepatic impairment.

Renal Impairment

A GFR level greater than 50 mL/minute, does not require dose modification.

A GFR level between 31 and 50 mL/minute requires dose reduction to 200 mg twice daily for tablets.

The drug has not been studied in patients with severe renal impairment (GFR level lower than 30 mL/minute).

Elderly

No dose adjustment is required.

Neratinib

Dosage

240 mg once daily for 1 year (https://www.accessdata.fda.gov/scripts/cder/daf/index.cfm) [1, 8, 9].

The recommended neratinib dose reductions for toxicity are first 200 mg once daily and then 160 mg and 120 mg once daily.

If toxicity does not recover to less than grade 1 level, if toxicities that result in a treatment delay of more than 3 weeks occur, or if patients are unable to tolerate the 120-mg once-daily dose; discontinue neratinib.

- Routine antidiarrheal prophylaxis with loperamide is recommended during the first 2 cycles of therapy; initiate with the first neratinib dose. Titrate to 1 to 2 bowel movements/day.
- Grade 1, grade 2 (lasting in 5 days), or grade 3 diarrhea (lasting in 2 days) do not require dose modification. Routine diarrhea management is recommended.
- If diarrhea has life-threatening consequences, permanently discontinue neratinib.

Hepatic Impairment

No dose modification is required for mild and moderate hepatic impairment (Child-Pugh class A or B).

Dosage at severe impairment (Child-Pugh class C) is 80 mg once daily.

Renal Impairment

No dose modification is recommended.

Dosage in the Elderly

No dose modification is recommended.

Lapatinib

Dosage

Oral 1,250 mg once daily in combination with capecitabine, 1,500 mg once daily in combination with letrozole, and 1,000 mg once daily in combination with trastuzumab [10–12].

Dose Modifications at Toxicity

Cardiac toxicity

Left ventricular ejection fraction level decreased to more than lower level of normal: hold the drug for at least 2 weeks.

LVEF recovers to normal value and patient is asymptomatic: Lapatinib may be restarted at 1,000 mg once daily (for capecitabine combined regimen) or 1,250 mg once daily (for letrozole combined regimen).

Dermatologic Toxicity

Erythema multiforme, Stevens-Johnson syndrome, or toxic epidermal necrolysis: discontinue the drug.

Diarrhea

Grade 3 diarrhea or grade 1 or 2 diarrhea with complicating features requires interruption of the drug until toxicity resolves to ≤ grade 1. Then resume the drug at the recommended lower dose (1,250 mg once daily or 1,000 mg once daily).

Diarrhea requiring hospitalization or life threatening toxicity (Grade 4 diarrhea): Discontinue the drug permanently.

Pulmonary Toxicity

Patient has severe symptoms with limiting self-care activities and needs oxygen therapy (Grade 3 toxicitiy): Discontinue the drug.

Renal Impairment

No dose modificaiton is needed.

Hepatic Impairment

Mild or moderate preexisting impairment (Child-Pugh class A or B) requires no dosage adjustments.

Severe preexisting impairment (Child-Pugh class C): Although there are no clinical data associated with the adjustments, dose reduction to 750 mg (capecitabine combined form) or 1,000 mg (letrozole combined form) is reasonable.

Severe hepatotoxicity during treatment needs discontinuation of the drug permanently.

Dosage in the Elderly

No dose modification is needed.

Trastuzumab, Pertuzumab and T-DM1

Dosage dose modification of trastuzumab, pertuzumab and T-DM1, based on asymptomatic left ventricular ejection fraction decrease from baseline are shown in Tables 27.2, 27.3, and 27.4.

Table 27.2 Dosage dose modification of trastuzumab and pertuzumab combination based on asymptomatic left ventricular ejection fraction decrease from baseline

Left ventricular ejection fraction	Trastuzumab and pertuzumab		
	Action	LVEF at reassessment	Dose
<40% AND asymptomatic	Pause and repeat MUGA in 3 weeks	>45% OR 40–45% AND <10% ↓ from baseline	Restart
40–50%[a] AND ≥10% points below baseline AND asymptomatic		<40% OR 40–50%[a] AND ≥ 10% points below baseline OR symptomatic	Discontinue
Symptomatic	Consider discontinuing	Not applicable	Not applicable

[a]In the CLEOPATRA trial [13], trastuzumab and pertuzumab treatments were paused if LVEF was 40–45% and ≥10% below baseline and asymptomatic. At LVEF reassessment, pertuzumab and trastuzumab may be restarted if LVEF "≥46%" or "40–45% and <10% ↓ from baseline"; otherwise, discontinue

Table 27.3 Dosage dose modification of trastuzumab based on asymptomatic left ventricular ejection fraction decrease from baseline

Relationship of left ventricular ejection fraction (LVEF) to the lower limit of normal (LLN)	Trastuzumab dose modification based on asymptomatic LVEF decrease from baseline		
	≤10 percentage points	10–15 percentage points	≥15 percentage points
Within a facility's normal limits	Continue	Continue	Hold and repeat MUGA/ECHO after 4 weeks[a]
<6% below LLN	Continue[a]	Hold and repeat MUGA/ECHO after 4 weeks[a,b]	Hold and repeat MUGA/ECHO after 4 weeks[b,c]
≥6% below LLN	Continue and repeat MUGA/ECHO after 4 weeks[c]	Hold and repeat MUGA/ECHO after 4 weeks[b,c]	Hold and repeat MUGA/ECHO after 4 weeks[b,c]

[a]Consider cardiac assessment. Cardiotoxicity associated with trastuzumab typically responds to appropriate medical therapy but may be severe and lead to cardiac failure
[b]After 2 holds, consider permanent trastuzumab discontinuation
[c]Refer to cardiologist

Table 27.4 Dosage dose modification of T-DM1 based on asymptomatic left ventricular ejection fraction decrease from baseline [14]

Criteria	Left ventricular ejection fraction (LVEF)	Action	Action at LVEF reassessment
1	>45%	Continue and follow routine monitoring guidelines	Follow actions based on criteria
2	40–45% AND <10% below baseline and asymptomatic	Continue and repeat LVEF in 3 weeks	Discontinue permanently if no recovery. If improved to criterion # 1 (for # 2, 3 or 4) or # 2 (for # 3 or 4), treatment may be restarted; monitor closely
3	40–45% AND ≥10% below baseline, and asymptomatic	Pause and repeat LVEF in 3 weeks	
4	<40% and asymptomatic		
5	Symptomatic or confirmed CHF	Discontinue	Not applicable

References

1. Common Terminology Criteria for Adverse Events (CTCAE), Version 5.0. 2017, National Institutes of Health, National Cancer Institute.
2. Yardley DA, Noguchi S, Pritchard KI, Burris HA, Baselga J, Gnant M, et al. Everolimus plus exemestane in postmenopausal patients with HR+ breast cancer: BOLERO-2 final progression-free survival analysis. Adv Ther. 2013;30(10):870–84.
3. Child CG III, Turcotte JG. Surgery and portal hypertension. In: Child III CG, editor. The liver and portal hypertension. Philadelphia: W. B. Saunders; 1964. p. 50.
4. Finn RS, Crown JP, Ettl J, Schmidt M, Bondarenko IM, Lang I, et al. Efficacy and safety of palbociclib in combination with letrozole as first-line treatment of ER-positive, HER2-negative, advanced breast cancer: expanded analyses of subgroups from the randomized pivotal trial PALOMA-1/TRIO-18. Breast Cancer Res. 2016;18(1):67. https://doi.org/10.1186/s13058-016-0721-5.
5. Hortobagyi GN, Stemmer SM, Burris HA, Yap YS, Sonke GS, Paluch-Shimon S, et al. Updated results from MONALEESA-2, a phase III trial of first-line ribociclib plus letrozole versus placebo plus letrozole in hormone receptor-positive, HER2-negative advanced breast cancer. Ann Oncol. 2018. https://doi.org/10.1093/annonc/mdy155.
6. Goetz MP, Toi M, Campone M, Sohn J, Paluch-Shimon S, Huober J, et al. MONARCH 3: abemaciclib as initial therapy for advanced breast cancer. J Clin Oncol. 2017;35(32):3638–46. https://doi.org/10.1200/JCO.2017.75.6155.
7. Robson M, Im SA, Senkus E, Xu B, Domchek SM, Masuda N, et al. Olaparib for metastatic breast cancer in patients with a germline BRCA mutation. N Engl J Med. 2017;377(6):523–33.
8. Tiwari SR, Mishra P, Abraham J. Neratinib, a novel HER2-targeted tyrosine kinase inhibitor. Clin Breast Cancer. 2016;16(5):344–8.
9. Chan A, Delaloge S, Holmes FA, Moy B, Iwata H, Harvey VJ, et al. Neratinib after trastuzumab-based adjuvant therapy in patients with HER2-positive breast cancer (ExteNET): a multicenter, randomized, double-blind, placebo-controlled, phase 3 trial. Lancet Oncol. 2016;17(3):367–77.

10. Cameron D, Casey M, Oliva C, Newstat B, Imwalle B, Geyer CE. Lapatinib plus capecitabine in women with HER-2-positive advanced breast cancer: final survival analysis of a phase III randomized trial. Oncologist. 2010;15(9):924–34.
11. Bachelot T, Romieu G, Campone M, Diéras V, Cropet C, Dalenc F, et al. Lapatinib plus capecitabine in patients with previously untreated brain metastases from HER2-positive metastatic breast cancer (LANDSCAPE): a single-group phase 2 study. Lancet Oncol. 2013;14(1):64–71.
12. Tykerb (lapatinib) [prescribing information]; 2017. East Hanover, NJ: Novartis Pharmaceuticals Corporation.
13. Swain SM, Baselga J, Kim SB, Ro J, Semiglazov V, Campone M, CLEOPATRA Study Group, et al. Pertuzumab, trastuzumab, and docetaxel in HER2-positive metastatic breast cancer. N Engl J Med. 2015;372(8):724–34.
14. Verma S, Miles D, Gianni L, Krop IE, Welslau M, Baselga J, Pegram M, Oh D-Y, Diéras V, Guardino E, Fang L, Lu MW, Olsen S, Blackwell K. Trastuzumab Emtansine for HER2-Positive Advanced Breast Cancer. N Engl J Med. 2012;367(19):1783–91.

Index

A. Aydiner et al. (eds.), *Breast Cancer*, https://doi.org/10.1007/978-3-319-96947-3

MIX
Papier aus verantwortungsvollen Quellen
Paper from responsible sources
FSC® C105338

If you have any concerns about our products,
you can contact us on
ProductSafety@springernature.com

In case Publisher is established outside the EU,
the EU authorized representative is:
Springer Nature Customer Service Center GmbH
Europaplatz 3, 69115 Heidelberg, Germany

Printed by Libri Plureos GmbH
in Hamburg, Germany